The Microbiome and Cancer Treatment

The Microbiome and Cancer Treatment

Overcoming Resistance and Enhancing Efficacy

Edited by

Arun Kumar Singh
University School of Pharmaceutical Sciences, Rayat Bahara University, Mohali, Punjab, India

Meenakshi Dhanawat
Amity Institute of Pharmacy, Amity University, Gurugram, Haryana, India

Garima Malik
Chitkara College of Pharmacy, Chitkara University, Rajpura, Punjab, India

Sadhna Aggarwal
University of Texas, MD Anderson Cancer Center, Houston, Texas, United States

ELSEVIER

ACADEMIC PRESS
An imprint of Elsevier
elsevier.com/books-and-journals

Academic Press is an imprint of Elsevier

125 London Wall, London EC2Y 5AS, United Kingdom
50 Hampshire Street, 5th Floor, Cambridge, MA 02139, United States

ISBN: 978-0-443-33206-7

For Information on all Academic Press publications visit our website at https://www.elsevier.com/books-and-journals

Publisher: Megan Ball
Acquisitions Editor: Linda Buschman
Editorial Project Manager: Debarati Roy
Production Project Manager: Supali Acharya
Cover Designer: Mark Rogers

Working together to grow libraries in developing countries
www.elsevier.com • www.bookaid.org

Typeset by Aptara, New Delhi, India

Contents

Contributors

Bhavana Alaparthi
Department of Pharmaceutical Sciences, KVSR Siddhartha College of Pharmaceutical Sciences, Vijayawada, Andhra Pradesh, India

Shailaja Allani
Centre for Molecular Biology and Biotechnology, Florida Atlantic University, Boca Raton, FL, United States

Harshal S. Anwane Dhote
Department of Pharmaceutical Chemistry, SGBAU, Rajashri College of Pharmacy, Mehkar, Maharashtra, India

Ann Catherine Archer
Department of Microbiology, JSS Academy of Higher Education and Research, Mysuru, Karnataka, India

Jyotchna Devi Bade
Department of Biochemistry, Great Eastern Medical School and Hospital, Srikakulam, Andhra Pradesh, India

Shafia Bashir
Department of Pharmaceutical Sciences, University of Kashmir, Hazratbal, Srinagar, Jammu and Kashmir, India

Pankaj Bhatt
College of Pharmacy, COER University, Roorkee, Uttarakhand, India

Bhupinder Bhyan
School of Pharmaceutical Sciences, RIMT University, Mandi Gobindgarh, Punjab, India

Ajay Bommareddy
Department of Biomedical Science, Charles E Schmidt College of Medicine, Florida Atlantic University, Boca Raton, FL, United States

Neelima Byahut
Dr. B.R. Ambedkar Center for Biomedical Research (ACBR), University of Delhi, Delhi, India

Hardik Chaudhari
Department of Pharmacy, Collier Pharmacy, Naples, FL, United States

Isha Chawla
Department of Pharmacology, MM College of Pharmacy, Maharishi Markandeshwar (Deemed to be University), Ambala, Haryana, India

Wandeep Dagar
Chitkara College of Pharmacy, Chitkara University, Rajpura, Punjab, India

Meenakshi Dhanawat
Amity Institute of Pharmacy, Amity University Haryana, Gurugram, Haryana, India

Deepika Dwivedi
Dr. B.R. Ambedkar Center for Biomedical Research (ACBR), University of Delhi, Delhi, India

Jashan Girdhar
Teerthanker Mahaveer College of Pharmacy, Teerthanker Mahaveer University, Moradabad, Uttar Pradesh, India

Karan Goel
Department of Pharmacology, Chitkara College of Pharmacy, Chitkara University, Rajpura, Punjab, India

Sumeet Gupta
Department of Pharmacology, MM College of Pharmacy, Maharishi Markandeshwar (Deemed to be University), Ambala, Haryana, India

Paras Jain
Department of Pharmaceutical Sciences, Maharshi Dayanand University, Rohtak, Haryana, India

Sarita Jangra
Chitkara College of Pharmacy, Chitkara University, Rajpura, Punjab, India

Shazia Javeed
Department of Pharmaceutical Sciences, University of Kashmir, Hazratbal, Srinagar, India

Deepthi Joji
Department of Microbiology, JSS Academy of Higher Education and Research, Mysuru, Karnataka, India

Anna Knapinska
Department of Chemistry & Biochemistry, Florida Atlantic University, Boca Raton, FL, United States

Prashanth Kotthapalli
Department of Microbiology, JSS Academy of Higher Education and Research, Mysuru, Karnataka, India

Neema Kumari
Malla Reddy Institute of Medical Sciences, Malla Reddy Vishwavidyapeeth, Hyderabad, Telangana, India

Akash Malik
Dr. B.R. Ambedkar Center for Biomedical Research (ACBR), University of Delhi, Delhi, India

Garima Malik
Chitkara College of Pharmacy, Chitkara University, Rajpura, Punjab, India

Ashish Mishra
Apex Institute of Pharmacy, Mirzapur, Uttar Pradesh, India

Neeraj Mittal
Chitkara College of Pharmacy, Chitkara University, Rajpura, Punjab, India

Kanaka Durga Devi Nelluri
Department of Pharmaceutical Sciences, KVSR Siddhartha College of Pharmaceutical Sciences, Vijayawada, Andhra Pradesh, India

Sunjana Nelluri
Department of Biochemistry, Great Eastern Medical School and Hospital, Srikakulam, Andhra Pradesh, India

Sambit Kumar Parida
Amity Institute of Pharmacy, Amity University, Jaipur, Rajasthan, India

Picheswara Rao Polu
School of Pharmaceutical Sciences, Lovely Professional University, Phagwara, Punjab, India

Paresh Prajapati
Department of Pharmacy, Gujarat University, Ahmedabad, Gujarat, India

Salome Satya Vani Punuri
Department of Pharmacy Practice, Sri Venkateshwara College of Pharmacy, Hyderabad, Telangana, India

Abdul Rahaman
Department of Pharmaceutical Sciences, Vignan's Foundation for Science, Technology and Research, Guntur, Andhra Pradesh, India

Shilpa Rani
Department of Pharmacy, RIMT University Mandi Gobindgarh, Punjab, India

Sanjeev Kumar Sahu
School of Pharmaceutical Sciences, Lovely Professional University, Phagwara, Punjab, India

Meenakshi Sharma
Dr. B.R. Ambedkar Center for Biomedical Research (ACBR), University of Delhi, Delhi, India

Raj Kishor Sharma
Department of Chemistry, University of Delhi, Delhi, India

Sarita Sharma
Department of Pharmacology, Amity Institute of Pharmacy, Amity University, Gwalior, Madhya Pradesh, India

Nasir Ali Siddiqui
Department of Pharmacognosy, College of Pharmacy, King Saud University, Riyadh, Saudi Arabia

Iqubal Singh
School of Pharmaceutical Sciences, Lovely Professional University, Phagwara, Punjab, India

Prabhakar Kumar Verma
Department of Pharmaceutical Sciences, Maharshi Dayanand University, Rohtak, Haryana, India

Shirisha Vodnala
Department of Pharmacy Practice, Sri Venkateshwara College of Pharmacy, Hyderabad, Telangana, India

Vansh Vohra
M.M College of Pharmacy, Maharishi Markandeshwar (Deemed to be University), Ambala, Haryana, India

About the editors

Dr. Arun Kumar Singh completed his M.Pharm in Pharmaceutics from Galgotias University, Greater Noida, India. He currently serves as Assistant Professor in the Department of Pharmacy at Rayat Bahra University, India, where he is involved in teaching and research. His research interests include pharmaceutical sciences, nanotechnology, cancer biology, neuroscience, artificial intelligence, machine learning, blockchain technology, the Internet of Things (IoT), and big data analytics. Dr. Singh has contributed to scholarly publications, books, and edited volumes, with a particular interest in interdisciplinary approaches that integrate healthcare, technology, and pharmaceutical research.

Dr. Meenakshi Dhanawat is Associate Professor at the Amity Institute of Pharmacy, Amity University Haryana, India. She specializes in medicinal chemistry and pharmaceutical sciences. She earned her master's degree from NIPER Mohali and completed her PhD at IIT (BHU), Varanasi, where her research focused on central nervous system drug delivery. Her research interests include CNS therapeutics, medicinal and heterocyclic chemistry, nanotechnology, drug delivery systems, prodrug design, polymer chemistry, and herbal drug research. Dr. Dhanawat is actively involved in teaching, research, scientific publishing, and academic service within the pharmaceutical sciences community.

Garima Malik is a Research Scholar at the Chitkara College of Pharmacy, Chitkara University, Punjab, India. She completed her B.Pharm from Vaish Institute of Pharmaceutical Education and Research, Rohtak, and her M.Pharm from Chandigarh College of Pharmacy, Landran. Her academic and research interests focus on nanotechnology, biomaterials, hydrogels, and advanced drug delivery systems. Prior to her doctoral research, she worked in academia and in pharmaceutical quality control. Her research activities center on the development and evaluation of innovative pharmaceutical formulations and their applications in improving therapeutic outcomes.

Dr. Sadhna Aggarwal received her PhD in Biotechnology from the All India Institute of Medical Sciences (AIIMS), New Delhi, India, with research focused on tumor immunology. She is currently engaged in cancer research at the University of Texas MD Anderson Cancer Center, Houston, USA. Her work focuses on cancer immunology, the tumor microenvironment, spatial multi-omics, biomarker discovery, and precision oncology. Dr. Aggarwal's research aims to advance understanding of mechanisms underlying cancer progression and treatment response, with particular emphasis on translational approaches that support the development of improved therapeutic strategies and personalized cancer.

About the editors

1

Understanding the microbiome: Microbiome and immune system interactions

Karan Goel[a], Isha Chawla[b], Sarita Sharma[c], Nasir Ali Siddiqui[d] and Sumeet Gupta[b,*]

[a]DEPARTMENT OF PHARMACOLOGY, CHITKARA COLLEGE OF PHARMACY, CHITKARA UNIVERSITY, RAJPURA, PUNJAB, INDIA [b]DEPARTMENT OF PHARMACOLOGY, MM COLLEGE OF PHARMACY, MAHARISHI MARKANDESHWAR (DEEMED TO BE UNIVERSITY), AMBALA, HARYANA, INDIA [c]DEPARTMENT OF PHARMACOLOGY, AMITY INSTITUTE OF PHARMACY, AMITY UNIVERSITY, GWALIOR, MADHYA PRADESH, INDIA [d]DEPARTMENT OF PHARMACOGNOSY, COLLEGE OF PHARMACY, KING SAUD UNIVERSITY, RIYADH, SAUDI ARABIA

*CORRESPONDING AUTHOR: SUMEETGUPTA25@GMAIL.COM

1.1 Introduction

The microbiome is a diverse collection of microorganisms such as bacteria, fungi, viruses, and archaea. Studies over the last two decades have highlighted their crucial role in the regulation and support of various bodily functions, such as those related to digestive, metabolic, immune, and psychological health. The main bacterial groups that constitute the microbiome are Firmicutes, Bacteroidetes, Actinobacteria, and Proteobacteria, and each of them performs specific functions in the body (Gilbert et al., 2018; Hou et al., 2022). *Candida* species and other fungi matter to keep the diversity and the balance of host-microbe interactions. The virome, comprising bacteriophages and different viruses, has a significant impact on both the composition and the function of the microbiome's bacterial community (Bertolini & Dongari-Bagtzoglou, 2019). Methanogenic archaea are involved in metabolic pathways that release methane. The microbiome serves as the platform for the growth and instruction of the immune system and is indispensable for general well-being (Volmer et al., 2023). It helps prevent autoimmune diseases and inflammation by promoting the secretion of cytokines such as interleukin-10 (IL-10) and encouraging the growth of regulatory T-cells. In addition to producing energy and ensuring good gastrointestinal health, the bacteria in your gut also have anti-inflammatory qualities via vitamin synthesis and the synthesis of short-chain fatty acids (SCFAs) (Pham et al., 2021). The gut epithelium is one physical

The Microbiome and Cancer Treatment: Overcoming Resistance and Enhancing Efficacy.
DOI: https://doi.org/10.1016/B978-0-443-33206-7.00010-8

barrier that commensal bacteria help to maintain by fighting with other bacteria for space and resources, creating antimicrobial peptides, and generally keeping illnesses at bay (Shi et al., 2017). Significant evidence shows that the microbiome regulates neuroimmune responses and is associated with systemic immunity via the gut-brain axis. It may impact treatment results because of its effects on medication metabolism, immunotherapy, and vaccination efficacy. There is great potential for therapies based on bacteria to revolutionize healthcare (Gopalakrishnan et al., 2018; Shi et al., 2017).

1.2 The immune system: Overview and functions

The immune system functions as the body's defense against damaging infections (bacteria, viruses, fungi, parasites), toxins, and abnormal cells such as cancer. It comprises organs, cells, and proteins that work to recognize and remove threats while sustaining tissue tolerance (Kogut et al., 2020). The immune system can distinguish between self and non-self-entities while still being tolerant of harmless environmental antigens and normal microbiota. It can be divided structurally and functionally into innate and adaptive components (González et al., 2014; Tang et al., 2025). As the first line of defense, innate immunity includes skin, mucous membranes, antimicrobial peptides, and gastric acid as physical and chemical barriers. Moreover, it involves cellular defenses such as macrophages, neutrophils, dendritic cells, and natural killer (NK) cells that attack infections quickly but generally without specificity (Afshar & Gallo, 2013; Şenel, 2021). On the other hand, adaptive immunity is slower but yields more specific and longer-lasting responses via B cells producing antibodies and T cells, which lead and orchestrate immune responses and directly kill infected or cancerous cells. Immune responses are regulated through complex crosstalk among immune cells and signaling molecules such as cytokines, chemokines, and antibodies (Lee et al., 2024; Madan et al., 2025; Wang et al., 2024). Antigen-presenting cells, especially dendritic cells and macrophages, are very important in connecting the innate and adaptive immune responses by processing antigens and stimulating T cells. Primary lymphoid organs which consist of bone marrow and thymus, are responsible for the generation and engineering of immune cells. Secondary lymphoid organs, such as lymph nodes, spleen, and mucosal-associated lymphoid tissue (MALT), are involved in immune surveillance and immune responses at the systemic and mucosal levels (Akhand & Ahsan, 2023; Hughes et al., 2016). The immune system can protect the body from potential pathogens effectively through immune activation. However, to prevent the development of excessive inflammation and autoimmunity, immune activation needs to be tightly regulated. This is done by regulatory T cells, anti-inflammatory cytokines such as IL-10, and immune checkpoint pathways that maintain tolerance and balance in the immune system. When these regulatory mechanisms are disrupted, it can lead to chronic inflammatory conditions, autoimmune disorders, allergies, or even a compromised antitumor immune response (Bhol et al., 2024; Rocamora-Reverte et al., 2021). Moreover, a healthy immune system is in constant communication with the microbiome, especially at mucosal surfaces like the gut. Microbial antigens and metabolites influence immune cell differentiation, cytokine production, and immunity mechanisms, emphasizing that the immune system is a constantly evolving and adaptable defense network. Hence, the immune system not only provides protection against pathogens and cancers but also helps maintain internal balance through its continual interaction with the microbiome. As such, it plays a vital role in health, vulnerability to disease, and reactions to treatments (Bhol et al., 2024; Kogut et al., 2020; Shi et al., 2017).

The immune system can be basically categorized into two branches: innate and adaptive immunity. Innate immunity, the first line of defense, is immediate, generic, and nondiscriminative, and it acts against pathogens through the recognition of conserved molecular patterns. Classic examples are infection, induced fever, and the very swift inflammatory reactions. On the other hand, adaptive immunity is capable of mounting highly antigen-specific responses and producing immune memory, e.g., after measles vaccination. Although adaptive responses take from days to weeks to reach the peak level, they ensure long-lasting, frequently lifelong protection via memory B cells and T cells (Alexander et al., 2014). The immune system comprises several layers of protective barriers. First, physical barriers like skin and mucous membranes act as the first line of defense against pathogen invasion, and chemical barriers such as gastric acid, salivary enzymes, and antimicrobial peptides work toward eliminating the invading microbes. Second, biological barriers, especially the gut and skin microbiota, compete with the pathogens and support the epithelial integrity by producing metabolites such as butyrate. Also, if these barriers are compromised or disrupted, for instance, through a skin cut or microbiome imbalance, the risk of infection goes up (Takiishi et al., 2017). Apart from these physical and chemical barriers, the immune system also relies on innate immune cells, including macrophages, neutrophils, dendritic cells, and NK cells, which together form the first line of defense. These cells come into play at different stages to protect the body from pathogens. For instance, macrophages engulf bacteria and also release substances that cause inflammation. Neutrophils are the first immune cells to arrive at the infection site; dendritic cells are responsible for linking innate and adaptive immunity by presenting antigens, and NK cells kill virus-infected or tumor cells. However, while neutrophils are key players in the early stage of infection, their overactivation can lead to tissue damage, which is characteristic of sepsis (Thaiss et al., 2016). Adaptive immune cells comprise B cells (β-cells), helper T cells ($CD4^+$), and cytotoxic T cells ($CD8^+$). B cells secrete antibodies specific to antigens, helper T cells coordinate the immune response, and cytotoxic T cells kill infected or abnormal cells directly. For example, helper T cells stimulate B cells during influenza infection, and cytotoxic T cells kill virus-infected cells. HIV, in particular, attacks $CD4^+$ T cells, resulting in a severe loss of the immune system's adaptive ability (Russo et al., 2016). Immune function arises through major molecules such as antibodies (IgG, IgA, IgM, IgE, IgD), cytokines, and complement proteins. Antibodies can directly neutralize the pathogen or attract other cells for destruction, while immunoglobulin A plays a protective role at mucosal surfaces. Furthermore, cytokines are involved in modulating the immune response, and complement proteins are part of the innate immunity that assists in creating membrane attack complexes. Nevertheless, an overproduction of cytokines, referred to as a cytokine storm, may result in uncontrollable inflammation such as that seen in COVID-19 (Abeles & Pride, 2014). Immune organs can be subdivided into primary and secondary lymphoid organs. Primary organs, which are the bone marrow and thymus, produce and mature immune cells. Secondary organs like lymph nodes, spleen, and mucosal-associated lymphoid tissue are the places where antigen presentation and immune activation occur. Lymph nodes, for example, become swollen when the body is fighting an infection, and Peyer's patches are involved in intestinal immunosurveillance. Individuals without a spleen are more susceptible to bacterial infections and, therefore, vaccination is advisable (Anwar et al., 2020). Critical immune processes are phagocytosis, antigen presentation, and inflammation. Through phagocytosis, macrophages and neutrophils can engulf and break down pathogens, whereas antigen presentation triggers T cells that start the adaptive immune response. Inflammation results in increased blood flow and attracts more immune cells to the infection sites, thus facilitating pathogen killing and tissue healing. On the other hand, prolonged inflammation is believed to be a major factor in the development of arthritis, diabetes, and heart disease (Santa, 2023). Immune dysregulation symptoms may largely be in the form of heightened or diminished immune responses. Pathological overactivation of immunity is causative of autoimmune diseases (such as lupus and type 1 diabetes) and also of allergic diseases such as asthma and hay fever. On the other hand, immunodeficiency diseases such as HIV/AIDS and SCID (severe combined immunodeficiency) become vulnerable to infection and cancer. Therapies comprise the use of immunosuppressants to treat autoimmune diseases and the use of immunostimulatory agents to reverse immune deficiencies (Zou et al., 2021). In the end, immune manipulation approaches are directed at improving or reestablishing immune homeostasis. Vaccination leads to the formation of protective immune memory. Probiotics and prebiotics are beneficial to the gut microbiota and, consequently, the immune system, while immunotherapies such as CAR-T cells and immune checkpoint inhibitors help stimulate immune responses against cancer. To illustrate, vaccination against influenza is a measure that helps in preventing seasonal flu. Probiotics nurturing a healthy gut immune environment and checkpoint blocker therapy are useful in managing melanoma. Microbiome-based therapies and personalized immunotherapies that are able to fine-tune immune responses better are among the subjects being studied currently (Kazemifard et al., 2022).

1.3 Interactions between the microbiome and immune system

The millions of microbes comprising the human microbiome, particularly those residing in the gut, play a central role in the development and modulation of immune responses. The immune-microbiome interactions are increasingly studied for deeper insights, emerging applications, and research trends (Di Simone et al., 2023). The microbiome and the immune system are in a dynamic, bidirectional, and mutually supportive relationship that is vital for immune homeostasis and overall health. Microbial colonization from the very beginning of life plays a pivotal role in immune education, which equips the immune system to differentiate between harmful pathogens and harmless antigens, such as dietary components and commensal microbes (Ullah et al., 2024; Wang et al., 2025). Microbiota-derived signals direct the development and functions of both innate and adaptive immune cells, thus affecting immune tolerance, inflammatory responses, and immune memory over the long term. Gut microbes constantly regulate immune responses by producing various bioactive metabolites such as SCFAs, tryptophan-derived compounds, bacteriocins, and polysaccharides (Negi et al., 2019; Wang et al., 2024; Zheng et al., 2020). In particular, SCFAs, such as butyrate, acetate, and propionate, stimulate Treg differentiation, increase the secretion of anti-inflammatory cytokines like IL-10, and inhibit excessive proinflammatory signaling. Besides, these metabolites play a part in gut barrier function by promoting tight junctions and mucus formation, thus preventing pathogens from crossing the gut lining and causing systemic inflammation (Duan et al., 2023; Venegas et al., 2019). The microbiome still contributes to immune defense by defeating pathogens in the fight for nutrients and binding sites, releasing antimicrobial peptides, and regulating antigen presentation. Unharmful bacteria are involved in setting the proportions of different T helper cell populations (Th1, Th2, and Th17), maintaining immune responses to infections while preventing, at the same time, autoimmunity and allergies. Microbes activating B cells help in increasing immunoglobulin A (IgA) production, which is the mainstay of mucosal immunity and the protection of epithelial surfaces (Wu & Wu, 2012; Seo et al., 2024). Figuring out the disruption of this delicately balanced interaction called dysbiosis, immune dysregulation happens, leading to weakened barrier function, cytokine imbalance, chronic inflammation, and increased susceptibility to autoimmune diseases, allergies, infections, and cancer. Alternatively, microbial population restoring therapies such as probiotics, prebiotics, dietary modifications, or fecal microbiota transplantation (FMT) have been proven quite effective in rebalancing the immune system. The microbiome-immune system partnerships represent a fundamental physiological route that governs immune maturation, disease outcomes, and responses to treatments, particularly in immune-mediated and inflammatory disorders (Mousa et al., 2022; Shen et al., 2025). The complex interactions between the microbiome and the immune system are one of the most elaborate and carefully regulated symbiotic relationships in human biology. Such a mutualistic partnership is essential for immune homeostasis, protection against infection, and the limitation of chronic inflammation. The gut microbiota, mainly comprised of Bacteroidetes and Firmicutes at the phylum level, continually "talks" to immune cells of the host through microbial-associated molecular patterns, metabolites, and structural elements of the microbe. One of the key immunomodulatory players among these components are SCFAs such as acetate, propionate, and butyrate. These metabolites are produced by the fermentation of dietary fibers and help immune cells get differentiated, maintain the epithelial barrier, and control local inflammation. By inducing Treg cell growth and lowering the release of proinflammatory cytokines, the microbiome serves as an active mechanism that prevents autoimmune diseases and chronic inflammatory conditions (Hooper et al., 2012). The notion of immune education highlights how pivotal early-life microbial colonization is for the immune system's ability to function properly in the long run. In the very first stage of life, infants receive signals from microbes that are indispensable for their immune systems to learn how to tell the difference between dangerous pathogens and innocuous environmental or food antigens. Experiments with germ-free animals reveal that they suffer from major immune system flaws, such as lymphoid tissues being poorly developed, lowered IgA secretion, and T-cell differentiation being compromised, etc. It has been found that the very first microbial disruptions, for example, cesarean section, formula feeding, or heavy use of antibiotics, are linked to a higher risk of developing allergic diseases, asthma, and autoimmune disorders later on in life. Hence, the microbiome has an essential role in immune tolerance, and microbiome-targeted interventions during early life might be a means to lower the risk of immune-mediated diseases in the future (De Luca & Shoenfeld, 2019). Besides immune education, the microbiome also helps to reinforce the barrier defense mechanisms of mucosal surfaces. The intestinal epithelium is a key frontline host-environment interface. Microbes like *Lactobacillus* and *Bifidobacterium* help to maintain the barrier by generating lactic acid and SCFAs that result in lower luminal pH, prevention of pathogen adhesion, and stimulation of tight junction protein expression. Besides that, commensal bacteria encourage the production of mucus as well as the secretion of antimicrobial peptides, thus forming a defensive multilayered shield. This barrier-augmenting role carries major therapeutic ramifications, especially in the context of gastrointestinal disorders manifesting epithelial lesions, e.g., inflammatory bowel disease (IBD) (Abeles & Pride, 2014). Cytokine modulation is yet another major route through which the microbiome exerts its impact on the immune system. SCFAs influence immune cells in an epigenetic and receptor-mediated manner, including the suppression of histone deacetylases and the triggering of G-protein-coupled receptors such as GPR41 and GPR43. Through these conduits, Treg differentiation and IL-10 production are increased, and proinflammatory mediators like IL-6 and tumor necrosis factor alpha (TNFα) are inhibited. Such cytokine-balancing mechanisms are vital for the avoidance of chronic inflammatory disorders, e.g., rheumatoid arthritis (RA) and IBD, and serve as the groundwork for microbiota-based therapy approaches that are presently being explored (Anwar et al., 2020).

Microbial antigens also play a role in regulating the adaptive immune system. A few specific taxa, such as *Bacteroides fragilis* (*B. fragilis*) and certain *Clostridia* species, secrete immunologically active molecules that lead to Treg expansion and help to develop tolerance. Polysaccharide A (PSA) of *B. fragilis* is a thoroughly studied example that can generate IL-10, produce T cells, and prevent inflammatory pathology in animal model colitis cases. These discoveries have encouraged scientists to look at microbial components as immune adjuvants and modulators of vaccine efficacy, thus providing new avenues for protective immunity enhancement while avoiding immune overactivation (Hsieh & Allen, 2020; Santa, 2023). The microbiota is also instrumental in pathogen defense through competitive exclusion and antimicrobial production. Commensal organisms not only compete with pathogens for nutrients but also for epithelial binding sites, thus helping to limit pathogen colonization. These beneficial bacteria produce bacteriocins and antimicrobial peptides that can directly kill such pathogens as *Clostridioides difficile and Salmonella.* This protective function underlies the use of FMT, which has shown spectacular results in curing repeated *C. difficile* infections, and now the procedure is being tried for immune-related and metabolic disorders (Kazemifard et al., 2022). Furthermore, microbial regulation of T-cell differentiation serves as another example of the intricate microbiome-immune crosstalk. For instance, segmented filamentous bacteria are well-known for stimulating Th17 cell differentiation, thus strengthening mucosal protection against extracellular pathogens. On the other hand, high Th17 activity may lead to autoimmune disorders, for which balanced microbial signaling is vital. In fact, a diverse and stable microbiome fosters the coexistence of proinflammatory Th1/Th17 cells and regulatory T cells, which is the mechanism for maintaining immune tolerance and preventing immune-mediated damage (Di Simone et al., 2023). Disarrangement of microbial homeostasis or dysbiosis is even more connected to the development of autoimmune diseases, allergic disorders, and asthma. The reports have demonstrated that patients with RA and Crohn's disease show a lowered level of anti-inflammatory bacteria such as *Faecalibacterium prausnitzii* (*F. prausnitzii*) *and B. fragilis*. Similarly, a decrease in microbial diversity in early life is associated with a higher risk of asthma and food allergies. The discovery of the aforementioned has raised an interest in the administration of probiotics and prebiotics to renormalize the microbial ecosystem and decrease immune dysregulation (De Luca & Shoenfeld, 2019; Hooper et al., 2012; Riiser, 2015). Moreover, the microbiome imparts the ability to the host to withstand infectious diseases by regulating innate immunity and adaptive immunity. It has been demonstrated that probiotic strains such as *Lactobacillus rhamnosus* are capable of lowering the incidence of respiratory tract infections and enhancing antiviral immunity against viruses like norovirus and rotavirus. Among others, the mechanisms of these phenomena involve increased production of IgA, enhanced barrier functions, and regulation of dendritic cell activity (Wiertsema et al., 2021). The microbiome has recently gained recognition as one of the main oncologic features determining immune surveillance and response to therapy. Certain bacterial strains are found to impact tumor recognition by the immune system, T-cell infiltration, and even the effectiveness of checkpoint inhibitors. For instance, the genera *Bacteroides and Firmicutes* were shown to correlate with better responses to immunotherapies like anti-PD-1 (Heilbronner et al., 2021; Sepich-Poore et al., 2021). SCFAs and other metabolites produced by bacteria influence the tumor microenvironment mainly through their effects on cytokine secretion and immune cell differentiation. Therefore, cancer therapies that target or include the microbiome, such as dietary changes, probiotics, and FMT, are being developed not only to improve immunotherapy effects but also to counteract resistance (Mann et al., 2024; Xu et al., 2022). As the main mediators of immune regulation, SCFAs are certainly the most prominent microbial metabolites. SCFAs not only encourage the differentiation of Treg cells but also affect the phenotype of macrophages and block the overactivation of inflammatory signaling pathways. Supplementation with SCFAs is at the moment being tested in clinical trials for inflammatory diseases. Also, gut microbial catabolism of tryptophan leads to the production of several compounds, including kynurenine, which are capable of activating the aryl hydrocarbon receptor and, thereby, contribute to immune tolerance and control of inflammation (Gao et al., 2018). Currently, interventions directed at tryptophan metabolism are considered a new approach for cancer immunotherapy that may also help to reestablish immune homeostasis. In total, these complex situations indicate that the microbiome is deeply involved in controlling immune system development, the maintenance of stability, defense against pathogens, and drug response. The two-way communication between the microbial communities and immune cells is, on the one hand, the factor that determines vulnerability to immune-mediated diseases. On the other hand, it also provides very good chances for new microbiome-targeted approaches to be used in the fields of infectious diseases, autoimmunity, and cancer (Li et al., 2019).

1.4 The gut microbiome and immune system crosstalk

The gut microbiota has a major influence on the immune system, and the two systems interact in a very dynamic and symbiotic way. Immune cells during their proper maturation in early infancy learn through experience to differentiate between harmful infections and friendly antigens; thus, the chance of overreactions is reduced (Li et al., 2019). In addition to that, butyrate and other SCFAs promote immunological tolerance by their anti-inflammatory effect and also by the induction of regulatory T cells (Tregs) proliferation (Luu et al., 2018). The microbiome helps keep hazardous substances and germs out of the bloodstream by making chemicals that fortify tight junctions and encourage mucus production, which in turn strengthens the intestinal barrier (Corrêa-Oliveira et al., 2016; Luu & Visekruna, 2019). To maintain a healthy equilibrium between proinflammatory and anti-inflammatory reactions, microbial metabolites, such as SCFAs, control cytokine synthesis. SCFAs suppress proinflammatory cytokines like IL-6 and TNF-α while enhancing the production of IL-10 and other anti-inflammatory cytokines (Gonçalves et al., 2018; Ratajczak et al., 2019). The development of diverse subsets of T cells, such as regulatory Tregs, Th1, Th2, and Th17 cells, is facilitated by the intestinal microbiota, which in turn affects immunological responses. Also, they help activate β-cells, which means more IgA is made (Gonçalves et al., 2018; Luu & Visekruna, 2019; Ratajczak et al., 2019; Schwarz et al., 2017). IgA is crucial for mucosal defense because it prevents pathogens from sticking to mucosal surfaces and neutralizes toxins. To prevent illnesses, commensal bacteria compete with pathogens for food, water, and other resources. Bacteriocins and antimicrobial peptides, produced by species such as *Bacteroides* and *Lactobacillus*, help keep the microbiome balanced and lower the likelihood of infections, as illustrated in Fig. 1.1 (Gonçalves et al., 2018; Haase et al., 2018; Luu & Visekruna, 2019).

Dysbiosis, or microbial imbalance, is linked to various inflammatory diseases, allergies, and autoimmune disorders (Levy et al., 2017). Reduced microbial diversity during early life is associated with a higher risk of asthma, eczema, and food allergies (Riiser, 2015). The depletion of beneficial bacteria, such as *F. prausnitzii* and *B. fragilis*, is observed in IBDs like Crohn's disease and ulcerative colitis (Zhang et al., 2017). A disruption of immunological homeostasis, caused by dysbiosis, raises the risk of autoimmune diseases, such as type 1 diabetes and RA (Paun et al., 2016). Success in addressing a variety of illnesses has been shown when microbial equilibrium is restored by the use of probiotics, prebiotics, or FMT.

Neurodegenerative diseases and multiple sclerosis (MS) are associated with changes in the gut microbiota, which in turn influence systemic and neuroimmune responses, such as microglial activation and neuroinflammation (Menees et al., 2022; Weiner, 2025). Cancer immunotherapy may be made more successful by altering the gut microbiota's impact on immune surveillance. Some species, like *B. fragilis* and *Akkermansia muciniphila* (*A. muciniphila*), have shown promise in enhancing the effectiveness of immune checkpoint inhibitors in the treatment of cancers, such as lung and melanoma (Russo et al., 2016; Sepich-Poore et al., 2021; Weiner, 2025).

Microbiome engineering is a relatively new field of study and provides a strategy to recreate natural microbiomes to generate specific SCFAs that can modulate the immune system (Gopalakrishnan et al., 2018). One approach to treatment being explored is modulating the gut

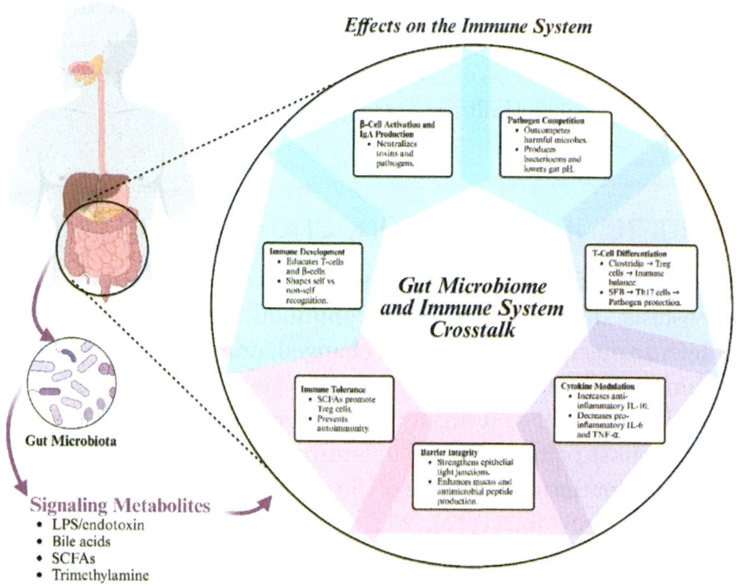

FIGURE 1.1 Gut microbiome and immune system crosstalk. The gut microbiome and immune system interact through the crosstalk of signaling metabolites, facilitating communication with host organs and tissues. The gut microbiome interacts with the immune system of the host through various microbial signaling molecules and metabolites, among which are short-chain fatty acids (SCFAs), bile acids, lipopolysaccharides (LPS), and trimethylamine. These signals originating from microbes govern major immune functions such as the maturation of immune cells, T- and B-cell differentiation, production of IgA, balancing cytokines, and immune tolerance. Beneficial microbes assist in keeping the gut barrier intact by increasing the strength of epithelial tight junctions, promoting mucus secretion, and triggering the generation of antimicrobial peptides, all of which effectively prevent pathogen translocation. Meanwhile, microbial competition limits pathogen colonization by means of bacteriocin production and pH alteration. Together, this bidirectional communication preserves immune homeostasis, helps the immune system to fight pathogens, and prevents excessive inflammation and autoimmunity, thus illustrating the essential role of the gut microbiome in immune modulation. *IgA*, immunoglobin A.

microbiome, a constituent of the gut system that plays a role in immune function (Li et al., 2019). Researchers are creating probiotics and prebiotics to enhance the effectiveness of vaccines, reduce inflammation, and prevent infections. FMT is a treatment under investigation for autoimmune disorders and neurological disorders, in addition to infections (Menees et al., 2022; Weiner, 2025).

Thymic output is complemented by the stimulation of immunological tolerance and the mutuality of interactions between gut and immune cells, and as such, the gut microbiome plays a complex and essential role in the early development of the immune system (Alexander et al., 2014; Ratajczak et al., 2019). For cancer patients, the gut microbiome composition has an impact on immunotherapy. This helps prevent systemic inflammation and the progression of diseases, keeping the intestinal barrier intact and the body in homeostasis. Researchers are examining novel gut health treatment options by modulating the microbiome, such as FMT (Xu et al., 2022). One of the latest studies shows that FMT by oral capsules, which are cheekily named crapsules, could be beneficial for insomnia, Parkinsons disease, allergy, bowel disorders, and even cancer. The gut microbiome is also influenced by environmental factors (Hsieh & Allen, 2020). Being in nature might have a positive effect on our immune system as well as on the diversity of microbes in our bodies (Anwar et al., 2020; Heilbronner et al., 2021).

1.5 Microbiome, inflammation, and immune homeostasis

The microbiome is central and irreplaceable in the control of inflammation and the maintenance of immune homeostasis. This is through being a continuous source of immunological signals that keep the host's defense mechanisms adjusted, changed, or modified, thus preventing excessive utilization and damage from the immune system. It is generally understood that a diverse and balanced community of microbes forms a symbiotic relationship with the host, the immune system is effective against pathogens, and inflammation is kept at a minimum. This kind of equilibrium is essential for the maintenance of the normal state of tissues, metabolic health, and immune tolerance over time (Mousa et al., 2022; Seo et al., 2024).

Host immune cells meticulously monitor microbial signals through pattern recognition receptors such as toll-like receptors and NOD-like receptors that are present on intestinal epithelial cells, macrophages, and dendritic cells. When these receptors are properly controlled during the interaction with commensal microbes, it triggers low-level immune activation, which primes immune readiness without causing pathological inflammation. Such low-level signaling is necessary for immune cell development, mucosal immune homeostasis, and controlling excessive immune responses to harmless antigens. A major way the microbiome affects inflammatory processes is via the generation of microbial metabolites, with SCFAs having a prominent role among them, especially butyrate, acetate, and propionate. These metabolites arise because beneficial gut bacteria ferment dietary fibers and then communicate with immune cells through G-coupled receptors as well as by epigenetic mechanisms. The net effect is the promotion of T regulatory cells (Tregs) and suppression of pro-inflammatory T helper 17 (Th17) responses. One of the most outstanding properties of butyrate is its ability to inhibit histone deacetylases, which consequently leads to the increased expression of immune tolerance genes and the production of anti-inflammatory cytokines (Qing et al., 2022; Takeuchi & Akira, 2010; Wicherska-Pawłowska et al., 2021).

Besides that, the microbiome is one of the major players that decides the strength of the gut's physical barrier, which in turn contributes greatly to immune system homeostasis. Normal bacteria or commensals possess the ability not only to trigger the secretion of mucus but also to promote the expression of tight junction proteins between epithelial cells, thus preventing the entry of pathogens and microbial toxins into the bloodstream. This immune regulatory effect of the barrier function serves as a protective mechanism against systemic inflammation. When the barrier is damaged, a condition often referred to as "leaky gut," microbial products such as lipopolysaccharides can find their way into the blood, thus triggering the immune system and inflammation to be in a chronic state (Li et al., 2020; Lin & Zhang, 2017; Wiertsema et al., 2021).

The microbiome that is functioning properly works closely to actively maintain the regulation of cytokine networks for balanced immune responses. To this end, it helps the promotion of anti-inflammatory cytokines and lowers the production of pro-inflammatory cytokines; thus it is assisting in the resolution of inflammation that happens after immune activation. It is very important that the resolution phase should be there to prevent the steady state of inflammation, which can cause tissue damage and diseases. Besides, macrophage polarization is entirely under the influence of microbial cues, which results in the generation of anti-inflammatory phenotypes that are capable of helping tissue repair and immune resolution. Microbial imbalance or dysbiosis is a condition that means the failure of the regulatory mechanisms that normally maintain immune homeostasis. It is characterized by a decrease in microbial diversity, the disappearance of beneficial metabolite bacteria, and the overgrowth of proinflammatory organisms. Consequently, there is defective Treg formation, excessive Th17-driven inflammation, cytokine imbalance, and weakened barrier functions. Therefore, a condition of chronic low-grade inflammation is initiated, which leads to the development of autoimmune diseases, allergies, metabolic disorders, neuroinflammatory diseases, and cancer (Hou et al., 2022; Juarez et al., 2022; Kushkevych et al., 2025; Mazziotta et al., 2023). The microbial restoration through a therapeutic mindset is a very attractive idea to reset the immune system and reduce inflammation. Both probiotics and prebiotics help the good bacteria to flourish, and consequently, the production of metabolites also increases. At the same time, fiber and polyphenol-rich diets contribute to anti-inflammatory microbial pathways. In very severe cases of dysbiosis, FMT may totally resettle microbial diversity and immune balance. These combined points indicate that the microbiota is the major player in controlling inflammation and immune homeostasis. The microbiome ensures immune homeostasis through well-learned microbial recognition, immune modulation through metabolites, preservation of the barrier, and cytokine balance. If these mechanisms fail, chronic inflammation and immune-mediated diseases ensue. However, precise microbiome strategies may provide a therapeutic solution for the restoration of immune balance and thus better health outcomes (Dahiya & Nigam, 2023; Latif et al., 2023; Zhou et al., 2024).

1.6 Dysbiosis and immune system dysfunction

If dysbiosis occurs (an imbalance in the gut microbiome characterized by an increase in harmful bacteria and a decrease in beneficial bacteria), this dysbiosis and the immune system may malfunction. Such disturbance could be due to reduced microbial diversity, increased pathogen bacteria, or the absence of beneficial bacteria. Any disturbances to the fragile balance of the gut flora and immune system may have consequences for the human race in general (Belizário et al., 2018; Logan et al., 2016; Petersen & Round, 2014).

Impaired intimate connections between epithelial cells are one of the main outcomes of dysbiosis, which is the breakdown of the intestinal barrier. Because of this defect, potentially dangerous bacteria and poisons may enter the circulation; this is known as a "leaky gut." This disorder causes inflammation throughout the body and an overactive immune system (Christovich et al., 2022; Kinashi & Hase, 2021). The development of cytokine dysregulation is characterized by an upregulation of cytokines that promote inflammation, including IL-6, TNF-α, and IL-17, and a downregulation of cytokines that inhibit inflammation, like IL-10 (Lemme-Dumit et al., 2022). When cytokine production is out of whack, it weakens the immune system and makes chronic inflammation worse. Autoimmunity and tissue damage may be exacerbated when dysbiosis interrupts T-cell development, leading to an increase in Th17 cells and a reduction in regulatory T-cells (Tregs) (Christovich et al., 2022; Lemme-Dumit et al., 2022; Petersen & Round, 2014). Furthermore, dysbiosis impacts IgA, the dominant mucosal antibody, and dysbiosis affects β-cell activity and production. Mucosal immunity is compromised (IgA is quite low); infections are more likely to be successful (Yu et al., 2021).

These immune dysfunctions have significantly impacted IBD, autoimmune diseases (like RA, MS, type 1 diabetes, among many others), increased sensitivity to allergies, and cancer susceptibility (Logan et al., 2016; Paun et al., 2016). In addition, the gut-brain axis can modify neuroinflammation in peripheral conditions, and changes in microbiota may contribute to neurodegenerative diseases related to Alzheimer's and Parkinsons. Several treatment approaches aimed at counteracting the consequences of dysbiosis are the focus of active investigation (Menees et al., 2022; Weiner, 2025). Antibiotic stewardship, FMT, microbial metabolite therapy, omega-3 fatty acid-rich plant-based diets, and probiotics are all examples of this genetic category. Understanding how dysbiosis affects the immune system and how it is tied to diseases like IBD, RA, allergies, and cancer can help with therapy programs to restore bacterial balance and boost immune health (Lemme-Dumit et al., 2022; Yu et al., 2021).

1.6.1 Inflammatory bowel disease

Bacteria that produce SCFAs, such as *F. prausnitzii* and *B. fragilis,* are significantly reduced. These SCFAs help maintain the integrity of the intestinal barrier and regulate the immune response. The loss of these SCFA-producing bacteria leads to a leaky gut, which enables pathogens to come in, and hence, chronic inflammation ensues in IBD patients. This imbalance leads to an overproduction of cytokines like IL-6 and TNF-α, darkening the scenario and further worsening the illness due to skewing of the immune system toward a pro-inflammatory state. FMT or probiotics have shown promising results in reducing inflammation and inducing remission in patients with IBD after restoring a balanced microbiome (Lal et al., 2022; Matsuoka & Kanai, 2015).

1.6.2 Rheumatoid arthritis

RA is a condition in which the immune system mistakenly attacks the joints. Dysbiosis can be seen in this study published by Van De Wiele et al., 2016 found that the gut microbiome of people with RA is significantly less diverse in terms of the types of microbes present. Firmicutes, a type of bacteria linked to inflammation, are down, and Proteobacteria are up. An aberrant immunological response triggered by this microbial imbalance could lead to stiffness, inflammation, and chronic pain. In addition, dysbiosis enhances the activation of proinflammatory Th17 cells and inhibits the generation of regulatory T-cells (Tregs) that regulate immunological responses. This aggravates the autoimmune response (Van De Wiele et al., 2016).

1.6.3 Allergic diseases

Dysbiosis has been linked to the incidence of allergic diseases such as food allergies, eczema, and asthma. Infants born into homes with few microbes experience more allergies. *Lactobacillus* and *Bacteroides* are two types of beneficial bacteria that help build resistance to infection, and their absence increases vulnerability. The same children who are at risk of developing allergies may benefit from taking probiotic supplements. Researchers have demonstrated the potential of probiotics as an early intervention to manage immune responses and reduce the prevalence of allergic diseases (Pascal et al., 2018).

1.6.4 Cancer and immunotherapy

Research on the microbiome's contribution to cancer and the efficacy of immunotherapy is an emerging area of study. When the microbiome is healthy, immune checkpoint inhibitors that train the immune system to target cancer cells work better. A study found that anti-PD-1 medications were more effective for cancer patients whose gut microbiomes were diverse and contained high levels of certain types of bacteria, including *A. muciniphila* and *B. fragilis*. These beneficial bacteria activate immunological cells such as T-cells and dendritic cells, which enhance the immune response. Those whose microbiomes were damaged had weaker immunological surveillance and poorer tumor suppression. Our data suggest that dietary modifications or probiotics might impact the microbiome in a way that promotes immunity, as noted, thus enhancing cancer immunotherapy response (Fessler et al., 2019; Mann et al., 2024; Roviello et al., 2022). Immune system dysfunction resulting from dysbiosis provides a clear example of how microbiome-based interventions could be implemented for disease occurrence reduction. It has been demonstrated in a number of studies that tactics targeted at restoring the microbial balance not only improve immunological health but also ease the symptoms of different diseases. The evidence concerning microbiome composition and its links with the immune system is so extensive that personalized microbiome intervention will probably become the distinguishing feature of 21st-century medicine. This kind of way forward may open up new possibilities for overcoming autoimmune diseases, allergies, infections, and cancer (Lal et al., 2022; Levy et al., 2017; Roviello et al., 2022).

1.7 Microbiome and cancer immunology

The microbiome is known as one of the leading factors in cancer immunology, thus affecting the tumor's initiation, development, immune surveillance, and the efficiency of anticancer therapies. Some microbial populations, particularly those living in the gut, influence local as well as systemic immune responses through microbial antigens, metabolites, and immune-modulatory signaling pathways. An equilibrium microbiome supports effective antitumor immunity, the promotion of dendritic cell maturation, T-cell activation, and cytotoxic immune responses; immune surveillance against tumor cells is thereby strengthened (Gopalakrishnan et al., 2018; Zhao et al., 2023; Zitvogel et al., 2016). SCFAs, secondary bile acids, and tryptophan-derived compounds, among other microbial metabolites, impact the tumor immune microenvironment by regulating cytokine production, immune cell differentiation, and epigenetic programming of immune cells. These metabolites can inhibit chronic inflammation, which is the main cause of carcinogenesis; at the same time, they support the immune regulatory mechanisms that prevent immune exhaustion. On the contrary, dysbiosis generates a proinflammatory environment that is characterized by elevated levels of such cytokines as IL-6 and TNF, loss of barrier integrity, and reduced antitumor immune activity, all of which would promote tumor growth and immune evasion (Duan et al., 2025; Luo et al., 2025; Zhang et al., 2024). The microbiome is tremendously important for determining whether cancer immunotherapy, especially immune checkpoint inhibitors against PD-1, PD-L1, and CTLA-4, will be successful. Some bacterial taxa, notably *A. muciniphila* and *B. fragilis*, have been correlated with a more favorable response to checkpoint blockers by helping T-cells to penetrate and become functionally activated in tumors. In contrast, the use of antibiotics or a poor diet causing microbiome changes has been associated with lowered drug efficacy and a rise in resistance to treatment. Cancer microbiome influence goes beyond immunotherapy by changing drug metabolism, toxicity, and systemic immunity. Microbiota enzymes can convert chemotherapy drugs into more active or less active forms, thereby modulating both their efficacy and their side effects. Therefore, the multiple strands of evidence point to the microbiome as a key player in cancer immunology and a promising therapeutic target. Altering the microbial community through probiotics, dietary changes, or FMT might pave the way for novel approaches to enhance antitumor immunity, overcome resistance, and increase the overall efficacy of cancer treatments (Choudhry, 2021; Davar & Zarour, 2022; Zarour & Trinchieri, 2025).

1.8 Techniques for studying microbiome-immune system interactions

The relationship between the microbiota and the immune system is extremely complicated; only advanced computational, cellular, and molecular methods will be able to identify it. More specifically, the use of molecular, cellular, computational, and experimental techniques should be synergized to disclose the complex, ever-changing nature of the microbiome and immune system interactions. Currently, various multiplex methods such as 16S rRNA gene profiling, shotgun metagenomics, and meta-transcriptomics are the most common methods used to reveal microbial diversity, composition, and functional capacity. These techniques allow an in-depth analysis of microbial communities and their genetic pathways, as well as the association of these microbial communities with immune regulation and diseases (Dakal et al., 2025; Hooper et al., 2012; Ma et al., 2024). In addition to this, meta-transcriptomics analysis not only complements the first level of data by providing insights into microbial gene expression but also allows one to link microbial activities with immune signaling and host responses. However, microbial genomics is not the only aspect of metabolomics in microbial and host metabolism interaction studies. Metabolomics is the science that traces the expression of microbial genes back to the metabolites, including SCFAs, bile acids, and tryptophan metabolites, which impact not only the immune system components such as immune cell differentiation and cytokine production but also the epithelial barrier's integrity. Experimental setups of gnotobiotic and germ-free animals provide a controlled and isolated environment to first inoculate test animals with a well-characterized microbial community and then dissect the immunological impact of each microbial component in vivo (Jovel et al., 2022; Lu et al., 2025; Patridge et al., 2024). Such a study is essentially a metaphor for immunological microbiota variation being an immune response, as corresponding dance moves. Furthermore, on the cellular level, single-cell RNA sequencing and flow cytometry give an unmatched detailed description of the diversity of immune cells, different activation states, and cytokine production triggered by microbial signals. Thus, the immune responses are traced with great accuracy back to even anatomical locations in complex tissues like the intestine. Additionally, 3D cultures and microfluidic chips simulate actual physiological microenvironments and thus are a great help for carrying out microbiome and immune interaction studies in a more controlled and human physiology-like setting. Therefore, bioinformatics, systems biology, and machine learning methods are applied to the integration of multiomics data and to the unraveling of the complex regulatory networks connecting bacterial functionalities with immune responses and disease phenotypes. These interdependent methodologies provide a solid base for grasping the communication pathways between the microbiome and the immune system, thereby resulting in microbiome-based personalized therapies and novel immunomodulatory strategies (Stubbington et al., 2017; Vegh & Haniffa, 2018). Unlocking the intricate and two-way communication network between the microbiome and the immune system is a challenge that calls for a unified strategy. This strategy should incorporate a spectrum of advanced methodologies such as high-throughput sequencing technologies, metabolite profiling, sophisticated in vivo models, spatial mapping tools, and computational biology. Microbiome-immune interactions are complex, spanning multiple biological layers: genomic, transcriptomic, proteomic, metabolomic, cellular, and tissue levels, which makes it impossible for one method to unravel the entire complexity. Hence, multiomics integration has been recognized as the ultimate method for a thorough mechanistic understanding and successful translation to humans. Metagenomics, by allowing culture-independent examination of microbial communities, has been the stepping stone of microbiome research. In most cases, 16S rRNA gene sequencing has been employed to distinguish the bacterial taxa and determine their relative abundance within a sample, thereby revealing the shifts in microbial diversity that are linked to immune-mediated diseases. Yet, 16S profiling only provides a limited picture of the functionality. To break down this limitation, whole-genome shotgun metagenomics sequences all microbial DNA found in a sample, thus it can uncover strain-level variation, gene content, virulence factors, antibiotic resistance genes, and metabolic potential. These methods have identified microbial patterns specific to IBD, RA, metabolic syndrome, and varying responses to cancer immunotherapy. Metagenomics significantly adds to compositional data by offering predictive functional pathways, which in turn allow the deduction of the immune and modulatory features that may be hidden within microbial genomes (Qin et al., 2010; Turnbaugh et al., 2007). Metagenomics uncovers what microbes are there and what genes they have, whereas meta-transcriptomics, on the other hand, reveals which genes are being actively expressed under specific physiological conditions. This procedure, through sequencing community-wide RNA transcripts, essentially takes a snapshot of the microbial activities and their responses to the host immune signals in real time. Additionally, with RNA, Seq platforms and bioinformatics tools such as HUMAnN2 and DESeq2, researchers can identify the metabolic and signaling pathways that are most active during conditions like inflammation, infection, or therapeutic intervention. For example, metatranscriptomic studies have identified a heightened microbial expression of pathways dealing with reactive oxygen species and immune evasion mechanisms in chronic inflammatory diseases. This added dimension of analysis is thus essential for understanding that there are dormant microbes with genetic potential that could modulate the immune system and those that are already actively engaged in the immune modulatory processes (Franzosa et al., 2014). Metabolomics reflects a functional endpoint of the cells by determining the concentration of the small molecules that are directly involved in host-microbe crosstalk. Several microbial metabolites, such as SCFAs, secondary bile acids, indole derivatives, trimethylamine, and fragments of lipopolysaccharides, have an extremely potent influence on immune cell differentiation, macrophage polarization, the integrity of the epithelial barrier, and cytokine networks. By applying mass spectrometry (MS) and nuclear magnetic resonance (NMR) spectroscopy, metabolomics provides very detailed detection of these molecules in biological fluids and tissues. Most notably, metabolomic patterns usually show a stronger correlation with the immune phenotypes than the mere taxonomic composition. For instance, the levels of SCFAs are associated with the expansion of regulatory T cells, whereas the changed profiles of bile acids affect the differentiation of Th17 cells. Consequently, metabolomics is the link between microbial activity and immune function; thus, it enables the identification of biomarkers of dysbiosis, inflammatory conditions, and immune therapy response (Nicholson et al., 2012). There is no doubt that gnotobiotic models are required for the experimental validation of microbiome-immune interactions. In these models, germ-free animals are used to provide a sterile immunological baseline, which makes it possible to accurately colonize them with a known microbial consortium. Such models have revealed the essential roles of gut microbiota in the immune system's development; the absence of microbiota leads to underdeveloped Peyer's patches, lowered IgA production, impaired Treg differentiation, and changed cytokine profiles. Through the introduction of specific bacterial strains or synthetic microbial communities, the scientists can pinpoint the cause of the host's immune response changes (Faith et al., 2010; Gray et al., 2017). For instance, segmented filamentous bacteria colonization triggers the production of Th17 cells, whereas some *Clostridia* species can increase Treg numbers. This is the type of mechanistic insight that is essential for the productive use of associative human data. scRNA, Seq has revolutionized the field of immunology by allowing the detection of the degree of heterogeneity among the immune cells. Instead of looking at the response of the whole tissue, scRNA, Seq permits the examination of each immune cell at the level of resolution at which the cells were exposed to the microbial signals. This method not only helps to identify the distinct activation states of the immune cells but also their differentiation trajectories, cytokine expression patterns, and metabolic programs in T cells, dendritic cells, macrophages, and innate lymphoid cells (Stubbington et al., 2017). In the tumor microenvironment, single-cell studies have led to the discovery of the signature of immune exhaustion linked to the microbiome, thus opening up new perspectives for understanding immunotherapy resistance.

Flow cytometry has been the basis of a complete immune phenotyping and functional validation tool. By using fluorescently labeled antibodies against surface markers and intracellular cytokines, immune players can be quantified, their activation markers can be checked, and the secretion of cytokines can be measured by flow cytometry. Multiplex instruments such as Luminex allow the simultaneous quantification of multiple inflammatory mediators (Bellais et al., 2022). Flow cytometry yields quantitative and functional immune readouts in both experimental models and clinical samples, thus complementing omics-based discoveries. Emerging three-dimensional culture systems, especially organoids, have generated physiologically relevant in vitro platforms for studying microbiome-immune interactions. Intestinal organoids differentiated from stem cells mimic epithelial architecture, mucus production, and barrier function. In fact, the coculture of immune cells and defined microbial strains with these organoids allows for dissecting epithelial, microbial, and immune crosstalk in a controlled manner (Shelkey et al., 2022). Since they capture patient heterogeneity, organoids become a tool for patient-specific inflammatory response modeling, infection dynamics, and therapeutic intervention, thus paving the way for personalized medicine. Spatial transcriptomics adds a new feature by retaining the structure of the tissue while locating patterns of gene expression. Instruments like 10x Genomics Visium combine transcriptomic data with histological information and thus make it possible to see the location of immune cells with respect to microbial colonization sites (Mayassi et al., 2024). This method is extremely useful for characterizing microenvironments of localized inflammation, tumor-immune-microbiome interactions, and the disruptions of the intestinal barrier. The integration of multiomics data sets necessitates the use of advanced bioinformatics and systems biology frameworks. For example, taxonomic analysis can be achieved with tools like QIIME2 and Kraken2, while machine learning algorithms can help discover predictive microbial signatures linked to immune phenotypes. Network modeling and AI methods are utilized to associate microbial metabolic pathways with cytokine networks, T-cell polarization, and clinical outcomes. In fact, these computational methodologies are gaining popularity to forecast the response of patients to immunotherapies and to develop microbiome-targeted strategies (Peñalver Bernabé et al., 2018).

Organ-on-a-chip technologies depict a new wave in translational modeling. These microfluidic devices recreate physiological conditions like peristalsis, vascular perfusion, and epithelial barrier function. Gut-on-a-chip models make it possible to witness microbial colonization, immune cell migration, and metabolite diffusion in real time under precisely regulated mechanical and biochemical conditions. Such devices provide a more dynamic and human, relevant method compared to animal models, especially when investigating the gut-brain-immune axis (Moysidou & Owens, 2021; Puschhof et al., 2021). High-throughput culturing, also known as culturomics, complements sequencing-based methods by allowing the isolation and functional characterization of previously unculturable microorganisms. The deployment of sophisticated anaerobic culturing techniques has significantly increased the variety of microbes known, at the same time allowing functional studies to identify the immunomodulatory features of rare bacterial strains (Yadav et al., 2023).

Functional metagenomics boosts discovery even more by inserting environmental DNA into expression vectors and looking for genes regulating immune responses. This method helps to spot new enzymes, signaling molecules, and antimicrobial compounds that together alter host immunity (Sardar et al., 2024). By associating gene function with immune modulation, functional metagenomics quickens the pace of finding therapeutic targets. Lastly, genetically modified probiotics are a translational application of microbiome research. Synthetic biology tools make it possible to change probiotic strains like *Lactobacillus* so that they produce anti-inflammatory cytokines, deliver tumor-targeting agents, or secrete immune-modulating metabolites (Mishra et al., 2022). These designed bacteria are a new and innovative way of precisely and locally controlling the immune system in inflammatory diseases and cancer. All these technological innovations lead to a well-rounded and multidimensional set of instruments for the study of the microbiome-immune system interplay. The combination of genomic, transcriptomic, metabolomic, cellular, spatial, and computational analyses goes beyond just increasing the mechanistic knowledge; it also brings about a faster realization of precise microbiome-based therapies that help immune homeostasis and improve disease outcomes.

1.9 Impact of microbiome on immune-mediated diseases

This extensive study delves into how the microbiome influences immune system-related diseases, offering details on a few disorders, the microbiome variations linked with them, the mechanisms involved, and the treatment possibilities. The presence of a healthy and varied microbiota is able to help immune tolerance by the generation of regulatory T cells, keeping the epithelial barrier intact, as well as the proper secretion of both pro- and anti-inflammatory cytokines. Whereas a dysbiotic situation characterized by low microbial diversity, disappearance of the good bacteria, and an increase in harmful species may bring about immune system defects, chronic inflammation, and greater susceptibility to illness (Oyovwi & Ajayi, 2025; Zhang et al., 2024). Autoimmunity, such as IBD, RA, MS and type 1 diabetes, the disturbed microbiota compromises the metabolism of SCFAs and causes a change in T-cell differentiation toward inflammatory Th1 and Th17 cells along with a decrease in regulatory T cells. As a result, the imbalance continues the inflammatory cycle and is the cause of the damage to the tissues. Likewise, in allergic conditions such as asthma, atopic dermatitis, and food allergies, the microbial perturbation of the early years leads to the loss of immune tolerance, thus resulting in Th2 predominance and increased IgE synthesis. It has been suggested that failure to get microbial exposure in early life can result in allergic sensitivity and immune overreaction. The microbiome is also among the most significant factors affecting cancer occurrence and treatment success (Bhutta et al., 2024; Rasouli-Saravani et al., 2023). Some microbial communities boost immune surveillance and increase the effectiveness of cancer immunotherapies, like immune checkpoint inhibitors, by promoting dendritic cell activation and T-cell responses. On the other hand, dysbiosis can limit tumor immunity, trigger carcinogenesis due to inflammation, and make cancer cells less sensitive to treatment. Furthermore, immune malfunction induced by the microbiome is a major factor in the development of metabolic and cardiovascular diseases, where low-grade chronic inflammation is the main cause. The accumulated data have shown that the microbiome is one of the main factors determining the risk, progression, and treatment response of immune-mediated diseases. Therapies aimed at correcting the microbial imbalance with the help of probiotics, prebiotics, diet modification, or FMT could be excellent ways of adjusting immune responses and thus treating immune-mediated diseases more personally and effectively, as illustrated in Table 1.1 (Chen et al., 2026; Lei et al., 2025; Zhao et al., 2024).

1.10 Therapeutic approaches targeting the microbiome-immune system axis

Therapeutic strategies targeting the microbiome-immune system axis are among the latest discoveries in medicine. The main idea is to restore the immune system's balance, increase the effectiveness of therapy, and directly counteract resistance to treatment, especially in immune-mediated and inflammatory diseases such as cancer. Such interventions aim to alter the microbiota composition, change the microbial community's function, and regulate metabolite production to coordinate immune responses safely and beneficially. Probiotics, prebiotics, synbiotics, and postbiotics are some basic microbiome-related therapies (Christina et al., 2025; Han et al., 2025; Nazir et al., 2025). Probiotics are live beneficial bacteria that can improve the mucosal layer function, thus controlling the production of cytokines and regulating the differentiation of T regulatory cells. Prebiotics serve as food for beneficial bacteria and thus only selectively increase their population, while synbiotics employ a combination of both components to perform the maximal synergistic effects. Postbiotics consist of microbial metabolites such as SCFAs and bioactive peptides that can directly modulate immune signaling pathways without the need for the presence of live microorganisms, which can thus improve safety and lead to more consistent outcomes (Ali et al., 2025; Mazziotta et al., 2023; Simon et al., 2021). During FMT, the microbial community of a healthy donor is transferred to a patient with a disturbed microbial community to restore microbial community diversity. It is one of the most powerful therapeutic approaches. Besides the proven success of FMT in treating recurrent *C. difficile* infection, it is also being considered for use in IBD, autoimmune disorders, metabolic syndromes, and cancer immunotherapy as an adjuvant. To enhance the safety and reproducibility of FMT, standardized preparations such as capsule-based and synthetic FMT are being developed. Considerable changes in the field of engineered and next-generation probiotics have made it possible to create microbial strains that can be utilized to deliver therapeutic molecules, produce immunomodulatory metabolites, or even target inflammatory pathways selectively. Such engineered microbes provide a very fine level of control over the immune response and thus are expected to usher in the era of personalized immunotherapy and optimization of cancer treatment (Liu et al., 2025; Suchitra, 2024; Yadegar et al., 2023).

Both dietary and lifestyle habits significantly impact the microbiome-immune system interplay. Consumption of foods that are high in dietary fiber, polyphenols, and omega-3 fatty acids leads to enhanced production of SCFAs and thus decreased chronic inflammation, whereas consumption of processed foods and repeated use of antibiotics exacerbates dysbiosis and immune dysfunction. Individual microbiome-based personalized nutritional approaches are gaining popularity as the most potent additional therapies. Recently, there have been some fresh

Table 1.1 Impact of microbiota on immune-mediated diseases.

Immune-mediated disease	Microbiome alterations	Mechanisms	Potential interventions	References
Inflammatory bowel disease (IBD), (Crohn's disease, Ulcerative colitis)	Decreased *Faecalibacterium prausnitzii*. Increased *Proteobacteria* and *Enterobacteriaceae*.	Loss of SCFA-producing bacteria disrupts gut epithelial integrity. Dysbiosis triggers pro-inflammatory cytokine production (e.g., TNF-α, IL-6).	FMT SCFA supplementation. Probiotic therapy (*Bifidobacterium*).	Mishra et al. (2022)
Type 1 diabetes (T1D)	Reduced microbial diversity. Increased *Bacteroides* and reduced *Firmicutes*.	Microbial metabolites influence T-cell differentiation, favoring Th1/Th17 proinflammatory responses.	Prebiotic and probiotic supplementation. FMT in early disease stages.	Paun et al. (2016)
Rheumatoid arthritis (RA)	Enrichment of *Prevotella copri*. Depletion of SCFA-producing bacteria.	Microbial antigens trigger systemic autoimmunity via molecular mimicry and Th17 activation.	Probiotic therapy (*Lactobacillus* species). Dietary modulation to restore SCFAs.	Van De Wiele et al. (2016)
Multiple sclerosis (MS)	Increased *Akkermansia muciniphila, Methanobrevibacter*, and *Clostridia*.	Dysbiosis alters gut permeability, promoting systemic inflammation. Tregs reduced, favoring autoimmunity.	Prebiotics enhance Treg populations. Probiotic strains modulating gut-immune homeostasis.	Haase et al. (2018)
Allergic diseases (Asthma, Eczema)	Reduced gut microbial diversity. Lower abundance of *Bifidobacterium* and *Lactobacillus*.	Dysbiosis skews Th1/Th2 balance toward Th2, promoting IgE production and allergic responses.	Early-life probiotic supplementation. Targeted gut microbiota modulation.	Riiser (2015)
Psoriasis	Increased *Firmicutes* to *Bacteroidetes* ratio.	Dysbiosis enhances the IL-23/Th17 axis, promoting keratinocyte hyperproliferation.	Topical probiotics. Dietary fiber for SCFA production.	Kapoor et al. (2022)

(*continued on next page*)

Systemic lupus erythematosus (SLE)	Enrichment of *Lactobacillus reuteri* and reduction of *Butyrate-producing bacteria*.	An altered microbiome increases gut permeability and activates systemic inflammation via IFN-γ pathways.	Probiotic therapy targeting microbial imbalances.	Katz-Agranov and Zandman-Goddard (2017)
Obesity and metabolic syndrome	Reduced microbial diversity. Increase in *Firmicutes/Bacteroidetes* ratio.	Dysbiosis promotes low-grade systemic inflammation via lipopolysaccharides and cytokine production.	Prebiotic dietary fibers. Probiotic strains (*Lactobacillus rhamnosus*).	Belizário et al. (2018)
Cancer (Colorectal cancer, CRC)	Enrichment of proinflammatory bacteria (e.g., *Fusobacterium nucleatum, Escherichia coli*).	Microbial toxins (e.g., colibactin) induce DNA damage. SCFA depletion reduces anti-inflammatory pathways.	FMT combined with checkpoint inhibitors. Anti-inflammatory prebiotics.	Fessler et al. (2019)
Cardiovascular diseases (CVD)	Increased *Trimethylamine-producing bacteria* (e.g., *Firmicutes*).	Microbial metabolism produces trimethylamine-N-oxide (TMAO), contributing to atherosclerosis.	Dietary modification reducing TMAO precursors. Probiotic strains targeting TMAO producers.	Kazemian et al. (2020)

FMT, fecal microbiota transplantation; *IgE*, immunoglobulin E; *IL-6*, interleukin-6; *LPS*, lipopolysaccharides; *Th1/Th17*, T helper 1/T helper 17; *SCFA*, short-chain fatty acids; *TNF-α*, tumor necrosis factor alpha.

methods like microbiome-based vaccines, immune adjuvants, and metabolite therapies, which use the microbes' signals to increase the efficiency of vaccines and the body's immune response to tumors. All these therapy methods emphasize the microbiome as a key natural regulator of immune functions and mark a revolutionary approach in precision medicine that can challenge the present medical norms and keep the door open for improving the treatment results of a very broad range of immune-mediated diseases (Meiners et al., 2025; Rondinella et al., 2026; Zhang, 2022).

Treatments that target the microbiome and the immune system have the potential to improve health, modulate immunological responses, and restore microbial balance in cases of immune-mediated illnesses (Gopalakrishnan et al., 2018; Logan et al., 2016). Among the most important therapies are metabolic engineering, organoids, microbial-targeted medicines, synbiotics, FMT, probiotics, prebiotics, dietary adjustments, and personalized medicine (Logan et al., 2016; Lemme-Dumit et al., 2022). When used to treat IBD, RA, and MS, FMT restores microbiome balance by delivering healthy donor feces into the gastrointestinal tract. Intestinal probiotics aid in the treatment of IBD, RA, allergies, and other gastrointestinal disorders by stimulating the growth of beneficial gut bacteria (Lemme-Dumit et al., 2022; Van De Wiele et al., 2016; Xu et al., 2022) In contrast to prebiotics, which support a healthy gut microbiota and immunological responses that fight inflammation, processed meals, sugar, and bad fats may lead to dysbiosis, which compromises the immune system. Therapeutics that target microorganisms, such as pharmaceutical enzymes, synthetic probiotics, and metabolites produced by microbes, alter immune responses (Corrêa-Oliveira et al., 2016; Shi et al., 2017). Both the gut's beneficial microbes and immunological regulation are improved by synthetic microbes. By manipulating the microbiota to increase immunity to illnesses or drugs, microbiome-based vaccines make use of the microbiome's immune-modulating properties (Takiishi et al., 2017). Organoids are being studied to better understand the immune-microbiome interactions that are unique to each patient and to anticipate successful treatments (Puschhof et al., 2021). Patients suffering from immune system illnesses may find new hope in tailored medications that target the microbiome, which has the potential to transform precision medicine (Levy et al., 2017).

1.11 Future directions in microbiome research

Microbiota research can fully turn healthcare upside down through the application of novel technology, further therapeutic uses, and the unraveling of the complicated relationship between bacteria and our immune system, leading to personalized treatments tailored to the specific needs of each individual (Gotschlich et al., 2019; Kiousi et al., 2023). Future microbiome investigations are set to drastically change the healthcare system as we gain a deeper understanding of host-microbe interactions and apply this knowledge to create personalized, mechanism-based therapies. One of the paths full of promise is the rollout of precision microbiome-based therapies, the use of an individual's microbial profile for the design of tailored, made-to-order probiotics, prebiotics, synbiotics, and diet plans. By combining powerful instruments such as ultra-high-throughput sequencing and multiomics with artificial intelligence and machine learning, we will

Table 1.2 Future directions in microbiome research.

Research area	Focus	Applications	Emerging innovations	Challenges	References
Precision microbiome-based therapies	Personalized probiotics and synthetic microbiomes. Microbiome sequencing for targeted interventions.	Tailored treatments for IBD, metabolic disorders, and mental health. Restore microbial balance through engineered microbial communities.	Engineered microbes designed to produce SCFAs and beneficial metabolites. AI-driven microbiome modeling for individualized therapies.	High interindividual variability in microbiomes. Lack of long-term safety data for engineered microbes.	Mishra et al. (2022), Kiousi et al. (2023)
Gut-brain axis research	Impact of gut microbiome on neuroinflammation. Gut-brain communication via SCFAs and neurotransmitters.	Treatments for Alzheimer's, Parkinson's, MS, depression, and anxiety	Development of psychobiotics for mental health. Novel probiotics targeting the vagus nerve and blood–brain barrier	Limited understanding of gut-brain communication mechanisms. Challenges in delivering probiotics across the BBB.	Chang et al. (2022)
Fecal microbiota transplantation (FMT)	Broader applications beyond infections. Development of synthetic FMT	Treatment for autoimmune diseases, metabolic disorders, and cancer. Safer, standardized FMT methods.	Capsule-based FMT for noninvasive administration. Synthetic microbial consortia to replicate donor microbiomes.	Regulatory hurdles. Risk of pathogen transmission from donors.	Xu et al. (2022), Lemme-Dumit et al. (2022)
Microbiome and cancer	Influence on cancer immunotherapy. Microbial metabolites as potential cancer treatments.	Enhance the efficacy of immune checkpoint inhibitors. Biomarkers for cancer progression and therapy response.	Use of butyrate and SCFA analogs to modulate the tumor microenvironment. Predictive microbiome-based biomarkers.	Complex interactions between gut microbes and cancer therapies. Potential off-target effects of microbiome modulation.	Gopalakrishnan et al. (2018), Li et al. (2019)

(*continued on next page*)

Table 1.2 Future directions in microbiome research—cont'd

Research area	Focus	Applications	Emerging innovations	Challenges	References
Microbiome and metabolic health	Gut microbiota modulation for obesity and diabetes. Role of SCFAs and prebiotics in metabolic regulation.	Improve glucose metabolism, reduce inflammation, and combat metabolic syndrome.	Designer prebiotics targeting specific bacterial pathways. Therapeutic use of novel strains like *Akkermansia muciniphila*.	Difficulties in maintaining stable microbiome changes. Variability in individual dietary responses.	Haase et al. (2018), Nicholson et al. (2012)
Microbiome-immune interactions	Vaccine response modulation. Role in allergies, autoimmunity, and antimicrobial resistance.	Design microbiome-based vaccine adjuvants. Reduce immune dysfunction and chronic inflammation.	Microbiota-informed vaccine development for improved immunization. Engineered probiotics reducing antibiotic resistance.	Lack of standardization in microbiome-immune interaction studies. Risk of unintended immune overactivation.	Di Simone et al. (2023), Sardar et al. (2024)
Diet and microbiome interaction	Personalized nutrition to optimize microbial diversity. Effects of plant-based diets and phytochemicals.	Promote SCFA production, prevent dysbiosis, and improve long-term health.	Microbiome-based diet apps provide personalized dietary recommendations. Functional foods targeting gut health.	Challenges in scaling personalized nutrition approaches. Difficulties in identifying universally beneficial foods.	Mann et al. (2024)
Environmental and early-life influences	Microbiome seeding for cesarean-born infants. Managing antibiotic overuse and urbanization impacts	Restore microbial diversity in early life. Prevent immune dysfunction and chronic diseases.	Vaginal microbiota transfer (VMT) for restoring infant microbiomes. Rewilding strategies to boost environmental microbiota exposure.	Ethical concerns around VMT. Lack of controlled studies on rewilding and microbiome restoration methods.	Dong and Gupta (2019)

(*continued on next page*)

Next-generation probiotics and prebiotics	Novel strains (*Akkermansia muciniphila, Faecalibacterium prausnitzii*). Designer prebiotics and synbiotics.	Enhance beneficial bacteria, promote gut health, and reduce chronic disease risks.	Postbiotics as direct therapeutic agents. Synergistic synbiotics combining probiotics and prebiotics for optimized effects.	Limited understanding of new probiotic strains. Safety concerns for widespread prebiotic use.	
Microbiome in drug development	Pharmacogenomics of microbiome-drug interactions. Microbiota's role in drug metabolism.	Develop microbiome-compatible drugs. Improve drug efficacy and reduce side effects.	Microbiome-responsive drugs targeting microbial metabolism. Identification of microbiota-enhancing chemotherapy outcomes.	Complexity in predicting microbiome-drug interactions. Risk of unanticipated changes in microbiota with drug therapies.	Mimee et al. (2016)

IBD, inflammatory bowel disease; MS, multiple sclerosis; *SCFA*, short-chain fatty acids.

be able to predict the risk of diseases, the response to treatments, and even a person's long-term health prognosis based on the composition and functional role of the microbiome. Microbiome engineering and synthetic biology, two fascinating future areas, will develop probiotics that are capable not only of delivering therapeutic molecules but also of modulating the immune system or resulting in the formation of beneficial substances such as SCFAs (Kashyap et al., 2017; Yaqub et al., 2025; Zhang, 2022). Conventional FMT can be replaced by a synthetic version using genetically modified microbial consortia, thus standardized, which will be able to solve problems of safety, reproducibility, and acceptance by regulatory bodies. These strategies are mainly intended for immune system disorders, metabolic diseases, and cancer treatment. The microbiome-cancer immunotherapy relationship is a very popular research area that will be followed continuously. Determining microbial signatures that reveal how well a patient responds to immune checkpoint inhibitors and other cancer treatments may be the basis for microbiome-derived biomarkers and cotreatments, i.e., treatments that can increase the effectiveness of therapy and decrease its side effects. Furthermore, research on the gut-brain-immune axis may lead to groundbreaking discoveries related to neuroinflammatory and neurodegenerative diseases, which in turn can be a great help in the development of psychobiotics and microbiome-targeted treatments for the nervous system. Despite these technological breakthroughs, major hurdles such as diverse individual responses, potential long-term effects of genetically modified microorganisms, ethical issues, and obtaining uniform regulations are still there. To solve these problems, running more animal/human studies well and collaborating globally will be necessary steps. Overall, the upcoming microbiome investigations are set to change the preventive and therapeutic aspects of medicine radically by combining microbiome studies with immunology, oncology, neuroscience, and personalized healthcare approaches, as illustrated in Table 1.2 (Quiroga-Centeno et al., 2025; Sahle et al., 2024; Yadegar et al., 2024; Yu et al., 2025).

1.12 Conclusion

The microbiota regulates the immune system, metabolism, and neuroinflammation and thus is a major determinant of health. Immune system interactions are essential for the detection and treatment of autoimmune disorders and cancer. To reverse the increasing dysbiosis, the use of probiotics, prebiotics, and FMT becomes necessary. Microbial metabolites influence cytokine production, T-cell polarization, and immune tolerance, thereby providing the microbiome with a direct connection to the immune system. The microbiome contributes to systemic health by strengthening the intestinal epithelium, which is a physical barrier that prevents infections. The susceptibility to infections, mucosal immunity, and chronic inflammation may be aggravated by dysbiosis, which is an imbalance of the microbiome. Recent evidence indicates that the microbiota may modulate immunotherapy, vaccination, and drug metabolism. Certain gut bacteria like *A. muciniphila* and *B. fragilis* make immune checkpoint inhibitors more efficient in cancer therapy by promoting immune surveillance and T-cell activation. Therapeutic solutions should be geared toward altering the microbiome because a disturbed microbiota can lead to a reduced therapy response. Therapies centering around the microbiome are redefining modern medicine. The combination of FMT with prebiotics and probiotics could be one of the ways to bring back a normal microbiota. In addition to its efficacy in treating chronic *C. difficile* infections, FMT has shown promise in the management of inflammatory, immunological, and neuropsychiatric disorders. Accelerated microbiome research and new information on microbial communities have resulted from recent advances in single-cell sequencing, metabolomics, and metagenomics. Individualized treatment based on genetic and microbiome profiles is made possible by improving microbiome prediction using AI and ML. Potentially revolutionizing cancer therapy and autoimmune disease prevention, the microbiome is reshaping the healthcare industry. By harnessing the power of the microbiome, we can enhance health, quality of life, and the treatment of complex illnesses.

References

Abeles, S. R., & Pride, D. T. (2014). Molecular bases and role of viruses in the human microbiome. *Journal of Molecular Biology, 426*(23), 3892–3906. https://doi.org/10.1016/j.jmb.2014.07.002.

Afshar, M., & Gallo, R. L. (2013). Innate immune defense system of the skin. *Veterinary Dermatology, 24*(1), 32. https://doi.org/10.1111/j.13653164.2012.01082.x.

Akhand, A. A., & Ahsan, N. (2023). *Cells and organs of the immune system immunology for dentistry* (pp. 1–12). Wiley. https://doi.org/10.1002/9781119893035.ch1.

Alexander, K. L., Targan, S. R., & Elson, C. O. (2014). Microbiota activation and regulation of innate and adaptive immunity. *Immunological Reviews, 260*(1), 206–220. https://doi.org/10.1111/imr.12180.

Ali, S., Hamayun, M., Siraj, M., Khan, S. A., Kim, H. o-Y., & Lee, B. (2025). Recent advances in prebiotics: Classification, mechanisms, and health applications. *Future Foods, 12*, 100680. https://doi.org/10.1016/j.fufo.2025.100680.

Anwar, H., Irfan, S., Hussain, G., Naeem Faisal, M., Muzaffar, H., Mustafa, I., Mukhtar, I., Malik, S., & Ullah, M. I. (2020). *Gut microbiome: A new organ system in body*. IntechOpen https://doi.org/10.5772/intechopen.89634.

Belizário, J., Faintuch, J., & Garay-Malpartida, M. (2018). Gut microbiome dysbiosis and immunometabolism: New frontiers for treatment of metabolic diseases. *Mediators of Inflammation, 2018*, 1–12. https://doi.org/10.1155/2018/2037838.

Bellais, S., Nehlich, M. é, Ania, M., Duquenoy, A., Mazier, W., van den Engh, G., Baijer, J., Simone Treichel, N., Clavel, T., Belotserkovsky, I., & Thomas, V. (2022). Species-targeted sorting and cultivation of commensal bacteria from the gut microbiome using flow cytometry under anaerobic conditions. *Microbiome, 10*(1). https://doi.org/10.1186/s40168-021-01206-7.

Bertolini, M., & Dongari-Bagtzoglou, A. (2019). The relationship of *Candida albicans* with the oral bacterial microbiome in health and disease. *Advances in Experimental Medicine and Biology, 1197*, 69–78. https://doi.org/10.1007/978-3-030-28524-1_6.

Bhol, N. K., Bhanjadeo, M. M., Singh, A. K., Dash, U. C., Ojha, R. R., Majhi, S., Duttaroy, A. K., & Jena, A. B. (2024). The interplay between cytokines, inflammation, and antioxidants: Mechanistic insights and therapeutic potentials of various antioxidants and anti-cytokine compounds. *Biomedicine and Pharmacotherapy, 178*. https://doi.org/10.1016/j.biopha.2024.117177.

Bhutta, N. K., Xu, X., Jian, C., Wang, Y., Liu, Y., Sun, J., Han, B., Wu, S., & Javeed, A. (2024). Gut microbiota mediated T cells regulation and autoimmune diseases. *Frontiers in Microbiology, 15*. https://doi.org/10.3389/fmicb.2024.1477187.

Chang, L., Wei, Y., & Hashimoto, K. (2022). Brain–gut–microbiota axis in depression: A historical overview and future directions. *Brain Research Bulletin, 182*, 44–56. https://doi.org/10.1016/j.brainresbull.2022.02.004.

Chen, Y., Fang, Y., Lyu, Z., Tian, Y., Niu, S., Li, Y. R., & Yang, L. (2026). Microbiome modulation of tumorigenesis and immune responses. *Journal of Biomedical Science, 33*(1). https://doi.org/10.1186/s12929-025-01208-9.

Choudhry, H. (2021). The microbiome and its implications in cancer immunotherapy. *Molecules, 26*(1), 206. https://doi.org/10.3390/molecules26010206.

Christina, B., Poongkuzhali, S., Muninathan, N., Bhaskaran, K., & Suresh, A. (2025). The mechanisms and therapeutic potential of the microbiome-immune interface in cancer. *Discover Biotechnology, 2*(1). https://doi.org/10.1007/s44340-025-00031-0.

Christovich, A., Luo, X. M., & Microbiota, G. (2022). Leaky gut, and autoimmune diseases. *Frontiers in Immunology, 13*. https://doi.org/10.3389/fimmu.2022.946248.

Corrêa-Oliveira, R., Fachi, J. L., Vieira, A., Sato, F. T., & Vinolo, M. A. R. (2016). Regulation of immune cell function by short-chain fatty acids. *Clinical and Translational Immunology, 5*(4). https://doi.org/10.1038/cti.2016.17.

Dahiya, D., & Nigam, P. S. (2023). Biotherapy using probiotics as therapeutic agents to restore the gut microbiota to relieve gastrointestinal tract inflammation, IBD, IBS and prevent induction of cancer. *International Journal of Molecular Sciences, 24*(6), 5748. https://doi.org/10.3390/ijms24065748.

Dakal, T. C., Xu, C., & Kumar, A. (2025). Advanced computational tools, artificial intelligence and machine-learning approaches in gut microbiota and biomarker identification. *Frontiers in Medical Technology, 6*. https://doi.org/10.3389/fmedt.2024.1434799.

Davar, D., & Zarour, H. M. (2022). Facts and hopes for gut microbiota interventions in cancer immunotherapy. *Clinical Cancer Research, 28*(20), 4370–4384. https://doi.org/10.1158/1078-0432.CCR-21-1129.

De Luca, F., & Shoenfeld, Y. (2019). The microbiome in autoimmune diseases. *Clinical and Experimental Immunology, 195*(1), 74–85. https://doi.org/10.1111/cei.13158.

Di Simone, S. K., Rudloff, I., Nold-Petry, C. A., Forster, S. C., & Nold, M. F. (2023). Understanding respiratory microbiome–immune system interactions in health and disease. *Science Translational Medicine, 15*(678). https://doi.org/10.1126/scitranslmed.abq5126.

Dong, T. S., & Gupta, A. (2019). Influence of early life, diet, and the environment on the microbiome. *Clinical Gastroenterology and Hepatology, 17*(2), 231–242. https://doi.org/10.1016/j.cgh.2018.08.067.

Duan, H., Wang, L., Huangfu, M., & Li, H. (2023). The impact of microbiota-derived short-chain fatty acids on macrophage activities in disease: Mechanisms and therapeutic potentials. *Biomedicine & Pharmacotherapy, 165*, 115276. https://doi.org/10.1016/j.biopha.2023.115276.

Duan, H., Xu, B., Luo, P., Chen, T., & Zou, J. (2025). Microbial metabolites and their influence on the tumor microenvironment. *Frontiers in Immunology, 16*. https://doi.org/10.3389/fimmu.2025.1675677.

Faith, J. J., Rey, F. E., O'Donnell, D., Karlsson, M., McNulty, N. P., Kallstrom, G., Goodman, A. L., & Gordon, J. I. (2010). Creating and characterizing communities of human gut microbes in gnotobiotic mice. *ISME Journal, 4*(9), 1094–1098. https://doi.org/10.1038/ismej.2010.110.

Fessler, J., Matson, V., & Gajewski, T. F. (2019). Exploring the emerging role of the microbiome in cancer immunotherapy. *Journal for ImmunoTherapy of Cancer, 7*(1). https://doi.org/10.1186/s40425-019-0574-4.

Franzosa, E. A., Morgan, X. C., Segata, N., Waldron, L., Reyes, J., Earl, A. M., Giannoukos, G., Boylan, M. R., Ciulla, D., Gevers, D., Izard, J., Garrett, W. S., Chan, A. T., & Huttenhower, C. (2014). Relating the metatranscriptome and metagenome of the human gut. *Proceedings of the National Academy of Sciences, 111*(22). https://doi.org/10.1073/pnas.1319284111.

Gao, J., Xu, K., Liu, H., Liu, G., Bai, M., Peng, C., Li, T., & Yin, Y. (2018). Impact of the gut microbiota on intestinal immunity mediated by tryptophan metabolism. *Frontiers in Cellular and Infection Microbiology, 8*. https://doi.org/10.3389/fcimb.2018.00013.

Gilbert, J. A., Blaser, M. J., Caporaso, J. G., Jansson, J. K., Lynch, S. V., & Knight, R. (2018). Current understanding of the human microbiome. *Nature Medicine, 24*(4), 392–400. https://doi.org/10.1038/nm.4517.

Gonçalves, P., Araújo, J. R., & Di Santo, J. P. (2018). A cross-talk between microbiota-derived short-chain fatty acids and the host mucosal immune system regulates intestinal homeostasis and inflammatory bowel disease. *Inflammatory Bowel Diseases, 24*(3), 558–572. https://doi.org/10.1093/ibd/izx029.

González, S., González-Rodríguez, A. P., López-Soto, A., Huergo-Zapico, L., López-Larrea, C., & Suárez-Álvarez, B. (2014). Conceptual aspects of self and nonself discrimination. *Self/Nonself, 2*(1), 19–25. https://doi.org/10.4161/self.2.1.15094.

Gopalakrishnan, V., Helmink, B. A., Spencer, C. N., Reuben, A., & Wargo, J. A. (2018). The influence of the gut microbiome on cancer, immunity, and cancer immunotherapy. *Cancer Cell, 33*(4), 570–580. https://doi.org/10.1016/j.ccell.2018.03.015.

Gotschlich, E. C., Colbert, R. A., & Gill, T. (2019). Methods in microbiome research: Past, present, and future. *Best Practice & Research Clinical Rheumatology, 33*(6), 101498. https://doi.org/10.1016/j.berh.2020.101498.

Gray, J., Oehrle, K., Worthen, G., Alenghat, T., Whitsett, J., & Deshmukh, H. (2017). Intestinal commensal bacteria mediate lung mucosal immunity and promote resistance of newborn mice to infection. *Science Translational Medicine, 9*(376). https://doi.org/10.1126/scitranslmed.aaf9412.

Haase, S., Haghikia, A., Wilck, N., Müller, D. N., & Linker, R. A. (2018). Impacts of microbiome metabolites on immune regulation and autoimmunity. *Immunology, 154*(2), 230–238. https://doi.org/10.1111/imm.12933.

Han, Q., Li, J., Li, Z., Aishajiang, R., & Yu, D. (2025). Novel therapeutic strategies and recent advances in gut microbiota synergy with nanotechnology for colorectal cancer treatment. *Materials Today Bio, 31*, 101601. https://doi.org/10.1016/j.mtbio.2025.101601.

Heilbronner, S., Krismer, B., Brötz-Oesterhelt, H., & Peschel, A. (2021). The microbiome-shaping roles of bacteriocins. *Nature Reviews Microbiology, 19*(11), 726–739. https://doi.org/10.1038/s41579-021-00569-w.

Hooper, L. V., Littman, D. R., & Macpherson, A. J. (2012). Interactions between the microbiota and the immune system. *Science, 336*(6086), 1268–1273. https://doi.org/10.1126/science.1223490.

Hou, K., Wu, Z. X., Chen, X. Y., Wang, J. Q., Zhang, D., Xiao, C., Zhu, D., Koya, J. B., Wei, L., Li, J., & Chen, Z. S. (2022). Microbiota in health and diseases. *Signal Transduction and Targeted Therapy, 7*(1). https://doi.org/10.1038/s41392-022-00974-4.

Hsieh, S. A., & Allen, P. M. (2020). Immunomodulatory roles of polysaccharide capsules in the intestine. *Frontiers in Immunology, 11*. https://doi.org/10.3389/fimmu.2020.00690.

Hughes, C. E., Benson, R. A., Bedaj, M., & Maffia, P. (2016). Antigen-presenting cells and antigen presentation in tertiary lymphoid organs. *Frontiers in Immunology, 7*. https://doi.org/10.3389/fimmu.2016.00481.

Jovel, J., Nimaga, A., Jordan, T., O'Keefe, S., Patterson, J., Thiesen, A., Hotte, N., Bording-Jorgensen, M., Subedi, S., Hamilton, J., Carpenter, E. J., Lauga, B. é, Elahi, S., Madsen, K. L., Wong, G. K. a-S., & Mason, A. L. (2022). Metagenomics versus metatranscriptomics of the murine gut microbiome for assessing microbial metabolism during inflammation. *Frontiers in Microbiology, 13*. https://doi.org/10.3389/fmicb.2022.829378.

Juarez, V. M., Montalbine, A. N., & Singh, A. (2022). Microbiome as an immune regulator in health, disease, and therapeutics. *Advanced Drug Delivery Reviews, 188*, 114400. https://doi.org/10.1016/j.addr.2022.114400.

Kapoor, B., Gulati, M., Rani, P., & Gupta, R. (2022). Psoriasis: Interplay between dysbiosis and host immune system. *Autoimmunity Reviews, 21*(11), 103169. https://doi.org/10.1016/j.autrev.2022.103169.

Kashyap, P. C., Chia, N., Nelson, H., Segal, E., & Elinav, E. (2017). Microbiome at the frontier of personalized medicine. *Mayo Clinic Proceedings, 92*(12), 1855–1864. https://doi.org/10.1016/j.mayocp.2017.10.004.

Katz-Agranov, N., & Zandman-Goddard, G. (2017). The microbiome and systemic lupus erythematosus. *Immunologic Research, 65*(2), 432–437. https://doi.org/10.1007/s12026-017-8906-2.

Kazemian, N., Mahmoudi, M., Halperin, F., Wu, J. C., & Pakpour, S. (2020). Gut microbiota and cardiovascular disease: Opportunities and challenges. *Microbiome, 8*(1). https://doi.org/10.1186/s40168-020-00821-0.

Kazemifard, N., & Dehkohneh, A. (2022). Shaghayegh Baradaran Ghavami, Probiotics and probiotic-based vaccines: A novel approach for improving vaccine efficacy. *Frontiers in Medicine, 9*. https://doi.org/10.3389/fmed.2022.940454.

Kinashi, Y., & Hase, K. (2021). Partners in Leaky Gut syndrome: Intestinal dysbiosis and autoimmunity. *Frontiers in Immunology, 12*. https://doi.org/10.3389/fimmu.2021.673708.

Kiousi, D. E., Kouroutzidou, A. Z., Neanidis, K., Karavanis, E., Matthaios, D., Pappa, A., & Galanis, A. (2023). The role of the gut microbiome in cancer immunotherapy: Current knowledge and future directions. *Cancers, 15*(7), 2101. https://doi.org/10.3390/cancers15072101.

Kogut, M. H., Lee, A., & Santin, E. (2020). Microbiome and pathogen interaction with the immune system. *Poultry Science, 99*(4), 1906–1913. https://doi.org/10.1016/j.psj.2019.12.011.

Kushkevych, I., Dvořáková, M., Dordevic, D., Futoma-Kołoch, B., Gajdács, M., Al-Madboly, L. A., & El-Salam, M. A. (2025). Advances in gut microbiota functions in inflammatory bowel disease: Dysbiosis, management, cytotoxicity assessment, and therapeutic perspectives. *Computational and Structural Biotechnology Journal, 27*, 851–868. https://doi.org/10.1016/j.csbj.2025.02.026.

Lal, S., Kandiyal, B., Ahuja, V., Takeda, K., & Das, B. (2022). In *Gut microbiome dysbiosis in inflammatory bowel disease: 192* (pp. 179–204). Elsevier BV. https://doi.org/10.1016/bs.pmbts.2022.09.003.

Latif, A., Shehzad, A., Niazi, S., Zahid, A., Ashraf, W., Iqbal, M. W., Rehman, A., Riaz, T., Aadil, R. M., Khan, I. M., Özogul, F., Rocha, J. M., Esatbeyoglu, T., & Korma, S. A. (2023). Probiotics: Mechanism of action, health benefits and their application in food industries. *Frontiers in Microbiology, 14*. https://doi.org/10.3389/fmicb.2023.1216674.

Lee, J. H., Shin, S. J., Lee, J. H., Knowles, J. C., Lee, H. H., & Kim, H. W. (2024). Adaptive immunity of materials: Implications for tissue healing and regeneration. *Bioactive Materials, 41*, 499–522. https://doi.org/10.1016/j.bioactmat.2024.07.027.

Lei, W., Zhou, K., Lei, Y., Li, Q., & Zhu, H. (2025). Gut microbiota shapes cancer immunotherapy responses. *npj Biofilms and Microbiomes, 11*(1). https://doi.org/10.1038/s41522-025-00786-8.

Lemme-Dumit, J. M., Song, Y., Lwin, H. W., Hernandez-Chavez, C., Sundararajan, S., Viscardi, R. M., Ravel, J., Pasetti, M. F., & Ma, B. (2022). Altered gut microbiome and fecal immune phenotype in early preterm infants with leaky gut. *Frontiers in Immunology, 13*. https://doi.org/10.3389/fimmu.2022.815046.

Levy, M., Kolodziejczyk, A. A., Thaiss, C. A., & Elinav, E. (2017). Dysbiosis and the immune system. *Nature Reviews Immunology, 17*(4), 219–232. https://doi.org/10.1038/nri.2017.7.

Li, W., Deng, Y., Chu, Q., & Zhang, P. (2019). Gut microbiome and cancer immunotherapy. *Cancer Letters, 447*, 41–47. https://doi.org/10.1016/j.canlet.2019.01.015.

Li, X., Liu, L., Cao, Z., Li, W., Li, H., Lu, C., Yang, X., & Liu, Y. (2020). Gut microbiota as an "invisible organ" that modulates the function of drugs. *Biomedicine & Pharmacotherapy, 121*, 109653. https://doi.org/10.1016/j.biopha.2019.109653.

Lin, L., & Zhang, J. (2017). Role of intestinal microbiota and metabolites on gut homeostasis and human diseases. *BMC Immunology, 18*(1). https://doi.org/10.1186/s12865-016-0187-3.

Liu, Y., Li, X., Chen, Y., Yao, Q., Zhou, J., Wang, X., Meng, Q., Ji, J., Yu, Z., & Chen, X. (2025). Fecal microbiota transplantation: Application scenarios, efficacy prediction, and factors impacting donor-recipient interplay. *Frontiers in Microbiology, 16*. https://doi.org/10.3389/fmicb.2025.1556827.

Logan, A. C., Jacka, F. N., & Prescott, S. L. (2016). Immune-microbiota interactions: Dysbiosis as a global health issue. *Current Allergy and Asthma Reports, 16*(2), 1–9. https://doi.org/10.1007/s11882-015-0590-5.

Lu, J., Zhang, W., He, Y., Jiang, M., Liu, Z., Zhang, J., Zheng, L., Zhou, B., Luo, J., He, C., Shan, Y., Zhang, R., Fan, K. L., Fang, B., & Wan, C. (2025). Multi-omics decodes host-specific and environmental microbiome interactions in sepsis. *Frontiers in Microbiology, 16*. https://doi.org/10.3389/fmicb.2025.1618177.

Luo, W., Li, R., Pan, C., & Luo, C. (2025). Gut microbiota–derived metabolites in immunomodulation and gastrointestinal cancer immunotherapy. *Frontiers in Immunology, 16*. https://doi.org/10.3389/fimmu.2025.1710880.

Luu, M., & Visekruna, A. (2019). Short-chain fatty acids: Bacterial messengers modulating the immunometabolism of T cells. *European Journal of Immunology, 49*(6), 842–848. https://doi.org/10.1002/eji.201848009.

Luu, M., Weigand, K., Wedi, F., Breidenbend, C., Leister, H., Pautz, S., Adhikary, T., & Visekruna, A. (2018). Regulation of the effector function of CD8+ T cells by gut microbiota-derived metabolite butyrate. *Scientific Reports, 8*(1). https://doi.org/10.1038/s41598-018-32860-x.

Ma, Z., Zuo, T., Frey, N., & Rangrez, A. Y. (2024). A systematic framework for understanding the microbiome in human health and disease: From basic principles to clinical translation. *Signal Transduction and Targeted Therapy, 9*(1). https://doi.org/10.1038/s41392-024-01946-6.

Madan, A., Ashique, S., Arora, D., Kumar Satapathy, M., & Gupta, S. (2025). *Tissue engineering paradigms stem cell therapeutics* (pp. 541–573). Wiley. https://doi.org/10.1002/9781394313785.ch12.

Mann, E. R., Lam, Y. K., & Uhlig, H. H. (2024). Short-chain fatty acids: Linking diet, the microbiome and immunity. *Nature Reviews Immunology, 24*(8), 577–595. https://doi.org/10.1038/s41577-024-01014-8.

Matsuoka, K., & Kanai, T. (2015). The gut microbiota and inflammatory bowel disease. *Seminars in Immunopathology, 37*(1), 47–55. https://doi.org/10.1007/s00281-014-0454-4.

Mayassi, T., Li, C., Segerstolpe, Å., Brown, E. M., Weisberg, R., Nakata, T., Yano, H., Herbst, P., Artis, D., Graham, D. B., & Xavier, R. J. (2024). Spatially restricted immune and microbiota-driven adaptation of the gut. *Nature, 636*(8042), 447–456. https://doi.org/10.1038/s41586-024-08216-z.

Mazziotta, C., Tognon, M., Martini, F., Torreggiani, E., & Rotondo, J. C. (2023). Probiotics mechanism of action on immune cells and beneficial effects on human health. *Cells., 12*(1), 184. https://doi.org/10.3390/cells12010184.

Meiners, F., Ortega-Matienzo, A., Fuellen, G., & Barrantes, I. (2025). Gut microbiome-mediated health effects of fiber and polyphenol-rich dietary interventions. *Frontiers in Nutrition, 12*. https://doi.org/10.3389/fnut.2025.1647740.

Menees, K. B., Otero, B. A., & Tansey, M. G. (2022). Microbiome influences on neuro-immune interactions in neurodegenerative disease. *International Review of Neurobiology, 167*, 25–57. https://doi.org/10.1016/bs.irn.2022.07.006.

Mimee, M., Citorik, R. J., & Lu, T. K. (2016). Microbiome therapeutics — Advances and challenges. *Advanced Drug Delivery Reviews, 105*, 44–54. https://doi.org/10.1016/j.addr.2016.04.032.

Mishra, J., Stubbs, M., Kuang, L., Vara, N., Kumar, P., Kumar, N., & Subramanian, V. S. (2022). Inflammatory bowel disease therapeutics: A focus on probiotic engineering. *Mediators of Inflammation, 2022*, 1–15. https://doi.org/10.1155/2022/9621668.

Mousa, W. K., Chehadeh, F., & Husband, S. (2022). Microbial dysbiosis in the gut drives systemic autoimmune diseases. *Frontiers in Immunology, 13*. https://doi.org/10.3389/fimmu.2022.906258.

Moysidou, C. M., & Owens, R. M. (2021). Advances in modelling the human microbiome-gut-brain axis in vitro. *Biochemical Society Transactions, 49*(1), 187–201. https://doi.org/10.1042/BST20200338.

Nazir, A., Hussain, F. H. N., Nadeem Hussain, T. H., Al Dweik, R., & Raza, A. (2025). Therapeutic targeting of the host-microbiota-immune axis: Implications for precision health. *Frontiers in Immunology, 16*. https://doi.org/10.3389/fimmu.2025.1570233.

Negi, S., Das, D. K., Pahari, S., Nadeem, S., & Agrewala, J. N. (2019). Potential role of gut microbiota in induction and regulation of innate immune memory. *Frontiers in Immunology, 10*. https://doi.org/10.3389/fimmu.2019.02441.

Nicholson, J. K., Holmes, E., Kinross, J., Burcelin, R., Gibson, G., Jia, W., & Pettersson, S. (2012). Host-gut microbiota metabolic interactions. *Science, 336*(6086), 1262–1267. https://doi.org/10.1126/science.1223813.

Oyovwi, M. O., & Ajayi, A. F. (2025). A comprehensive review on immunological mechanisms and gut-brain pathways linking gut health and neurological disorders. *Discover Medicine, 2*(1). https://doi.org/10.1007/s44337-025-00495-3.

Pascal, M., Perez-Gordo, M., Caballero, T., Escribese, M. M., Longo, M. N. L., Luengo, O., Manso, L., Matheu, V., Seoane, E., Zamorano, M., Labrador, M. és, & Mayorga, C. (2018). Microbiome and allergic diseases. *Frontiers in Immunology, 9*. https://doi.org/10.3389/fimmu.2018.01584.

Patridge, E., Gorakshakar, A., Molusky, M. M., Ogundijo, O., Janevski, A., Julian, C., Hu, L., Vuyisich, M., & Banavar, G. (2024). Microbial functional pathways based on metatranscriptomic profiling enable effective saliva-based health assessments for precision wellness. *Computational and Structural Biotechnology Journal, 23*, 834–842. https://doi.org/10.1016/j.csbj.2024.01.018.

Paun, A., Yau, C., & Danska, J. S. (2016). Immune recognition and response to the intestinal microbiome in type 1 diabetes. *Journal of Autoimmunity, 71*, 10–18. https://doi.org/10.1016/j.jaut.2016.02.004.

Peñalver Bernabé, B., Cralle, L., & Gilbert, J. A. (2018). Systems biology of the human microbiome. *Current Opinion in Biotechnology, 51*, 146–153. https://doi.org/10.1016/j.copbio.2018.01.018.

Petersen, C., & Round, J. L. (2014). Defining dysbiosis and its influence on host immunity and disease. *Cellular Microbiology, 16*(7), 1024–1033. https://doi.org/10.1111/cmi.12308.

Pham, V. T., Dold, S., Rehman, A., Bird, J. K., & Steinert, R. E. (2021). Vitamins, the gut microbiome and gastrointestinal health in humans. *Nutrition Research, 95*, 35–53. https://doi.org/10.1016/j.nutres.2021.09.001.

Puschhof, J., Pleguezuelos-Manzano, C., & Clevers, H. (2021). Organoids and organs-on-chips: Insights into human gut-microbe interactions. *Cell Host & Microbe, 29*(6), 867–878. https://doi.org/10.1016/j.chom.2021.04.002.

Qin, J., Li, R., Raes, J., Arumugam, M., Burgdorf, K. S., Manichanh, C., Nielsen, T., Pons, N., Levenez, F., Yamada, T., Mende, D. R., Li, J., Xu, J., Li, S., Li, D., Cao, J., Wang, B., Liang, H., Zheng, H., … Zoetendal, E. (2010). A human gut microbial gene catalogue established by metagenomic sequencing. *Nature, 464*(7285), 59–65. https://doi.org/10.1038/nature08821.

Qing, F., Xie, T., Xie, L., Guo, T., & Liu, Z. (2022). How gut microbiota are shaped by pattern recognition receptors in colitis and colorectal cancer. *Cancers, 14*(15), 3821. https://doi.org/10.3390/cancers14153821.

Quiroga-Centeno, A. C., Atanasova, K., Ebert, M. P., Thomann, A. K., & Reindl, W. (2025). Emerging microbiome-directed therapies in inflammatory bowel disease: Beyond diet modification and FMT. *Seminars in Immunopathology, 47*(1). https://doi.org/10.1007/s00281-025-01066-5.

Rasouli-Saravani, A., Jahankhani, K., Moradi, S., Gorgani, M., Shafaghat, Z., Mirsanei, Z., Mehmandar, A., & Mirzaei, R. (2023). Role of microbiota short-chain fatty acids in the pathogenesis of autoimmune diseases. *Biomedicine & Pharmacotherapy, 162*, 114620. https://doi.org/10.1016/j.biopha.2023.114620.

Ratajczak, W., Rył, A., Mizerski, A., Walczakiewicz, K., Sipak, O., & Laszczyńska, M. (2019). Immunomodulatory potential of gut microbiome-derived short chain fatty acids (SCFAs). *Acta Biochimica Polonica, 66*(1), 1–12. https://doi.org/10.18388/abp.2018_2648.

Riiser, A. (2015). The human microbiome, asthma, and allergy. *Allergy, Asthma & Clinical Immunology, 11*(1). https://doi.org/10.1186/s13223-015-0102-0.

Rocamora-Reverte, L., Melzer, F. L., Würzner, R., & Weinberger, B. (2021). The complex role of regulatory T cells in immunity and aging. *Frontiers in Immunology, 11*. https://doi.org/10.3389/fimmu.2020.616949.

Rondinella, D., Margarita, E., Raoul, P. C., Galli, F. S., Severino, A., Porcari, S., Mele, M. C., Gasbarrini, A., Cammarota, G., Rinninella, E., & Ianiro, G. (2026). The impact of diet on gut microbiome composition: Implications for immune-mediated diseases. *Clinical Immunology Communications, 9*, 1–11. https://doi.org/10.1016/j.clicom.2025.12.001.

Roviello, G., Francesco Iannone, L., Bersanelli, M., Mini, E., & Catalano, M. (2022). The gut microbiome and efficacy of cancer immunotherapy. *Pharmacology & Therapeutics, 231*, 107973. https://doi.org/10.1016/j.pharmthera.2021.107973.

Russo, E., Taddei, A., Ringressi, M. N., Ricci, F., & Amedei, A. (2016). The interplay between the microbiome and the adaptive immune response in cancer development. *Therapeutic Advances in Gastroenterology, 9*(4), 594–605. https://doi.org/10.1177/1756283X16635082.

Sahle, Z., Engidaye, G., Shenkute Gebreyes, D., Adenew, B., & Abebe, T. A. (2024). Fecal microbiota transplantation and next-generation therapies: A review on targeting dysbiosis in metabolic disorders and beyond. *SAGE Open Medicine, 12*. https://doi.org/10.1177/20503121241257486.

Santa, K. (2023). *Macrophages: Phagocytosis, antigen presentation, and activation of immunity*. IntechOpen https://doi.org/10.5772/intechopen.110832.

Sardar, P., Almeida, A., & Pedicord, V. A. (2024). Integrating functional metagenomics to decipher microbiome–immune interactions. *Immunology and Cell Biology, 102*(8), 680–691. https://doi.org/10.1111/imcb.12798.

Schwarz, A., Bruhs, A., & Schwarz, T. (2017). The short-chain fatty acid sodium butyrate functions as a regulator of the skin immune system. *Journal of Investigative Dermatology, 137*(4), 855–864. https://doi.org/10.1016/j.jid.2016.11.014.

Şenel, S. (2021). An overview of physical, microbiological and immune barriers of oral mucosa. *International Journal of Molecular Sciences, 22*(15), 7821. https://doi.org/10.3390/ijms22157821.

Seo, H., Kim, S., Beck, S., & Song, H. o-Y. (2024). Perspectives on microbiome therapeutics in infectious diseases: A comprehensive approach beyond immunology and microbiology. *Cells, 13*(23), 2003. https://doi.org/10.3390/cells13232003.

Sepich-Poore, G. D., Zitvogel, L., Straussman, R., Hasty, J., Wargo, J. A., & Knight, R. (2021). The microbiome and human cancer. *Science, 371*(6536). https://doi.org/10.1126/science.abc4552.

Shelkey, E., Oommen, D., Stirling, E. R., Soto-Pantoja, D. R., Cook, K. L., Lu, Y., Votanopoulos, K. I., & Soker, S. (2022). Immuno-reactive cancer organoid model to assess effects of the microbiome on cancer immunotherapy. *Scientific Reports, 12*(1). https://doi.org/10.1038/s41598-022-13930-7.

Shen, Y., Fan, N., Ma, S.-X., Cheng, X., Yang, X., & Wang, G. (2025). Gut microbiota dysbiosis: Pathogenesis, diseases, prevention, and therapy. *MedComm., 6*(5). https://doi.org/10.1002/mco2.70168.

Shi, N., Li, N., Duan, X., & Niu, H. (2017). Interaction between the gut microbiome and mucosal immune system. *Military Medical Research, 4*(1). https://doi.org/10.1186/s40779-017-0122-9.

Simon, E., Călinoiu, L. F., Mitrea, L., & Vodnar, D. C. (2021). Probiotics, prebiotics, and synbiotics: Implications and beneficial effects against irritable bowel syndrome. *Nutrients, 13*(6), 2112. https://doi.org/10.3390/nu13062112.

Stubbington, M. J. T., Rozenblatt-Rosen, O., Regev, A., & Teichmann, S. A. (2017). Single-cell transcriptomics to explore the immune system in health and disease. *Science, 358*(6359), 58–63. https://doi.org/10.1126/science.aan6828.

Suchitra, M. R. (2024). Fecal microbiota transplantation: A revolutionary approach to treating gut-related disorders. *SBV Journal of Basic, Clinical and Applied Health Science, 7*(3), 131–134. https://doi.org/10.4103/sbvj.sbvj_48_24.

Takeuchi, O., & Akira, S. (2010). Pattern recognition receptors and inflammation. *Cell., 140*(6), 805–820. https://doi.org/10.1016/j.cell.2010.01.022.

Takiishi, T., Fenero, C. I. M., & Câmara, N. O. S. (2017). Intestinal barrier and gut microbiota: Shaping our immune responses throughout life. *Tissue Barriers, 5*(4), e1373208. https://doi.org/10.1080/21688370.2017.1373208.

Tang, M. H., Ligthart, I., Varga, S., Lebeer, S., van Overveld, F. J., & Rijkers, G. T. (2025). Mutual interactions between microbiota and the human immune system during the first 1000 days of life. *Biology, 14*(3). https://doi.org/10.3390/biology14030299.

Thaiss, C. A., Zmora, N., Levy, M., & Elinav, E. (2016). The microbiome and innate immunity. *Nature, 535*(7610), 65–74. https://doi.org/10.1038/nature18847.

Turnbaugh, P. J., Ley, R. E., Hamady, M., Fraser-Liggett, C. M., Knight, R., & Gordon, J. I. (2007). The human microbiome project. *Nature, 449*(7164), 804–810. https://doi.org/10.1038/nature06244.

Ullah, H., Arbab, S., Tian, Y., Chen, Y., Liu, C., Li, Q., & Li, K. (2024). Crosstalk between gut microbiota and host immune system and its response to traumatic injury. *Frontiers in Immunology, 15*. https://doi.org/10.3389/fimmu.2024.1413485.

Van De Wiele, T., Van Praet, J. T., Marzorati, M., Drennan, M. B., & Elewaut, D. (2016). How the microbiota shapes rheumatic diseases. *Nature Reviews Rheumatology, 12*(7), 398–411. https://doi.org/10.1038/nrrheum.2016.85.

Vegh, P., & Haniffa, M. (2018). The impact of single-cell RNA sequencing on understanding the functional organization of the immune system. *Briefings in Functional Genomics, 17*(4), 265–272. https://doi.org/10.1093/bfgp/ely003.

Venegas, D. P., De la Fuente, M. K., Landskron, G., González, M., Quera, R., Dijkstra, G., Harmsen, H. J. M., Faber, K. N., & Hermoso, M. A. (2019). Short chain fatty acids (SCFAs)-mediated gut epithelial and immune regulation and its relevance for inflammatory bowel diseases. *Frontiers in Immunology, 10*. https://doi.org/10.3389/fimmu.2019.00277.

Volmer, J. G., McRae, H., & Morrison, M. (2023). The evolving role of methanogenic archaea in mammalian microbiomes. *Frontiers in Microbiology, 14*. https://doi.org/10.3389/fmicb.2023.1268451.

Wang, Q., Meng, Q., Chen, Y., Liu, Y., Li, X., Zhou, J., Ma, Y., Yu, Z., & Chen, X. (2025). Interaction between gut microbiota and immunity in health and intestinal disease. *Frontiers in Immunology, 16*. https://doi.org/10.3389/fimmu.2025.1673852.

Wang, R., Lan, C., Benlagha, K., Camara, N. O. S., Miller, H., Kubo, M., Heegaard, S., Lee, P., Yang, L., Forsman, H., Li, X., Zhai, Z., & Liu, C. (2024a). The interaction of innate immune and adaptive immune system. *MedComm, 5*(10). https://doi.org/10.1002/mco2.714.

Wang, X., Peng, J., Cai, P., Xia, Y., Yi, C., Shang, A., Atim Akanyibah, F., & Mao, F. (2024b). The emerging role of the gut microbiota and its application in inflammatory bowel disease. *Biomedicine & Pharmacotherapy, 179*, 117302. https://doi.org/10.1016/j.biopha.2024.117302.

Weiner, H. L. (2025). Immune mechanisms and shared immune targets in neurodegenerative diseases. *Nature Reviews Neurology, 21*(2), 67–85. https://doi.org/10.1038/s41582-024-01046-7.

Wicherska-Pawłowska, K., Wróbel, T., & Rybka, J. (2021). Toll-like receptors (TLRs), NOD-like receptors (NLRs), and RIG-I-like receptors (RLRs) in innate immunity. TLRs, NLRs, and RLRs ligands as immunotherapeutic agents for hematopoietic diseases. *International Journal of Molecular Sciences, 22*(24), 13397. https://doi.org/10.3390/ijms222413397.

Wiertsema, S. P., van Bergenhenegouwen, J., Garssen, J., & Knippels, L. M. J. (2021). The interplay between the gut microbiome and the immune system in the context of infectious diseases throughout life and the role of nutrition in optimizing treatment strategies. *Nutrients, 13*(3), 1–14. https://doi.org/10.3390/nu13030886.

Wu, H. J., & Wu, E. (2012). The role of gut microbiota in immune homeostasis and autoimmunity. *Gut Microbes, 3*(1). https://doi.org/10.4161/gmic.19320.

Xu, H., Cao, C., Ren, Y., Weng, S., Liu, L., Guo, C., Wang, L., Han, X., Ren, J., & Liu, Z. (2022). Antitumor effects of fecal microbiota transplantation: Implications for microbiome modulation in cancer treatment. *Frontiers in Immunology, 13*. https://doi.org/10.3389/fimmu.2022.949490.

Yadav, A., Ahlawat, S., & Sharma, K. K. (2023). Culturing the unculturables: Strategies, challenges, and opportunities for gut microbiome study. *Journal of Applied Microbiology, 134*(12). https://doi.org/10.1093/jambio/lxad280.

Yadegar, A., Bar-Yoseph, H., Monaghan, T. M., Pakpour, S., Severino, A., Kuijper, E. J., Smits, W. K., Terveer, E. M., Neupane, S., Nabavi-Rad, A., Sadeghi, J., Cammarota, G., Ianiro, G., Nap-Hill, E., Leung, D., Wong, K., & Kao, D. (2024). Fecal microbiota transplantation: Current challenges and future landscapes. *Clinical Microbiology Reviews, 37*(2). https://doi.org/10.1128/cmr.00060-22.

Yadegar, A., Pakpour, S., Ibrahim, F. F., Nabavi-Rad, A., Cook, L., Walter, J., Seekatz, A. M., Wong, K., Monaghan, T. M., & Kao, D. (2023). Beneficial effects of fecal microbiota transplantation in recurrent *Clostridioides difficile* infection. *Cell Host & Microbe, 31*(5), 695–711. https://doi.org/10.1016/j.chom.2023.03.019.

Yaqub, M. O., Jain, A., Joseph, C. E., & Edison, L. K. (2025). Microbiome-driven therapeutics: From gut health to precision medicine. *Gastrointestinal Disorders, 7*(1). https://doi.org/10.3390/gidisord7010007.

Yu, G., Ji, X., Huang, J., Liao, A., Pan, L., Hou, Y., Hui, M., & Guo, W. (2021). Immunity improvement and gut microbiota remodeling of mice by wheat germ globulin. *World Journal of Microbiology and Biotechnology, 37*(4). https://doi.org/10.1007/s11274-021-03034-1.

Yu, H., Zhang, Y., Yang, D., Luo, H., & Zhou, Y. (2025). Advances in capsule-based fecal microbiota transplantation: Clinical applications and innovations. *Journal of Translational Medicine, 23*(1). https://doi.org/10.1186/s12967-025-07407-0.

Zarour, H. M., & Trinchieri, G. (2025). Harnessing the microbiome in cancer immunotherapy: Regulation, prediction, and therapeutic targeting. *Annual Review of Immunology*. https://doi.org/10.1146/annurev-immunol-082323-114522.

Zhang, P. (2022). Influence of foods and nutrition on the gut microbiome and implications for intestinal health. *International Journal of Molecular Sciences, 23*(17), 9588. https://doi.org/10.3390/ijms23179588.

Zhang, S. L., Wang, S. N., & Miao, C. Y. (2017). Influence of microbiota on intestinal immune system in Ulcerative colitis and its intervention. *Frontiers in Immunology, 8*. https://doi.org/10.3389/fimmu.2017.01674.

Zhang, Y., Tang, N., Zhou, H., & Zhu, Y. (2024a). The role of microbial metabolites in endocrine tumorigenesis: From the mechanistic insights to potential therapeutic biomarkers. *Biomedicine & Pharmacotherapy, 172*, 116218. https://doi.org/10.1016/j.biopha.2024.116218.

Zhang, Y., Wang, H., Sang, Y., Liu, M., Wang, Q., Yang, H., & Li, X. (2024b). Gut microbiota in health and disease: Advances and future prospects. *MedComm, 5*(12). https://doi.org/10.1002/mco2.70012.

Zhao, B., Zhou, B., Li, Q., Su, C., Ma, J., & Yang, L. i (2024). Harnessing the gut microbiome to enhance cancer immunotherapy: Current advances and future directions in microbiota-based therapeutic strategies. *MedComm - Future Medicine, 3*(4). https://doi.org/10.1002/mef2.70006.

Zhao, L. Y., Mei, J. X., Yu, G., Lei, L., Zhang, W. H., Liu, K., Chen, X. L., Kołat, D., Yang, K., & Hu, J. K. (2023). Role of the gut microbiota in anticancer therapy: From molecular mechanisms to clinical applications. *Signal Transduction and Targeted Therapy, 8*(1). https://doi.org/10.1038/s41392-023-01406-7.

Zheng, D., Liwinski, T., & Elinav, E. (2020). Interaction between microbiota and immunity in health and disease. *Cell Research, 30*(6), 492–506. https://doi.org/10.1038/s41422-020-0332-7.

Zhou, P., Chen, C., Patil, S., & Dong, S. (2024). Unveiling the therapeutic symphony of probiotics, prebiotics, and postbiotics in gut-immune harmony. *Frontiers in Nutrition, 11*. https://doi.org/10.3389/fnut.2024.1355542.

Zitvogel, L., Ayyoub, M., Routy, B., & Kroemer, G. (2016). Microbiome and anticancer immunosurveillance. *Cell, 165*(2), 276–287. https://doi.org/10.1016/j.cell.2016.03.001.

Zou, J., Liu, C., Jiang, S., Qian, D., Duan, J., & Richardson, A. R. (2021). Cross talk between gut microbiota and intestinal mucosal immunity in the development of ulcerative colitis. *Infection and Immunity, 89*(9). https://doi.org/10.1128/iai.00014-21.

2

The microbiome: Its impact on cancer development and therapeutic responses

Sanjeev Kumar Sahu[a], Picheswara Rao Polu[a], Iqubal Singh[a] and Sambit Kumar Parida[b]

[a]SCHOOL OF PHARMACEUTICAL SCIENCES, LOVELY PROFESSIONAL UNIVERSITY, PHAGWARA, PUNJAB, INDIA [b]AMITY INSTITUTE OF PHARMACY, AMITY UNIVERSITY, JAIPUR, RAJASTHAN, INDIA

2.1 Introduction and overview of the human microbiome

2.1.1 Definition and composition of the microbiome

Human microbiome refers to the total genomic content of microorganisms that occupy the human body and thus create a complex ecosystem existing in a dynamic interaction with the host. It is a microbial community consisting of bacteria, archaea, viruses, fungi, and protozoa that inhabit different anatomical locations, forming unique ecological niches that have unique compositions and functions (Marchesi & Ravel, 2025). The microbiome contains about 38 trillion microbial cells, which is about the same as the human cells, and its genetic contribution is much greater than the human genome, at least 150 times more (Sender et al., 2016). The microbiome was given the name by Joshua Lederberg to denote the ecological community of commensal, symbiotic, and pathogenic microorganisms that exist in our body space, and has been virtually ignored as a cause of disease and health.

The human microbiome is incredibly diverse and variable among people and is dependent on some factors such as age, diet, genetics, environmental exposures, and medical interventions. The emergence of culture-free methodologies, especially next-generation sequencing methodologies of bacterial 16S rRNA gene and whole-genome shotgun metagenomic sequencing, has transformed our perception of the complexity of the microbiome (Knight et al., 2018). These new methods have demonstrated that the human microbiome includes more than 1000 bacterial species, and the most common phyla are *Firmicutes, Bacteroidetes, Actinobacteria, and Proteobacteria*. This microbial diversity helps the formation of a functional core microbiome that is needed to offer vital metabolic functions, even though there may be taxonomic differences among individuals.

The Microbiome and Cancer Treatment: Overcoming Resistance and Enhancing Efficacy.
DOI: https://doi.org/10.1016/B978-0-443-33206-7.00007-8

2.1.2 Major microbial communities in the human body

The human body contains different microbial communities in different organs or anatomical locations, with each having different compositions that determine the physiological condition of the site or organs. The gastrointestinal tract hosts the most abundant and diverse microbial community, which is home to about 70percent of the human microbiota (Sekirov et al., 2010). It is a complex ecosystem exhibiting a gradient of rising bacterial density along the intestinal tract, with the highest count in the distal colon (10^3–10^5 cells/g) and the lowest count in the stomach (10^{11}–10^{12} cells/g). This ecosystem is dominated by anaerobic bacteria, which are represented by the Bacteroidetes and Firmicutes phyla (Donaldson et al., 2016). The large surface area of the gut lining is an area that provides close contact between the host and microbiota and thus is able to support the important metabolic interaction and immunological communication with a great impact on the overall well-being of the system.

The second largest microbial community is the skin microbiome, which shows impressive site-specific diversity that reflects the variation in the level of moisture, sebum, and temperature among the different skin regions. The second most varied microbiome is found in the oral cavity; communities live on the teeth, the gingival sulcus, tongue, cheek, and palate. These oral microorganisms play important functions in ensuring oral health, although in cases of dysregulation, they cause diseases like periodontal disease. Microbial density in the respiratory tract microbiota is decreasing in a gradient toward the lower airways, and recently, the lower respiratory tract has been recognized to have a sparse but functionally important microbiota (Dickson et al., 2016). Similarly, site-specific microbial communities can be found in the female reproductive tract, where lactobacilli prevail in the vaginal microbiome, and which help protect against pathogenic colonization, shifting to *Lactobacilli* at the vagina and *Lactobacilli, Staphylococcus,* and *Esophricoccus* toward the fallopian tubes and ovaries, respectively. The urinary tract, which was believed to be sterile, has been found to have a resident microbiome that can affect the health of the urology.

2.1.3 Core functions in health and homeostasis

The human microbiome plays a crucial role in maintaining homeostasis and supporting overall health. The first one is the fact that it has a large metabolic capacity, which completes human metabolism by extracting the energy contained in the otherwise indigestible elements of the diet, synthesizing vital vitamins (especially B vitamins and vitamin K), and forming short-chain fatty acids (SCFAs) like butyrate, propionate, and acetate (Koh et al., 2016). These SCFAs act as sources of energy to colonic cells, control pH levels within the intestinal tract, and have an anti-inflammatory effect, which maintains the integrity of gut barriers. Also, the microbiome is involved in xenobiotic metabolism, meaning that it enhances biotransformation of environmental chemicals, pollutants, and pharmaceuticals, in this way affecting their bioavailability and potential toxicity.

The microbiome is also very important in regulating and developing the immune system in addition to its metabolic roles. Microbial colonization during early life influences the development of gut-associated lymphoid tissues and predetermines the development of immune tolerance (Gensollen et al., 2016). The microbiota keeps on training the immune system with the help of pattern-recognition receptors (PPRs), which stimulate regulatory T cells and balance proinflammatory and anti-inflammatory reactions (Thaiss et al., 2016). This immunomodulatory effect avoids overreaction of inflammations and still has the effect of defense against pathogens. The microbiome also renders colonization resistance to pathogenic microorganisms by direct competition for nutrients and attachment sites, antimicrobial compound production, and the activation of the host defense mechanisms (Pickard et al., 2017). Further, there is a growing body of evidence that there is a complex two-way communication system between the gut microbiome and the central nervous system, known as the microbiome-gut-brain axis, that has an impact on neurodevelopment, behavior, and cognitive processes.

2.1.4 Emerging significance in cancer biology

The appreciation of the significant effect of the microbiome on human health has extended to cancer biology, where a growing body of research has suggested microbial dysbiosis as the cause of carcinogenesis, tumor progression, and therapeutic responses (Zitvogel et al., 2017). The microbiome can also cause cancer in several ways, including direct genotoxicity, chronic inflammation, metabolic production, and immune modulation. *Helicobacter pylori (H. pylori)* has also been identified as an oncogenic driver in gastric cancer, human papillomavirus in cervical cancer, and enterotoxin *Bacteroides fragilis* (ETBF) in colorectal cancer (CRC). These pathogenic microorganisms may directly cause damage to DNA or activate oncogenic signaling pathways or provide a proinflammatory microenvironment, which allows genetic instability and tumor formation (Irrazábal et al., 2014).

In addition to direct carcinogenicity, the microbiome has proven to have a strong association with different types of cancer and can be used as a diagnostic and prognostic biomarker. Different microbial signatures of colorectal, pancreatic, breast, lung, and prostate cancers are identified, and this may indicate the potential of microbiome profiling in cancer early detection and risk stratification (Sepich-Poore et al., 2021). As an example, the population of *Fusobacterium nucleatum* in the tumor tissues of CRC is related to higher development stages and worse prognosis, which indicates their involvement in tumor development (Bullman et al., 2017). Moreover, the microbiome has become a highly important factor in cancer treatment effectiveness, affecting responses to chemotherapy, radiotherapy, and immunotherapy. Innovative research has shown that the gut microbiota composition can forecast and control the reactions to immune checkpoint inhibitors (ICIs) in melanoma and other cancers, and distinct bacterial species can increase the therapeutic effects.

The growing understanding of the role of the microbiome in oncogenesis has opened new opportunities for innovative treatment approaches. Dietary intervention, probiotics, prebiotics, antibiotics, and fecal microbiota transplantation (FMT) are potential methods to supplement existing cancer therapeutic strategies and mitigate the side effects (Wong & Yu, 2019). The creation of microbial-based biomarkers to identify cancer at its initial stages and to select the optimal treatment option for a patient also highlights the potential of microbiome research in oncology to be used in clinical practice (Zitvogel et al., 2018). With the ever-changing nature of the research on microbiome-cancer interactions, the implementation of microbiome evaluation into regular cancer treatment can contribute greatly to the precision of oncology and better patient outcomes.

2.2 Microbiome dysbiosis and mechanisms of carcinogenesis

Human microbiome and its relationship with cancer development have become an essential field of study in oncology, particularly due to the complex nature of the relationship between the two. Dysbiosis, which is a change in microbial composition, diversity, and activity, is a major deviation from the homeostatic condition of the microbiome that can result in carcinogenesis (Levy et al., 2017). Although the presence of links between microorganisms and particular cancers was long-established, including the connection between gastric cancer and the related *H. pylori,* or gastric cancer, and the presence of dysbiosis in microbial communities and their role in cancer initiation and progression are complex issues that have been identified in recent studies. The paper presents the complex nature of how microbiome dysbiosis promotes carcinogenesis, including direct genotoxic, indirect inflammatory, metabolite-driven, and microbial species involved in the process.

2.2.1 Direct mechanisms: Genotoxicity and oncogenic pathways

Direct involvement of microorganisms in carcinogenesis involves multiple genotoxic pathways that destroy host DNA and initiate oncolytic pathways. Some types of bacteria cause genotoxins, which directly cause damage to DNA, causing genomic instability and possible malignant transformation (Gagnaire et al., 2017). One such notable example is colibactin, which is a polyketide-peptide genotoxin secreted by selected strains of *Escherichia coli (E. coli)* that carry a pks genomic island. Colibactin causes broken strands of DNA as well as interstrand cross-linkages, which produce specific mutation patterns found in CRC samples (Colibactin Causes Colorectal Cancer-Associated Mutational Signature, 2020). It has been shown that *in vitro* and *in vivo* colibactin-producing *E. coli* facilitate colorectal carcinogenesis through the induction of DNA damage and chromosomal aberration in intestinal epithelial cells, followed by the mutation process (Wilson et al., 2019).

Equally, some strains of the genus *Bacteroides fragilis* produce *B. fragilis* toxin (BFT), associated with carcinogenesis of the colorectum. BFT disassembles E-catenin, impairs epithelial barrier activity, and triggers 2-catenin signaling, a pathway commonly dysregulated during CRC (Wu et al., 2009). The result of this activation is an increase in cellular proliferation and oncogene expression, including c-Myc, which is a proven carcinogen of the human body, making use of several direct pathways to induce gastric carcinogenesis. Its virulence factor CagA enters gastric epithelial cells and disrupts many of the cell polarity, cell proliferation, and cell differentiation pathways. Moreover, VacA toxin of *H. pylori* induces mitochondrial dysfunction and cellular apoptosis, a process that may result in the chronic damage-repair process, which can result in malignant transformation (Junaid et al., 2016).

In addition to bacteria, oncogenic viruses combine their own DNA with that of a host and thus directly modify the cellular functions by expressing viral oncoproteins. E6 and E7 human papillomavirus (HPV) proteins inactivate human tumor suppressor proteins p53 and retinoblastoma protein (pRb), respectively, interfering with cell-cycle regulation and inducing genomic instability (McBride, 2022). Likewise, the hepatitis B virus (HBV) also expresses HBx protein that disrupts the repair of DNA and supports hepatocarcinogenesis. These direct genotoxic effects underscore the ability of the microorganisms to trigger the carcinogenic process through direct interference with the integrity and regulation of the genome and the cell.

2.2.2 Indirect mechanisms: Chronic inflammation and immune dysregulation

Chronic inflammation is one of the most important indirect processes by which dysbiosis of the microbiome leads to carcinogenesis. The chronic microbial dysbiosis may interfere with the operation of the epithelial barrier, allowing the establishment of microbial translocation and the subsequent activation of the PRRs, including toll-like receptors (TLRs) and NOD-like receptors (NLRs) (Grivennikov et al., 2010). This stimulates inflammatory signaling pathways, including nuclear factor-B (NF–B) and signal transducer and activator of transcription 3 (STAT3), and results in the generation of proinflammatory cytokines, chemokines, and growth factors that give rise to a tumor-promoting microenvironment (Elinav et al., 2013).

The inflammatory condition leads to a continuous production of reactive oxygen and nitrogen species (ROS and RNS), which induce oxidative damage to the DNA, which further increases genomic instability. Also, chronic inflammation enhances epigenetic changes, such as the DNA methylation profiles and histone modifications that can either silence tumor suppressors or activate oncogenes. Inflammatory microenvironment also promotes cellular proliferation, angiogenesis, and tissue remodeling, which can also be hijacked in the process of carcinogenesis to facilitate tumor growth and progression.

Dysbiosis of the microbiome also helps in carcinogenesis through the regulation of immune surveillance. Having a balanced microbiome is crucial to maintain normal immune growth and function, such as the development of gut-associated lymphoid tissue and optimization of innate and adaptive immune responses (Schirmer et al., 2016). Dysbiosis may affect the growth and activity of immune cell subsets that play a crucial role in tumor surveillance, including natural killer (NK) cells, cytotoxic T lymphocytes, and dendritic cells (Matson et al., 2018). An example is certain commensal bacteria that have been found to increase production of IL-12 by dendritic cells, which favor the Th1 type of immune response that is required to develop antitumor immunity. Disturbance of these advantageous microbial communities may undermine these protective mechanisms, thereby providing permissive environments for tumor growth.

In addition, there are specific microorganisms that actively prevent antitumor immunity by a number of different mechanisms. By binding the TIGIT immune inhibitory receptor on NK and T cells via its Fap2 protein, *Fusobacterium nucleatum*, enriched in CRC tissues, inhibits tumor-infiltrating lymphocyte activity by blocking immune evasion (Gur et al., 2015). Equally, dysbiosis of microbes can foster the growth of immunosuppressive cell types, including myeloid-derived suppressor cells and regulatory T cells, further undermining antitumor immunity. These results highlight the severe importance of the microbiome-mediated immune dysregulation in establishing the conditions favorable to carcinogenesis.

2.2.3 Metabolite-mediated effects on host cells

The microbiome is capable of producing a huge number of metabolites that may have a profound effect on the physiology of host cells and lead to carcinogenesis when uncontrolled. Butyrate, propionate, and acetate are SCFAs that are produced during the fermentation of dietary fiber by the commensal bacteria and usually have protective effects against CRC in a variety of ways (Louis et al., 2014). Specifically, butyrate acts as a histone deacetylase inhibitor, inducing the expression of genes that regulate cell-cycle arrest and apoptosis in cancerous colonocytes and inducing cell growth in normal colonocytes. In turn, these protective effects can be diminished by dysbiosis, which is characterized by decreased SCFA-producing gut bacteria and can lead to colorectal carcinogenesis.

Other microbial metabolites, on the other hand, have been found to support carcinogenesis. The secondary bile acids are the products of the deconjugation and dihydroxylation of primary bile acids that are produced by gut bacteria and which are shown to disrupt cellular membranes, produce reactive oxygen species, cause DNA damage and mutations (Ridlon et al., 2016). In one study of deoxycholic acid (DCA) specifically, and lithocholic acid (LCA), in particular, both of them activate epidermal growth factor receptor and cyclooxygenase-2 (COX-2) pathways linked to cellular proliferation and inflammation. Empirical evidence has indicated an increase in the level of secondary bile acids in patients with colorectal adenomas and carcinomas and thus provides evidence of their contributory effect on colorectal oncogenesis.

Another possible carcinogenic metabolite, H_2S, which is a product of sulphate-reducing bacteria like *Bilophila wadsworthia* and *Desulfovibrio* spp., is produced. H_2S may also cause cytochrome C oxidase inhibition, mitochondrial dysfunction, and free radical formation, which cause DNA damage at high concentrations (Attene-Ramos et al., 2006). Additionally, some bacterial species break down foodstuff ingredients to produce genotoxins. As an example, a large amount of protein being taken may cause a rise in bacterial synthesis of N-nitroso compounds and heterocyclic amines, both of which are mutagenic. On the same note, gut microbiota metabolism of alcohol produces acetaldehyde, a well-known carcinogen that reacts with DNA to create DNA adducts and disrupts the DNA repair process (Seitz & Stickel, 2007). These effects mediated by metabolites highlight the multifaceted processes through which microbiome dysbiosis may rearrange the biochemical landscape of tissues, which may result in or contribute to carcinogenesis.

2.2.4 Key microbial species implicated in carcinogenesis

The microbial species have been specifically attributed to carcinogenesis in different types of cancer. The best-characterized microbial carcinogen is still *H. pylori*, which is classified as a Group 1 carcinogen by the International Agency for Research on Cancer because it causes gastric adenocarcinoma and mucosa-associated lymphoid tissue lymphoma. In addition to the direct and inflammatory actions as mentioned above, *H. pylori* infection leads to aberrant patterns of

DNA methylation, which remain after elimination of bacteria, thus possibly resulting in the field cancerization effect in gastric oncogenesis (Maeda et al., 2017).

In CRC, *Fusobacterium nucleatum* has become an important carcinogen. Being enriched in colorectal tumor tissues compared to the adjacent normal mucosa, the tumorigenic-promoting activity of *F. nucleatum* is enhanced in several mechanisms. Its FadA adhesin interacts with E- cadherin and thus triggers β-catenin signaling and induces the expression of oncogenes and inflammatory genes (Rubinstein et al., 2013). Another alteration that occurs is that *F. nucleatum* also regulates the immune microenvironment in cancer by suppressing T-cell and NK cells, as well as recruiting myeloid-derived suppressor cells. Moreover, increased prevalence of the abundance of *F. nucleatum* in CRC tissues is associated with particular molecular characteristics, such as microsatellite instability and CpG island methylator phenotype, which indicate the possible interactions of genetic and epigenetic pathways of colorectal carcinogenesis.

Another major species that is involved in the pathogenesis of colorectal carcinoma is the ETBF. In addition to the direct effects of the BFT mentioned above, ETBF colonization induces an inflammatory response of T helper type 17(Th17) dominance (high IL-17 and IL-23) that fosters the formation of colorectal tumors in murine models (Orberg et al., 2017). Likewise, pks and *E. coli* strains are significantly enriched in cancer tissues of the colon and play a role in carcinogenesis through the genotoxic effects of colibactin.

Microbiota perturbation and intestinal microbial product translocation to the liver play a role in carcinogenesis in hepatocellular carcinoma (HCC), especially when a liver disease is present, such as nonalcoholic steatohepatitis and alcoholic liver disease. Gram-negative bacterial lipopolysaccharide triggers TLR4 signaling in hepatic stellate cells and the Kupffer cells, which facilitates inflammation, fibrosis, and eventually hepatocarcinogenesis (Dapito et al., 2012). Also, certain bacterial species, such as the *Helicobacter hepaticus* species, have been identified to contribute to liver cancer growth by direct colonization as well as inflammatory pathways.

There are also emerging indications of possible functions of certain microorganisms in pancreatic, breast, and prostate cancers. Oral pathogens, including those that are unique to the pancreatic microenvironment, including, but not limited to, *Porphyromonas gingivalis*, have been implicated in carcinogenesis and progression of pancreatic cancer (Gaiser et al., 2019). The research on the breast microbiome has shown that there are unique microbial profiles present in breast cancer tissues compared to the normal breast tissue, and certain bacteria, such as *E. coli* and *Staphylococcus epidermidis*, are enriched (O'Toole et al., 2017). On the same note, the change in urinary and intestinal microbiome has been associated with the development and progression of prostate cancer. These data on different types of cancer underline the potentially general nature of microbiome dysbiosis in carcinogenesis and the importance of further research on these complicated interactions (Table 2.1).

2.3 Microbiome signatures across different cancer types

The revelation that distinct microbial signatures are associated with various cancer types has transformed our understanding of tumor biology and created new opportunities for cancer

Table 2.1 Key microbial species and their carcinogenic mechanisms.

Microbial species	Primary mechanism	Associated cancer type(s)	Key pathways/toxins	Clinical evidence level
H. pylori	Direct genotoxicity, chronic inflammation	Gastric adenocarcinoma, MALT lymphoma	CagA protein, VacA toxin, IL-8 pathway	Strong (WHO Group 1 carcinogen)
Fusobacterium nucleatum	Immune evasion, tumor promotion	Colorectal cancer	Wnt/β-catenin, FadA adhesin	Moderate-Strong
Bacteroides fragilis	Enterotoxin production	Colorectal cancer	BFT toxin, Wnt pathway activation	Moderate
E. coli (pks+)	Genotoxic metabolites	Colorectal cancer	Colibactin, DNA double-strand breaks	Moderate
Porphyromonas gingivalis	Chronic inflammation	Oral, pancreatic cancer	Gingipains, IL-1β, TNF-α	Limited-Moderate
Salmonella spp.	Chronic inflammation, DNA damage	Gallbladder, hepatobiliary	Typhoid toxin, ROS production	Limited
Streptococcus bovis	Biofilm formation, inflammation	Colorectal cancer	IL-1β, COX-2 pathway	Moderate
Peptostreptococcus anaerobius	Immune suppression	Colorectal cancer	PCDC protein, cholesterol metabolism	Emerging

diagnosis, prognosis, and treatment. Advanced sequencing technologies have enabled researchers to characterize the microbiome composition across diverse cancer types, revealing site-specific microbial communities that may contribute to carcinogenesis, influence disease progression, and affect treatment outcomes. These cancer-associated microbiome signatures often differ significantly from those found in healthy tissues, suggesting potential roles in disease pathogenesis or as consequences of the altered tumor microenvironment (Nejman et al., 2020). This chapter explores the characteristic microbiome profiles associated with various cancer types, including gastrointestinal malignancies, hormone-related cancers, respiratory tract tumors, and other cancer types, while also examining the emerging evidence for pan-cancer microbial patterns and the role of the microbiome in cancer progression and metastasis.

2.3.1 Gastrointestinal tract cancers

The gastrointestinal tract harbors the largest and most diverse microbial communities in the human body, creating a complex ecosystem that significantly influences cancer development within this organ system. CRC represents the most extensively studied malignancy in relation to the microbiome, with substantial evidence supporting distinct microbial signatures associated with carcinogenesis (Wirbel et al., 2019). Multiple studies have demonstrated enrichment of specific bacterial taxa in CRC tissues compared to adjacent normal mucosa, particularly *Fusobacterium nucleatum, Bacteroides fragilis, E. coli, Streptococcus gallolyticus,* and *Peptostreptococcus anaerobius* (Ahn et al., 2013). These bacteria employ various mechanisms to promote carcinogenesis, as discussed in the previous chapter 1. Beyond individual species, broader dysbiotic patterns characterized by reduced microbial diversity, decreased abundance of beneficial butyrate-producing bacteria (such as *Faecalibacterium prausnitzii* and *Roseburia* species), and increased representation of proinflammatory and genotoxic organisms have been consistently observed in CRC patients (Feng et al., 2015).

The temporal relationship between microbiome alterations and colorectal carcinogenesis has been investigated through studies of the adenoma-carcinoma sequence. Research indicates that microbial dysbiosis occurs progressively along this sequence, with certain changes detectable in early adenomas and becoming more pronounced in advanced adenomas and carcinomas. For example, *F. nucleatum* abundance correlates with adenoma progression to carcinoma, suggesting its potential role in promoting this transition. These findings have stimulated interest in developing microbiome-based biomarkers for CRC screening, with several studies demonstrating that fecal microbial signatures can detect CRC with sensitivity and specificity comparable to established screening methods (Zeller et al., 2014).

Gastric cancer exhibits a well-established relationship with *H. pylori*, with approximately 90% of noncardia gastric cancers attributable to this infection. However, recent research indicates that *H. pylori* does not act in isolation but within the context of the broader gastric microbiome. Studies have revealed progressive changes in gastric microbiota composition along the Correa cascade of gastric carcinogenesis, from chronic gastritis to intestinal metaplasia, dysplasia, and finally adenocarcinoma (Coker et al., 2018). Gastric cancer is associated with reduced microbial diversity and enrichment of certain bacterial genera, including *Lactobacillus, Streptococcus,* and

Veillonella, while some Proteobacteria species are depleted. These alterations may contribute to carcinogenesis through promoting inflammation, modulating *H. pylori* virulence, or producing carcinogenic metabolites such as N-nitroso compounds.

Pancreatic ductal adenocarcinoma (PDAC) has been linked to distinctive microbiome signatures in both the intestinal and pancreatic tissues. Despite traditionally being considered a sterile organ, evidence now suggests that the pancreas harbors a low-biomass microbiome that becomes altered in PDAC (Geller et al., 2017). Studies have reported enrichment of specific oral bacterial species in PDAC tissues, including Fusobacterium, Porphyromonas, and Actinobacteria, suggesting potential translocation from the oral cavity. Concurrently, gut microbiome alterations characterized by increased abundance of Proteobacteria and decreased representation of Bacteroidetes and Firmicutes have been observed in PDAC patients (Ren et al., 2017). These dysbiotic patterns may influence pancreatic carcinogenesis through various mechanisms, including modulation of inflammation, immune responses, and metabolism of carcinogens. Furthermore, specific gut microbial signatures have been associated with PDAC risk, raising the possibility of microbiome-based strategies for early detection of this typically late-diagnosed malignancy.

2.3.2 Hormone-related cancers

Emerging evidence indicates that the microbiome may influence hormone-related cancers, particularly breast and prostate cancers, through modulation of steroid hormone metabolism and immune function. The female breast, previously considered sterile, has been shown to harbor a diverse microbiome that differs between healthy and cancerous tissues (Hieken et al., 2016). Studies have identified distinct breast cancer-associated microbial signatures characterized by enrichment of specific taxa, including *E. coli, Staphylococcus epidermidis,* and members of the *Enterobacteriaceae* family. These microorganisms possess β-glucuronidase activity, which can deconjugate estrogens in the breast tissue, potentially increasing local estrogenic concentrations and promoting carcinogenesis in hormone-responsive tumors.

Additionally, the gut microbiome influences systemic estrogen levels through the enterohepatic circulation of estrogens. The "estrobolome"—the collective genomic content of the gut microbiota capable of metabolizing estrogens—can significantly impact estrogen homeostasis (Kwa et al., 2016). Gut microbiome profiles characterized by increased β-glucuronidase activity have been associated with elevated systemic estrogen levels and increased breast cancer risk, particularly in postmenopausal women. Furthermore, specific gut microbial patterns have been linked to clinical outcomes in breast cancer patients, suggesting potential prognostic applications. These findings highlight the complex interplay between microbial communities at local and distant sites in influencing breast cancer development and progression.

Prostate cancer similarly demonstrates associations with specific microbiome signatures across multiple anatomical sites. The prostate itself harbors a low-biomass microbiome that differs between benign and malignant tissues (Cavarretta et al., 2017). Studies have identified enrichment of specific genera, including *Propionibacterium, Escherichia,* and *Staphylococcus,* in prostate cancer tissues compared to benign prostatic hyperplasia or healthy prostate tissues. Furthermore, urinary microbiome alterations characterized by increased bacterial diversity and abundance of specific taxa, such as *Escherichia, Lactococcus,* and *Streptococcus,* have been reported in prostate cancer patients. The gut microbiome also demonstrates associations with prostate cancer, with specific microbial signatures linked to disease risk and aggressiveness. Mechanistically, these microbiome alterations may influence prostate carcinogenesis through modulation of androgen metabolism, regulation of inflammatory responses, and production of oncogenic metabolites. The multisite microbiome associations with prostate cancer underscore the systemic nature of microbiome-cancer interactions and suggest potential for integrated microbiome-based approaches in prostate cancer management.

2.3.3 Lung cancer and respiratory tract malignancies

The relationship between the respiratory microbiome and lung cancer has gained increasing attention, challenging the traditional view of the lower respiratory tract as sterile. Studies utilizing culture-independent sequencing methods have revealed that lung cancer tissues harbor distinct microbial communities compared to adjacent nonmalignant tissues or healthy lungs (Lee et al., 2016). These cancer-associated microbiome signatures are characterized by increased abundance of specific taxa, including *Streptococcus, Veillonella, Prevotella,* and *Neisseria,* with corresponding decreases in other commensal bacteria. Interestingly, these enriched genera include many taxa typically associated with the oral microbiome, suggesting potential aspiration or translocation of oral bacteria to the lower respiratory tract.

The lung cancer microbiome also demonstrates associations with histological subtypes, with different microbial compositions observed between adenocarcinoma, squamous cell carcinoma, and small cell lung cancer (Peters et al., 2019b). Furthermore, specific microbial signatures have been linked to clinical outcomes, including response to therapy and survival. Mechanistically, the respiratory microbiome may influence lung carcinogenesis through various pathways, including induction of chronic inflammation, production of genotoxic metabolites, and modulation of host immune responses (Tsay et al., 2018). Additionally, the lung microbiome may interact with environmental factors, such as tobacco smoke, potentially amplifying their carcinogenic effects.

Beyond the local lung microbiome, evidence suggests that the gut microbiome may also influence lung cancer development and progression through systemic effects on immunity and inflammation, exemplifying the concept of interorgan microbiome-mediated effects (Gui et al., 2015). This gut-lung axis represents a potential avenue for therapeutic intervention, with studies exploring the impact of gut microbiome modulation on lung cancer outcomes. The evolving understanding of respiratory microbiome signatures in lung cancer offers new perspectives on disease pathogenesis and opportunities for microbiome-based diagnostic and therapeutic approaches for these aggressive malignancies.

2.3.4 Other cancer types and pan-cancer microbiome patterns

Microbiome signatures have been identified in numerous other cancer types beyond the gastrointestinal, hormone-related, and respiratory malignancies. HCC demonstrates associations with altered gut microbial communities, characterized by reduced beneficial taxa such as *Bifidobacterium* and enrichment of proinflammatory species (Ren et al., 2019). These gut microbiome alterations may contribute to HCC pathogenesis through increased translocation of bacterial products to the liver, promoting inflammation and fibrosis. Similarly, specific oral microbiome profiles have been linked to head and neck squamous cell carcinomas, with enrichment of certain taxa, including *Fusobacterium, Peptostreptococcus*, and *Prevotella*.

Hematological malignancies also exhibit associations with the microbiome, particularly through the interaction between gut microbiota and the bone marrow microenvironment. Studies in acute myeloid leukemia and multiple myeloma have demonstrated altered gut microbiome compositions that may influence disease progression and treatment responses (Taur et al., 2014). Furthermore, emerging evidence suggests associations between microbiome signatures and skin cancers, bladder cancer, and central nervous system tumors, highlighting the potentially universal role of microbiome dysbiosis in cancer.

Recent comprehensive analyses across multiple cancer types have identified potential pan-cancer microbial signatures—microbial patterns that transcend specific cancer types and may represent common features of carcinogenesis. These studies have identified tissue-specific microbial signatures as well as a core set of microbial features shared across diverse tumor types. For instance, a comprehensive analysis of over 17,000 samples across 33 cancer types identified cancer type-specific microbial signatures and a pan-cancer microbial signature characterized by specific viral and bacterial associations (Robinson et al., 2017). These findings suggest that certain microbial patterns may represent fundamental features of the cancer microenvironment or common mechanisms of microbiome-cancer interactions.

The identification of microbial signatures across diverse cancer types has significant implications for cancer diagnosis and monitoring. Several studies have demonstrated the potential of microbiome-based biomarkers for early cancer detection, with promising results for colorectal, gastric, pancreatic, and liver cancers. These noninvasive approaches, primarily utilizing stool or saliva samples, offer advantages over traditional screening methods and could significantly improve early detection rates for various malignancies. Furthermore, microbiome signatures have demonstrated prognostic value across multiple cancer types, with specific microbial patterns associated with disease progression, treatment response, and survival outcomes.

2.3.5 Role in cancer progression and metastasis

Beyond cancer initiation, the microbiome plays significant roles in disease progression and metastasis across various cancer types. Specific microbial signatures have been associated with advanced disease stages, tumor invasiveness, and metastatic potential. For instance, increased abundance of *Fusobacterium nucleatum* in CRC tissues correlates with advanced disease stage, lymph node metastasis, and poorer prognosis. Mechanistically, *F. nucleatum* promotes cancer cell proliferation and invasion through activation of the autophagy pathway and stimulation of TLRs 4 signaling (Zhang et al., 2019).

The microbiome influences cancer progression through multiple mechanisms, including modulation of the tumor microenvironment, promotion of epithelial-to-mesenchymal transition (EMT), and facilitation of angiogenesis. Certain bacteria can remodel the tumor extracellular matrix, enhancing cancer cell invasion and migration. For example, *B. fragilis* can degrade E-cadherin through its toxin BFT, disrupting cell–cell junctions and facilitating tumor cell invasion. Similarly, specific microbial species induce matrix metalloproteinases that degrade extracellular matrix components, creating pathways for cancer cell migration.

Microbial influences on cancer progression extend to local and distant metastasis. The liver, a common site for CRC metastasis, demonstrates distinct microbiome signatures in metastatic lesions compared to primary tumors, suggesting microbial adaptation to or selection within the metastatic microenvironment. Furthermore, specific gut microbial communities have been associated with enhanced development of liver metastasis in CRC animal models. These findings highlight the potential role of the microbiome in creating premetastatic niches or favorable conditions for metastatic colonization.

The relationship between the microbiome and cancer progression represents a promising avenue for therapeutic intervention. Targeting specific cancer-promoting microorganisms or their metabolites could potentially inhibit disease progression and metastasis. Additionally, microbiome modulation could enhance responses to conventional therapies, as specific microbial communities have been associated with improved outcomes across various treatment modalities. As research in this field continues to advance, integrating microbiome assessment into cancer staging and prognostication may provide valuable information for treatment planning and risk stratification, ultimately improving patient outcomes through more personalized approaches to cancer management (Table 2.2).

2.4 Microbiome influence on cancer therapeutics

The human microbiome is a dynamic ecosystem of microorganisms that live in the human body, and new evidence shows that they have a significant impact on the development of cancer and the response to therapeutic measures. Current technological progress has allowed the description of the specifics of these complex communities and metabolic activities, which demonstrate complex interactions between the microbial populations and treatment effects in cancer patients (Dzutsev et al., 2017). The chapter examines the role played by the microbiome in regulating the outcome of different cancer therapies, which provides an insight into new strategies to improve the efficacy of appropriate therapeutic agents and reduce their side effects.

2.4.1 Impact on chemotherapy efficacy and toxicity

Gut microbiome plays a major role in determining the efficacy and toxicity profile of chemotherapeutic agents in a series of pathways. Several bacterial species catabolize chemotherapy agents, thereby directly affecting their bioavailability and pharmacologic activity. Iida et al. (2013) showed that germ-free or antibiotic-treated mice had weakened reactions to oxaliplatin and had inferior tumor regression compared to mice that had preserved microbiota.

Table 2.2 Microbiome signatures across major cancer types.

Cancer type	Increased taxa	Decreased taxa	Alpha diversity	Key biomarker species	Diagnostic potential
Colorectal cancer	*Fusobacterium, Bacteroides fragilis, Peptostreptococcus*	*Faecalibacterium, Roseburia, Blautia*	Reduced	*F. nucleatum, pks+ E. coli*	High (AUC: 0.80–0.85)
Gastric cancer	*H. pylori, Lactobacillus, Streptococcus*	*Prevotella, Veillonella*	Markedly reduced	*H. pylori* CagA+ strains	Very High (AUC: >0.90)
Pancreatic cancer	*Porphyromonas, Aggregatibacter, Fusobacterium*	*Neisseria, Granulicatella*	Reduced	*P. gingivalis, A. actinomycetem comitans*	Moderate (AUC: 0.70–0.75)
Breast cancer	*Methylobacterium, Sphingomonas, Pseudomonas*	*Lactococcus, Streptococcus*	Variable	*Methylobacterium radiotolerans*	Low-Moderate (AUC: 0.65–0.70)
Lung cancer	*Granulicatella, Abiotrophia, Streptococcus*	*Veillonella, Megasphaera*	Reduced	*Granulicatella adiacens*	Moderate (AUC: 0.72–0.78)
Prostate cancer	*Propionibacterium, Corynebacterium, Staphylococcus*	*Faecalibacterium, Eubacterium*	Variable	*P. acnes, E. coli*	Low (AUC: 0.60–0.65)
Hepatocellular cancer	*Klebsiella, Haemophilus, Enterobacteriaceae*	*Bifidobacterium, Faecalibacterium*	Reduced	*K. pneumoniae, E. coli*	Moderate (AUC: 0.75–0.80)
Oral cancer	*Fusobacterium, Prevotella, Porphyromonas*	*Neisseria, Haemophilus*	Reduced	*F. nucleatum, P. gingivalis*	High (AUC: 0.85–0.90)

This was explained by the fact that microbiome-dependent effects on the myeloid-derived cell functions in the tumor microenvironment attenuated this, thus highlighting the significance of bacterial communities in enhancing the effects of chemotherapeutics.

Some microorganisms catalyze the conversion of prodrugs into their therapeutically active forms. As an example, Bacteroides species deactivate irinotecan through 2-glucuronidase enzymes, which increases the cytotoxic activity on malignant cells at the expense of increasing intestinal toxicity. On the other hand, Alexander et al. (2017) found a negative relationship between the abundance of *Ruminococcus* and the occurrence of mucositis induced by 5-fluorouracil, a finding which implied a protective effect of this group on the chemotherapy-induced gastrointestinal damage (Wallace et al., 2010). Another essential issue is microbial dysbiosis after chemotherapy. Cyclophosphamide causes impairment of the intestinal barrier, which allows commensal bacteria to translocate and activate useful antitumor immunity. However, the same process can trigger pathological inflammation and sepsis in neutropenic patients, which underscores the fragility of beneficial and harmful microbiome-mediated outcomes when undergoing chemotherapy (Wallace et al., 2010).

2.4.2 Influence on radiation therapy outcomes

Radiation therapy activity is also dependent on the composition and activity of the microbiome. According to Alexander et al. (2017), it was found that mice kept germ-free showed higher radiation resistance as compared to traditionally kept counterparts; recolonization returned radiation sensitivity (Alexander et al., 2017). It is a phenomenon that is affected by the microbiome through the control of DNA damage response pathways and apoptotic pathways in tumor cells.

The gut microbiota has strong effects on radiation-induced gastrointestinal poisoning, which is a prevalent dose-limiting side effect. *Lactobacillus* species are radioprotective in small intestinal mucosal settings and potent in reducing mucosal inflammation and repairing the tissue after radiation. Such results have inspired clinical trials to examine probiotic intervention to prevent radiation enteropathy in cancer patients. The microbiome is also the intermediary in systemic radiation therapy inflammatory reactions. The excessive production of proinflammatory cytokines, which leads to fatigue and other systemic manifestations common in patients, is a result of postradiation gut dysbiosis. Homeostasis of the microbiome in radiotherapy could therefore improve the quality of life and tolerance to the treatment (Touchefeu et al., 2014).

2.4.3 Role in immunotherapy response and resistance

The most remarkable impact microorganisms have on cancer treatment is, perhaps, related to immunotherapy responses, specifically, to ICIs. Historical literature has indicated that patients with melanoma who respond to anti-PD-1 therapy have had a different gut microbial composition than those who do not respond. Particularly, the favorable clinical responses are linked with enrichment of *Faecalibacterium* and *Bifidobacterium*, and the resistance trends are linked with the prevalence of *Bacteroidales*.

Mechanistically, these bacteria augment the functions of dendritic cells and CD8-T-cell priming, which increases systemic antitumor immune responses in response to checkpoint blockade. There is causal evidence that microbiome-mediated immunotherapy effects were acquired with FMT of responding patients into germ-free mice alongside anti-PD-1 therapy (Routy et al., 2018).

The application of antibiotics shortly before or during immunotherapy is a very vital confounding variable that negatively impacts the outcomes. There are several reports of highly decreased progression-free and overall survival in cancer patients who are treated with antibiotics in parallel with ICIs (Pinato et al., 2019). The presented findings hint at the necessity of antimicrobial stewardship in the course of immunotherapy and indicate the possible injury of unjustified exposure to antibiotics in this group.

2.4.4 Microbiome as a predictor of treatment outcomes

The patterns of microbiome composition that are specific to treatment response have generated much enthusiasm for microbial signatures as predictive biomarkers. Peters et al. (2019a) designed a classifier using the microbiome that could predict immunotherapy responses in patients with advanced melanoma with 80% accuracy. Similar methods have been explored in chemotherapy and radiation therapy, which may allow an individual to select personalized treatment regimens depending on microbiome profiles.

Prognostic data are further given by longitudinal observation of the microbiome throughout the therapy. Significant changes in diversity and community arrangement can be found before clinical changes or desirable reactions, indicating an application of real-time readjustment of treatment plans. Combining microbiome data with other biomarkers, e.g., tumor genomics and immune parameters, can improve predictive accuracy and clinical relevance even more.

2.4.5 Drug metabolism and bioavailability

The broad spectrum of the metabolic activity of the gut microbiome has a significant impact on the mechanisms of drug pharmacokinetics and pharmacodynamics. Drug metabolites discharged into bile are deconjugated by bacterial 2-glucuronidases and reinstated into the enterohepatic circulation. Many anticancer agents, such as irinotecan, doxorubicin, and tamoxifen, are influenced by this mechanism.

Compounds that interact with host drug-metabolizing enzymes can be produced as a result of microbial metabolism. As an example, the expression of cytochrome P450 in hepatocytes is regulated by bacterial-derived LCA, which indirectly influences the metabolism of many chemotherapeutic agents (Scott et al., 2017). Besides, drug molecules may undergo direct reactions of microbial reduction, hydrolysis, and acetylation, thus modifying their therapeutic effects. Fig. 2.1 shows the dual role the microbiome plays in the outcome of cancer therapy. Microbial communities may increase the efficacy of treatment by drug metabolism and immune modulation or increase treatment resistance and toxicity. The microbes and the complex interaction between microbes and cancer treatment responses are illustrated in terms of effects presented in three major therapeutic modalities: chemotherapy, radiation therapy, and immunotherapy.

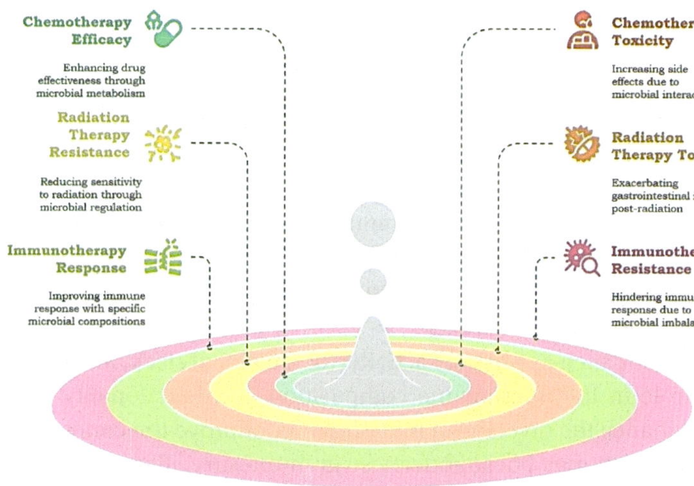

FIGURE 2.1 Microbiome influence on cancer treatment. The microbiome significantly influences cancer treatment by modulating immune responses, affecting drug metabolism, shaping tumor microenvironment interactions, and ultimately impacting therapeutic efficacy and toxicity.

2.5 Microbiome-targeted strategies in cancer management

With the new insights into the complex interaction between the microbiome and cancer, specific interventions directed at altering microbial communities have become possible as promising adjunctive options in cancer treatment. The proposed strategies capitalize on the effects of the microbiome on cancer progression and reaction to treatment with the view of enhancing treatment outcomes and reducing toxicity. This chapter discusses many types of microbiome-targeted interventions, including dietary changes and high-tech biotechnological ones, their mechanistic principles, and applications in the management of cancer.

2.5.1 Dietary and lifestyle interventions

Diet is one of the most readily available and most potent channels for regulating the gut microbiome. Diets have a strong effect on microbial profile and metabolism that can mediate the development and responses to treatment of cancer. The Mediterranean diet, which is marked by a large intake of vegetable foods, olive oil, and low intake of red meat, has been linked to favorable microbiome composition, which is correlated to low cancer risks and better therapeutic response (Garcia-Mantrana et al., 2018). Singh et al. (2017) established that change toward a Mediterranean diet enhanced the concentration of beneficial bacteria, such as *Faecalibacterium prausnitzii* and *Bifidobacterium* species, amongst them, which are associated with improved immune response to immunotherapy.

Dietary fiber is an important feedstock on which fermentation by bacteria occurs to produce SCFAs, including butyrate, propionate, and acetate. These metabolites have a strong anti-inflammatory and antineoplastic effect due to the following mechanisms: histone deacetylase inhibition and stimulation of regulatory T cells. Byndloss et al. (2017), in a landmark study, showed that butyrate inhibits cancer-promoting inflammation by stimulating the peroxisome proliferator-activated receptor gamma pathway in intestinal epithelial cells, which gives mechanistic consideration to the protective effect of fiber against CRC.

Intermittent fasting and caloric restriction are new diet strategies with a bright potential for microbiome composition and cancer prognosis. Preclinical models reveal that changes in the microbiome caused by fasting increase the cancer therapy effects and prevent the toxicity of normal tissues. Such advantages seem to be mediated by the changes in bile acid metabolism and intestinal permeability, and the fact that host metabolic condition, microbial ecosystem, and responses to cancer treatment are complex.

Other lifestyle factors, such as physical activity, the quality of sleep, and stress management, also play a major role in the microbiome composition and functionality, beyond nutrition. Routine activities enhance the diversity of microbes and improve the concentration of bacteria that generate SCFA, which may boost anticancer immune surveillance (Allen et al., 2018). On the other hand, long-term psychological stress and circadian rhythm disruption cause dysbiosis, which is manifested by reduced beneficial commensals and enhanced pathobionts, leading to the development of a proinflammatory microenvironment that could predispose to cancer.

2.5.2 Probiotics, prebiotics, and synbiotics

A direct way of microbiome modulation in cancer treatment is probiotics, which are live microorganisms that provide health benefits when taken in sufficient quantities. Certain probiotic strains exhibit anticancer effects with such mechanisms as inhibition of pathogenic organisms, the improvement of the barrier effect, immunomodulation, and the destabilization of carcinogens (Hibberd et al., 2017). Within the context of surgery among patients with CRC, the use of *Bifidobacterium longum* and *Lactobacillus johnsonii* in perioperative showed significant decrease in postoperative infectious complications and decreased hospitalization.

Probiotics could help reduce adverse effects of treatment during cancer therapy and even improve treatment efficacy. Wang et al. (2017) conducted a randomized controlled trial to prove the reduction of incidence and severity of diarrhea in patients undergoing chemotherapy using 5-fluorouracil by *Lactobacillus rhamnosus* GG supplementation. Let me say likewise, a certain combination of *Lactobacillus* has been shown to have radiation prevention of radiation-induced enteritis, though the correct choice of strains, dose, and timing is still among the important research questions.

Prebiotics are food materials that do not undergo digestion and that selectively promote beneficial microorganisms, which provide an indirect method of modulating the microbiome. Fructo-oligosaccharides, galacto-oligosaccharides, and resistant starch specifically feed on the good bacteria, such as *Bifidobacterium* and *Lactobacillus* species, so increasing the production of SCFA and improving the gut barrier (Gibson et al., 2017). Prebiotics administration in animal models of CRC decreased tumor burden via pathways of bile acid metabolism and antitumor immunity.

The combination of probiotics and prebiotics, synbiotics, may have superior benefits, which may be complementary in nature. A recent clinical study of patients with CRC showed that a synbiotic mixture consisting of *Bifidobacterium* lactis and oligofructose-enriched inulin had a significant reduction in cancer biomarkers and enhanced mucosal immune activity relative to either of the two interventions separately.

2.5.3 Fecal microbiota transplantation

FMT, the transfer of processed feces of healthy donors to the recipient, is the most holistic method of restoration of the microbiome. After impressive results in the treatment of *Clostridioides difficile* (*C. difficile*) infection, FMT has been of interest in cancer therapy, especially in improving immunotherapy. A pioneering phase I trial by Davar et al. (2021) has shown that immunotherapy responder FMT can overcome anti-PD-1-resistant melanoma patients, and that clinical responses are associated with positive changes in the microbiome composition and augmented CD8 +T cell effect.

In addition to immunotherapy, fecal microbial transplantation shows potential in the treatment of toxicities related to treatments. In steroid-resistant immune checkpoint inhibitor-associated colitis patients, FMT demonstrated high clinical remission rates relative to conventional immunosuppressive management and resulted in fewer adverse events (Wang et al., 2018). Despite such promising findings, there are still significant issues to deal with in terms of donor screening, standardization, and the selection of the most suitable routes and timing of administration to achieve the greatest therapeutic effects and reduce the possible risks.

2.5.4 Small molecule approaches targeting microbial pathways

Targeted microbiome manipulation in cancer treatment with small molecules provides an accurate approach to microbial metabolic pathway control. The bacterial 2-glucuronidases represent good targets because they reactivate glucuronidated drug metabolites in the intestine, which contributes to chemotherapy-induced toxicity. The inhibitors of these enzymes have also shown exceptional efficacy in the inhibition of irinotecan-induced diarrhea without affecting the antitumor effect in preclinical models.

Another recent approach is to target bacterial formyl peptide receptors. Wallace et al. (2018) have discovered the small molecules that selectively block these receptors and, therefore, decelerate the inflammation-mediated carcinogenesis of the colon in murine models. Correspondingly, cancer-related inflammation and tumor growth have also been suppressed in humans using inhibitors of bacterial polyamine transport systems with a modulation in host-microbe metabolic interactions.

The selective depletion of tumor-promoting bacteria with antimicrobial agents is another possible solution. Specific eradication of the *Fusobacterium nucleatum* that induces chemoresistance in CRC by activating autophagy increased the effects of 5-fluorouracil in preclinical models (Yu et al., 2017). These strategies require thorough optimization to prevent the disturbance of useful commensals and, at the same time, without fail eliminating pathogenic species.

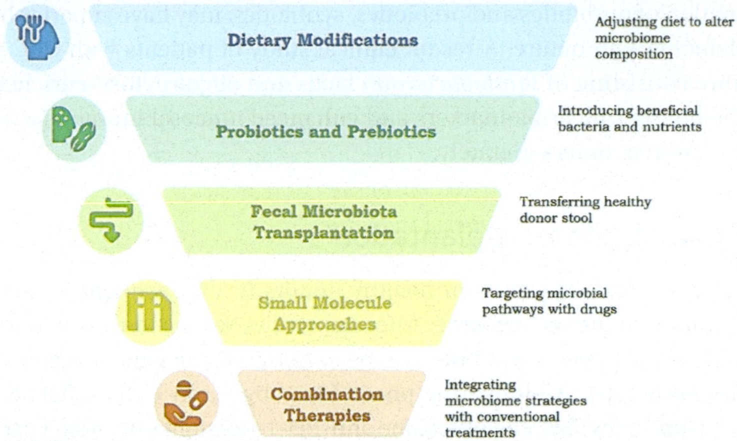

FIGURE 2.2 Microbiome modulation in cancer management. Microbiome modulation in cancer management involves strategically altering the composition and function of the gut and tumor-associated microbiota to enhance therapeutic efficacy, reduce treatment-related toxicity, and improve overall patient outcomes.

2.5.5 Combination approaches with conventional cancer therapies

A microbiome-specific intervention in combination with standard cancer treatments is one of the promising areas in cancer treatment. The addition of probiotics to checkpoint inhibitor immunotherapy has shown a synergistic antitumor effect in preclinical models, increased infiltration of CD8 3 T cells in tumors, and decreased populations of regulatory T-cells (Sivan et al., 2015). There have been positive results in respect to safety and initial signs of efficacy in early-stage clinical trials in melanoma and lung cancer with this approach.

Dietary changes might help improve the effectiveness and reduce the toxicity of chemotherapy by being rational. Intermittent fasting or ketogenic diets given between treatment regimens seem to enhance the delivery to tumors of drugs and safeguard normal tissues in mechanisms that depend on the microbiome. The strategies can be highly beneficial in agents whose therapeutic index is extremely small, and may, perhaps, allow an increase in dose with a reduction in toxicity.

The therapeutic interventions of microbiome modulation in cancer treatment provide five major strategies mentioned in Fig. 2.2 with hierarchical order, namely, dietary modification in response to composition changes, microbial introduction (probiotics and prebiotics) to introduce beneficial microorganisms, comprehensive repair of the microbiome by fecal transplantation, small-molecule-based targeting of microbial pathways, and combination therapies combining microorganism interventions with traditional cancer therapies.

2.6 Methodological approaches and clinical applications

The translation of microbiome studies into clinical implementations is an innovative change in precision oncology. As our insight into the interactions of hosts and microbes in cancer grows, so do the methodological tools used to study these complex interactions and their associated clinical applications.

2.6.1 Advanced technologies in microbiome research

Next-generation sequencing technologies have transformed the microbiome research field and allowed the characterization of microbial communities in a more comprehensive way than ever before. 16S rRNA gene amplicon sequencing has been used extensively as a fundamental technique to give a taxonomic representation of bacterial communities by targeting the amplification of this highly conserved gene. Though it is inexpensive and available, the technique has a low level of resolution of species and strain, where species-specific differences of functional importance to cancer pathophysiology can be observed. To overcome these shortcomings, shotgun metagenomic sequencing has recently gained more popularity, which is able to capture the entire genomic content of microbial communities and allow resolving them at the strain-level and analyzing their functional pathways (Quince et al., 2017).

In addition to genomics, there are also the multiomic technologies that have proved to be potent in the interpretation of the microbiome functionality in cancer. Metatranscriptomics is the active expression of genes, and it gives information about the activity of the microbes and not their presence (Gibson et al., 2017). Metaproteomics and metabolomics go further to describe the protein expression and metabolite production, respectively. Lloyd-Price et al. (2019) showed the strength of combined multiomic analysis with inflammatory bowel disease patients and identified microbial signatures that indicated disease activity and response to treatment, and the results had significant implications for inflammation-related cancer.

Another important development is culturomics, which allows isolating and characterizing previously unculturable microorganisms by the use of specialized growth conditions. The net effect of this has increased our list of cultivable gut microbes by a factor of about 30 to cover more than 70 in recent years. The manipulation of such organisms in laboratories enables mechanistic investigations that are essential in comprehending their role in carcinogenesis and treatment reactions.

More recent spatial technologies can now visualize microbe-host interactions in the tumor microenvironment at subcellular resolution. Fluorescence in situ hybridization (FISH) and multiplexed immunofluorescence have shown the existence of specific microbial niches in colorectal tumors, with certain bacterial colocalizations with immune cell populations-discoveries which have wide implications for the study of local immunomodulation. Likewise, microfluidic models and advanced microfluidics systems offer confined microbiome-cancer interaction studies, which have benefits over more conventional animal models in throughput and human relevance (Williamson et al., 2018).

2.6.2 From bench to bedside: Challenges in clinical translation

Although there have been impressive advancements in the comprehension of the possibility that there is an association between microbiomes and cancer, it has been challenging to apply the knowledge practically in clinical settings. The first one is the vast inter-individual microbiome variation in terms of composition, functionality, and response to interventions. The resulting heterogeneity, which is influenced by genetics, diet, the use of medications, and exposure to the environment, makes it more complex to formulate therapeutic methods that are applicable to everyone (Zmora et al., 2016). Such approaches that consider this variation, such as the design of interventions that are specific to a person and grounded in baseline microbiome features, are opportunities for the future.

Clinical translation is also compromised by methodological inconsistencies in the analysis of microbiomes. Variability arises due to the differences in sample collection, storage, DNA extraction, sequencing platforms, and bioinformatic pipelines, which complicate cross-study comparisons and meta-analyses. The International Human Microbiome Standards Project has achieved significant steps in the direction of the standardization of protocols, but they have not been adopted in full. Similarly, there is also a difficulty in determining causality in microbiome-cancer relationships, and numerous studies have only been done based on correlative findings. To fill this gap, a complex of experimental methods (such as gnotobiotic animal models, transplantation of bacterial strains in a systematic way, and intervention studies with strict controls) is needed (Walter et al., 2020).

The regulatory aspect also presents several complexities whereby microbiome-based therapeutics, in most cases, fail to comply with traditional drug classification systems. Live biotherapeutic products such as characterized bacterial consortia face unique regulatory challenges associated with safety evaluation, stability, and manufacturing reproducibility (O'Toole et al., 2017). Regardless of these challenges, recent FDA approvals of microbiome-based products to treat the use of microbiomes against the infection of *C. difficile* have set precedents that could facilitate the use of microbiomes in oncology in the future.

2.6.3 Current clinical trials and emerging applications

Clinical trials that focus on the microbiome as treatment in oncology have grown exponentially over the past few years, with an extremely broad range of interventions and types of tumor represented. Combination immunotherapy approaches deserve some special consideration in the wake of preclinical findings of microbiome modulation of checkpoint-inhibitor reactions. A Phase 1 trial (NCT03341143) established that FMT based on immunotherapy responders had the ability to overcome resistance in patients with PD-1-refractory melanoma, and clinical response to FMT was associated with positive changes in gut microbial composition. Similar strategies are currently in development in colorectal, lung, and renal-cell carcinoma.

The use of probiotic interventions alongside traditional methods of cancer treatment is another ongoing active field of clinical research. PRIMAGE (NCT03782428) is a trial that is assessing the efficacy of a specified probiotic combination to prevent mucositis caused by chemotherapy in CRC patients; the results of which are encouraging, as both the occurrence and severity of mucositis are observed to decrease (Danis et al., 2022). In addition to controlling the symptoms, other studies like NCT04107168 are exploring the possibility of using particular strains of probiotics to improve chemotherapy efficacy due to the immunomodulatory effects of probiotics.

Dietary interventions on the microbiome, in the treatment of cancer, have also found their way into clinical testing. The PRIME trial (NCT04645680) tests whether a plant-based diet rich in fiber and immunotherapy in patients with advanced melanoma can be improved by modulating the microbiome, and the interim analysis of the project demonstrates that the method shows promising changes in the composition of the gut microbiome and metabolite production. Their attractiveness lies specifically in the fact that such approaches are easy to access, and they can be integrated into standard care practices.

2.6.4 Diagnostic and prognostic biomarker development

The unique patterns of microbiome disturbance in different types of tumors have prompted the desire to pursue microbial signatures as diagnostic and prognostic biomarkers. In lower digestive tract cancer (colorectal cancer), metagenomic classifiers involving the use of the bacterial species, including *Fusobacterium nucleatum, Parvimonas micra,* and others, are sensitive and specific (more than 90%) in the detection of early-stage disease. These strategies would have some possible benefits compared with the traditional screening techniques, such as being noninvasive, low-priced, and even possible early diagnosis.

In addition to diagnosis, microbiome signatures are promising to be prognostic and predictive of treatment response. Peters et al. (2019b) created a microbiome-based classifier that achieved 80% accuracy in predicting immunotherapy outcomes in melanoma patients. Combining the taxonomic characteristics and functional pathways, the classifier was more effective than the conventional biomarkers, including tumor mutational burden and PD-L1 expression. Chemotherapy and radiation therapy have been studied using similar methodologies, which may allow therapeutic decision-making based on microbiome profiles.

Longitudinal monitoring of the microbiome during treatment is an additional source of prognostic data. The clinical deterioration or good responses are often preceded by dramatic changes in diversity and community structure, which is why real-time treatment adjustment is a valuable tool (Derosa et al., 2018). The microbiome data can be combined with other biomarkers, such as tumor genomics and immune parameters, and potentially, this will increase predictive accuracy and clinical utility.

2.6.5 Personalized medicine approaches

The exceptional interindividual differences in the structure and activity of microbiomes are both a challenge to personalized oncology and an opportunity. There is a growing body of evidence indicating that inherent microbiome phenotypes can be used to predict a response to a particular intervention and thus guide rational choice of therapy. As an example, Gopalakrishnan et al. established that patients with melanoma and a high concentration of the species of the genus *Faecalibacterium* responded better to anti-PD-1 therapy than those controlled by the species of the genus *Bacteroidales* (Gopalakrishnan et al., 2018).

The same idea applies to the microbiome-targeted interventions per se, where response to probiotics, prebiotics, and dietary interventions differs based on baseline microbiome characteristics. The idea of microbiome profiling to identify a responder has become a solution in an attempt to optimize the effect of interventions. Moreover, patient-specific nutritional prescriptions based on microbiome specifics can be viewed as a convenient method of microbiome-based interventions that can improve the results of cancer-therapy interventions and reduce their side effects (Kolodziejczyk et al., 2019).

With the development of technologies, more sophisticated personalized techniques are possible. These may include engineered bacterial consortia specific to host and tumor features, tailored prebiotic formulations to achieve selective promotion of desirable commensals, and diet-microbiome-drug interaction models that provide accurate therapeutic remodeling with regard to individual pharmacomicrobiomics.

2.7 Future perspectives

The fast-moving oncology microbiome research specialty is at a critical crossroads, where several fundamental research findings start to be converted into clinical solutions with disruptive potential. The final chapter concepts and directions of research, how microbiome data may be integrated with other omics methods, implications of microbiomes in precision oncology, challenges and opportunities facing this area, and offers a synthesis of the major concepts with a perspective on what will happen in the future. The microbiome may have a major role in mediating the process of cancer, its treatment, and survival, as we learn more about host-microbe interactions in cancer, and this presents new opportunities to intervene at different stages of the cancer-care continuum.

2.7.1 Emerging concepts and research directions

On the horizon of microbiome-oncology studies, several paradigm-shifting ideas are underway. The cancer-microbiome axis is now understood as a two-way process, where tumors shape their microbial community as microbes respond to tumor growth and progression. Specific microbial communities live in different types of tumors, and they have tissue-specific signatures that can potentially regulate local immune responses and metabolic processes. This intertumoral microbiome represents a new aspect to explore with fundamental consequences on the concept of tumor heterogeneity and resistance to treatment.

The microbial biogeography idea of the geographic distribution of microorganisms in body sites and tissues has become prominent with the development of technologies that facilitate site-specific sampling and analysis. There are also discrete microbial niches between different major body compartments and even within single tissues and single tumors, and they form microenvironments that have distinct functional characteristics (Korem et al., 2015). The explanation of these spatial relationships could be the reason behind such phenomena as organ-specific metastatic topography and area differences in treatment response.

New studies have also found microbial dark matter, the neglected parts of the microbiome, such as bacteriophages, fungi, archaea, and protozoa, as important contributors to the biology of cancer. Specifically, the virome has appeared as an important controller of bacterial community form and functionality by predator-prey interactions and horizontal gene transfer. Bacteriophage populations have been shown to experience radical changes throughout colorectal carcinogenesis, which may be used as a preliminary indicator of malignancy (Shkoporov & Hill, 2019). Also, the mycobiome (fungal constituent) regulates inflammation and immune responses pertaining to cancer development, but it is still being studied in its infancy.

One of the boundaries with an immediate clinical impact is the nascent field of pharmacomicrobiomics, which focuses on the effects of the variation or microbiome on the disposition and pharmacodynamic actions of drugs. With respect to drug biotransformation, many significant therapeutic agents have been found through systematic characterization of the metabolic capabilities of intestinal microorganisms, e.g., anticancer agents are bio-transformed by the action of bacterial enzymes through a variety of chemical reactions. A clear understanding of these interactions can potentially clarify confounding inter-individual differences in drug efficacy and toxicity, potentially leading to microbiome-based dosing regimens and the creation of new strategies to overcome undesirable phenomena.

2.7.2 Integration with other "Omics" approaches

The future of microbiome studies in cancer biology depends on their incorporation with other omics systems to attain a global systems-wide view of cancer biology. Multiomic approaches integrating microbiome analyses with genomics, transcriptomics, proteomics, metabolomics, and immunomics offer the best understanding of the intricate interactions between host, microbiome, and tumor. This method has proven effective in inflammatory bowel disease as demonstrated by the work of Lloyd-Price et al. (2019), who combined microbiome, metatranscriptome, proteome, metabolome, and immunome data to identify molecular networks linked to disease activity results that have profound implications in inflammation-related cancer.

Multiomic data integration algorithms are one of the leading fields of development. Machine-learning and artificial-intelligence systems that can identify more complex patterns in non-homogeneous data have been demonstrated to have the potential to extract insights of clinical utility from a high-dimensional dataset. A computational framework designed by Pasolli et al. (2016) involved combining information about metagenomics and metabolomics to identify microbial signatures that correlate with CRC and display greater predictive power than either of the two modalities independently.

The spatial multiomic methods that record the molecular data on a spatial scale are especially promising in understanding microbiome-tumor interactions. Some of the technologies that, when combined with microbiome profiling, may demonstrate the effects of particular bacterial communities on the tumor microenvironment at microscopic scales are spatial transcriptomics and imaging mass spectrometry. Such methods can be used to explain the intratumor heterogeneity of therapeutic response and the pattern of immune infiltration, which have long baffled oncologists.

2.7.3 Implications for precision oncology

The introduction of microbiome science to precision oncology models is a rational move that could lead to the optimization of treatment choice and patient-betterment outcomes. The microbiome profile has the potential to be an effective biomarker that can be used to supplement traditional tumor-genomic and immunophenotypic measures. Gopalakrishnan et al. showed that baseline gut microbiome composition was a stronger predictor of response to ICIs in melanoma patients compared with tumor mutational burden, and microbiome analysis could help to better stratify patients to ICIs (Gopalakrishnan et al., 2018).

In addition to biomarker discovery, microbiome regulation can enhance the action of an already existing treatment with a synergistic effect. The integration of microbiome-targeted interventions with traditional oncologic forms presents a future research direction that can be described as rational. The efficacy of this strategy is supported by preliminary clinical trials that have shown promising outcomes of FMT with checkpoint inhibitors that have been reported in immunotherapy-refractory melanoma patients.

In the future, microbiome-specific interventions that are personalized based on the characteristics of the patient and tumor could be the sole parts of precision oncology. The design of particular diets, probiotic formulations, or engineered bacterial consortia to optimize the therapeutic outcome could be informed by computational models that combine host genetics, microbiome composition, tumor attributes, and environmental exposures (Zeevi et al., 2015). These interventions can be particularly useful in resistance to current treatment and the treatment-related toxicity.

2.7.4 Challenges and opportunities in the field

Although a lot of progress has been made, there are still several obstacles that stall the process of translating microbiome research into clinical practice. The persistent problem is that methodological standardization, because sample collection, processing, sequencing, and analytical workflows differ between studies, makes cross-study comparisons and meta-analyses difficult. Some initiatives like the Microbiome Quality Control Project are significant steps toward the harmonization of protocols, but the complete implementation has not been accomplished (Sinha et al., 2017).

Another milestone challenge is to establish causality in the microbiome-cancer associations. Most of these studies are only correlative, restricting their translational application. Such a gap in knowledge needs complex experimental methods, such as gnotobiotic animal models, transplantation of bacterial strains, and systematically and tightly controlled intervention studies. Walter et al. (2020) suggested a pattern of determining causality in microbiome studies that can be used in subsequent studies and the evidence base for clinical translation.

The regulatory issues are challenges and opportunities because microbiome-based therapeutics are currently moving to clinical application. Such interventions often cannot fit into existing drug classification paradigms, and new ways of assessing safety, proving efficacy, and establishing manufacturing criteria are needed. Recent FDA instructions on live biotherapeutic products and approval of microbiome-based products to treat *C. difficile* infection provide precedents that can be used to enable further oncology uses.

Most importantly, the development of microbiome-based oncology applications will necessitate even more intensive interdisciplinary collaboration between microbiology, immunology, oncology, bioinformatics, and clinical medicine. Research projects and training programs that are made to go beyond traditional disciplinary lines are key investments toward the development of the field. Similarly, the creation of biobanks that can provide standardized samples of the microbiome with detailed clinical information will hasten the identification and confirmation of microbiome-related biomarkers and therapeutic targets.

2.8 Conclusion

The discovery of the microbiome in cancer biology comprises one of the most impactful paradigm shifts in the modern field of oncology, outlining four principles that will guide future research and clinical practice. The microbiome can have a variety of effects on carcinogenesis, such as inflammation, metabolism, immune regulation, and direct genotoxicity, where different types of cancers have unique microbial signatures with potential diagnostic and prognostic applications. On clinical grounds, the microbiome has a significant impact on all primary treatment modalities, including chemotherapy, radiation, and immunotherapy, as an undetected but powerful predictor of treatment success or failure. These understandings have led to microbiome-specific interventions such as dietary changes to design bacterial communities, which make them promising approaches to improve efficacy and reduce adverse outcomes.

It seems that the concept of microbiome science entering the practice of oncology is an ever-growing inevitability as the evidence of clinical significance keeps piling in. Near-term applications are targeted at microbiome profiling to select a treatment option or predict responses, especially in immunotherapy settings where the effects of microbes are well understood, and complementary approaches to optimize the microbiome during therapy are being developed based on current clinical trials. Other, more advanced interventions, such as defined bacterial consortia and engineered probiotics that transfer therapeutic payloads directly to tumors, are longer-term possibilities with transformative potential. However, there are still major barriers to the application of microbiome science in the bedside, which require methodological standardization, causal relationship (not correlation) establishment, and scalable intervention development via long-term research investment and interdisciplinary cooperation.

References

Ahn, J., Sinha, R., Pei, Z., Dominianni, C., Wu, J., Shi, J., Goedert, J. J., Hayes, R. B., & Yang, L. (2013). Human gut microbiome and risk for colorectal cancer. *Journal of the National Cancer Institute, 105*(24), 1907–1911. https://doi.org/10.1093/jnci/djt300.

Alexander, J. L., Wilson, I. D., Teare, J., Marchesi, J. R., Nicholson, J. K., & Kinross, J. M. (2017). Gut microbiota modulation of chemotherapy efficacy and toxicity. *Nature Reviews. Gastroenterology & Hepatology, 14*(6), 356–365. https://doi.org/10.1038/nrgastro.2017.20.

Allen, J. M., Mailing, L. J., Niemiro, G. M., Moore, R., Cook, M. D., White, B. A., Holscher, H. D., & Woods, J. A. (2018). Exercise alters gut microbiota composition and function in lean and obese humans. *Medicine and Science in Sports and Exercise, 50*(4), 747–757. https://doi.org/10.1249/MSS.0000000000001495.

Attene-Ramos, M. S., Wagner, E. D., Plewa, M. J., & Rex Gaskins, H. (2006). Evidence that hydrogen sulfide is a genotoxic agent. *Molecular Cancer Research: MCR, 4*(1), 9–14.

Bullman, S., Pedamallu, C. S., Sicinska, E., Clancy, T. E., Zhang, X., Cai, D., Neuberg, D., Huang, K., Guevara, F., Nelson, T., Chipashvili, O., Hagan, T., Walker, M., Ramachandran, A., Diosdado, B., Serna, G., Mulet, N., Landolfi, S., Ramon Y Cajal, S., … Meyerson, M. (2017). Persistence and antibiotic response in colorectal cancer. *Science (New York, N.Y.), 358*(6369), 1443–1448. https://doi.org/10.1126/science.aal5240.

Byndloss, M. X., Olsan, E. E., Rivera-Chávez, F., Tiffany, C. R., Cevallos, S. A., Lokken, K. L., Torres, T. P., Byndloss, A. J., Faber, F., Gao, Y., Litvak, Y., Lopez, C. A., Xu, G., Napoli, E., Giulivi, C., Tsolis, R. M., Revzin, A., Lebrilla, C. B., & Bäumler, A. J. (2017). Microbiota-activated PPAR-γ signaling inhibits dysbiotic Enterobacteriaceae expansion. *Science (New York, N.Y.), 357*(6351), 570–575. https://doi.org/10.1126/science.aam9949.

Cavarretta, I., Ferrarese, R., Cazzaniga, W., Saita, D., Lucianò, R., Ceresola, E. R., Locatelli, I., Visconti, L., Lavorgna, G., Briganti, A., Nebuloni, M., Doglioni, C., Clementi, M., Montorsi, F., Canducci, F., & Salonia, A. (2017). The microbiome of the prostate tumor microenvironment. *European Urology, 72*(4), 625–631.

Coker, O. O., Dai, Z., Nie, Y., Zhao, G., Cao, L., Nakatsu, G., Wu, W. K., Wong, S. H., Chen, Z., Sung, J. J. Y., & Yu, J. (2018). Mucosal microbiome dysbiosis in gastric carcinogenesis. *Gut, 67*(6), 1024–1032. https://doi.org/10.1136/gutjnl-2017-314281.

Colibactin Causes Colorectal Cancer-Associated Mutational Signature. Cancer Discovery. 2020 10(5):635. https://doi.org/10.1158/2159-8290.CD-RW2020-037.

Danis, R., Mego, M., Antonova, M., Stepanova, R., Svobodnik, A., Hejnova, R., & Wawruch, M. (2022). Orally administered probiotics in the prevention of chemotherapy (± radiotherapy)-induced gastrointestinal toxicity: A systematic review with meta-analysis of randomized trials. *Integrative Cancer Therapies, 21*. https://doi.org/10.1177/15347354221144309.

Dapito, D. H., Mencin, A., Gwak, G.-Y., Pradere, J.-P., Jang, M.-K., Mederacke, I., Caviglia, J. M., Khiabanian, H., Adeyemi, A., Bataller, R., Lefkowitch, J. H., Bower, M., Friedman, R., Sartor, R. B., Rabadan, R., & Schwabe, R. F. (2012). Promotion of hepatocellular carcinoma by the intestinal microbiota and TLR4. *Cancer Cell, 21*(4), 504–516. https://doi.org/10.1016/j.ccr.2012.02.007.

Davar, D., Dzutsev, A. K., McCulloch, J. A., Rodrigues, R. R., Chauvin, J.-M., Morrison, R. M., Deblasio, R. N., Menna, C., Ding, Q., Pagliano, O., Zidi, B., Zhang, S., Badger, J. H., Vetizou, M., Cole, A. M., Fernandes, M. R., Prescott, S., Costa, R. G. F., Balaji, A. K., … Zarour, H. M. (2021). Fecal microbiota transplant overcomes resistance to anti-PD-1 therapy in melanoma patients. *Science (New York, N.Y.), 371*(6529), 595–602. https://doi.org/10.1126/science.abf3363.

Derosa, L., Hellmann, M. D., Spaziano, M., Halpenny, D., Fidelle, M., Rizvi, H., Long, N., Plodkowski, A. J., Arbour, K. C., Chaft, J. E., Rouche, J. A., Zitvogel, L., Zalcman, G., Albiges, L., Escudier, B., & Routy, B. (2018). Negative association of antibiotics on clinical activity of immune checkpoint inhibitors in patients with advanced renal cell and non-small-cell lung cancer. *Annals of Oncology, 29*(6), 1437–1444. https://doi.org/10.1093/annonc/mdy103.

Dickson, R. P., Erb-Downward, J. R., Martinez, F. J., & Huffnagle, G. B. (2016). The microbiome and the respiratory tract. *Annual Review of Physiology, 78*, 481–504. https://doi.org/10.1146/annurev-physiol-021115-105238.

Donaldson, G. P., Lee, S. M., & Mazmanian, S. K. (2016). Gut biogeography of the bacterial microbiota. *Nature Reviews. Microbiology., 14*(1), 20–32. https://doi.org/10.1038/nrmicro3552.

Dzutsev, A., Badger, J. H., Perez-Chanona, E., Roy, S., Salcedo, R., Smith, C. K., & Trinchieri, G. (2017). Microbes and cancer. *Annual Review of Immunology, 35*, 199–228. https://doi.org/10.1146/annurev-immunol-051116-052133.

Elinav, E., Nowarski, R., Thaiss, C. A., Hu, B., Jin, C., & Flavell, R. A. (2013). Inflammation-induced cancer: Crosstalk between tumours, immune cells and microorganisms. *Nature reviews. Cancer., 13*(11), 759–771. https://doi.org/10.1038/nrc3611.

Feng, Q., Liang, S., Jia, H., Stadlmayr, A., Tang, L., Lan, Z., Zhang, D., Xia, H., Xu, X., Jie, Z., Su, L., Li, X., Li, X., Li, J., Xiao, L., Huber-Schönauer, U., Niederseer, D., Xu, X., Yousuf Al-Aama, J., … Wang, J. (2015). Gut microbiome development along the colorectal adenoma-carcinoma sequence. *Nature Communications, 6.* https://doi.org/10.1038/ncomms7528.

Gagnaire, A., Nadel, B., Raoult, D., Neefjes, J., & Gorvel, J.-P. (2017). Collateral damage: Insights into bacterial mechanisms that predispose host cells to cancer. *Nature Reviews. Microbiology., 15*(2), 109–128. https://doi.org/10.1038/nrmicro.2016.171.

Gaiser, R. A., Halimi, A., Alkharaan, H., Lu, L., Davanian, H., Healy, K., Hugerth, L. W., Ateeb, Z., Valente, R., Moro, C. F., Chiaro, M. D., & Chen, M. S. (2019). Enrichment of oral microbiota in early cystic precursors to invasive pancreatic cancer. *Gut, 68*(12), 2186–2194. https://doi.org/10.1136/gutjnl-2018-317458.

Garcia-Mantrana, I., Selma-Royo, M., Alcantara, C., & Collado, M. C. (2018). Shifts on gut microbiota associated to Mediterranean diet adherence and specific dietary intakes on general adult population. *Frontiers in Microbiology, 9.* https://doi.org/10.3389/fmicb.2018.00890.

Geller, L. T., Barzily-Rokni, M., Danino, T., Jonas, O. H., Shental, N., Nejman, D., Gavert, N., Zwang, Y., Cooper, Z. A., Shee, K., Thaiss, C. A., Reuben, A., Livny, J., Avraham, R., Frederick, D. T., Ligorio, M., Chatman, K., Johnston, S. E., Mosher, C. M., … Straussman, R. (2017). Potential role of intratumor bacteria in mediating tumor resistance to the chemotherapeutic drug gemcitabine. *Science (New York, N.Y.), 357*(6356), 1156–1160. https://doi.org/10.1126/science.aah5043.

Gensollen, T., Iyer, S. S., Kasper, D. L., & Blumberg, R. S. (2016). How colonization by microbiota in early life shapes the immune system. *Science (New York, N.Y.), 352*(6285), 539–544. https://doi.org/10.1126/science.aad9378.

Gibson, G. R., Hutkins, R., Sanders, M. E., Prescott, S. L., Reimer, R. A., Salminen, S. J., Scott, K., Stanton, C., Swanson, K. S., Cani, P. D., Verbeke, K., & Reid, G. (2017). Expert consensus document: The International Scientific Association for Probiotics and Prebiotics (ISAPP) consensus statement on the definition and scope of prebiotics. *Nature Reviews. Gastroenterology & Hepatology, 14*(8), 491–502. https://doi.org/10.1038/nrgastro.2017.75.

Gopalakrishnan, V., et al. (2018). Gut microbiome modulates response to anti–PD-1 immunotherapy in melanoma patients. *Science, 359*, 97–103. https://doi.org/10.1126/science.aan4236.

Grivennikov, S. I., Greten, F. R., & Karin, M. (2010). Immunity, inflammation, and cancer. *Cell, 140*(6), 883–899. https://doi.org/10.1016/j.cell.2010.01.025.

Gui, Q.-F., Lu, H.-F., Zhang, C.-X., Xu, Z.-R., & Yang, Y.-H. (2015). Well-balanced commensal microbiota contributes to anti-cancer response in a lung cancer mouse model. *Genetics and Molecular Research: GMR, 14*(2), 5642–5651. https://doi.org/10.4238/2015.May.25.16.

Gur, C., Ibrahim, Y., Isaacson, B., Yamin, R., Abed, J., Gamliel, M., Enk, J., Bar-On, Y., Stanietsky-Kaynan, N., Coppenhagen-Glazer, S., Shussman, N., Almogy, G., Cuapio, A., Hofer, E., Mevorach, D., Tabib, A., Ortenberg, R., Markel, G., Miklić, K., … Mandelboim, O. (2015). Binding of the Fap2 protein of *Fusobacterium nucleatum* to human inhibitory receptor TIGIT protects tumors from immune cell attack. *Immunity, 42*(2), 344–355. https://doi.org/10.1016/j.immuni.2015.01.010.

Hibberd, A. A., Lyra, A., Ouwehand, A. C., Rolny, P., Lindegren, H., Cedgård, L., & Wettergren, Y. (2017). Intestinal microbiota is altered in patients with colon cancer and modified by probiotic intervention. *BMJ Open Gastroenterology, 4*(1). https://doi.org/10.1136/bmjgast-2017-000145.

Hieken, T. J., Chen, J., Hoskin, T. L., Walther-Antonio, M., Johnson, S., Ramaker, S., Xiao, J., Radisky, D. C., Knutson, K. L., Kalari, K. R., Yao, J. Z., Baddour, L. M., Chia, N., & Degnim, A. C. (2016). The microbiome of aseptically collected human breast tissue in benign and malignant disease. *Scientific Reports, 6.* https://doi.org/10.1038/srep30751.

Iida, N., Dzutsev, A., Andrew Stewart, C., Smith, L., Bouladoux, N., Weingarten, R. A., Molina, D. A., Salcedo, R., Back, T., Cramer, S., Dai, R.-M., Kiu, H., Cardone, M., Naik, S., Patri, A. K., Wang, E., Marincola, F. M., Frank, K. M., Belkaid, Y., … Goldszmid, R. S. (2013). Commensal bacteria control cancer response to therapy by modulating the tumor microenvironment. *Science (New York, N.Y.), 342*(6161), 967–970. https://doi.org/10.1126/science.1240527.

Irrazábal, T., Belcheva, A., Girardin, S. E., Martin, A., & Philpott, D. J. (2014). The multifaceted role of the intestinal microbiota in colon cancer. *Molecular Cell, 54*(2), 309–320.

Junaid, M., Khine Linn, A., Bagher Javadi, M., Al-Gubare, S., Ali, N., & Katzenmeier, G. (2016). Vacuolating cytotoxin A (VacA) - A multi-talented pore-forming toxin from *Helicobacter pylori. Toxicon: Official Journal of the International Society on Toxinology, 118*, 27–35.

Knight, R., Vrbanac, A., Taylor, B. C., Aksenov, A., Callewaert, C., Debelius, J., Gonzalez, A., Kosciolek, T., McCall, L.-I., McDonald, D., Melnik, A. V., Morton, J. T., Navas, J., Quinn, R. A., Sanders, J. G., Swafford, A. D., Thompson, L. R., Tripathi, A., Xu, Z. Z., … Dorrestein, P. C. (2018). Best practices for analysing microbiomes. *Nature Reviews. Microbiology., 16*(7), 410–422. https://doi.org/10.1038/s41579-018-0029-9.

Koh, A., De Vadder, F., Kovatcheva-Datchary, P., & Bäckhed, F. (2016). From dietary fiber to host physiology: Short-chain fatty acids as key bacterial metabolites. *Cell, 165*(6), 1332–1345.

Kolodziejczyk, A. A., Zheng, D., & Elinav, E. (2019). Diet-microbiota interactions and personalized nutrition. *Nature Reviews. Microbiology., 17*(12), 742–753. https://doi.org/10.1038/s41579-019-0256-8.

Korem, T., Zeevi, D., Suez, J., Weinberger, A., Avnit-Sagi, T., Pompan-Lotan, M., Matot, E., Jona, G., Harmelin, A., Cohen, N., Sirota-Madi, A., Thaiss, C. A., Pevsner-Fischer, M., Sorek, R., Xavier, R. J., Elinav, E., & Segal, E. (2015). Growth dynamics of gut microbiota in health and disease inferred from single metagenomic samples. *Science, 349*(6252), 1101–1106. https://doi.org/10.1126/science.aac4812.

Kwa, M., Plottel, C. S., Blaser, M. J., & Adams, S. (2016). The intestinal microbiome and estrogen receptor-positive female breast cancer. *Journal of the National Cancer Institute, 108*(8). https://doi.org/10.1093/jnci/djw029.

Lee, S. H., Sung, J. Y., Yong, D., Chun, J., Kim, S. Y., Song, J. H., Chung, K. S., Kim, E. Y., Jung, J. Y., Kang, Y. A., Kim, Y. S., Kim, S. K., Chang, J., & Park, M. S. (2016). Characterization of microbiome in bronchoalveolar lavage fluid of patients with lung cancer comparing with benign mass like lesions. *Lung Cancer, 102*, 89–95. https://doi.org/10.1016/j.lungcan.2016.10.016.

Levy, M., Kolodziejczyk, A. A., Thaiss, C. A., & Elinav, E. (2017). Dysbiosis and the immune system. *Nature Reviews. Immunology., 17*(4), 219–232. https://doi.org/10.1038/nri.2017.7.

Lloyd-Price, J., Arze, C., Ananthakrishnan, A. N., Schirmer, M., Avila-Pacheco, J., Poon, T. W., Andrews, E., Ajami, N. J., Bonham, K. S., Brislawn, C. J., Casero, D., Courtney, H., Gonzalez, A., Graeber, T. G., Hall, A. B., Lake, K., Landers, C. J., Mallick, H., Plichta, D. R., … Huttenhower, C. (2019). Multi-omics of the gut microbial ecosystem in inflammatory bowel diseases. *Nature, 569*(7758), 655–662. https://doi.org/10.1038/s41586-019-1237-9.

Louis, P., Hold, G. L., & Flint, H. J. (2014). The gut microbiota, bacterial metabolites and colorectal cancer. *Nature Reviews. Microbiology., 12*(10), 661–672. https://doi.org/10.1038/nrmicro3344.

Maeda, M., Moro, H., & Ushijima, T. (2017). Mechanisms for the induction of gastric cancer by *Helicobacter pylori* infection: Aberrant DNA methylation pathway. *Gastric Cancer: Official Journal of the International Gastric Cancer Association and the Japanese Gastric Cancer Association, 20*(Suppl 1), 8–15. https://doi.org/10.1007/s10120-016-0650-0.

Marchesi, J. R., & Ravel, J. (2025). The vocabulary of microbiome research: A proposal. *Microbiome, 31*(1), 1–3. https://doi.org/10.1186/s40168-015-0094-5.

Matson, V., Fessler, J., Bao, R., Chongsuwat, T., Zha, Y., Alegre, M.-L., Luke, J. J., & Gajewski, T. F. (2018). The commensal microbiome is associated with anti-PD-1 efficacy in metastatic melanoma patients. *Science (New York, N.Y.), 359*(6371), 104–108. https://doi.org/10.1126/science.aao3290.

McBride, A. A. (2022). Human papillomaviruses: Diversity, infection and host interactions. *Nature Reviews. Microbiology., 20*(2), 95–108. https://doi.org/10.1038/s41579-021-00617-5.

Nejman, D., Livyatan, I., Fuks, G., Gavert, N., Zwang, Y., Geller, L. T., Rotter-Maskowitz, A., Weiser, R., Mallel, G., Gigi, E., Meltser, A., Douglas, G. M., Kamer, I., Gopalakrishnan, V., Dadosh, T., Levin-Zaidman, S., Avnet, S., Atlan, T., Cooper, Z. A., … Straussman, R. (2020). The human tumor microbiome is composed of tumor type-specific intracellular bacteria. *Science (New York, N.Y.), 368*(6494), 973–980. https://doi.org/10.1126/science.aay9189.

O'Toole, P. W., Marchesi, J. R., & Hill, C. (2017). Next-generation probiotics: The spectrum from probiotics to live biotherapeutics. *Nature Microbiology, 2*. https://doi.org/10.1038/nmicrobiol.2017.57.

Pasolli, E., Truong, D. T., Malik, F., Waldron, L., & Segata, N. (2016). Machine learning meta-analysis of large metagenomic datasets: Tools and biological insights. *PLoS Computational Biology, 12*(7). https://doi.org/10.1371/journal.pcbi.1004977.

Peters, B. A., Wilson, M., Moran, U., Pavlick, A., Izsak, A., Wechter, T., Weber, J. S., Osman, I., & Ahn, J. (2019a). Relating the gut metagenome and metatranscriptome to immunotherapy responses in melanoma patients. *Genome Medicine, 11*(1). https://doi.org/10.1186/s13073-019-0672-4.

Peters, B. A., Hayes, R. B., Goparaju, C., Reid, C., Pass, H. I., & Ahn, J. (2019b). The microbiome in lung cancer tissue and recurrence-free survival. *Cancer Epidemiology, Biomarkers & Prevention: A Publication of the American Association for Cancer Research, Cosponsored by the American Society of Preventive Oncology, 28*(4), 731–740. https://doi.org/10.1158/1055-9965.EPI-18-0966.

Pickard, J. M., Zeng, M. Y., Caruso, R., & Núñez, G. (2017). Gut microbiota: Role in pathogen colonization, immune responses, and inflammatory disease. *Immunological Reviews, 279*(1), 70–89. https://doi.org/10.1111/imr.12567.

Pinato, D. J., Howlett, S., Ottaviani, D., Urus, H., Patel, A., Mineo, T., Brock, C., Power, D., Hatcher, O., Falconer, A., Ingle, M., Brown, A., Gujral, D., Partridge, S., Sarwar, N., Gonzalez, M., Bendle, M., Lewanski, C., Newsom-Davis, T., … Bower, M. (2019). Association of prior antibiotic treatment with survival and response to immune checkpoint inhibitor therapy in patients with cancer. *JAMA Oncology, 5*(12), 1774–1778. https://doi.org/10.1001/jamaoncol.2019.2785.

Quince, C., Walker, A. W., Simpson, J. T., Loman, N. J., & Segata, N. (2017). Shotgun metagenomics, from sampling to analysis. *Nature Biotechnology, 35*(9), 833–844. https://doi.org/10.1038/nbt.3935.

Ren, Z., Jiang, J., Xie, H., Li, A., Lu, H., Xu, S., Zhou, L., Zhang, H., Cui, G., Chen, X., Liu, Y., Wu, L., Qin, N., Sun, R., Wang, W., Li, L., Wang, W., & Zheng, S. (2017). Gut microbial profile analysis by MiSeq sequencing of pancreatic carcinoma patients in China. *Oncotarget, 8*(56), 95176–95191. https://doi.org/10.18632/oncotarget.18820.

Ren, Z., Li, A., Jiang, J., Zhou, L., Yu, Z., Lu, H., Xie, H., Chen, X., Shao, L., Zhang, R., Xu, S., Zhang, H., Cui, G., Chen, X., Sun, R., Wen, H., Lerut, J. P., Kan, Q., Li, L., & Zheng, S. (2019). Gut microbiome analysis as a tool towards targeted non-invasive biomarkers for early hepatocellular carcinoma. *Gut, 68*(6), 1014–1023. https://doi.org/10.1136/gutjnl-2017-315084.

Ridlon, J. M., Wolf, P. G., & Rex Gaskins, H. (2016). Taurocholic acid metabolism by gut microbes and colon cancer. *Gut Microbes, 7*(3), 201–215. https://doi.org/10.1080/19490976.2016.1150414.

Robinson, K. M., Crabtree, J., Mattick, J. S. A., Anderson, K. E., & Hotopp, J. C. D. (2017). Distinguishing potential bacteria-tumor associations from contamination in a secondary data analysis of public cancer genome sequence data. *Microbiome, 5*(1). https://doi.org/10.1186/s40168-016-0224-8.

Routy, B., Chatelier, E. L., Derosa, L., Duong, C. P. M., Alou, M. T., Daillère, R., Fluckiger, A., Messaoudene, M., Rauber, C., Roberti, M. P., Fidelle, M., Flament, C., Poirier-Colame, V., Opolon, P., Klein, C., Iribarren, K., Mondragón, L., Jacquelot, N., Qu, B., … Zitvogel, L. (2018). Gut microbiome influences efficacy of PD-1-based immunotherapy against epithelial tumors. *Science (New York, N.Y.), 359*(6371), 91–97. https://doi.org/10.1126/science.aan3706.

Rubinstein, M. R., Wang, X., Liu, W., Hao, Y., Cai, G., & Han, Y. W. (2013). *Fusobacterium nucleatum* promotes colorectal carcinogenesis by modulating E-cadherin/β-catenin signaling via its FadA adhesin. *Cell Host & Microbe, 14*(2), 195–206. https://doi.org/10.1016/j.chom.2013.07.012.

Schirmer, M., Smeekens, S. P., Vlamakis, H., Jaeger, M., Oosting, M., Franzosa, E. A., Horst, R. T., Jansen, T., Jacobs, L., Bonder, M. J., Kurilshikov, A., Fu, J., Joosten, L. A. B., Zhernakova, A., Huttenhower, C., Wijmenga, C., Netea, M. G., & Xavier, R. J. (2016). Linking the human gut microbiome to inflammatory cytokine production capacity. *Cell, 167*(4).

Scott, T. A., Quintaneiro, L. M., Norvaisas, P., Lui, P. P., Wilson, M. P., Leung, K.-Y., Herrera-Dominguez, L., Sudiwala, S., Pessia, A., Clayton, P. T., Bryson, K., Velagapudi, V., Mills, P. B., Typas, A., Greene, N. D. E., & Cabreiro, F. (2017). Host-microbe co-metabolism dictates cancer drug efficacy in *C. elegans*. *Cell, 169*(3).

Seitz, H. K., & Stickel, F. (2007). Molecular mechanisms of alcohol-mediated carcinogenesis. *Nature Reviews. Cancer., 7*(8), 599–612.

Sekirov, I., Russell, S. L., Caetano M Antunes, L., & Brett Finlay, B. (2010). Gut microbiota in health and disease. *Physiological Reviews, 90*(3), 859–904. https://doi.org/10.1152/physrev.00045.2009.

Sender, R., Fuchs, S., & Milo, R. (2016). Revised estimates for the number of human and bacteria cells in the body. *PLoS Biology, 14*(8). https://doi.org/10.1371/journal.pbio.1002533.

Sepich-Poore, G. D., Zitvogel, L., Straussman, R., Hasty, J., Wargo, J. A., & Knight, R. (2021). The microbiome and human cancer. *Science, 371*(6536). https://doi.org/10.1126/science.abc4552.

Shkoporov, A. N., & Hill, C. (2019). Bacteriophages of the human gut: The "Known Unknown" of the microbiome. *Cell Host & Microbe, 25*(2), 195–209.

Singh, R. K., Chang, H.-W., Yan, D., Lee, K. M., Ucmak, D., Wong, K., Abrouk, M., Farahnik, B., Nakamura, M., Zhu, T. H., Bhutani, T., & Liao, W. (2017). Influence of diet on the gut microbiome and implications for human health. *Journal of Translational Medicine, 15*(1). https://doi.org/10.1186/s12967-017-1175-y.

Sinha, R., Abu-Ali, G., Vogtmann, E., Fodor, A. A., Ren, B., Amir, A., Schwager, E., Crabtree, J., Ma, S., Abnet, C. C., Knight, R., White, O., & Huttenhower, C. (2017). Assessment of variation in microbial community amplicon sequencing by the Microbiome Quality Control (MBQC) project consortium. *Nature Biotechnology, 35*(11), 1077–1086. https://doi.org/10.1038/nbt.3981.

Sivan, A., Corrales, L., Hubert, N., Williams, J. B., Aquino-Michaels, K., Earley, Z. M., Benyamin, F. W., Lei, Y. M., Jabri, B., Alegre, M. L., Chang, E. B., & Gajewski, T. F. (2015). Commensal *Bifidobacterium* promotes antitumor immunity and facilitates anti-PD-L1 efficacy. *Science, 350*(6264), 1084–1089. https://doi.org/10.1126/science.aac4255.

Taur, Y., Jenq, R. R., Perales, M.-A., Littmann, E. R., Morjaria, S., Ling, L., No, D., Gobourne, A., Viale, A., Dahi, P. B., Ponce, D. M., Barker, J. N., Giralt, S., Brink, M., & Pamer, E. G. (2014). The effects of intestinal tract bacterial diversity on mortality following allogeneic hematopoietic stem cell transplantation. *Blood, 124*(7), 1174–1182. https://doi.org/10.1182/blood-2014-02-554725.

Thaiss, C. A., Zmora, N., Levy, M., & Elinav, E. (2016). The microbiome and innate immunity. *Nature, 535*(7610), 65–74. https://doi.org/10.1038/nature18847.

Orberg, E. T., Fan, H., Tam, A. J., Dejea, C. M., Destefano Shields, C. E., Wu, S., Chung, L., Finard, B. B., Wu, X., Fathi, P., Ganguly, S., Fu, J., Pardoll, D. M., Sears, C. L., & Housseau, F. (2017). The myeloid immune signature of enterotoxigenic *Bacteroides fragilis*-induced murine colon tumorigenesis. *Mucosal Immunology, 10*(2), 421–433. https://doi.org/10.1038/mi.2016.53.

Touchefeu, Y., Montassier, E., Nieman, K., Gastinne, T., Potel, G., Bruley des Varannes, S., Le Vacon, F., & de La Cochetière, M. F. (2014). Systematic review: The role of the gut microbiota in chemotherapy- or radiation-induced gastrointestinal mucositis – Current evidence and potential clinical applications. *Alimentary Pharmacology & Therapeutics, 40*(5), 409–421. https://doi.org/10.1111/apt.12878.

Tsay, J.-C. J., Wu, B. G., Badri, M. H., Clemente, J. C., Shen, N., Meyn, P., Li, Y., Yie, T.-A., Lhakhang, T., Olsen, E., Murthy, V., Michaud, G., Sulaiman, I., Tsirigos, A., Heguy, A., Pass, H., Weiden, M. D., Rom, W. N., Sterman, D. H., … Segal, L. N. (2018). Airway microbiota is associated with upregulation of the PI3K pathway in lung cancer. *American Journal of Respiratory and Critical Care Medicine, 198*(9), 1188–1198. https://doi.org/10.1164/rccm.201710-2118OC.

Wallace, B. D., Wang, H., Lane, K. T., Scott, J. E., Orans, J., Koo, J. S., Venkatesh, M., Jobin, C., Yeh, L.-A., Mani, S., & Redinbo, M. R. (2010). Alleviating cancer drug toxicity by inhibiting a bacterial enzyme. *Science (New York, N.Y.), 330*(6005), 831–835. https://doi.org/10.1126/science.1191175.

Wallace, J. L., Motta, J.-P., & Buret, A. G. (2018). Hydrogen sulfide: An agent of stability at the microbiome-mucosa interface. *American Journal of Physiology. Gastrointestinal and Liver Physiology, 314*(2). https://doi.org/10.1152/ajpgi.00249.2017.

Walter, J., Armet, A. M., Brett Finlay, B., & Shanahan, F. (2020). Establishing or exaggerating causality for the gut microbiome: Lessons from human microbiota-associated rodents. *Cell, 180*(2), 221–232.

Wang, Y., Deng, H., Li, Z., Tan, Y., Han, Y., Wang, X., Du, Z., Liu, Y., Yang, R., Bai, Y., Bi, Y., & Zhi, F. (2017). Safety evaluation of a novel strain of *Bacteroides fragilis. Frontiers in Microbiology, 8.* https://doi.org/10.3389/fmicb.2017.00435.

Wang, Y., Wiesnoski, D. H., Helmink, B. A., Gopalakrishnan, V., Choi, K., DuPont, H. L., Jiang, Z.-D., Abu-Sbeih, H., Sanchez, C. A., Chang, C.-C., Parra, E. R., Francisco-Cruz, A., Raju, G. S., Stroehlein, J. R., Campbell, M. T., Gao, J., Subudhi, S. K., Maru, D. M., Blando, J. M., … Jenq, R. R. (2018). Fecal microbiota transplantation for refractory immune checkpoint inhibitor-associated colitis. *Nature Medicine, 24*(12), 1804–1808. https://doi.org/10.1038/s41591-018-0238-9.

Williamson, I. A., Arnold, J. W., Samsa, L. A., Gaynor, L., DiSalvo, M., Cocchiaro, J. L., Carroll, I., Andrea Azcarate-Peril, M., Rawls, J. F., Allbritton, N. L., & Magness, S. T. (2018). A high-throughput organoid microinjection platform to study gastrointestinal microbiota and luminal physiology. *Cellular and Molecular Gastroenterology and Hepatology, 6*(3), 301–319. https://doi.org/10.1016/j.jcmgh.2018.05.004.

Wilson, M. R., Jiang, Y., Villalta, P. W., Stornetta, A., Boudreau, P. D., Carrá, A., Brennan, C. A., Chun, E., Ngo, L., Samson, L. D., Engelward, B. P., Garrett, W. S., Balbo, S., & Balskus, E. P. (2019). The human gut bacterial genotoxin colibactin alkylates DNA. *Science, 363*(6428). https://doi.org/10.1126/science.aar7785.

Wirbel, J., Pyl, P. T., Kartal, E., Zych, K., Kashani, A., Milanese, A., Fleck, J. S., Voigt, A. Y., Palleja, A., Ponnudurai, R., Sunagawa, S., Coelho, L. P., Schrotz-King, P., Vogtmann, E., Habermann, N., Niméus, E., Thomas, A. M., Manghi, P., Gandini, S., … Zeller, G. (2019). Meta-analysis of fecal metagenomes reveals global microbial signatures that are specific for colorectal cancer. *Nature Medicine, 25*(4), 679–689. https://doi.org/10.1038/s41591-019-0406-6.

Wong, S. H., & Yu, J. (2019). Gut microbiota in colorectal cancer: Mechanisms of action and clinical applications. *Nature Reviews. Gastroenterology & Hepatology, 16*(11), 690–704. https://doi.org/10.1038/s41575-019-0209-8.

Wu, S., Rhee, K.-J., Albesiano, E., Rabizadeh, S., Wu, X., Yen, H.-R., Huso, D. L., Brancati, F. L., Wick, E., McAllister, F., Housseau, F., Pardoll, D. M., & Sears, C. L. (2009). A human colonic commensal promotes colon tumorigenesis via activation of T helper type 17 T cell responses. *Nature Medicine, 15*(9), 1016–1022. https://doi.org/10.1038/nm.2015.

Yu, T. C., Guo, F., Yu, Y., Sun, T., Ma, D., Han, J., Qian, Y., Kryczek, I., Sun, D., Nagarsheth, N., Chen, Y., Chen, H., Hong, J., Zou, W., & Fang, J.-Y. (2017). *Fusobacterium nucleatum* promotes chemoresistance to colorectal cancer by modulating autophagy. *Cell., 170*(3).

Zeevi, D., Korem, T., Zmora, N., Israeli, D., Rothschild, D., Weinberger, A., Ben-Yacov, O., Lador, D., Avnit-Sagi, T., Lotan-Pompan, M., Suez, J., Mahdi, J. A., Matot, E., Malka, G., Kosower, N., Rein, M., Zilberman-Schapira, G., Dohnalová, L., Pevsner-Fischer, M., … Segal, E. (2015). Personalized nutrition by prediction of glycemic responses. *Cell, 163*(5), 1079–1094.

Zeller, G., Tap, J., Voigt, A. Y., Sunagawa, S., Kultima, J. R., Costea, P. I., Amiot, A., Böhm, J., Brunetti, F., Habermann, N., Hercog, R., Koch, M., Luciani, A., Mende, D. R., Schneider, M. A., Schrotz-King, P., Tournigand, C., Nhieu, J. T. V., Yamada, T., … Bork, P. (2014). Potential of fecal microbiota for early-stage detection of colorectal cancer. *Molecular Systems Biology, 10*(11). https://doi.org/10.15252/msb.20145645.

Zhang, S., Yang, Y., Weng, W., Guo, B., Cai, G., Ma, Y., & Cai, S. (2019). *Fusobacterium nucleatum* promotes chemoresistance to 5-fluorouracil by upregulation of BIRC3 expression in colorectal cancer. *Journal of Experimental & Clinical Cancer Research: CR, 38*(1). https://doi.org/10.1186/s13046-018-0985-y.

Zitvogel, L., Daillère, R., Roberti, M. P., Routy, B., & Kroemer, G. (2017). Anticancer effects of the microbiome and its products. *Nature Reviews. Microbiology., 15*(8), 465–478. https://doi.org/10.1038/nrmicro.2017.44.

Zitvogel, L., Ma, Y., Raoult, D., Kroemer, G., & Gajewski, T. F. (2018). The microbiome in cancer immunotherapy: Diagnostic tools and therapeutic strategies. *Science (New York, N.Y.), 359*(6382), 1366–1370. https://doi.org/10.1126/science.aar6918.

Zmora, N., Zeevi, D., Korem, T., Segal, E., & Elinav, E. (2016). Taking it personally: Personalized utilization of the human microbiome in health and disease. *Cell Host & Microbe, 19*(1), 12–20.

3

Microbiome dynamics in cancer treatment: Impact of chemotherapy on the microbiome

Akash Malik[a], Neelima Byahut[a], Deepika Dwivedi[a], Raj Kishor Sharma[b] and Meenakshi Sharma[a]

[a]DR. B.R. AMBEDKAR CENTER FOR BIOMEDICAL RESEARCH (ACBR), UNIVERSITY OF DELHI, DELHI, INDIA [b]DEPARTMENT OF CHEMISTRY, UNIVERSITY OF DELHI, DELHI, INDIA

3.1 Introduction

The human microbiome, which consists of trillions of microorganisms, such as bacteria, viruses, fungi, and archaea, is currently recognized as an integral part of the human physiological landscape and is no longer regarded as just a mere assembly of commensals. The microbial populations can be found on almost every surface of the human body, including the skin, oral, respiratory, and genitourinary tracts. Of these, the gastrointestinal (GI) tract is home to the most dense and active microbial community. In particular, the role of the gut microbiota has been the subject of recent intense research interest due to its profound impact on the host.

The interaction between the host and the microbial community is an active, well-coordinated, and integrated one, which is deeply involved in normal physiological processes. In fact, microbial populations take part in immunogenesis, metabolic regulation, nutrient absorption, vitamin synthesis, and maintaining the integrity of the mucosal surface, among others (Gopalakrishnan et al., 2018). In constant communication with the host's immune system, the microbial community is responsible for maintaining immune tolerance and simultaneously retains the ability to defend against microbial invasion. This subtle balance is what keeps the entire system in homeostasis. However, when such a balance is disrupted, which is referred to as dysbiosis, it can set the stage for the onset of several disease states, ranging from inflammatory, metabolic, autoimmune, and cancerous disorders, among others.

During the last decade or so, the relationship between the microbial community and cancer has been one of the most dominant themes in biomedical research. Initially, studies focused on particular disease-causing microorganisms associated with different forms of cancer. However,

The Microbiome and Cancer Treatment: Overcoming Resistance and Enhancing Efficacy.
DOI: https://doi.org/10.1016/B978-0-443-33206-7.00006-6

recent studies have begun to reveal the role of microbial communities and their functional impact on cancer. It is currently well accepted that the microbial community is not only involved in the onset and progression of cancer but also in the outcome of cancer therapy (Montassier et al., 2015). Alterations in the microbial community and its metabolic activity have been linked with chronic inflammation, genomic instability, and uncontrolled immune responses, which are all hallmarks of cancerous transformations.

At the same time, anticancer therapy also affects microbial populations. Among anticancer agents, chemotherapy is a commonly practiced treatment modality for a variety of cancer types. Chemotherapeutic agents have been known to affect rapidly dividing cancer cells. However, it is also known to affect host cells, resulting in a variety of effects. Since the GI tract is an area of rapid cell division, it is more susceptible to the effects of chemotherapeutic agents.

Chemotherapeutic agents can have a significant impact on microbial populations, quantity, and productivity. This can result in a decrease in the population of beneficial microbes, whereas opportunistic pathogens can flourish. This can compromise epithelial cell layer integrity, tight junction proteins, and gut permeability. This can result in the entry of microbial products into systemic circulation, resulting in systemic inflammatory response syndrome and compromise of the immune system (Kenneth et al., 2025). Clinical manifestations of such effects can include mucositis, diarrhea, GI discomfort, and secondary infection, particularly in immunocompromised patients. Thus, chemotherapy can have a significant impact on microbial populations, resulting in systemic effects apart from local effects.

Apart from being responsible for treatment-induced toxicity, the microbiome can also influence treatment efficacy. The microbiome can modulate host-microbe interactions, which can influence drug metabolism, immune system activation, and inflammation. Such interactions can significantly influence treatment outcomes (Alexander et al., 2017). The microbiome can either activate antitumor immunity by activating dendritic cell maturation and cytotoxic T-cell activation or compromise it, making it difficult for tumors to be eliminated. Recent studies suggest the existence of distinct microbial patterns in patients who either respond or do not respond to chemotherapy. Such studies suggest the potential of microbiome profiling in treatment outcome prediction (Gopalakrishnan et al., 2018). By identifying microbial patterns in cancer patients before treatment initiation, it may be possible to predict treatment response and potential toxicity.

Traditionally, the microbiome has been given relatively little consideration in classical oncology studies. Initial studies were mostly restricted to digestion and nutrient metabolism, with little questioning of its immunological and oncogenic aspects. With the introduction of next-generation sequencing technologies and advanced multiomics platforms, this position has been changed forever. With metagenomic, metabolomic, and transcriptomic studies, researchers can now have the ability to not only define microbial composition but also to probe functional prowess. Recent data show that microbial metabolites have the potential to regulate oncogenic signaling pathways, affect epigenetic changes, and shape host immune homeostasis (Li et al., 2024). The microbiome's composition tends to fluctuate depending on the nature and progression of cancer and its location within the body, thereby forming a disease-specific signature (Fig. 3.1). To exemplify this, "*Fusobacterium nucleatum* and *Enterococcus faecalis*" have been

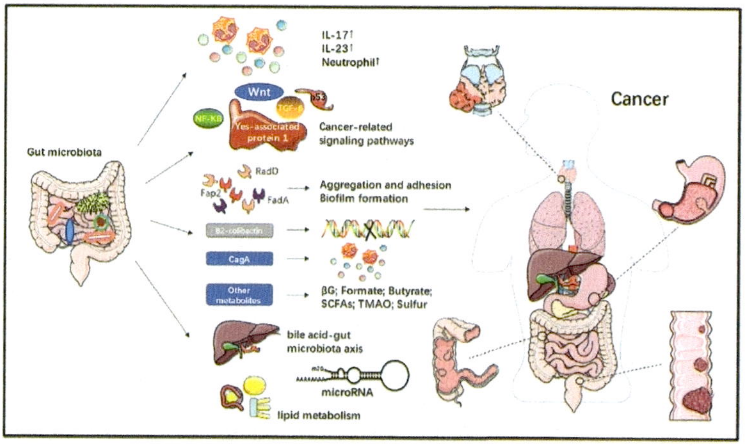

FIGURE 3.1 The possible mechanisms of the gut microbiota in the occurrence and development of cancer. The possible mechanisms by which gut microbiota contribute to the initiation, progression, immune modulation, inflammation, metabolic reprogramming, and therapeutic response in cancer development. *Source: From Li et al. (2023) under an open access license.*

found to accumulate within colorectal and pancreatic cancer, and they are implicated in the establishment of a proinflammatory tumor microenvironment (Yang et al., 2023). The aforementioned statements and findings point to the notion that perhaps the dysregulation of the microbiome could act as a potential cause for oncogenesis, progression, and the dissemination of cancer.

Most importantly, the establishment of the microbiome within the tumor before the administration of treatment tends to have a determining effect on the efficacy of chemotherapy and immunotherapy. The establishment and maintenance of a well-balanced and diversified microbiome, including the aforementioned *Bifidobacterium, Faecalibacterium prausnitzii,* and *Akkermansia muciniphila,* have been found to correlate with enhanced survival rates and efficacy with immune checkpoint inhibitors (Routy et al., 2018). The aforementioned microbiome maintains the integrity of the mucosa, produces anti-inflammatory metabolites such as short-chain fatty acids (SCFAs), and mounts a potent antitumor immune response. Conversely, the disruption of a well-diversified microbiome, particularly with antibiotics prior to and during chemotherapy, has been implicated in reduced tumor control, relapse rates, and toxicity (Dahiya & Nigam, 2023).

The results show that the effectiveness of the therapy can easily be disrupted by the disruption of the microbiota. The depletion of commensal flora caused by antibiotics can impair immune system priming and weaken the immune response to anticancer agents. On the other hand, the disruption of the microbiome by chemotherapy can cause a proinflammatory environment, which increases toxicity and diminishes antitumor immunity. This two-way interaction shows that the microbiome plays an active role rather than a passive role in the process of treatment. Therefore, the evidence presented makes the microbiome the interface between oncologic biology, immune regulation, and treatment responsiveness. This interaction between chemotherapy and microbial ecosystems provides a rationale for effective interaction (Rajak et al., 2026). The modes of intervention that have been put under scrutiny include probiotic supplements, diet modulation, specific manipulation of microbial metabolites, and fecal microbiome transplantation, which have been used as an adjunct to increase treatment adherence and effectiveness.

It is this understanding that provides a paradigm shift to a more integrative and precision-oriented paradigm rather than the traditional oncology paradigm. The treatment of cancer can no longer be viewed as a war against cancerous cells but as a complex interaction between tumor genomics, immune response, and the tumor's metabolism and microbiome. With microbiome analysis becoming a part of clinical decision-making, in the future, clinicians will be able to base therapeutic regimens on factors beyond just tumor characteristics, microbial composition, and functional activity as well.

With the ongoing research that seeks to establish the mechanistic connections between the dynamics of the microbiome and oncologic therapy, it is becoming clear that microbial homeostasis might be essential to maximize clinical performance. Microbiome science integration into oncology will boost the treatment efficacy, reduce toxicity, and eventually enhance patient survival and quality of life in patients receiving cancer treatment. The interaction of chemotherapy with the microbiome is also influenced by a variety of host factors, including antibiotic use, diet, genetic factors, lifestyle, and disease status, all of which play a crucial role in the composition and function of the gut microbiome (Mafe & Büsselberg, 2025). These factors, taken together, play an essential role in the resilience or susceptibility of the microbiome to chemotherapy.

For example, the use of broad-spectrum antibiotics can lead to a decrease in the number of commensal microbes, resulting in a reduction of microbial diversity. This weakening of colonization resistance can also lead to an increased susceptibility to opportunistic pathogens. Thus, the use of antibiotics before or even with chemotherapy can lead to an increased severity of dysbiosis, GI complications, and instability of the immune response. The weakening of the microbiome can also lead to a decrease in the production of SCFAs, resulting in an inflammatory response (Alexander et al., 2017).

Dietary habits also play a crucial role in the function of the microbiome. For example, a diet rich in dietary fibers can support the growth of SCFA-producing microbes, thus providing a healthy mucosal surface and immune response. However, a diet rich in fat can imbalance the microbiome, resulting in an inflammatory response. Chemotherapy already puts a host under a lot of stress, and dietary habits can play a crucial role in the tolerance of chemotherapy. Nutrient intake can also play a crucial role in supporting the function of the microbiome (Zhang, 2022).

Genetic variability between individuals also moderates host-microbe interactions. Differences in genes regulating immune responses, inflammatory signaling pathways, and drug metabolism may have an influence on the way in which the microbiome responds to cytotoxic stress. Some people may have genetic predispositions that allow them to more efficiently repair microbial balance after it has been disrupted, while others may be predisposed to a longer state of dysbiosis. The nature of the malignancy and the level of disease burden also play an important role in determining microbial composition. As such, these issues introduce another level of complexity in the treatment-induced changes (Chu, 2017). In light of these multifactorial issues, there is an emerging scientific interest in developing strategies that are focused on maintaining microbiome homeostasis during oncologic treatment.

Instead of treating the adverse effects of chemotherapy-induced microbial imbalance as an inevitable consequence of treatment, there is an interest in developing targeted approaches that are focused on reducing the level of microbial imbalance and enhancing treatment outcomes. These include microbiota-directed approaches such as the use of probiotics, prebiotics, fecal microbiota transplantation (FMT), and dietary approaches. These approaches are focused on maintaining microbial diversity, improving gut integrity, and modulating immune responses during treatment. By reducing the adverse effects of chemotherapy on the GI system through these approaches, treatment efficacy may be enhanced. An important issue is the conceptual integration of microbiome-targeting approaches with the larger context of precision oncology. This chapter offers an overview of the microbiome dynamics with respect to cancer therapy, with a special emphasis on chemotherapy. It aims to highlight the mechanisms through which chemotherapy agents affect the microbiome, the consequences of this effect, and emerging strategies for microbiome modulation to improve patient outcomes. By examining the intricate interplay between the host, microbiome, and chemotherapy agents, this discussion aims to highlight the potential benefits of microbiome-based therapies to cancer patients.

3.2 Chemotherapy and its impact on the host

Chemotherapy is one of the most important modalities in cancer treatment, and it remains one of the most commonly used forms of treatment today for cancer, including both solid tumors and hematologic cancers. Chemotherapy follows the principle of targeting rapidly dividing cells, which eventually leads to the destruction of cancer cells that divide and proliferate in an uncontrolled manner. However, this approach is not very selective, and other rapidly dividing normal tissues, such as those in the GI tract, bone marrow, and hair follicles, are also damaged. Chemotherapy, thus, leads to changes in the body that are far beyond just cancer cell destruction. Chemotherapy not only causes damage to tissues but also affects the immune response, endocrine balance, and microbial flora in the body (Table 3.1) (Pouncey et al., 2018; Sharma et al., 2024).

Since chemotherapy is a systemic form of treatment, it is not possible to study it in isolation. When chemotherapy is given, there is a complex interplay of cellular stress, inflammation, and the microbial flora of the body. One of the most important mechanisms involved in the host response to chemotherapy is the excessive production of reactive oxygen species (ROS). Although the production of ROS is involved in the apoptosis of cancer cells and the induction of DNA damage in cancer tissues, it is also responsible for injury to normal tissues. An increase in ROS production leads to lipid peroxidation, mitochondrial dysfunction, protein oxidation, and genetic instability in normal tissues, which in turn activates an inflammatory response and leads to the production of proinflammatory cytokines (Böhm et al., 2025).

The GI tract is particularly susceptible to oxidative damage. The epithelial cells lining the GI tract have a high turnover rate and require precise regulation of mitochondrial function.

Table 3.1 Systemic and localized effects of chemotherapy on the host: Mechanisms, agents, consequences, and evidence.

Affected system	Mechanism of chemotherapy impact	Examples	Clinical consequences	References
Gastrointestinal mucosa	Chemotherapy damages rapidly dividing intestinal epithelial cells, initiates ROS production and NF-κB-mediated inflammation, and upregulates IL-1β and TNF-α.	5-Fluorouracil, Irinotecan, Methotrexate	Severe diarrhea, mucositis, pain, increased gut permeability, and microbial translocation	Akbarali et al. (2022), Alcorta et al. (2024)
Bone marrow / Hematopoietic system	Myelosuppression due to targeting of rapidly dividing stem/progenitor cells; decreasedWBCs, RBCs, and platelets	Cyclophosphamide, Doxorubicin, Carboplatin	Neutropenia, anemia, thrombocytopenia febrile neutropenia, bleeding, transfusion need	Li et al. (2024), Jameus et al. (2021)
Immune system	Lymphopenia, neutropenia, depletion of dendritic cells and T-lymphocytes, impaired antigen presentation, and cytokine signaling	Fludarabine, Cytarabine, Rituximab	Immunosuppression, poor pathogen clearance, increased infection susceptibility, reduced vaccine efficacy	Prasad et al. (2022), Gassner et al. (2011)
Oral mucosa	Similar to GI mucosa – epithelial apoptosis via ROS and cytokine amplification; microbial dysbiosis enhances lesion severity	Methotrexate, Cisplatin	Painful oral ulcers, dysphagia, poor nutritional intake, secondary fungal/bacterial infections	Chen et al. (2020), Basile et al. (2019)

(*continued on next page*)

Table 3.1 Systemic and localized effects of chemotherapy on the host: Mechanisms, agents, consequences, and evidence—cont'd

Affected system	Mechanism of chemotherapy impact	Examples	Clinical consequences	References
Peripheral nervous system	Mitochondrial dysfunction, axonal injury, demyelination, neuroinflammation via IL-6 and TNF-α	Paclitaxel, Vincristine, Oxaliplatin	Chemotherapy-induced peripheral neuropathy (CIPN), chronic pain, gait instability	Zajaczkowską et al. (2019), Trecarichi and Flatters (2019)
Central nervous system	Disruption of the blood-brain barrier, cytokine-induced inflammation, and white matter volume loss	Methotrexate, 5-FU, Cytarabine	Cognitive impairment ("chemo brain"), memory issues, reduced executive function	Was et al. (2022), Ren et al. (2019)
Metabolic/Endocrine system	Altered insulin sensitivity, adipokine release, cortisol imbalance, and oxidative stress	Doxorubicin, Tamoxifen, Cisplatin	Fatigue, weight gain or cachexia, metabolic syndrome, steroid-induced diabetes	Hutchison et al. (2023), Tangvarasittichai (2015)
Microbiome-immune crosstalk	Loss of Treg-promoting and SCFA-producing microbes; decreased IL-10, increased gut permeability, and systemic LPS	Most chemotherapies (indirect effect) + antibiotics	Dysbiosis, systemic inflammation, impaired antitumor immunity, increased GVHD risk	Campbell et al. (2023), Biennier et al. (2024)
Liver and detoxification systems	Hepatocyte stress due to reactive metabolites; impaired detox enzyme expression	Cyclophosphamide, Methotrexate	Transaminitis, drug-induced liver injury (DILI), and altered metabolism of other drugs	Schmidt et al. (2022), Villanueva-Paz et al. (2021)
Skin and appendages	Impact on keratinocytes and dermal matrix; cytokine-driven damage	Paclitaxel, Capecitabine	Alopecia, rash, nail changes, and hand-foot syndrome	Miller et al. (2014), Sibaud et al. (2016)

GI, gastrointestinal; *IL-6*, interleukin-6; *IL-10*, interleukin-10; *LPS*, lipopolysaccharides; *ROS*, reactive oxygen species; *SCFAs*, short-chain fatty acids; *TNF-α*, tumor necrosis factor alpha.

High concentrations of ROS impair the functioning of the epithelial cells. The tight junction proteins are critical for maintaining epithelial function. However, when they are disordered due to high concentrations of ROS, the permeability of the intestine increases. The increased permeability allows the entry of luminal bacteria and their products into the systemic circulation, thereby initiating an inflammatory cascade. It can be seen that oxidative stress not only causes damage to the host but also disrupts the normal microbial community, thereby creating a favorable condition for dysbiosis and opportunistic infections. Apart from oxidative stress, there are other factors that are equally responsible for the damage caused by chemotherapy. Chemotherapy agents have a profound effect on the endocrine and metabolic pathways. Chemotherapy is known to have a profound effect on insulin signaling pathways, carbohydrate metabolism, lipid metabolism, and hormone balance. The effect of chemotherapy on cancer cells is not confined to the cancer cells alone but affects the entire organism (Li et al., 2025).

Since microbes rely on host-derived substrates, it is logical to conclude that chemotherapy-induced changes in nutrient availability will have a profound impact on the composition of the microbiome. For example, chemotherapy-induced changes in carbohydrate metabolism can fuel the growth of certain microbial populations, whereas changes in lipid metabolism can affect microbial composition and function. Thus, chemotherapy can have a profound impact on the composition and function of the microbiome. Chemotherapy can decrease the availability of substrates for microbial metabolism, thus affecting SCFA production and weakening the host's mucosal defense mechanism. Chemotherapy can also affect lipid metabolism, thus altering the inflammatory response. These changes, in a vicious cycle, can result in a situation where systemic physiological stress can fuel microbial imbalance, and microbial imbalance can fuel systemic inflammatory response. The human immune system constitutes another interface that is affected by chemotherapy. Cytotoxic drugs, for instance, can impair bone marrow function, resulting in neutropenia and lymphocytopenia (Li et al., 2024a). This compromises the host's ability to fight off diseases, hence disrupting the microbiota equilibrium. In a normal host, there is a balance between microbes, and opportunistic pathogens are kept at bay by the host's immune system. However, when this balance is disrupted, there is a decrease in microbiota diversity, and pathobionts overgrow. Concurrently, there is increased susceptibility to opportunistic infections, which are typically of enteric origin. As such, chemotherapy-induced changes in the host's immune system and microbiota are two sides of the same coin. Recent studies have shed new light on host-specific factors that influence chemotherapy-induced toxicity and microbiota response. For instance, sex and age differences are critical host-specific factors that influence chemotherapy-induced microbiota changes. In elderly women, notably postmenopausal women, there is delayed mucosal healing and prolonged microbiota imbalance following chemotherapy exposure (Özdemir et al., 2022). This could be attributed to reduced estrogen levels, lower regenerative capacity, and immunosenescence, all of which result in delayed healing of the epithelial barrier and microbiota diversity. In contrast, cancer-affected children may display different microbiota changes following chemotherapy exposure. In this case, although there is significant microbiota dysbiosis during the initial phase of chemotherapy, there is remarkable microbiota resilience and recovery following chemotherapy completion (Rotz & Dandoy, 2020). This could be explained by enhanced regenerative capacity, immune recovery, and inherent microbiota diversity. As such, chemotherapy-induced changes do not occur in all host populations. Instead, there is a complex interplay of host-specific factors, including physiological, immunological, hormonal, nutritional, and microbiota factors.

Genetic background is another factor that further influences the host's response. The differences in the expression of genes related to inflammation, antioxidants, and drug metabolism can affect the risk of oxidative stress and dysbiosis. Nutritional status is another major factor that plays an important role in determining the host's resilience. Nutritional deficiency can impair the healing of the epithelial barrier and the immune system, which can increase the risk of chemotherapy-induced complications. Antibiotics administered before chemotherapy can alter the baseline microbiota composition, which might reduce the diversity of the microbiota and thereby increase the risk of severe dysbiosis. All these factors related to the host's response indicate that chemotherapy is administered in a highly individualized biological context. The biological effects of chemotherapy involve oxidative stress, metabolism, immune suppression, and disruption of the microbiota. The interplay of all these factors determines the efficacy and toxicity of chemotherapy. Understanding the complex effect of chemotherapy on the host's biological system is very important for developing new individualized chemotherapy protocols. The inclusion of microbiota analysis in chemotherapy protocols can give us new insights regarding individualized risk factors and protective mechanisms. As oncology is shifting toward individualized medicine, chemotherapy protocols clearly need to be individualized to take into consideration the tumor's biology as well as the host's biology (Chrysostomou et al., 2023). Understanding the effect of chemotherapy on the host's biological system is the foundation of new chemotherapy protocols that can maintain the balance of the biological system while maintaining the antitumor effect of chemotherapy.

3.3 Chemotherapy-induced dysbiosis

Chemotherapy, being one of the most commonly used anticancer treatments, has profound effects not only on the rapidly proliferating tumor cells but also on the resident microbial flora of the host. Though chemotherapy is specifically designed to target rapidly proliferating tumor cells, it is inevitable that it will have some effect on the normal tissues and the resident microbial flora of the body. Amongst these, the gut microbiota is particularly susceptible to chemotherapy-induced alterations. Recent findings have confirmed that chemotherapy can cause alterations in microbial diversity, composition, and metabolism, leading to a condition known as dysbiosis (Ciernikova et al., 2021;Roggiani et al., 2023). The key characteristics of chemotherapy-induced dysbiosis include a decrease in the populations of beneficial microorganisms, a decrease in microbial diversity, and an increase in the populations of opportunistic/pathogenic microorganisms. The decrease in the populations of beneficial microorganisms, which play an important role in the production of SCFAs, maintenance of the mucosal barrier, and immune system modulation, can be associated with chemotherapy-induced dysbiosis. On the other hand, the populations of opportunistic/pathogenic microorganisms, which have the potential to cause inflammatory responses and can take advantage of the compromised immune system of the patient, can be associated with chemotherapy-induced dysbiosis (Markowiak-Kopeć & Śliżewska, 2020). These changes can result in an imbalance of the intestinal barrier, thus increasing the permeability of the gut, allowing lipopolysaccharides (LPS) to penetrate the bloodstream, resulting in an exaggerated inflammatory response.

Most importantly, it has been recognized that dysbiosis is not merely a side effect of damage to the epithelium but rather a factor that plays a role in determining the toxicities and efficacy of chemotherapy. An imbalance in the microbiota can alter immune function, potentially influencing the regulation of antitumor immunity. It can also play a role in the severity of chemotherapy-induced GI toxicities such as diarrhea and mucositis. It can impair the efficacy of chemotherapy by impacting the activation and metabolism of the immune cells. Chemotherapy-induced dysbiosis, therefore, plays a role in determining the outcome of patients receiving chemotherapy. The degree and nature of dysbiosis can vary greatly between individuals. The reasons for this are varied and include the nature of the chemotherapeutic agent used, the dose of the chemotherapeutic agent, the period for which the chemotherapy is administered, and the dose of the chemotherapeutic agent. The nature and degree of effect of different classes of chemotherapeutic agents on the microbiota are varied. Some agents can preferentially target anaerobic bacteria, while some can influence bile metabolism and oxidative stress. Host factors can also play an integral role in determining the effect of chemotherapy-induced dysbiosis. Age is an important factor, especially in older individuals, who have low baseline microbial diversity and reduced intestinal regenerative capacity (Mollaei et al., 2021). Nutritional status can affect the availability of substrates for microbial metabolism, while immune competence can play an integral role in determining the ability of the patient to maintain microbial balance. The effect of antibiotics can significantly exacerbate the risk of chemotherapy-induced dysbiosis. In some cases, specific types of dysbiosis have been correlated with specific chemotherapy regimens, which implies that the microbiota can be used as a biomarker to predict chemotherapy efficacy and toxicity. The identification of such biomarkers can be used to stratify patients according to risk factors before the administration of chemotherapy. Patients with specific types of microbiota can be targeted to receive supportive care to maintain the balance of the microbiota. The knowledge of chemotherapy-induced dysbiosis is essential for the assessment of the patient's outcome (Dahiya & Nigam, 2023). Moreover, the description of the changes occurring in the microbial flora is not only helpful for a deeper knowledge of the interactions occurring within the host–drug–microbe system but also for the development of a more precise treatment strategy, as described in Table 3.2 . Indeed, the integration of microbiome analysis within oncological treatment is a crucial step for the development of more precise treatment modalities, accepting dysbiosis as a condition to be managed, rather than a condition to be considered unavoidable.

Intestinal homeostasis and mucosal integrity are primarily governed and maintained by the gut microbiome, which varies in different populations and individuals according to their genetic, dietary, environmental, and health conditions. Generally, a healthy gut microbiome is usually characterized by high microbial diversity, redundancy, and colonization resistance

Table 3.2 Chemotherapy-induced dysbiosis – mechanisms, microbial changes, and clinical relevance.

Aspect	Details	Mechanisms and microbial examples	Clinical relevance	References
Microbial diversity	Significant decline in both α-diversity (within-sample richness) and β-diversity (between-sample variation)	Loss of beneficial species (*Lactobacillus, Bifidobacterium, Faecalibacterium*) due to epithelial damage, ROS exposure, and nutrient shifts	Impaired gut homeostasis, reduced colonization resistance, increased infection risk	Kerstens and Joyce (2024), Checa-Ros et al. (2021)
Loss of commensal microbes	Depletion of beneficial taxa with immunoregulatory functions	Decrease in *Clostridium* cluster IV/XIVa, *Akkermansia muciniphila*, and butyrate producers	↓ IL-10 production, ↓ Treg differentiation, ↑ and mucosal inflammation	Cohen et al. (2021), Kujawa et al. (2023)
Overgrowth of pathobionts	Bloom of opportunistic and potentially pathogenic bacteria	Overrepresentation of *Enterococcus faecalis, Klebsiella, Escherichia coli*, and *Clostridium difficile* during mucosal vulnerability	Associated with bacteremia, mucositis, and nosocomial infections	Atarashi et al. (2017), Fiore et al. (2019)
Chemotherapy-specific microbiome disruption	Varies by drug class (e.g., alkylating agents versus antimetabolites)	Cyclophosphamide ↑ gut permeability and translocation of Gram+ bacteria; 5-FU causes mucositis and microbiota depletion	Immunopathology (e.g., TH17 skewing), worsening of chemotherapy side effects	Wei et al. (2021), Yin et al. (2022)
Intestinal mucosal damage	Damage to rapidly proliferating epithelial cells	Mucosal thinning, goblet cell loss, compromised barrier proteins (e.g., ZO-1)	Facilitates bacterial translocation, systemic inflammation (endotoxemia)	Nie et al. (2024), Chen et al. (2025)

(*continued on next page*)

Table 3.2 Chemotherapy-induced dysbiosis – mechanisms, microbial changes, and clinical relevance—cont'd

Aspect	Details	Mechanisms and microbial examples	Clinical relevance	References
Temporal microbiome dynamics	Distinct microbiome shifts over the treatment timeline	1–3 d: loss of strict anaerobes; 1–2 wk: enrichment of facultative anaerobes; recovery *often incomplete*	Persistent dysbiosis may affect long-term immune function and quality of life	Derrien et al. (2019), Patangia et al. (2022)
Antibiotic use during chemotherapy	Common during neutropenic episodes, but exacerbates dysbiosis	Broad-spectrum antibiotics ↓ commensals, ↑ MDROs, and *Clostridium difficile* risk; disrupt SCFA production	Delayed microbiome recovery, poor immune reconstitution, ↑, and treatment complications	Rashidi and Weisdorf (2020), Xu et al. (2022b)
Immune modulation by microbiota	Dysbiosis alters immune cell priming and cytokine secretion	↓ DC maturation, ↓ CD8+ T cell recruitment, and ↓ memory T cell formation	Reduced chemotherapy efficacy and impaired antitumor immunity	Rad et al. (2024), Zhuang et al. (2023)
Microbial Metabolite depletion	Reduced SCFAs, tryptophan metabolites, and inosine	Loss of butyrate and propionate leads to ↑ permeability, ↓ anti-inflammatory signaling	Associated with GI toxicity, systemic inflammation, and fatigue	Lange et al. (2023), Morris et al. (2017)

(*continued on next page*)

Biomarkers and predictive value	Microbiome signatures can predict outcomes	High pretreatment diversity → better response; domination by *Enterococcus* → worse prognosis	Potential for personalized microbiome-based treatment stratification	Meade et al. (2023), Al Radi et al. (2024)
Host and environmental modulators	Age, diet, prior antibiotics, baseline microbiome, and genetics	Elderly and malnourished patients show more severe dysbiosis and delayed recovery	Refers to the need for personalized microbiome support (diet, prebiotics, etc.)	Berding et al. (2021), Safarchi et al. (2025)

GI, gastrointestinal; *IL-10*, interleukin-10; *ROS*, reactive oxygen species; *SCFAs*, short-chain fatty acids.

against invading pathogens. However, during cancer treatment, the administration of conventional chemotherapeutic agents often disrupts this microbiome balance, leading to gut dysbiosis with reduced beneficial commensals and increased opportunistic and pathogenic microbiota (Cohen et al., 2021;Roggiani et al., 2023).

The disruption of the mucosal integrity during chemotherapy triggers a series of proinflammatory reactions. The impairment of epithelial cell junctions increases intestinal permeability, allowing pathogenic bacteria and their products, such as LPS, to spread into the bloodstream (Berding et al., 2021;Rad et al., 2024). This leads to a strong proinflammatory immune response, contributing to GI toxicity and, in severe cases, bacteremia and infections. Moreover, microbiota-induced changes in the intestinal microbiome also affect critical metabolic pathways such as nucleotide synthesis, mitochondrial energy metabolism, and vitamin production, which further impair mucosal repair and immune function. GI mucositis, which includes inflammation and ulceration of mucous membranes, is one of the most common and debilitating side effects of chemotherapy and radiotherapy agents (Akbarali et al., 2022).

Recent advances in metagenomic sequencing technologies have also enabled the longitudinal analysis of microbial communities in cancer patients undergoing chemotherapy. For example, chemotherapy with 5-fluorouracil and irinotecan has been reported to cause decreased levels of beneficial microbes such as Bacteroides fragilis and *Lactobacillus reuteri*, which are involved in the maintenance of homeostasis of the mucosal surfaces of the body and the regulation of local immunological responses, respectively (Roggiani et al., 2023). On the other hand, opportunistic pathogens such as *Clostridium difficile* and *Enterococcus faecalis* may also overproliferate in the bodies of cancer patients undergoing chemotherapy with these two drugs, thereby leading to increased risks of antibiotic-associated diarrhea, enterocolitis, and systemic infections.

The interaction between microbiota and the metabolome is also important in chemotherapy. For example, SCFAs such as acetate and butyrate are important microbial metabolites that are generated through the microbial fermentation of dietary fiber. SCFAs are involved in the regulation of epithelial barrier functions by regulating tight junction proteins such as occludin and zonula occludens-1 (ZO-1), thereby enhancing these functions. SCFAs are also involved in the regulation of immunological functions. For example, chemotherapy-induced decreased levels of SCFA-producing microbes impair epithelial functions, leading to increased levels of endotoxemia. In addition, chemotherapy-induced dysbiosis also leads to decreased activation of dendritic cells, antigen presentation, and recruitment of cytotoxic T lymphocytes to the tumor sites, leading to immunosuppression (Al-Qadami et al., 2022; Eiman et al., 2025).

Some of the recent studies have highlighted the potential usefulness of microbial biomarkers in predicting therapeutic response and clinical prognosis. Microbial signatures have been identified to predict good or bad prognosis in a range of cancers, and the composition of gut microbiota has been implicated as both a predictive and prognostic marker. Discovery of such biomarkers; provides clinicians with a guideline on how to stratify and predict the adverse effects on a patient and design patient-specific treatment regimens (Villanueva-Paz et al., 2021Zhuang et al., 2023). Outside the oncology domain, the gut microbiota has a significant effect on the systemic physiological functions, especially neuro-immune regulation. New signs define the hyperirritability of the central nervous system to microbial disturbances. The changes in the gut microbial composition can adjust the brain activity, influence the mood, and cognitive processing. Rodent models continuously show that microbiota-host interaction disturbance alters the enteric nervous system, triggers neuro-immune signaling, and influences brain development and behavioral consequences (Ciernikova et al., 2021).

Microbiota-gut-brain axis is a complex, two-way network of communication that involves the central nervous system, endocrine, immune, and metabolic signaling cascades. This axis connects the emotional and cognitive spheres of the brain and the peripheral intestinal activity through the mediation of a combination of neural, hormonal, and immunological intermediates. Within the framework of chemotherapy-induced dysbiosis, disruptions in this axis could be the cause of the fatigue, mood changes, and cognitive impairment that cancer patients often complain about (Kerstens & Joyce, 2024). Taken together, these observations highlight the fact that chemotherapy-induced dysbiosis does not have localized GI effects. It is echoed through systemic immunity, metabolic balance, infectious vulnerability, and neurocognitive performance. An in-depth understanding of these mutually supportive relationships is essential in creating strategies that protect microbial homeostasis in oncological therapy and eventually improve the overall patient outcomes.

3.4 Microbiome and chemotherapy side effects

Chemotherapy, beyond a doubt, has dramatically altered the face of cancer treatment, allowing for increased survival and disease remission for millions of patients worldwide. The systemic nature of chemotherapy allows for the targeting of cancer cells that may have metastasized to other areas of the body. However, this systemic nature also leads to the unwanted side effect of damaging healthy cells. The side effects of chemotherapy have been well documented for many decades to be a result of the direct toxicity to rapidly dividing cells. However, emerging evidence suggests that many of the debilitating and uncomfortable side effects, including nausea, diarrhea, fatigue, increased susceptibility to infections, and inflammation, are directly related to disruptions within the human microbiome (Karagiannis et al., 2018). The once-untapped role of the microbiome has been recognized to play a significant role in the toxicities associated with chemotherapy and the resilience of patients to the treatments they are receiving. The interaction between chemotherapy and the microbiome can be complex and individualized. The types and combinations of drugs used, the dose and total dose received, and the duration and schedule of the treatment can have a significant effect on the disruption of the microbiome. The administration methods, including intravenous, oral, and topical administration, can have a significant effect on the degree to which the microbiome is altered. However, host factors, including diet, genetic factors, immune status, comorbidities, antibiotic use, and environmental factors, can also have a significant effect on the baseline state and susceptibility to chemotherapy-induced alterations to the microbiome (Fernandes et al., 2024). These layered interactions explain why patients receiving similar regimens often experience markedly different toxicity profiles.

3.4.1 Effect of chemotherapy on human microbiome

The gut microbiota is an intricate ecosystem composed of various microbes such as bacteria, viruses, fungi, and archaea. These microbes play an important role in maintaining host homeostasis. They are involved in nutrient metabolism, vitamin production, bile acid sequestration, immune modulation, epithelial integrity maintenance, and protection against pathogenic invasion. Under physiological conditions, an intricate equilibrium is maintained between the host immune system and the microbes (Pickard et al., 2017).

This equilibrium ensures that the host is not invaded by these microbes but is protected against pathogenic invasion. Chemotherapeutic agents are potent agents that target rapidly proliferating cancer cells. In the process, these agents disrupt the intricate equilibrium maintained between the host immune system and the microbes. Most chemotherapeutic agents have antimicrobial properties. They either directly damage microbial DNA or indirectly affect the microbial community by damaging the epithelial cells of the gut, leading to increased oxidative stress and immune suppression. This disrupts the microbial community composition significantly. This disruption is termed dysbiosis. Under dysbiotic conditions, the microbial community richness is significantly reduced. There is also an increased number of opportunistic microbes. Most importantly, dysbiosis is not an indirect effect but is directly involved in chemotherapy-induced toxicity (Sun et al., 2024). In the case of chemotherapy-induced damage, the GI tract is significantly affected because of the presence of rapidly proliferating cells in the epithelium. When the epithelial cells are damaged, there is reduced mucus production. In addition, the tight junction proteins, such as occludin and claudins, are also damaged. This leads to increased intestinal permeability. At the same time, the nutrient concentration in the gut is increased, leading to an increased microbial population (Pouncey et al., 2018).

3.4.2 Dysbiosis and its consequences

Chemotherapy-associated dysbiosis represents a fundamental shift in microbial ecology. A healthy gut ecosystem is marked by resilience, functional redundancy, and metabolic efficiency. When disturbed by cytotoxic therapy, several pathological consequences emerge (Pouncey et al., 2018).

3.4.3 Loss of microbial diversity

Reduced diversity diminishes ecosystem stability and compromises colonization resistance. A less diverse microbiome is more susceptible to pathogen overgrowth and slower to recover after stress. This loss of resilience contributes to prolonged GI complications.

3.4.4 Depletion of beneficial commensals

Chemotherapy frequently reduces populations of SCFA-producing bacteria (Winter & Bäumler, 2023). SCFAs such as butyrate and acetate are critical for epithelial repair, regulation of inflammation, and energy supply to colonocytes. Their depletion weakens mucosal defense and predisposes patients to mucositis and diarrhea.

3.4.5 Overgrowth of pathobionts

Opportunistic organisms may proliferate disproportionately during dysbiosis (Petersen & Round, 2014). These pathobionts activate proinflammatory signaling pathways and produce metabolites that exacerbate tissue injury. Overgrowth increases susceptibility to antibiotic-associated diarrhea, enterocolitis, and systemic infections.

3.4.6 Impaired gut barrier function

Chemotherapy-induced epithelial damage leads to increased intestinal permeability, often referred to as a "leaky gut" (Jansen et al., 2024). This allows bacterial components such as LPS to enter systemic circulation, triggering immune activation and cytokine release. Systemic inflammation arising from endotoxemia contributes to fatigue, malaise, and immune dysregulation.

3.4.7 Gastrointestinal toxicity

Nausea, vomiting, diarrhea, abdominal pain, and mucositis are among the most frequent chemotherapy-related adverse effects. Inflammation driven by microbial imbalance amplifies epithelial injury, creating a feedback loop that worsens symptoms. GI mucositis reflects the combined impact of direct epithelial damage and microbial-driven immune activation.

3.4.8 Cognitive impairment

Alterations in gut microbial composition have been increasingly linked to cognitive disturbances commonly described as "chemo brain." Patients may experience memory deficits, reduced attention span, and mental fatigue. Dysbiosis influences neuroinflammatory pathways and alters neurotransmitter synthesis via immune and metabolic signaling networks.

3.4.9 Increased infection risk

Chemotherapy-induced immunosuppression, compounded by microbial imbalance, increases vulnerability to infections. As the gut represents a major immunological interface, barrier dysfunction facilitates bacterial translocation into the bloodstream, potentially leading to bacteremia or sepsis.

3.4.10 Inflammation and fatigue

Chronic low-grade systemic inflammation resulting from dysbiosis contributes significantly to persistent fatigue, one of the most debilitating symptoms during chemotherapy. Elevated inflammatory mediators disrupt metabolic homeostasis and impair tissue repair.

3.4.11 Altered drug metabolism and toxicity

The gut microbiome participates directly in the metabolism of various chemotherapeutic agents (Li et al., 2024b). Changes in microbial enzyme activity can modify drug activation, detoxification, or reactivation. Some bacterial enzymes convert inactive metabolites back into toxic forms, intensifying side effects and prolonging tissue injury. Collectively, these consequences illustrate that dysbiosis is not merely a byproduct of chemotherapy but an active driver of symptom severity and therapeutic variability.

3.4.12 Neuroimmune and metabolic complications

The effects of chemotherapy-induced dysbiosis are not limited to the GI system and are also known to affect neuroimmune and metabolic systems. Chemotherapy-induced neurotoxicity, commonly referred to as "chemo brain," includes cognitive impairment, anxiety, sleep problems, and fatigue. Current evidence suggests that microbiome-mediated neuroinflammation contributes to chemotherapy-induced neurotoxicity (Song & Bai, 2021).

The gut-brain axis represents a complex communication network between intestinal microbiota and the central nervous system through neural, endocrine, and immune pathways. Microbial metabolites such as tryptophan derivatives, indoles, and SCFAs are known to influence neurotransmitter production, microglial activity, and synaptic plasticity. Chemotherapy-induced dysregulation of these metabolites affects gut-brain axis communication, leading to cognitive impairment. Experimental studies have proven that microbiome imbalance activates microglial activity and alters synaptic connectivity. Chemotherapy-induced microbiome imbalance was treated with microbiome restoration therapy, which was found to be promising in animal studies. Chemotherapy-treated mice were given a mixture of probiotic strains such as *Lactobacillus plantarum* and *Bifidobacterium breve*, which reduced anxiety and improved memory performance (Kim, 2018).

Metabolic abnormalities represent another aspect of microbiome-mediated side effects. The gut microbiome contributes significantly to bile acid metabolism, lipid metabolism, and glucose metabolism. Chemotherapy-induced microbiome imbalance affects these metabolic pathways by changing the levels of SCFAs and bile acids. Increased levels of LPS in the body, resulting from increased intestinal permeability, are known to cause inflammation and insulin resistance. Chemotherapy-induced microbiome imbalance leads to increased levels of LPS, which cause metabolic abnormalities similar to those observed in metabolic syndrome, including glucose intolerance and dyslipidemia. These metabolic abnormalities contribute to fatigue and negatively impact cancer treatment outcomes. Chemotherapy-induced inflammation, which arises as a result of microbiome imbalance, negatively impacts immune-mediated cancer treatment (Juan et al., 2022; Wu et al., 2024).

3.4.13 Integrative perspective

Collectively, these findings situate the microbiome as an important regulator of GI, neuroimmune, and metabolic homeostasis during chemotherapy. The effects of chemotherapy on cancer cells are only one part of a much broader, more complex picture, in which multiple interconnected systems are impacted in ways that significantly influence patient well-being and treatment outcomes. The appreciation of the microbiome as an intermediary in chemotherapy-induced side effects offers promise for innovation in cancer treatment. Approaches to protect microbial diversity, promote beneficial microbial components, strengthen epithelial barriers, and modulate inflammation may help alleviate toxicity effects without compromising antitumor efficacy (Anand et al., 2023). To further advance supportive oncology medicine, it is necessary to integrate microbiome medicine into clinical practice. Further studies on host, microbiome, and drug interactions will help us appreciate how microbiome modulation can be exploited to improve treatment outcomes. As knowledge advances, it may become as important to target the microbiome as it is to target cancer cells in cancer treatment.

3.5 Modulating the microbes to enhance chemotherapy

The increasing knowledge of microbiome–drug interactions has ushered in a paradigm shift in the field of oncology by harnessing the potential of modulating the microbiome to enhance chemotherapy efficacy. What is now known is that the biological factor is an active regulator of drug metabolism, immune response, and systemic inflammation. The gut microbiota is known to play an integral role in determining the efficacy and toxicity of chemotherapy agents. This is especially so in aggressive cancers such as pancreatic ductal adenocarcinoma (PDAC), where chemotherapy resistance is a major clinical problem. Some bacteria have evolved specific enzymatic machinery to metabolize chemotherapeutic agents, thereby affecting drug metabolism, degradation, and bioavailability (Fu et al., 2021). These microbes may either increase or decrease drug efficacy. Certain microbes are known to transform prodrugs into active drugs, thus increasing the cytotoxic effect of chemotherapeutic drugs on cancer cells. Conversely, certain microbes may transform active chemotherapeutic drugs into inactive compounds, thus reducing their efficacy against cancer cells, leading to chemoresistance (Lehouritis et al., 2015). As illustrated by these examples, it is evident that the microbiome is not simply a passive occupant of the host's environment; instead, it plays an active role in chemotherapeutic dynamics. In addition, drug metabolism is not limited to the liver or tumor site, as previously described; it may also occur within the intestinal lumen or even within the tumor microenvironment.

In addition to direct interaction with chemotherapeutic drugs, microbes of the gut microbiome may produce a variety of metabolites that modulate host immune responses, systemic inflammatory pathways, and host metabolism. For instance, SCFAs, bile acid derivatives, and peptides may modulate systemic host immunity and tumor-associated inflammatory pathways. In this manner, microbes modulate systemic host responses to chemotherapy. As illustrated by this complex relationship between microbes and chemotherapeutic dynamics, it is evident that manipulation of this relationship may provide a compelling approach to modulating chemotherapeutic benefits. As illustrated by one of many examples, microbes may modulate chemotherapeutic efficacy by degrading chemotherapeutic drugs. For instance, cytidine deaminase, or CDD, is a bacterial enzyme that degrades gemcitabine, a chemotherapeutic drug used to treat PDAC. When CDD is upregulated, gemcitabine is rendered ineffective prior to its interaction with cancer cells. In fact, bacterial CDD inhibition has been shown to restore chemotherapeutic drug sensitivity, thus enhancing chemotherapeutic benefits (Geller et al., 2017; Preitakaitė et al., 2025).

Significantly, both intratumoral and intestinal microbiota play an important role in chemotherapy. Recent studies have identified microbial DNA in tumor tissues. This indicates that intratumoral microbes may directly interact with cancer cells. Elucidation of the roles of intratumoral microbes and intestinal microbes may help develop precise treatment modalities depending on the characteristics of the microbes in the tumor tissues.

Significant technological advancements are also underway in the field of cancer microbiome. Machine learning algorithms are now used to analyze the microbiome profile and identify predictive microbial signatures that are correlated with treatment response. These algorithms can analyze intricate relationships between microbial genes, metabolites, and host immune markers. This may help identify patterns that would otherwise go unnoticed. Low-biomass microbiome profiling technologies enable accurate detection of microbes in tumor tissues, regardless of the quantity of the microbes. Furthermore, patient-derived organoid models are also being used to develop precise laboratory models in which the interaction between microbes and cancer cells can be observed in real time.

Equally relevant is the aspect of chemotherapy-induced toxicity reduction by microbiome modulation. The more debilitating side effects of chemotherapy, such as nausea, vomiting, diarrhea, mucositis, and inflammation, are strongly correlated with chemotherapy-induced dysbiosis. The results of microbiome balance have been promising in preclinical and clinical trials. Environmental factors, diet, medications, and antibiotics can all affect the composition of the microbiome and have been found to play a role in chemotherapy efficacy.

Intestinal microbiota-directed therapies such as probiotics, prebiotics, and FMT have been found to be promising in the context of chemotherapy efficacy and toxicity reduction. Studies have found that probiotics can reduce inflammation, build immunity, and promote faster recovery in cancer patients. The results of a study by Zhang (2022) showed that the administration of probiotics reduced inflammation, improved immune status, and improved postoperative recovery in gastrectomy patients with gastric cancer. Similarly, the administration of *C. butyricum* has been found to prolong progression-free survival in metastatic renal cell carcinoma patients receiving nivolumab–ipilimumab combination therapy (Guo et al., 2023). Such findings suggest that microbiome-directed interventions may meaningfully improve both short-term tolerance and long-term outcomes.

3.5.1 Probiotics and prebiotics

Probiotics, which are live microorganisms that, when administered in adequate amounts, provide health benefits to the host, have been receiving considerable interest as supportive care agents in cancer therapy. Certain types of probiotics, such as *Lactobacillus rhamnosus* GG and *Bifidobacterium breve*, have been found to exert protective effects against irinotecan-induced diarrhea and support the maintenance of epithelial barrier function.

Prebiotics are nondigestible food ingredients that beneficially affect the host by serving as substrates for the stimulation of beneficial microorganisms. Prebiotics such as inulin, fructo-oligosaccharides, and resistant starch are known to increase the production of beneficial SCFA-producing microbes, which in turn increase butyrate and acetate production. SCFA production supports the integrity of tight junctions and reduces intestinal permeability and inflammation (Ciernikova et al., 2023).

Interest has also been directed toward postbiotics, which are bioactive microbial metabolites with therapeutic activities that are independent of live bacterial therapy. Butyrate and propionate, for instance, are known to serve as energy sources for colonocytes and HDAC inhibitors.

These metabolites, through epigenetic activity, decrease proinflammatory gene expression and enhance immune homeostasis. Postbiotic therapy has been seen as beneficial in immunocompromised individuals, where there are risks with live probiotic therapy (Balendra et al., 2024). Probiotic and prebiotic therapy, however, still needs to be validated at large levels. Variability in strain selection and dosing regimens, as well as individual factors, makes this therapy still in need of standardized guidelines. However, evidence supports their use as adjunctive therapy to increase tolerance to chemotherapy and stability in immune response.

3.5.2 Fecal microbiota transplantation

On the other hand, FMT is a more holistic approach to the problem of microbial diversity and functional capacity. FMT is an approach in which stool samples from screened donors are used to transfer a balanced and robust microbial ecosystem to a patient. Originally used to treat recurrent *Clostridioides difficile* infection, FMT is now being considered in the context of oncology. Studies conducted in patients with hematologic malignancies have revealed that FMT can correct antibiotic-induced dysbiosis, reduce infection, and hasten hematopoiesis following chemotherapy. The results of recent studies have revealed that FMT can improve the efficacy of chemotherapy by modifying immune cell infiltration and cytokine signaling in the tumor microenvironment. The improvement of microbial diversity can lead to better dendritic cell maturation, T cell recruitment, and immune activation (Xu et al., 2022a). However, there are some limitations to FMT, which have encouraged the use of synthetic microbiota consortia. The limitations of FMT have been the need to screen donors to prevent the transmission of infectious agents. The composition of the microbiota of donors can be heterogeneous and can affect the consistency of FMT. The limitations of FMT have encouraged the use of synthetic microbiota consortia.

3.5.3 Diet, phytochemicals, and lifestyle modulation

Dietary intake is considered to be an easy-to-modulate factor for the composition of the microbiome, particularly during chemotherapy. It is recommended to consume a diet rich in fiber, as this can promote microbial diversity and induce the production of SCFAs, thus facilitating epithelial repair and anti-inflammatory effects. Phytochemical compounds, such as polyphenols contained in green tea, curcumin, or resveratrol, have prebiotic properties. These compounds can support the growth of beneficial microorganisms, such as *Akkermansia muciniphila*, and inhibit the growth of *Enterobacteriaceae*, a family of microorganisms that can induce inflammatory effects. These compounds can indirectly modulate the immune response, thus facilitating the tolerance of chemotherapy. Exercise can also play a role in the modulation of the microbiome. Exercise can promote microbial diversity, thus increasing the production of SCFAs, thus facilitating metabolic stability. Exercise can also decrease the systemic inflammatory response. These nontraditional methods, combined with traditional chemotherapy, can be considered to be cost-effective and noninvasive (Boytar et al., 2022). In summary, it is recommended to modulate the microbiome to improve the efficacy of chemotherapy. This is a rapidly evolving area, particularly for the treatment of cancer. By modulating the composition of the microbiome, it is recommended to improve the efficacy of chemotherapy, thus reducing the toxic effects of chemotherapy.

3.6 Emerging trends and future directions

The rapid progress of metagenomic sequencing technologies and advances in computational biology are revolutionizing our understanding of the complex relationship between microbiomes, cancer biology, and chemotherapy. In previous decades, microbiome research was focused on identifying broad microbiome composition changes, including which bacterial populations increased or decreased during disease states. Although this type of research provided foundational knowledge, it was not sufficient to provide a functional understanding of microbiome changes. Today, advances in various omics technologies, including metagenomics, metabolomics, transcriptomics, and proteomics, provide a multidimensional, functional view of microbiomes. This type of research now provides scientists with the opportunity to look beyond microbiome composition and understand microbiome function, including changes in microbial gene expression patterns, which directly influence chemotherapy metabolism, immune system function, and cancer biology (Su et al., 2025). This type of research has shown that microbiome function may be more critical than microbiome presence. In two different patients, different microbiome compositions may be present, while changes in microbiome function, including differences in gene expression, may result in different chemotherapy outcomes. In fact, by analyzing changes in microbial enzyme function, including those involved in drug metabolism, inflammation, and immune system function, researchers are now identifying microbiome function signatures that predict increased drug efficacy or increased drug toxicity. Perhaps one of the most exciting advances in this field is the application of artificial intelligence and machine learning technologies to microbiome research. In fact, advances in microbiome sequencing technologies have created a need for sophisticated analytical tools to analyze complex microbiome sequencing data, including identifying subtle patterns within thousands of different microbial genes and metabolites. Machine learning algorithms can now analyze pretreatment microbiome composition and predict how a cancer patient is likely to respond to chemotherapy (Kim et al., 2024). These models can identify microbial configurations associated with favorable responses, treatment resistance, or high toxicity risk.

The implications for clinical practice are enormous. Instead of waiting for adverse reactions to occur, doctors could potentially use predictive microbiome analytics to stratify patients even before they start treatment. This implies that patients who are likely to have adverse reactions to treatment could potentially be treated differently. On the other hand, patients who are likely to have a poor response to treatment could potentially be helped to have a more successful response to immune activation. This is a paradigm shift from a reactive approach to cancer treatment to a proactive and preventive oncology care model. In addition to this, synthetic biology and microbial engineering are also providing new opportunities for microbiome science. This includes the exploration of the possibility of developing a genetically engineered bacterial strain that can function as a drug delivery system. This implies that the genetically engineered bacteria have the potential to be programmed to get to the tumor microenvironment, thereby delivering localized doses of cytotoxins to the tumor without causing systemic toxicity or adverse reactions (Bayley et al., 2019). This precision drug delivery system works on the principle of the natural tumor homing capacity of some types of bacteria, particularly to hypoxic or necrotic areas within tumors.

The engineered microbes can also function for detoxification purposes, which may become a problem during chemotherapy. Some chemotherapeutic agents have the potential to produce toxic metabolites, which may cause GI and systemic toxicity. By engineering the bacterial metabolism, it may be possible to inactivate this metabolite, thereby protecting the host. This shows how microbiome manipulation can advance from an adjunct therapy to a potentially integral part of cancer treatment. Along with this, there is a growing interest in the field of postbiotics and precision probiotics. The term "postbiotics" refers to bioactive substances derived from beneficial microbes, including SCFAs, peptides, and immunomodulators. Unlike probiotics, this does not have the problem of the viability of the microbes and the potential for infection in immunocompromised patients. The bioactive nature of this makes it an attractive option for further investigation.

Precision Probiotics is an extension of probiotics. Instead of using general microbial supplements, precision probiotics propose using specific microbial strains, which may be tailored according to the type of cancer, chemotherapy regimens, and microbiome types. For instance, microbial strains, which can activate dendritic cells or augment cytotoxic T cells, may be used in conjunction with chemotherapy to boost antitumor immunity. These advances mark an evolution from microbiome support to microbial intervention, which may be more in line with the immunobiology of cancer (Ahmad et al., 2025). As the development of microbiome-based therapy is progressing toward integration with clinical practice, ethical concerns have also come to the forefront. Questions regarding the screening of donors for FMT, the safety monitoring of engineered bacterial strains, and the standardization of microbial products have to be addressed. There is also a need to protect patient data, particularly with the development of microbiome sequencing. These issues have to be addressed to meet the challenges of translating microbiome research to routine cancer therapy. The idea of a "personalized microbiome diagnosis" is also gaining momentum. It is envisioned that, in the near future, microbial analysis will become as routine a part of cancer therapy as genomic sequencing or immunophenotyping. It is envisioned that the integration of microbiome data with genomic, transcriptomic, and immune data could potentially provide a multidimensional view of each patient's disease state. This may prove useful in developing a comprehensive treatment plan, not only based on the mutational status of the tumor, but also based on the interactions of the host microbiome and the effects of therapy.

The longitudinal assessment of microbiome changes during chemotherapy is another area of significant interest. As previously mentioned, it is understood that the microbiome is not static, meaning that changes do occur over time. The changes may be influenced by a number of different factors, including chemotherapy, diet, antibiotics, or immune response. It is envisioned that changes to the microbiome may prove useful in identifying signs of dysbiosis or immune compromise. In addition, it may prove useful in understanding how changes to the microbiome may be related to tumor response, recurrence, or resistance (Silva et al., 2025). The convergence of microbiome science and precision medicine in oncology represents a new paradigm for cancer therapy. Instead of focusing solely on cancer cells, cancer therapy of the near future may incorporate the host microbiome as a major player in cancer biology. Cancer therapy may be more effective, less toxic, and improve the quality of life for cancer patients by using advances in next-generation sequencing, artificial intelligence, synthetic biology, and diagnostic tests of personalized medicine. The promise of this new and exciting field of medicine does not only come from new advances in technology and medicine, but it is also from a new and holistic approach to cancer treatment. Cancer treatment today is understood to be a system-level problem, which means that there is a need to understand complex interactions between cancer cells, the immune system, metabolism, and microbiome. As this science continues to evolve and reveal new connections, microbiome cancer treatment could be a hallmark of next-generation cancer treatment.

3.7 Clinical trials related to microbiome-targeted interventions

In recent years, with the increasing knowledge about the role of the microbiome in cancer therapy, a number of clinical trials have been initiated to explore the effectiveness of microbiome-targeted interventions in cancer therapy. These trials have been conducted across a variety of geographic regions, covering a spectrum of cancer types, with a global interest in applying microbiome science to cancer therapy. These trials have focused on assessing whether microbiome modulation can help improve the tolerance, decrease the toxicity, and increase the efficacy of conventional anticancer therapy, such as chemotherapy and radiotherapy, in cancer patients (Table 3.3). A number of clinical trials have explored the use of probiotics as an adjunct therapy to chemotherapy. These trials have focused on a variety of outcomes, including the incidence of diarrhea, mucositis, infection, systemic inflammatory response, and quality of life. Preliminary data from a number of randomized clinical trials have suggested that certain probiotic strains can decrease GI toxicity and preserve epithelial barrier function. Moreover, probiotic therapy has also been shown to decrease systemic inflammatory response syndrome and immune parameters in patients with certain types of cancer.

Another set of interventions currently under investigation is prebiotics and synbiotics. Synbiotics are defined as the combination of probiotics and prebiotics. These are designed to foster beneficial microbial growth while simultaneously adding beneficial microbes. Early-stage clinical trials have shown that synbiotics may help boost microbial diversity while reducing inflammatory cytokines in cancer patients undergoing treatment. While these are still in the early stages of investigation, these approaches hold promise for maintaining microbiome resilience in cancer patients undergoing cytotoxic treatment. Another set of approaches currently under investigation is FMT. It is currently under clinical investigation in cancer patients with both hematologic and solid malignancies. Current investigations are focused on determining whether FMT may help in reversing antibiotic-induced microbiome damage while reducing infections in cancer

Table 3.3 List of clinical trials investigating microbiome-based interventions to improve chemotherapy efficacy and reduce treatment-related toxicities.

Trial id	Official title	Cancer type	Microbial intervention	Primary outcome measures	Location
NCT03358511	Engineering gut microbiome to target breast cancer	Breast cancer	Probiotic	Mean number of cytotoxic T lymphocytes (CD8+ cells)	USA
NCT03290651	Resetting the breast microbiome to lower inflammation and risk of cancer	Breast cancer	Probiotic natural health product: RepHresh Pro-B	Change in breast microbiota	Canada
NCT03072641	Using probiotics to reactivate tumor suppressor genes in colon cancer	Colon cancer	ProBion Clinica	Changes in microbiota composition after probiotic use	Sweden
ChiCTR-INQ-17014181	The effect of probiotics on preventing cancer-related cognitive impairment in breast cancer patients	Breast cancer	Probiotic capsules with *Bifidobacterium longum, Lactobacillus acidophilus*, and *Enterococcus faecalis*	Incidence of cancer-related cognitive impairment	China
NCT01410955	Prevention of irinotecan-induced diarrhea by probiotics: A Phase III study	Colorectal cancer	Probiotic	Prevention of grade 3–4 diarrhea in patients treated with irinotecan-based chemotherapy	Slovakia

(*continued on next page*)

Table 3.3 List of clinical trials investigating microbiome-based interventions to improve chemotherapy efficacy and reduce treatment-related toxicities—cont'd

Trial id	Official title	Cancer type	Microbial intervention	Primary outcome measures	Location
NCT01839721	Impact of probiotic BIFILACT® on diarrhea in patients treated with pelvic radiation	Prostate cancer and Gynecologic cancer	Probiotic: Bifilact®	The efficacy of probiotic Bifilact®	Canada
NCT04040712	FMT to treat diarrhea induced by tyrosine-kinase inhibitors in metastatic renal cell carcinoma	Renal cell cancer	FMT	Rate of patients experiencing resolution of diarrhea 4 wk after treatment	Italy
NCT03420443	Randomized clinical trial of the effects of synbiotics on intestinal microbiota in patients undergoing short-course preoperative radiotherapy for rectal cancer	Rectal cancer	Dietary supplement: Oat bran and blueberry husks	Action of synbiotics on irradiated GI mucosa in rectal cancer treatment	Sweden
NCT01549782	Effect of a mixture of inulin and fructo-oligosaccharide on *Lactobacillus* and *Bifidobacterium* in patients receiving radiotherapy	Endometrial neoplasms	Dietary supplement: Inulin, fructo-oligosaccharide, and maltodextrin	Changes in *Lactobacillus* and *Bifidobacterium* populations	Spain

FMT, fecal microbiota transplantation; *GI*, gastrointestinal.

patients undergoing chemotherapy. Exploratory investigations are also currently underway on using FMT in combination with immunotherapy. This is because of recent evidence showing that microbial diversity is correlated with immune checkpoint inhibitor response. While these are still in the early stages of investigation, these approaches hold promise for improving cancer treatment with minimal toxicities. In addition to these traditional approaches using microbes, new approaches are currently under investigation using engineered microbes. While these are still in the early stages of investigation, these approaches hold promise for the next generation of cancer treatment using microbiome-directed approaches. While these are still in the early stages of investigation, these approaches hold promise for the next generation of cancer treatment using microbiome-directed approaches. Collectively, these approaches hold promise for improving cancer treatment with minimal toxicities. While these are still in the early stages of investigation, these approaches hold promise for improving cancer treatment with minimal toxicities. As these approaches continue to evolve, the integration of microbiome-directed approaches in cancer treatment is expected to hold promise.

3.8 Conclusion

The interaction between cancer therapy and the human microbiome is intricate and dynamic, and is now recognized to have important clinical implications. Chemotherapy remains a mainstay of cancer treatment and continues to save many lives from a broad spectrum of cancers. However, due to its systemic nature, chemotherapy does not target cancer cells alone. Along with its anticancer properties, chemotherapy can have a profound effect on the intricate equilibrium of the microbiome. This disruption of the microbiome can cause a variety of side effects, including diarrhea, mucositis, infections, inflammation, and immunosuppression. Chemotherapy not only causes side effects due to its toxic nature but can also have a profound effect on the efficacy of the treatment by impacting the way the drugs are metabolized and the degree to which they are effective. The complex interaction between chemotherapy and the microbiome now presents a new window of opportunity for cancer therapy. Instead of regarding side effects as unavoidable side effects of cancer treatment, researchers are now exploring ways to maintain the equilibrium of the microbiome during chemotherapy. The promising results obtained with probiotics, prebiotics, dietary changes, and fecal microbiome transplantation have been promising and show great potential for the future. These treatments not only show great potential for minimizing side effects but also for improving the efficacy of the drugs and the immune system. The equilibrium of the microbiome can have a profound effect on the strength of the immune system and can help to prevent infections and inflammation.

Another promising area is in predictive microbiome profiling. Today, it is possible to obtain an in-depth profile of an individual's microbiome prior to treatment using advances in DNA sequencing and computer analysis. The future may see doctors being able to predict which patients are more likely to experience severe side effects or lack an adequate response to particular chemotherapy regimens. Such an ability may help doctors tailor treatment in ways that are more individualized. The combination of microbiome profiling, genome profiling, and immunological profiling is an important step toward precision medicine in cancer therapy. Despite all the advances made in this area, however, it is still not fully understood. How particular types of bacteria affect drug metabolism and immunity is still being researched. The variability between individuals, differences in diet, environmental factors, and the effects of antibiotics on the microbiome all contribute to making it difficult to interpret study results. Longitudinal studies are needed to determine how microbiome changes during treatment can be used to predict treatment outcome and toxicity. These studies may provide us with reliable markers of treatment outcome and response.

In the future, it is likely that it will be possible to monitor an individual's microbiome during chemotherapy. Such an ability may help doctors prevent potential complications before they arise. Such an approach may also help doctors provide more effective treatment regimens using both microbiome-targeting drugs and chemotherapy. As more is known about the microbiome, it is likely to be used not only as a predictor of cancer outcome but also as an ally in cancer treatment. The complex relationships between drugs, microbiomes, and human physiology highlight the importance of an interdisciplinary systems biology approach to cancer treatment. As more is known about the microbiome, it may be possible in the future to tailor cancer treatment in ways that not only help individuals survive their cancer but also live a good quality of life during treatment.

References

Ahmad, M. F., Ahmad, F. A., Alsayegh, A. A., Zeyaullah, M., Babalghith, A. O., Faidah, H., Ahmed, F., Khanam, A., Mozaffar, B., Kambal, N., & Bantun, F. (2025). Probiotics and cancer: Mechanistic insights and organ-specific impact. *Biomolecules, 15*(6). https://doi.org/10.3390/biom15060879.

Akbarali, H. I., Muchhala, K. H., Jessup, D. K., & Cheatham, S. (2022). Chemotherapy-induced gastrointestinal toxicities. *Advances in Cancer Research, 155*, 131–166. https://doi.org/10.1016/bs.acr.2022.02.007.

Al Radi, Z. M. A., Prins, F. M., Collij, V., Vich Vila, A., Festen, E. A. M., Dijkstra, G., Weersma, R. K., Klaassen, M. A. Y., & Gacesa, R. (2024). Exploring the predictive value of gut microbiome signatures for therapy intensification in patients with inflammatory bowel disease: A 10-year follow-up study. *Inflammatory Bowel Diseases, 30*(10), 1642–1653. https://doi.org/10.1093/ibd/izae064.

Alcorta, A., López-Gómez, L., Capasso, R., & Abalo, R. (2024). Vitamins and fatty acids against chemotherapy-induced intestinal mucositis. *Pharmacology & Therapeutics, 261*, 108689. https://doi.org/10.1016/j.pharmthera.2024.108689.

Alexander, J. L., Wilson, I. D., Teare, J., Marchesi, J. R., Nicholson, J. K., & Kinross, J. M. (2017). Gut microbiota modulation of chemotherapy efficacy and toxicity. *Nature Reviews Gastroenterology and Hepatology, 14*(6), 356–365. https://doi.org/10.1038/nrgastro.2017.20.

Al-Qadami, G. H., Secombe, K. R., Subramaniam, C. B., Wardill, H. R., & Bowen, J. M. (2022). Gut microbiota-derived short-chain fatty acids: Impact on cancer treatment response and toxicities. *Microorganisms., 10*(10), 2048. https://doi.org/10.3390/microorganisms10102048.

Anand, U., Dey, A., Chandel, A. K. S., Sanyal, R., Mishra, A., Pandey, D. K., De Falco, V., Upadhyay, A., Kandimalla, R., Chaudhary, A., Dhanjal, J. K., Dewanjee, S., Vallamkondu, J., & Pérez de la Lastra, J. M. (2023). Cancer chemotherapy and beyond: Current status, drug candidates, associated risks and progress in targeted therapeutics. *Genes and Diseases, 10*(4), 1367–1401. https://doi.org/10.1016/j.gendis.2022.02.007.

Atarashi, K., Suda, W., Luo, C., Kawaguchi, T., Motoo, I., Narushima, S., Kiguchi, Y., Yasuma, K., Watanabe, E., Tanoue, T., Thaiss, C. A., Sato, M., Toyooka, K., Said, H. S., Yamagami, H., Rice, S. A., Gevers, D.,

Johnson, R. C., Segre, J. A., … Honda, K. (2017). Ectopic colonization of oral bacteria in the intestine drives T H 1 cell induction and inflammation. *Science, 358*(6361), 359–365. https://doi.org/10.1126/science.aan4526.

Balendra, V., Rosenfeld, R., Amoroso, C., Castagnone, C., Rossino, M. G., Garrone, O., & Ghidini, M. (2024). Postbiotics as adjuvant therapy in cancer care. *Nutrients, 16*(15), 2400. https://doi.org/10.3390/nu16152400.

Basile, D., Nardo, P. D., Corvaja, C., Garattini, S. K., Pelizzari, G., Lisanti, C., Bortot, L., Ros, L. D., Bartoletti, M., Borghi, M., Gerratana, L., Lombardi, D., & Puglisi, F. (2019). Mucosal injury during anti-cancer treatment: From pathobiology to bedside. *Cancers., 11*(6), 857. https://doi.org/10.3390/cancers11060857.

Bayley, H., Harimoto, T., & Danino, T. (2019). Engineering bacteria for cancer therapy. *Emerging Topics in Life Sciences, 3*(5), 623–629. https://doi.org/10.1042/etls20190096.

Berding, K., Vlckova, K., Marx, W., Schellekens, H., Stanton, C., Clarke, G., Jacka, F., Dinan, T. G., & Cryan, J. F. (2021). Diet and the microbiota–gut–brain axis: Sowing the seeds of good mental health. *Advances in Nutrition, 12*(4), 1239–1285. https://doi.org/10.1093/advances/nmaa181.

Biennier, S., Fontaine, M., Duquenoy, A., Schwintner, C., Doré, J., & Corvaia, N. (2024). Narrative review: Advancing dysbiosis treatment in onco-hematology with microbiome-based therapeutic approach. *Microorganisms, 12*(11), 2256. https://doi.org/10.3390/microorganisms12112256.

Böhm, D., Russ, E., Guchelaar, H. J., Ziemons, J., Penders, J., Smidt, M. L., van Best, N., & Deenen, M. J. (2025). The role of the gut microbiota in chemotherapy response, efficacy and toxicity: A systematic review. *npj Precision Oncology, 9*(1). https://doi.org/10.1038/s41698-025-01034-0.

Boytar, A. N., Nitert, M. D., Morrision, M., Skinner, T. L., & Jenkins, D. G. (2022). Exercise-induced changes to the human gut microbiota and implications for colorectal cancer: A narrative review. *Journal of Physiology, 600*(24), 5189–5201. https://doi.org/10.1113/JP283702.

Campbell, C., Kandalgaonkar, M. R., Golonka, R. M., Yeoh, B. S., Vijay-Kumar, M., & Saha, P. (2023). Crosstalk between gut microbiota and host immunity: Impact on inflammation and immunotherapy. *Biomedicines., 11*(2). https://doi.org/10.3390/biomedicines11020294.

Checa-Ros, A., Jeréz-Calero, A., Molina-Carballo, A., Campoy, C., & Muñoz-Hoyos, A. (2021). Current evidence on the role of the gut microbiome in ADHD pathophysiology and therapeutic implications. *Nutrients, 13*(1), 1–32. https://doi.org/10.3390/nu13010249.

Chen, C., Zhang, Q., Yu, W., Chang, B., Le, A. D., & Mucositis, O. (2020). An update on innate immunity and new interventional targets. *Journal of Dental Research, 99*(10), 1122–1130. https://doi.org/10.1177/0022034520925421.

Chen, S., Shen, C., Zeng, X., Sun, L., Luo, F., Wan, R., Zhang, Y., Chen, X., Hou, Y., Wang, W., Zheng, Q., & Li, Y. (2025). Energy metabolism and the intestinal barrier: Implications for understanding and managing intestinal diseases. *Frontiers in Microbiology, 16*. https://doi.org/10.3389/fmicb.2025.1515364.

Chrysostomou, D., Roberts, L. A., Marchesi, J. R., & Kinross, J. M. (2023). Gut microbiota modulation of efficacy and toxicity of cancer chemotherapy and immunotherapy. *Gastroenterology, 164*(2), 198–213. https://doi.org/10.1053/j.gastro.2022.10.018.

Chu, H. (2017). Host gene–microbiome interactions: Molecular mechanisms in inflammatory bowel disease. *Genome Medicine, 9*(1). https://doi.org/10.1186/s13073-017-0459-4.

Ciernikova, S., Mego, M., & Chovanec, M. (2021). Exploring the potential role of the gut microbiome in chemotherapy-induced neurocognitive disorders and cardiovascular toxicity. *Cancers, 13*(4), 1–26. https://doi.org/10.3390/cancers13040782.

Ciernikova, S., Sevcikova, A., Drgona, L., & Mego, M. (2023). Modulating the gut microbiota by probiotics, prebiotics, postbiotics, and fecal microbiota transplantation: An emerging trend in cancer patient care. *Biochimica et Biophysica Acta (BBA) - Reviews on Cancer, 1878*(6), 188990. https://doi.org/10.1016/j.bbcan.2023.188990.

Cohen, I., Ruff, W. E., & Longbrake, E. E. (2021). Influence of immunomodulatory drugs on the gut microbiota. *Translational Research, 233*, 144–161. https://doi.org/10.1016/j.trsl.2021.01.009.

Dahiya, D., & Nigam, P. S. (2023). Antibiotic-therapy-induced gut dysbiosis affecting gut microbiota—brain axis and cognition: Restoration by intake of probiotics and synbiotics. *International Journal of Molecular Sciences, 24*(4). https://doi.org/10.3390/ijms24043074.

Derrien, M., Alvarez, A. S., & de Vos, W. M. (2019). The gut microbiota in the first decade of life. *Trends in Microbiology, 27*(12), 997–1010. https://doi.org/10.1016/j.tim.2019.08.001.

Eiman, L., Moazzam, K., Anjum, S., Kausar, H., Sharif, E. A. M., & Ibrahim, W. N. (2025). Gut dysbiosis in cancer immunotherapy: Microbiota-mediated resistance and emerging treatments. *Frontiers in Immunology, 16*. https://doi.org/10.3389/fimmu.2025.1575452.

Fernandes, C., Miranda, M. C. C., Roque, C. R., Paguada, A. L. P., Mota, C. A. R., Florêncio, K. G. D., Pereira, A. F., Wong, D. V. T., Oriá, R. B., & Lima-Júnior, R. C. P. (2024). Is there an interplay between environmental factors, microbiota imbalance, and cancer chemotherapy-associated intestinal mucositis? *Pharmaceuticals, 17*(8). https://doi.org/10.3390/ph17081020.

Fiore, E., Van Tyne, D., & Gilmore, M. S. (2019). Pathogenicity of enterococci. *Microbiology Spectrum, 7*(4). https://doi.org/10.1128/microbiolspec.GPP3-0053-2018.

Fu, C., Yang, J., Yu, J., & Wei, M. (2021). The interaction between gut microbiome and anti-tumor drug therapy. *American Journal of Cancer Research, 11*(12), 5812–5832.

Gassner, F. J., Weiss, L., Geisberger, R., Hofbauer, J. P., Egle, A., Hartmann, T. N., Greil, R., & Tinhofer, I. (2011). Fludarabine modulates composition and function of the T cell pool in patients with chronic lymphocytic leukaemia. *Cancer Immunology, Immunotherapy, 60*(1), 75–85. https://doi.org/10.1007/s00262-010-0920-3.

Geller, L. T., Barzily-Rokni, M., Danino, T., Jonas, O. H., Shental, N., Nejman, D., Gavert, N., Zwang, Y., Cooper, Z. A., Shee, K., Thaiss, C. A., Reuben, A., Livny, J., Avraham, R., Frederick, D. T., Ligorio, M., Chatman, K., Johnston, S. E., Mosher, C. M., … Straussman, R. (2017). Potential role of intratumor bacteria in mediating tumor resistance to the chemotherapeutic drug gemcitabine. *Science, 357*(6356), 1156–1160. https://doi.org/10.1126/science.aah5043.

Gopalakrishnan, V., Helmink, B. A., Spencer, C. N., Reuben, A., & Wargo, J. A. (2018). The influence of the gut microbiome on cancer, immunity, and cancer immunotherapy. *Cancer Cell, 33*(4), 570–580. https://doi.org/10.1016/j.ccell.2018.03.015.

Guo, C., Kong, L., Xiao, L., Liu, K., Cui, H., Xin, Q., Gu, X., Jiang, C., & Wu, J. (2023). The impact of the gut microbiome on tumor immunotherapy: From mechanism to application strategies. *Cell & Bioscience, 13*(1). https://doi.org/10.1186/s13578-023-01135-y.

Hutchison, A. L., Tavaglione, F., Romeo, S., & Charlton, M. (2023). Endocrine aspects of metabolic dysfunction-associated steatotic liver disease (MASLD): Beyond insulin resistance. *Journal of Hepatology, 79*(6), 1524–1541. https://doi.org/10.1016/j.jhep.2023.08.030.

Jameus, A., Kennedy, A. E., & Thome, C. (2021). Hematological changes following low dose radiation therapy and comparison to current standard of care cancer treatments. *Dose-Response, 19*(4). https://doi.org/10.1177/15593258211056196.

Jansen, S. A., Cutilli, A., de Koning, C., van Hoesel, M., Frederiks, C. L., Saiz Sierra, L., Nierkens, S., Mokry, M., Nieuwenhuis, E. E. S., Hanash, A. M., Mocholi, E., Coffer, P. J., & Lindemans, C. A. (2024). Chemotherapy-induced intestinal epithelial damage directly promotes galectin-9-driven modulation of T cell behavior. *iScience, 27*(6). https://doi.org/10.1016/j.isci.2024.110072.

Juan, Z., Chen, J., Ding, B., Yongping, L., Liu, K., Wang, L., Le, Y., Liao, Q., Shi, J., Huang, J., Wu, Y., Ma, D., Ouyang, W., & Tong, J. (2022). Probiotic supplement attenuates chemotherapy-related cognitive impairment in patients with breast cancer: A randomised, double-blind, and placebo-controlled trial. *European Journal of Cancer, 161*, 10–22. https://doi.org/10.1016/j.ejca.2021.11.006.

Karagiannis, G. S., Condeelis, J. S., & Oktay, M. H. (2018). Chemotherapy-induced metastasis: Mechanisms and translational opportunities. *Clinical and Experimental Metastasis, 35*(4), 269–284. https://doi.org/10.1007/s10585-017-9870-x.

Kenneth, M. J., Wu, C. C., Fang, C. Y., Hsu, T. K., Lin, I. C., Huang, S. W., Chiu, Y. C., & Hsu, B. M. (2025). Exploring the impact of chemotherapy on the emergence of antibiotic resistance in the gut microbiota of colorectal cancer patients. *Antibiotics, 14*(3). https://doi.org/10.3390/antibiotics14030264.

Kerstens, R., & Joyce, P. (2024). The gut microbiome as a catalyst and emerging therapeutic target for Parkinson's disease: A comprehensive update. *Biomedicines, 12*(8), 1738. https://doi.org/10.3390/biomedicines12081738.

Kim, C. H. (2018). Immune regulation by microbiome metabolites. *Immunology, 154*(2), 220–229. https://doi.org/10.1111/imm.12930.

Kim, D., Yu, Y., Jung, K. S., Kim, Y. H., & Kim, J. J. (2024). Tumor microenvironment can predict chemotherapy response of patients with triple-negative breast cancer receiving neoadjuvant chemotherapy. *Cancer Research and Treatment, 56*(1), 162–177. https://doi.org/10.4143/crt.2023.330.

Kujawa, D., Laczmanski, L., Budrewicz, S., Pokryszko-Dragan, A., & Podbielska, M. (2023). Targeting gut microbiota: New therapeutic opportunities in multiple sclerosis. *Gut Microbes, 15*(2). https://doi.org/10.1080/19490976.2023.2274126.

Lange, O., Proczko-Stepaniak, M., & Mika, A. (2023). Short-chain fatty acids—A product of the microbiome and its participation in two-way communication on the microbiome-host mammal line. *Current Obesity Reports, 12*(2), 108–126. https://doi.org/10.1007/s13679-023-00503-6.

Lehouritis, P., Cummins, J., Stanton, M., Murphy, C. T., McCarthy, F. O., Reid, G., Urbaniak, C., Byrne, W. L., & Tangney, M. (2015). Local bacteria affect the efficacy of chemotherapeutic drugs. *Scientific Reports, 5*(1). https://doi.org/10.1038/srep14554.

Li, Z., Ke, X., Zuo, D., Wang, Z., Fang, F., & Li, B. (2023). New insights into the relationship between gut microbiota and radiotherapy for cancer. *Nutrients, 15*(1), 48. https://doi.org/10.3390/nu15010048.

Li, S., Zhu, S., & Yu, J. (2024a). The role of gut microbiota and metabolites in cancer chemotherapy. *Journal of Advanced Research, 64*, 223–235. https://doi.org/10.1016/j.jare.2023.11.027.

Li, J., Wu, H., Yu, Z., Wang, Q., Zeng, X., Qian, W., Lu, S., Jiang, L., Li, J., Zhu, M., Han, Y., Gao, J., & Qian, P. (2024b). Hematopoietic stem and progenitor cell membrane-coated vesicles for bone marrow-targeted leukaemia drug delivery. *Nature Communications, 15*(1). https://doi.org/10.1038/S41467-024-50021-9.

Li, X., Jia, Y., Li, Y., Hei, H., Zhang, S., & Qin, J. (2025). Crosstalk between metabolic reprogramming and microbiota: Implications for cancer progression and novel therapeutic opportunities. *Frontiers in Immunology, 16*. https://doi.org/10.3389/fimmu.2025.1582166.

Mafe, A. N., & Büsselberg, D. (2025). Microbiome integrity enhances the efficacy and safety of anticancer drug. *Biomedicines, 13*(2). https://doi.org/10.3390/biomedicines13020422.

Markowiak-Kopeć, P., & Śliżewska, K. (2020). The effect of probiotics on the production of short-chain fatty acids by human intestinal microbiome. *Nutrients, 12*(4), 1107. https://doi.org/10.3390/nu12041107.

Meade, S., Kiow, J. L. C., Massaro, C., Kaur, G., Squirell, E., Bressler, B., & Lunken, G. (2023). Gut microbiome-associated predictors as biomarkers of response to advanced therapies in inflammatory bowel disease: A systematic review. *Gut Microbes, 15*(2). https://doi.org/10.1080/19490976.2023.2287073.

Miller, K. K., Gorcey, L., & McLellan, B. N. (2014). Chemotherapy-induced hand-foot syndrome and nail changes: A review of clinical presentation, etiology, pathogenesis, and management. *Journal of the American Academy of Dermatology, 71*(4), 787–794. https://doi.org/10.1016/j.jaad.2014.03.019.

Mollaei, M., Hassan, Z. M., Khorshidi, F., & Langroudi, L. (2021). Chemotherapeutic drugs: Cell death- and resistance-related signaling pathways. Are they really as smart as the tumor cells? *Translational Oncology, 14*(5). https://doi.org/10.1016/j.tranon.2021.101056.

Montassier, E., Gastinne, T., Vangay, P., Al-Ghalith, G. A., Bruley des Varannes, S., Massart, S., Moreau, P., Potel, G., de La Cochetière, M. F., Batard, E., & Knights, D. (2015). Chemotherapy-driven dysbiosis in the intestinal microbiome. *Alimentary Pharmacology & Therapeutics, 42*(5), 515–528. https://doi.org/10.1111/apt.13302.

Morris, G., Berk, M., Carvalho, A., Caso, J. R., Sanz, Y., Walder, K., & Maes, M. (2017). The role of the microbial metabolites including tryptophan catabolites and short chain fatty acids in the pathophysiology of immune-inflammatory and neuroimmune disease. *Molecular Neurobiology, 54*(6), 4432–4451. https://doi.org/10.1007/s12035-016-0004-2.

Nie, H. Y., Ge, J., Huang, G. X., Liu, K. G., Yue, Y., Li, H., Lin, H. G., Zhang, T., Yan, H. F., Xu, B. X., Sun, H. W., Yang, J. W., Si, S. Y., Zhou, J. L., & Cui, Y. (2024). New insights into the intestinal barrier through "gut-organ" axes and a glimpse of the microgravity's effects on intestinal barrier. *Frontiers in Physiology, 15*. https://doi.org/10.3389/fphys.2024.1465649.

Özdemir, B. C., Gerard, C. L., & Espinosa da Silva, C. (2022). Sex and gender differences in anticancer treatment toxicity: A call for revisiting drug dosing in oncology. *Endocrinology, 163*(6). https://doi.org/10.1210/endocr/bqac058.

Patangia, D. V., Anthony Ryan, C., Dempsey, E., Paul Ross, R., & Stanton, C. (2022). Impact of antibiotics on the human microbiome and consequences for host health. *MicrobiologyOpen, 11*(1). https://doi.org/10.1002/mbo3.1260.

Petersen, C., & Round, J. L. (2014). Defining dysbiosis and its influence on host immunity and disease. *Cellular Microbiology, 16*(7), 1024–1033. https://doi.org/10.1111/cmi.12308.

Pickard, J. M., Zeng, M. Y., Caruso, R., & Núñez, G. (2017). Gut microbiota: Role in pathogen colonization, immune responses, and inflammatory disease. *Immunological Reviews, 279*(1), 70–89. https://doi.org/10.1111/imr.12567.

Pouncey, A. L., Scott, A. J., Leslie Alexander, J., Marchesi, J., & Kinross, J. (2018). Gut microbiota, chemotherapy and the host: The influence of the gut microbiota on cancer treatment. *ecancermedicalscience, 12*. https://doi.org/10.3332/ecancer.2018.868.

Prasad, R. M., Srivastava, S., Wang, E., Liu, J. Z., Gami, R., Abdelgadir, A., Sharma, A., Rayamajhi, S., & Tikaria, R. (2022). Effect of immunosuppressive diseases and rituximab infusions on allowing COVID-19 infection to relapse. *Permanente Journal, 26*(1), 122–131. https://doi.org/10.7812/TPP/21.035.

Preitakaitė, V., Kazlauskas, A., Aučynaitė, A., Butkutė, K., Lapinskaitė, R., Urbelienė, N., Laurynėnas, A., & Meškys, R. (2025). Bacterial cytidine deaminases as versatile activators of fluoropyrimidine nucleoside prodrugs. *European Journal of Medicinal Chemistry, 296*, 117860. https://doi.org/10.1016/j.ejmech.2025.117860.

Rad, H. F., Tahmasebi, H., Javani, S., Hemati, M., Zakerhamidi, D., Hosseini, M., Alibabaei, F., Banihashemian, S. Z., Oksenych, V., & Eslami, M. (2024). Microbiota and cytokine modulation: Innovations in enhancing anticancer immunity and personalized cancer therapies. *Biomedicines, 12*(12), 2776. https://doi.org/10.3390/biomedicines12122776.

Rajak, M., Dash, D., & Koiri, R. K. (2026). Microbiota-derived metabolites in cancer: Dual roles in pathogenesis and opportunities for therapy. *Medicine in Drug Discovery, 29*, 100245. https://doi.org/10.1016/j.medidd.2025.100245.

Rashidi, A., & Weisdorf, D. J. (2020). Microbiota-based approaches to mitigate infectious complications of intensive chemotherapy in patients with acute leukemia. *Translational Research, 220*, 167–181. https://doi.org/10.1016/j.trsl.2020.03.011.

Ren, X., Boriero, D., Chaiswing, L., Bondada, S., Clair, D. K. S. t., & Butterfield, D. A. (2019). Plausible biochemical mechanisms of chemotherapy-induced cognitive impairment ("chemobrain"), a condition that significantly impairs the quality of life of many cancer survivors. *Biochimica et Biophysica Acta (BBA) - Molecular Basis of Disease, 1865*(6), 1088–1097. https://doi.org/10.1016/j.bbadis.2019.02.007.

Roggiani, S., Mengoli, M., Conti, G., Fabbrini, M., Brigidi, P., Barone, M., D'Amico, F., & Turroni, S. (2023). Gut microbiota resilience and recovery after anticancer chemotherapy. *Microbiome Research Reports, 2*(2), 16. https://doi.org/10.20517/mrr.2022.23.

Rotz, S. J., & Dandoy, C. E. (2020). The microbiome in pediatric oncology. *Cancer, 126*(16), 3629–3637. https://doi.org/10.1002/cncr.33030.

Routy, B., Le Chatelier, E., Derosa, L., Duong, C. P. M., Alou, M. T., Daillère, R., Fluckiger, A., Messaoudene, M., Rauber, C., Roberti, M. P., Fidelle, M., Flament, C., Poirier-Colame, V., Opolon, P., Klein, C., Iribarren, K., Mondragón, L., Jacquelot, N., Qu, B., … Zitvogel, L. (2018). Gut microbiome influences efficacy of

PD-1–based immunotherapy against epithelial tumors. *Science, 359*(6371), 91–97. https://doi.org/10.1126/science.aan3706.

Safarchi, A., Al-Qadami, G., Tran, C. D., & Conlon, M. (2025). Understanding dysbiosis and resilience in the human gut microbiome: Biomarkers, interventions, and challenges. *Frontiers in Microbiology, 16*. https://doi.org/10.3389/fmicb.2025.1559521.

Schmidt, S., Messner, C. J., Gaiser, C., Hämmerli, C., & Suter-Dick, L. (2022). Methotrexate-induced liver injury is associated with oxidative stress, impaired mitochondrial respiration, and endoplasmic reticulum stress *in vitro*. *International Journal of Molecular Sciences, 23*(23), 15116. https://doi.org/10.3390/ijms232315116.

Sharma, A., Jasrotia, S., & Kumar, A. (2024). Effects of chemotherapy on the immune system: Implications for cancer treatment and patient outcomes. *Naunyn-Schmiedeberg's Archives of Pharmacology, 397*(5), 2551–2566. https://doi.org/10.1007/s00210-023-02781-2.

Sibaud, V., Leboeuf, N. R., Roche, H., Belum, V. R., Gladieff, L., Deslandres, M., Montastruc, M., Eche, A., Vigarios, E., Dalenc, F., & Lacouture, M. E. (2016). Dermatological adverse events with taxane chemotherapy. *European Journal of Dermatology, 26*(5), 427–443. https://doi.org/10.1684/ejd.2016.2833.

Silva, C. A. C., Almonte, A. A., & Zitvogel, L. (2025). Oncobiomics: Leveraging microbiome translational research in immuno-oncology for clinical-practice changes. *Biomolecules, 15*(4), 504. https://doi.org/10.3390/biom15040504.

Song, B. C., & Bai, J. (2021). Microbiome-gut-brain axis in cancer treatment-related psychoneurological toxicities and symptoms: A systematic review. *Supportive Care in Cancer, 29*(2), 605–617. https://doi.org/10.1007/s00520-020-05739-9.

Su, F., Su, M., Wei, W., Wu, J., Chen, L., Sun, X., Liu, M., Sun, S., Mao, R., Bourgonje, A. R., & Hu, S. (2025). Integrating multi-omics data to reveal the host-microbiota interactome in inflammatory bowel disease. *Gut Microbes, 17*(1). https://doi.org/10.1080/19490976.2025.2476570.

Sun, Y., Wang, X., Li, L., Zhong, C., Zhang, Y., Yang, X., Li, M., & Yang, C. (2024). The role of gut microbiota in intestinal disease: From an oxidative stress perspective. *Frontiers in Microbiology, 15*. https://doi.org/10.3389/fmicb.2024.1328324.

Tangvarasittichai, S. (2015). Oxidative stress, insulin resistance, dyslipidemia and type 2 diabetes mellitus. *World Journal of Diabetes, 6*(3), 456. https://doi.org/10.4239/wjd.v6.i3.456.

Trecarichi, A., & Flatters, S. J. L. (2019). Mitochondrial dysfunction in the pathogenesis of chemotherapy-induced peripheral neuropathy. *International Review of Neurobiology, 145*, 83–126. https://doi.org/10.1016/bs.irn.2019.05.001.

Villanueva-Paz, M., Morán, L., López-Alcántara, N., Freixo, C., Andrade, R. J., Lucena, M. I., & Cubero, F. J. (2021). Oxidative stress in drug-induced liver injury (Dili): From mechanisms to biomarkers for use in clinical practice. *Antioxidants, 10*(3), 1–35. https://doi.org/10.3390/antiox10030390.

Was, H., Borkowska, A., Bagues, A., Tu, L., Liu, J. Y. H., Lu, Z., Rudd, J. A., Nurgali, K., & Abalo, R. (2022). Mechanisms of chemotherapy-induced neurotoxicity. *Frontiers in Pharmacology, 13*. https://doi.org/10.3389/fphar.2022.750507.

Wei, L., Wen, X. S., & Xian, C. J. (2021). Chemotherapy-induced intestinal microbiota dysbiosis impairs mucosal homeostasis by modulating toll-like receptor signaling pathways. *International Journal of Molecular Sciences, 22*(17). https://doi.org/10.3390/ijms22179474.

Winter, S. E., & Bäumler, A. J. (2023). Gut dysbiosis: Ecological causes and causative effects on human disease. *Proceedings of the National Academy of Sciences of the United States of America, 120*(50). https://doi.org/10.1073/pnas.2316579120.

Wu, J., Zhang, R., Yin, Z., Chen, X. u, Mao, R., Zheng, X., Yuan, M., Li, H., Lu, Y., Liu, S., Gao, X., & Sun, Q. (2024). Gut microbiota-driven metabolic alterations reveal the distinct pathogenicity of chemotherapy-induced cachexia in gastric cancer. *Pharmacological Research, 209*, 107476. https://doi.org/10.1016/j.phrs.2024.107476.

Xu, H., Cao, C., Ren, Y., Weng, S., Liu, L., Guo, C., Wang, L., Han, X., Ren, J., & Liu, Z. (2022a). Antitumor effects of fecal microbiota transplantation: Implications for microbiome modulation in cancer treatment. *Frontiers in Immunology, 13*. https://doi.org/10.3389/fimmu.2022.949490.

Xu, K., Cai, J., Xing, J., Li, X., Wu, B., Zhu, Z., & Zhang, Z. (2022b). Broad-spectrum antibiotics associated gut microbiome disturbance impairs T cell immunity and promotes lung cancer metastasis: A retrospective study. *BMC Cancer, 22*(1). https://doi.org/10.1186/s12885-022-10307-x.

Yang, X., An, H., He, Y., Fu, G., & Jiang, Z. (2023). Comprehensive analysis of microbiota signature across 32 cancer types. *Frontiers in Oncology, 13*. https://doi.org/10.3389/fonc.2023.1127225.

Yin, B., Wang, X., Yuan, F., Li, Y., & Lu, P. (2022). Research progress on the effect of gut and tumor microbiota on antitumor efficacy and adverse effects of chemotherapy drugs. *Frontiers in Microbiology, 13*. https://doi.org/10.3389/fmicb.2022.899111.

Zajaczkowską, R., Kocot-Kępska, M., Leppert, W., Wrzosek, A., Mika, J., & Wordliczek, J. (2019). Mechanisms of chemotherapy-induced peripheral neuropathy. *International Journal of Molecular Sciences, 20*(6). https://doi.org/10.3390/ijms20061451.

Zhang, P. (2022). Influence of foods and nutrition on the gut microbiome and implications for intestinal health. *International Journal of Molecular Sciences, 23*(17), 9588. https://doi.org/10.3390/ijms23179588.

Zhuang, Y. P., Zhou, H. L., Chen, H. B., Zheng, M. Y., Liang, Y. W., Gu, Y. T., Li, W. T., Qiu, W. L., & Zhou, H. G. (2023). Gut microbiota interactions with antitumor immunity in colorectal cancer: From understanding to application. *Biomedicine and Pharmacotherapy, 165*. https://doi.org/10.1016/j.biopha.2023.115040.

4

Microbiome as a modulator of immunotherapy: Synergistic effects of the microbiome in immunotherapy

Vansh Vohra[a], Garima Malik[b], Neeraj Mittal[b], Meenakshi Dhanawat[c] and Jashan Girdhar[d]

[a]M.M COLLEGE OF PHARMACY, MAHARISHI MARKANDESHWAR (DEEMED TO BE UNIVERSITY), AMBALA, HARYANA, INDIA [b]CHITKARA COLLEGE OF PHARMACY, CHITKARA UNIVERSITY, RAJPURA, PUNJAB, INDIA [c]AMITY INSTITUTE OF PHARMACY, AMITY UNIVERSITY HARYANA, GURUGRAM, HARYANA, INDIA [d]TEERTHANKER MAHAVEER COLLEGE OF PHARMACY, TEERTHANKER MAHAVEER UNIVERSITY, MORADABAD, UTTAR PRADESH, INDIA

4.1 Introduction

The human body contains microorganisms that are very important in sustaining our good health; they help us with digestion, produce substances that we cannot produce, and communicate with the host immune system (Falony et al., 2019; Fujimura et al., 2010; Jones et al., 2014). Often, the plausibility of the gut microbiota has been regarded with suspicion due to cultivation prejudices, and the fact that many of the gut bacteria estimated to occur in the colon were not cultivable by traditional methods was subsequently reported by early microbiologists (Falony et al., 2019). Nevertheless, molecular techniques like DNA sequencing have revolutionized the information about microbial diversity, thereby shedding new light on microbiome functions and relationships with health and disease (Falony et al., 2019). The microbiota refers to all the microorganisms that live in and on the human body, and the microbiome is a complex made up of all the genomes existing in these microorganisms today (Jones et al., 2014). Even though the human body has more microbial cells than human cells, approximately three times more, the gastrointestinal tract (GIT) is the main location of the majority of these microorganisms (Fujimura et al., 2010; Jones et al., 2014). Beyond its crucial role in metabolism and supporting the immune system, the gut microbiome also contributes to energy that can be harvested and stored, fermentation

The Microbiome and Cancer Treatment: Overcoming Resistance and Enhancing Efficacy.
DOI: https://doi.org/10.1016/B978-0-443-33206-7.00005-4

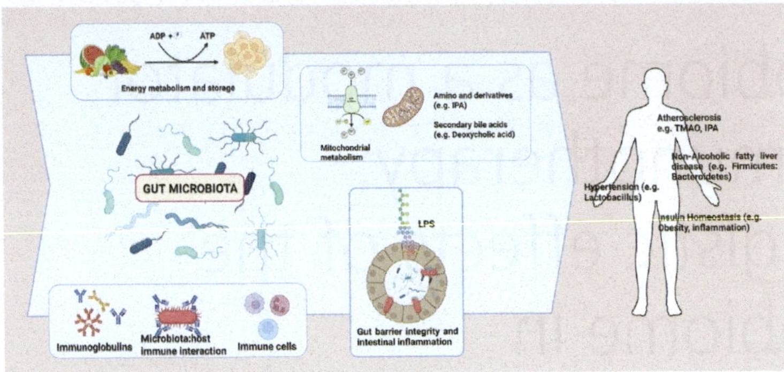

FIGURE 4.1 Modulatory effect of gut microbiota.

of indigestible carbohydrates, and the production of vitamins K and B, and the modulation of innate and cell-mediated immunity (Fujimura et al., 2010; Jones et al., 2014). Additionally, the gut microbiome helps maintain the intestinal barrier by breaking down mucosal polysaccharides and fermenting dietary fibers. This process produces SCFAs, which serve as an energy source for colon cells and play a key role in regulating immune responses (Jones et al., 2014).

By far, one of the key roles of the microbiome in the human health system is the relationship with the immune system, which regulates the development and maturation of the gut-associated lymphoid tissue (GALT) and indirectly influences cell types like T-regulatory (Treg) cells that help maintain immune homeostasis (Falony et al., 2019; Fujimura et al., 2010). Microbiota's ability to live harmoniously in the human body, even if the immune system is completely functional in eliminating invaders, is one of the most striking features of this symbiotic relationship; this is particularly true in the gastrointestinal tract, where microbial communities participate in the processing of food, metabolism, and the immune defense mechanism against proliferating pathogens there (Fujimura et al., 2010). The balance of the microbiome is formed by a number of elements, which include nutrition, the use of antibiotics, genetics, and environmental factors, showing great differences between humans (Falony et al., 2019; Fujimura et al., 2010; Jones et al., 2014). The immunity of the child in the earlier stages of life, together with the implementation of the immune resistance pathway through the mother's microbiota by means such as parturition, lactation, as well as exposure to vital elements such as pet ownership or farm—animal association, is a way of immune tolerance, and thus the risk of allergic diseases is reduced (Fujimura et al., 2010). The microbial flora, on the other hand, tend to decrease in number with more unnatural influences, such as antibiotic use; dietary changes; or environmental changes, which in turn, may lead to the state of dysbiosis, in which the microbial diversity is reduced, and the community structure is different from the previous states, and that, in turn, has been linked to the occurrence of some diseases like inflammatory bowel, metabolic problems, and the increased risk of infections (Falony et al., 2019; Fujimura et al., 2010; Jones et al., 2014) (Fig. 4.1).

The structure of microbial communities is directly related to health. For example, a wide variety of bacterial species has been observed in healthy individuals, whereas people who suffer from various diseases, such as obesity and inflammatory disorders, have different, diversified, and temporally stable populations of bacteria that they carry (Fujimura et al., 2010). The study of the microbiome's role in metabolism is a notable case, given the evidence that an excessive increase in the *Firmicutes/Bacteroidetes* ratio in obese individuals boosts the energy extraction capacity of food and contributes to the accumulation of fat, thus demonstrating the microbes' effect on the host and disease susceptibility (Fujimura et al., 2010). Furthermore, microbiome research has presented the microbiome as a dynamic system that responds to changes in diet and environmental exposure. It has highlighted that further investigation into this system is crucial for protecting human health and eventually preventing disease (Fujimura et al., 2010). Although the microbiome research area is gaining momentum, challenges still exist in translating findings into clinical practice. This is due to the influence of factors such as technical variability, study reproducibility, and standardization of methodologies (Falony et al., 2019). Understanding microbiome variation at the population level is key to identifying microbiome covariates and developing clinical applications (Falony et al., 2019).

Immunotherapy is one of the rapidly advancing fields in advanced cancer research that uses the immune system to identify and kill cancer cells with high specificity compared to chemotherapy, radiation, and surgery, which are the usual treatments (Bassiony et al., 2020; Oli et al., 2024; Yang et al., 2022). Thus, this method has already been very effective due to the potential for long-lasting treatment reactions, decreased side effects on the body, and higher survival rates, especially in cases where traditional treatments have proven ineffective or unsafe (Bassiony et al., 2020; Oli et al., 2024; Yang et al., 2022). Immune therapies, unlike chemotherapy, which affects anything that divides quickly (including normal host cells), are more selective and work by helping the organism's defenses to attack the cancer cells, leaving the rest of the body unharmed (Bassiony et al., 2020; Oli et al., 2024). The success of immunotherapy is largely due to advancements in tumor biology, especially our understanding of the complex interactions among cancer cells, immunity, and the tumor microenvironment (TME), which all play a decisive role in cancer development and immune evasion (Oli et al., 2024; Yang et al., 2022).

Various immunotherapeutic methods have been developed, such as immune checkpoint inhibitors (ICIs), adoptive cell therapy (ACT), cancer vaccines, cytokine-based therapies, monoclonal antibodies (MoAb), and oncolytic virus therapy, which are developed to help the immune system differentiate and kill cancer cells (Bassiony et al., 2020; Oli et al., 2024; Yang et al., 2022). ICIs include a chemical, for example, anti-PD-1, anti-PD-L1, and anti-CTLA-4 antibodies, which work by stopping the immune evasion pathways that tumors take advantage of, which aids in reversing the T-cell activity and thus can cause the tumors' shape to go away (Oli et al., 2024; Yang et al., 2022). The use of ICIs by blocking immune checkpoints with inhibitors such as ipilimumab, pembrolizumab, and nivolumab induces a promising alteration of the immune status in which the tumors are the target, but complications like immune-related adverse events (irAEs) and varying response rates are still present (Yang et al., 2022). The ACT process is the transfer of modified and reinfused patient-derived T cells that are specifically cytotoxic into the body of the patient in the next stage, after which they simulate an overwhelming attack on cancer cells (Oli et al., 2024; Yang et al., 2022). The list of innovative procancer immunotherapy methods that includes chimeric antigen receptor T (CAR-T) cells, tumor-infiltrating lymphocytes (TILs), and T cell receptor-modified T (TCR-T) cells proves these methods to be the most effective in anticancer exploration (Yang et al., 2022).

Cytokine-based therapies interact with the cells of the immune system, mainly the immune-modulating molecules IL-2 and interferon gamma (IFN-γ), to improve the functioning and the number of control immune system cells, giving rise, in the process, to antitumor activity. Cancer vaccines, on the other hand, teach the immune system cells to recognize antigens from tumor cells and then mount a direct immune response to kill cancer cells (Oli et al., 2024; Yang et al., 2022). Preventive vaccines such as those targeting human papillomavirus (HPV) for cervical cancer have been very potent, unlike therapeutic cancer vaccines, e.g., sipuleucel-T for prostate cancer, which have exhibited only poor clinical results in solid tumors (Yang et al., 2022). Oncolytic virus therapy is a method of using a specially designed virus to infect tumor cells and then cause their death. This method achieves two goals at the same time because it is capable of stimulating an immune response against cancer (Yang et al., 2022). Furthermore, MoAb play a vital role in the targeting of specific antigens on cancer cells. They help the immune system to recognize and destroy cancer cells (Bassiony et al., 2020).

Even though tumor immunotherapy has shown an unbelievable improvement, immune resistance, adverse immune-related side effects, and the complexity of the TME continue to be problems for the technology because of the immunosuppressive environment that the TME can create (Bassiony et al., 2020; Oli et al., 2024; Yang et al., 2022). Immunotherapy offers a good alternative to classical treatments, such as chemotherapy, radiotherapy, and surgeries, which have many side effects, toxicities, drug resistance, and a lack of long-term survival benefits, besides the fact that they are suitable for advanced tumor patients only (Bassiony et al., 2020; Yang et al., 2022). Some people may benefit a lot from immunotherapy treatment, yet, on the other hand, some may not because of immune system resistance or the differences in immune system-cancer cells interactions (Bassiony et al., 2020). The effectiveness of immunotherapy mostly lies in patient selection, since different types of tumors have different levels of immune response, and treating them with immune-evasion mechanisms can lead to a reduction in treatment efficacy (Bassiony et al., 2020). Furthermore, linking immunotherapy with other forms of treatment has been proven to be of help, and it is possible to increase treatment efficacy, reduce relapse rates, and improve patient survival in the long run. By opposing chemotherapy, which has a direct effect on the entire body, immunotherapy specifically directs immune cells, which in turn cause fewer side effects, but some patients may be susceptible to immune activation that may result in unfavorable reactions (Bassiony et al., 2020). Evidently, the viral way of infection is similar to the one in the development of cancer, as chronic viral infections can create a risk of cancer formation, and the cancer hallmarks are similar to the viral replication processes, which are indicative of studies on viral-based therapies and viral antigens in cancer immunology (Bassiony et al., 2020).

The gut microbiota shapes the immune system by influencing both innate and adaptive immune responses. This interaction can affect the effectiveness of ICIs, such as anti-PD-1 and anti-CTLA-4 therapies. Research suggests that certain beneficial bacteria like *Akkermansia muciniphila (A. muciniphila)*, *Bacteroides fragilis (B. fragilis)*, *Bifidobacterium*, and *Faecalibacterium prausnitzii (F. prausnitzii)* can enhance the immune response by stimulating T-cell activation, promoting the production of immune-boosting cytokines, and aiding dendritic cells in presenting antigens. These actions collectively lead to greater infiltration of cytotoxic T-cells into tumors, potentially improving cancer treatment outcomes (Inamura, 2020; Pham et al., 2021; Villemin et al., 2023). At the same time, an inappropriately developed bacterial kingdom (symptomatic of dysbiosis), an altered bacterial composition, differing from the typical microbiota diversity, is associated with reduced effectiveness of immunotherapy. Although antibiotic treatment may relieve symptoms in patients with non-small cell lung carcinoma (NSCLC), renal cell carcinoma (RCC), and urothelial carcinoma who do not respond to anti-PD-1 therapy, its benefits appear to be limited when not used in conjunction with immunotherapy (Inamura, 2020; Pham et al., 2021). Based on the data obtained from patients with metastatic melanoma, NSCLC, and RCC involved in the clinical study, a higher diversity of microbiota is directly proportional to better progression-free and overall survival (OS) in ICI-treated individuals, while patients with a predominance of *Bacteroidales* have significantly lower effectiveness and higher irAEs of their treatment (Pham et al., 2021).

The gut microbiota's effect on immunotherapy involves various ways, including microbial-associated molecular patterns(MAMPs) that are recognized by the pattern recognition receptors (PRRs), such as Toll-like receptors (TLRs) and nucleotide oligomerization domain (NOD)-like receptors; stimulation of immune response and proinflammatory mechanisms advantageous for tumor control are related to this (Villemin et al., 2023). Some commensal bacteria resemble tumor antigens, leading to cross-reactive CD8+ T cell activation of immunity against tumors, as shown by *Bifidobacterium breve* and *Enterococcus hirae*, which have epitopes analogous to tumor neoantigens. Additionally, microbial products such as SCFAs, inosine, and vitamin B derivatives alter immune cell metabolic pathways, cytokine production, and other intracellular signaling pathways, which in turn affect the efficacy (Villemin et al., 2023). The SCFAs, including butyrate and propionate, can significantly enhance cytotoxic activity and the apoptosis of T cells, but these compounds may also have alternative immunosuppressive effects, depending on their location and concentration (Pham et al., 2021; Villemin et al., 2023). Positive correlations between serum butyrate and propionate concentrations and poor immune checkpoint inhibitor (ICI) application, as well as high inosine levels produced by *Bifidobacterium pseudolongum (B. pseudolongum)*, reinforce antitumor immunity through CD8+ and CD4+ T cell activation via the adenosine A2A receptor and the immune receptor family (Villemin et al., 2023).

Fecal microbiota transplantation (FMT) from ICI responders to nonresponders has demonstrated potential in overcoming immunotherapy resistance in both experimental models and small clinical trials (Inamura, 2020; Pham et al., 2021; Villemin et al., 2023). Although this technique could offer some hope in managing cancer, the risks of possible infections and diseases remained (Pham et al., 2021). Besides this, there are other strategies for microbiome modulation, for example, prebiotics, probiotics, postbiotics, targeted antibiotic use, and bacteriophage therapy, that are also being investigated to optimize ICI effectiveness (Pham et al., 2021).

Selective antibiotics designed specifically to destroy bacteria that are fighting against the body are proposed as one of the potential methods, but the use of broad-spectrum antibiotics negatively enhances treatment effects by reducing the diversity of microbiota. Secondly, new probiotics like the *Bifidobacterium* and *Faecalibacterium* strains are being developed, which might be useful in giving ICI by modulating the activities of immune cells and the process of inflammation (Pham et al., 2021). Furthermore, bacteriophage therapy is indicated as a method to precisely destroy bacteria that cause immunotherapy failure through a series of comprehensive studies, in which it has been shown that phages can act as tumor antigens and activate immune responses (Pham et al., 2021). Another useful method might be the creation of live bacterial therapeutics(LBPs), which are microorganisms of known consortia or genetically designed strains, as they will also contribute to better therapy for ICI (Villemin et al., 2023).

Overall, growing evidence suggests that the human microbiome plays a crucial role in maintaining immune homeostasis and modulating cancer therapy outcomes (Pham et al., 2021). The identification of specific bacterial taxa and microbial metabolites as biomarkers for predicting ICI responses highlights the potential of microbiota-targeted interventions in improving immunotherapy success (Pham et al., 2021; Villemin et al., 2023).

4.2 The microbiome

The microbiome is an intricate community of microorganisms, which is composed of bacteria, archaea, fungi, protists, and viruses (mainly bacteriophages) that inhabit different parts of the body, with the gut microbiome being the most extensive and influential in regulating physiological functions (Keely et al., 2025; Kedia & Ahuja, 2023; Moges & Mengistu, 2024; Tannock, 2024). With trillions of microbes at its core, the microbiome is one of the most important systems in metabolism, immune modulation, and the overall health of an organism (Keely et al., 2025; Kedia & Ahuja, 2023). Bacteria are the major group in the gut microbiome, the mission of which is to carry out digestion, nutrient absorption, bile acid metabolism, vitamin synthesis, and SCFA production; consequently, host energy balance and metabolic health are promoted (Kedia & Ahuja, 2023; Keely et al., 2025; Tannock, 2024). The microbiome is also involved in the gut-brain axis by modulating mood, cognition, and neurological functions (Kedia & Ahuja, 2023; Keely et al., 2025). The key point of functional redundancy is that different microbial communities can operate in the same way, regardless of taxonomic differences, and thus connect with the notion that one's microbiome health depends even more on its function than on its species (Tannock, 2024).

The composition of the microbiome can differ from individual to individual, according to various factors such as diet, genetics, geography, lifestyle, and environmental exposures, including antibiotic use (Kedia & Ahuja, 2023; Keely et al., 2025; Moges & Mengistu, 2024; Tannock, 2024). While Western diets that are richer in fat and protein are not inherently harmful, they do, however, reduce the body's microbial diversity, which is in contrast to plant-based and traditional diets that have been proven to promote a healthier gut microbiome (Kedia & Ahuja, 2023). The findings from studies demonstrate that rural and high-altitude dwellers have the most distinct microbiome in comparison with urban area residents, as the environment is a key factor in microbial diversity (Kedia & Ahuja, 2023). The good health of athletes is mainly due to the presence of certain bacteria that have the ability to produce substances known as SCFAs, which improve pH levels, metabolism, and high performance (Keely et al., 2025). The composition of a gut microbiome undergoes significant changes during its development, namely: from the time it is established in the intestine at birth until it is stabilized in some adults, after which it changes in older age due to factors such as a weakening of the immune system and lifestyle (Kedia & Ahuja, 2023).

Obviously, the diversity of microbiomes is crucial for health since high α-diversity (species richness and evenness) is associated with a stable gut environment, and reduced α-diversity is associated with diseases such as inflammatory bowel disease (IBD), metabolic syndrome, and *Clostridioides difficile* infections (Kedia & Ahuja, 2023). The β-diversity index is a tool that allows microbial diversity measurement across individuals while at the same time distinguishing microbiomes across populations and disease states (Kedia & Ahuja, 2023). Dysbiosis, or microbial imbalance, as well as diseases like obesity, type 2 diabetes (T2D), cardiovascular conditions, gastrointestinal disorders, neurodegenerative diseases, and immune dysfunction (Kedia & Ahuja, 2023; Keely et al., 2025; Moges & Mengistu, 2024). Through fecal samples of microbiota, the microbiome is the line of defense for the host's gut that lets in only the most beneficial microorganisms, which can limit harmful microorganisms in their need for nutrients and space, and produce certain antimicrobial peptides (AMPs) that can assist gut homeostasis. (Moges & Mengistu, 2024). However, metabolites such as SCFAs and imidazole propionate that directly affect host metabolism are secondary bile acids (BAs), and their changes in these pathways have zoned them as metabolic diseases (Keely et al., 2025; Tannock, 2024).

Microbiome research has advanced due to metagenomics, that led to identifying the full spectrum of microbial species, the way they interact, and the resistance genes to antibiotics, as well as giving us insight into microbiome function in health and disease (Moges & Mengistu, 2024). The use of DNA sequencing techniques that include 16S rRNA sequencing and shotgun metagenomics, in addition to bioinformatics tools such as MetaPhlAn2, SILVA, and Greengenes, helps in taxonomic classification and functional profiling of microbial communities (Kedia & Ahuja, 2023). Metabolomics approaches are designed to analyze or study the activity of the microbial community, with specific metabolites like trimethylamine N-oxide (TMAO) linked with cardiovascular risk being indicative of the presence of the microorganisms (Tannock, 2024). Apart from the gut transit time, mucin degradation, and immune interactions, the level of secretory immunoglobulin A (S-IgA) coating bacteria is also an important biomarker to reveal microbiome health (Tannock, 2024).

4.3 Microbiome-immunotherapy relationship

According to numerous studies, there are a number of specific microbes, including their metabolites, that can either augment or discourage the power of ICIs, adoptive T-cell therapies, and cancer vaccines (Yang et al., 2024). Tumor ICIs like anti-PD-1/PD-L1 and anti-CTLA-4 therapies act by activating T-cells and thus reestablishing their ability to annihilate cancer cells. Nevertheless, their efficacy is very different from patient to patient, and among gut bacteria, the composition of the microbiota is an important factor in the response to treatment. Particular bacterial species, such as *A. muciniphila, B. fragilis,* and *Bifidobacterium* spp., have been related to better responses to ICIs due to the fact that these bacteria are able to promote antigen presentation and reinforce T-cell activation (Bibbò et al., 2023). The gut microbiome is balanced by a proper balance between commensal and pathogenic bacteria, thus leading to a decrease in systemic inflammation and an increase in the strength of the immune system (Humphries & Daud, 2018). Gut microbiota is responsible for the proper working of various immune cells, such as specialized cells like dendritic cells, which in turn act as a catalyst for the immune response by killing cancer cells. This innovation by the researchers plays a part in the creation of T-cell antitumor responses that are the primary targets of immune checkpoint therapy. Gut microbiota is the factor that not only has the power to influence this activity but could also emerge as the main determinant of the efficacy of the therapy, like ICIs (Rezasoltani et al., 2021).

The regulation of these immune cells by microbiome, as it can boost the immune system's ability to detect and eliminate tumor cells. Specific gut bacteria, like *Bifidobacterium* and *F. prausnitzii*, have been found to enhance the effectiveness of immunotherapy by stimulating the activity of these immune cells (Xie et al., 2024). Moreover, the composition of the gut microbiota has been shown to influence not only the immune system's ability to fight cancer but also the susceptibility of cancer cells to treatment. Some studies indicate that a diverse microbiota, rich in beneficial bacteria, may improve the response to therapies, while dysbiosis can impair therapeutic outcomes (Jiang et al., 2023). This finding is consistent with evidence showing that the microbiota affects tumor progression and the response to immunotherapy, indicating that a balanced microbiome is crucial for optimal treatment efficacy (Rezasoltani et al., 2021).

Microbial metabolites, like SCFAs, secondary BAs, and polyamines, have a significant effect on the immune system by modulating T-cell differentiation, Treg balance, and proinflammatory cytokine production. SCFAs, such as butyrate and propionate, are pro-inflammatory and, by controlling Foxp3+ Tregs, decrease autoimmune illnesses and irAEs in immunotherapy (Strouse et al., 2019). Furthermore, microbial-derived tryptophan metabolites have been found to regulate the aryl hydrocarbon receptor (AhR), which in turn functions as a tumor immunity and inflammation regulator (Said & Ibrahim, 2025). Moreover, these stocks do a great job at regulating the TME as they have the ability to affect the immune cell activation and the differentiation as well. SCFAs, in addition to having been found to bring about the success of immunotherapy, as they help in the formation of the permissive environment that will support the treatment efficacy (Yin et al., 2024). Gut microbiota further influences the production of inflammatory cytokines that can regulate the progression of cancer. Bacteria-induced swelling may be a boost to the effectiveness of immune therapy by creating a more permissive environment for biased immune cells to infiltrate tumors as well as fight malignancy.

An overactive inflammatory response that is set off by dysbiosis can bring about health problems, such as immune suppression that compromises the immunotherapy responses (Xie et al., 2024). So, it becomes clear that the balance between immune activation and suppression is a key indicator of the overall success of (cancer) immunotherapy. Due to the direct relation between the composition of the microbiota and the effectiveness of immunotherapy, FMT as a potential therapeutic strategy has recently come into the spotlight as a way to restore the beneficial microbial communities in nonresponding patients. FMT from immunotherapy to nonresponders has been proven successful clinically, and it facilitates the efficacy of ICI by enhancing antigen presentation, thus T-cell activation (Lin et al., 2025). New therapeutics focused on the gut microbiota as a target through immunotherapy treatments are the current research area. Probiotics, prebiotics, and FMT serve as the tools for affecting the gut microbial diversity and therefore permitting the restoration of the internal ecosystem balance that encourages the immune system's effectiveness in cancer therapies (Rezasoltani et al., 2021; Xie et al., 2024).

4.3.1 Microbial metabolites and immune modulation

SCFAs like butyrate, propionate, and acetate are produced as a result of the fermentation of dietary fibers by some bacterial species such as *Bacteroides*, *Clostridium, Bifidobacterium, Prevotella*, and *Ruminococcus* (Hosseinkhani et al., 2021; Kim, 2025; Kedia & Ahuja, 2023; Moges & Mengistu, 2024; Tannock, 2024; Zhang et al., 2024). SCFAs are also very important in immune regulation; they do this by, first of all, inhibiting histone deacetylases (HDACs) and, next, activating G-protein-coupled receptors (GPCRs) such as FFAR2, FFAR3, and HCAR2; thus, the process leads to the increase of Treg cell accumulation and the suppression of nuclear factor κB (NF-κB) signaling (Hosseinkhani et al., 2021; Kim, 2025; Kedia & Ahuja, 2023; Moges & Mengistu, 2024; Tannock, 2024; Zhang et al., 2024). They further secure the gut barrier, decrease the levels of the inflammatory cytokines, and fight against such diseases as IBD, T2D, and neuroinflammatory disorders (Hosseinkhani et al., 2021; Kedia & Ahuja, 2023; Moges & Mengistu, 2024; Zhang et al., 2024). Also, SCFAs leave an impact on adaptive immunity by the ways they help cytotoxic T lymphocyte (CTL) memory formation, promote cytotoxicity, and bring about the increase of IFN-γ production (Kim, 2025; Moges & Mengistu, 2024; Tannock, 2024; Zhang et al., 2024). Their lack has been proven to result in the buildup of PD-1+CD39+ exhausted CTLs, which are less capable of efficient tumor elimination (Kim, 2025; Tannock, 2024). The research denoted that butyrate supplementation could enhance antitumor CTL responses; in contrast, microbial dysbiosis declined SCFA levels, which in turn caused immune dysfunction (Kim, 2025; Moges & Mengistu, 2024; Tannock, 2024; Zhang et al., 2024) (Fig. 4.2).

Tryptophan metabolites, such as indole, indole-3-aldehyde, and kynurenine, operate with immune responses by means of the activation of the AhR, which in turn leads to IL-22 release to fortify the defense of gut mucosa (Hosseinkhani et al., 2021; Jia et al., 2024; Kim, 2025; Kedia & Ahuja, 2023; Moges & Mengistu, 2024; Tannock, 2024; Yang et al., 2024; Zhang et al., 2024). Through the pathos ILCs, *Lactobacillus reuteri (L. reuteri)* and *Lactobacillus johnsonii* form indole-3-aldehyde, a substance that serves to alleviate gut inflammation (Hosseinkhani et al., 2021; Kedia & Ahuja, 2023). Indole metabolites are also responsible for CTL differentiation and exhaustion (Jia et al., 2024; Kim, 2025; Tannock, 2024; Yang et al., 2024). Certain indoles like indole-3-propionic acid (IPA) work on exhausted T (Tpex) cell populations, thus boosting the effect of the ICIs, while others, like indole-3-lactic acid (ILA), induce dendritic cells to release IL-12A thus indirectly making it easier for CTL cells to be primed (Jia et al., 2024; Kim, 2025; Tannock, 2024; Yang et al., 2024). Nevertheless, an overdose of AhR caused by environmental ligands such as TCDD inhibits CTL function by repressing the repression of IFN-γ and Granzyme B levels, which depicts the dual role of indole metabolites in immune modulation (Jia et al., 2024; Kim, 2025; Tannock, 2024; Yang et al., 2024).

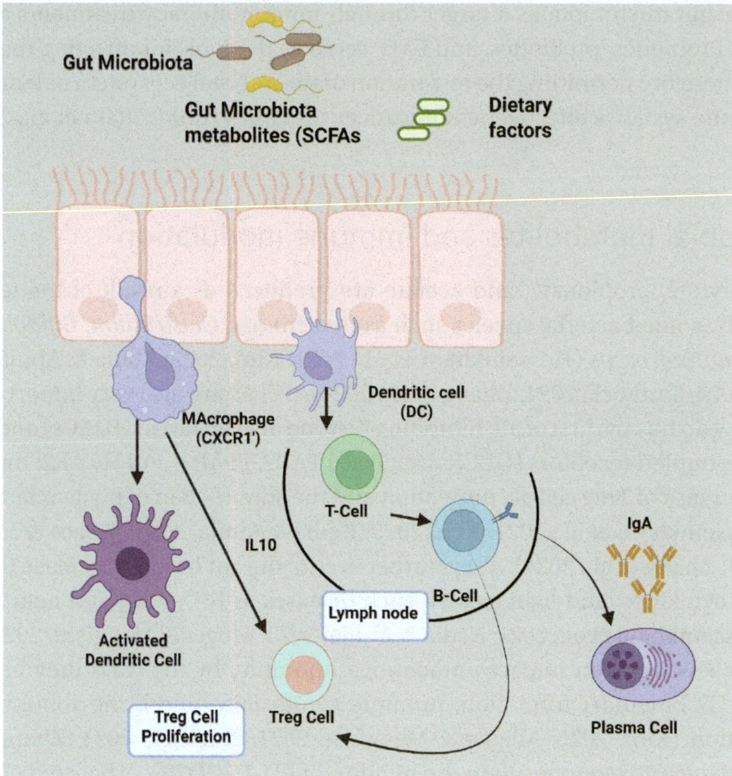

FIGURE 4.2 Microbial metabolites and immune modulation.

One of the other key microbial metabolites, TMAO, is derived from dietary choline through the microbial biosynthesis of *Clostridium cluster* XIVa, *Eubacterium*, and *Actinobacteria* (Hosseinkhani et al., 2021; Kedia & Ahuja, 2023). In addition to the NF-κB pathway, TMAO also works through GPCR pathways that, in turn, activate endothelial inflammation as a result of ROS production, thus triggering cardiovascular disease (CVD) and neurodegeneration (Kedia & Ahuja, 2023). TMAO also acts as a promoter of pathological IL-1β and TNF-α cytokine production in IBD (Hosseinkhani et al., 2021; Kedia & Ahuja, 2023).

Moreover, BAs regulate the immune system by interacting with farnesoid X receptor (FXR) and GPCR TGR5, among other mechanisms that lead to NF-κB inhibition (Hosseinkhani et al., 2021; Kim, 2025; Zhang et al., 2024). Deoxycholic acid (DCA) and lithocholic acid (LCA) diminish IL-1β, but at the same time, *Lactobacillus* and *Bacteroides* are active in the transformation of BAs (Hosseinkhani et al., 2021). IBD patients exhibit a decrease in secondary bile acid levels as a result of deficient bile salt hydrolase (BSH) activity; thus, the inflammation in the intestines is intensified (Hosseinkhani et al., 2021; Zhang et al., 2024). By the way, secondary BAs, as opposed to primary BAs, prevent CTL functioning and even assist in immune escape by tumors through NFAT2 inhibition, plasma membrane Ca^{2+}ATPase activation, and mitochondria ROS production

(Kim, 2025; Zhang et al., 2024). On the one hand, evidence shows that colorectal cancer patients with high bile acid levels are defective in CTL responses due to the increased calcium levels, while T cell activities are rescued by calcium supplementation (Kim, 2025; Zhang et al., 2024).

Polyamines, such as putrescine, spermidine, and spermine, have immunomodulatory effects by inhibiting TNF-α, IL-1β, and IL-6 production through the suppression of NF-κB and MAPK signaling pathways (Hosseinkhani et al., 2021; Zhang et al., 2024). Spermidine lowers neuroinflammation in multiple sclerosis models and promotes immune tolerance in the gut as well (Hosseinkhani et al., 2021). During cancer, polyamines are involved in memory CTL formation via autophagy boosting, which is fundamental for long-term immune responses (Kim, 2025; Zhang et al., 2024). So, while the polyamines are enhancing CTL survival and differentiation, which is also responsible for the tumor growth by stimulating epithelial cell proliferation, on the other hand, they are also stimulating epithelial cell proliferation. Treatment with spermidine could reverse cellular senescence and thus rejuvenate aged CTLs and restore function in elderly subjects, indicating a possibility for a new therapeutic strategy (Kim, 2025; Zhang et al., 2024).

Microbial derived like vitamin B and K as well are a crucial part of immunity regulation. Vitamin B3 suppresses IL-6 and TNF-α; vitamin B6 deficiency, however, increases IL-4 levels. In the case of vitamin K2, it also inhibits NF-κB-mediated inflammation (Hosseinkhani et al., 2021). The resulting vitamins are B and K2, which are synthesized by *Bifidobacterium* and *Lactobacillus*, while the microbiota in the gut has an important function in vitamin K2 production as a factor that regulates immune homeostasis (Hosseinkhani et al., 2021).

Dysbiosis of gut microbiota disrupts metabolite production and, in this way, affects immune modulation and the progression of disease (Hosseinkhani et al., 2021; Zhang et al., 2024). The link between dysregulated microbial metabolites and inflammatory diseases, metabolic syndromes, and neurodegenerative disorders was confirmed (Hosseinkhani et al., 2021). In cancer, dysbiosis is a consequence of the loss of SCFAs and indoles that are beneficial for health and an increase in the immunosuppressive ones such as DCA, the main promoter of tumor cells (Kim, 2025; Zhang et al., 2024). It is widely known that the balance of intestinal microbiota significantly impacts the efficacy of immunotherapy treatments since patients with diverse but beneficial bacteria, probably *Bifidobacterium* and *Akkermansia*, respond considerably better to immunotherapy, while antibiotic use makes it less efficient (Kim, 2025).

One way of making the beneficial microbes the stars is to supply them through dietary interventions, probiotics, or FMT, which has been applied to immune therapy. The availability of data suggests that the FMT of the bioresponder can improve CTL function in the nonresponders, and the supplementation with *A. muciniphila* can directly boost the antitumor immunity (Kim, 2025). Dietary fiber supplementation is a method of increasing SCFA production; the process of differentiation and memory formation of CTL is also supported (Kim, 2025; Zhang et al., 2024).

4.3.2 Interactions between microbes and immune cells

During the neonatal period, microbiota holds an extremely important position in the development of the immune system, which in turn survives on microbial ligands, antigens, and metabolites (Brown et al., 2025). The newborn immune system is very low-reactive to the processes of inflammation and infection, as this prevents the immune system from harming the body (Brown et al., 2025). Microbial ligands in the immune system tend to interact with immune cells that are connected with them and macrophages through TLRs and other PRRs on dendritic cells. This triggers the Treg induction, which is necessary for immune tolerance (Brown et al., 2025; Kogut et al., 2020). Gut microbiota and intestinal CD103^{+} dendritic cells, on the one hand, are important in this process, thus, the lights that are always on for cells which are induced to migrate to mesenteric lymph nodes, where they are then presented with microbial antigens, are the movements not only of engine components, like fun microtubules, but of the en-grow the vehicle of the enzymes participating in these processes (Brown et al., 2025). Intestinal SCFAs and tryptophan metabolites are the ones closely working with the Treg that enable cancer cells to die of natural causes and are perfect (Brown et al., 2025; Kogut et al., 2020). The breast milk and the anti-IgA and IgG are responsible for the reduction of the number of microbial of the pathogenic and nonpathogenic ones but either way of the early stage of immune development (Brown et al., 2025).

Microbial imbalances worsen with age, causing chronic inflammation and immune senescence. While beneficial bacteria, including *Bifidobacteriaceae*, are being lost, pathobionts such as *Enterobacteriaceae* are increasing, which results in the direct activation of antigen-presenting cells through TLR2 and TLR4 signaling (Brown et al., 2025). A deficiently functioning gut barrier is more permeable and allows the microbial components, such as lipopolysaccharides (LPS), to enter circulation, again and again, activating monocytes and neutrophils, and continuously increasing the chronic low-grade inflammation, which is referred to as "inflammaging." The hapless condition of the gut microbiome also causes the bone marrow hematopoiesis to be influenced, in which microbial TLR ligands boost the IL-1α/IL-1β signaling, and subsequently, the immune cell production is shifted to myeloid lineages at the expense of lymphoid cells. T cell dysfunction and the immune response to infections and vaccines are adversely affected (Brown et al., 2025).

Microbial interactions with immune cells have been shown to broadly affect disease development. For example, in IBD associated with diminished microbial-induced Treg differentiation, the disturbed immune system becomes excessively activated (Brown et al., 2025). In cancer, the imbalance of the microbiota results in an altered reaction of macrophages and T-cells, which in turn quenches the microenvironment and creates an immunosuppressive situation (Brown et al., 2025; Yang et al., 2024). In neurodegenerative diseases such as Alzheimer's disease, microbiota-derived metabolites produced from the breakdown of tryptophan and SCFAs alter microglial activation, leading to the aggravation of cognitive decline (Brown et al., 2025).

The immune system recognizes the microbes due to the PRRs, which are expressed on the intestinal epithelial cells, macrophages, and dendritic cells (Kogut et al., 2020). These receptors find MAMPs, including lipoproteins, carbohydrates, nucleic acids, peptidoglycan, flagellin, and LPS, expanded to have their room next to damage-associated molecular patterns (DAMPs) released during infections or cell damage, and they bind to them (Kogut et al., 2020). PRR amplification will bring cytokines into being, increase recruitment of immune cells, and increase the secretion of AMPs (Kogut et al., 2020). After uptake and processing of the microbial antigens by dendritic cells and macrophages, the same cells present the antigens to T cells in tertiary organs such as

Peyer's patches and cecal tonsils such that the differentiation of T-helper cells (Th1, Th2, Th17, and Tregs) and the stimulation of IgA-secreting plasma cells is fostered (Kogut et al., 2020). The intestinal epithelial lining has a double purpose. On the one hand, it is a physical obstacle, and on the other hand, it is a sensor that is active in immune processes (Geuking et al., 2014; Kogut et al., 2020).

The immune cells are directed by Commensal microbes, which produce metabolites that directly communicate with the immune cells (Kogut et al., 2020). SCFAs, such as butyrate, are the initial ones to facilitate the process of producing Treg cells, which are anti-inflammatories, and polysaccharide A (PSA) is the one that is responsible for Treg differentiation from *B. fragilis*. Moreover, bacteria's metabolism of tryptophan encountering indoles, and then enhancing epithelial barrier integrity, is a result of this (Kogut et al., 2020). The microbiome is discovered to control the innate immune system through PRRs. PRRs, including TLRs, Nod-like receptors (NLRs), RIG-I-like receptors (RLRs), and C-type lectin receptors (CLRs), which mediate inflammatory responses and coordinate adaptive immunity, are the majority of the modulators (Graham & Xavier, 2023). *A. muciniphila* produces examples in which the phospholipid interacts with TLR2-TLR1 on dendritic cells and surfaces of the immune tolerance, which is the exact expression of the induction or not, and the timing to take. Besides, *Bacteroidetes* and *Proteobacteria* are involved in distinctive cytokine responses, where *Bacteroidetes* will lead to IL-6, TNF-α, and IL-10, whereas *Proteobacteria* will also be the first to break off through stimulating IL-23 and IL-1β. Without the PRR signaling hedge, gut commensal-derived outer membrane vesicles (OMVs) go into the blood circulation and then take over IFN-α overproduction due to the cGAS-STING pathway, thus making the whole antiviral immunity activation (Graham & Xavier, 2023).

Microbiota influences tumor immunity through multiple mechanisms. Certain bacterial species enhance ICI efficacy by increasing cytotoxic T-cell infiltration into the TME and modulating checkpoint molecule expression (PD-1/PD-L1), improving responses to treatments like anti-PD-1 therapy (Yang et al., 2024). Microbial metabolites, such as SCFAs, influence inflammatory responses by interacting with NF-κB, impacting immune activation. Some bacteria promote tumor proliferation by inducing IL-6, IL-10, and TGF-β, which suppress cytotoxic T cells and NK cells, while others enhance antitumor immunity. The tumor microbiome also modifies the behavior of tumor-associated macrophages (TAMs), shifting between pro-inflammatory M1 and immunosuppressive M2 phenotypes, thereby influencing tumor progression (Yang et al., 2024).

Intestinal epithelium serves as a first-line defense by expressing PRRs that detect microbial signals and trigger immune responses. The mucus layer, which limits microbial contact, is formed by MUC2, which is manufactured by goblet cells and Paneth cells, which secrete AMPs like Reg3γ (Geuking et al., 2014). After that, the dendritic cells will sample microbial antigens, thus promoting immune tolerance or activation depending on microbial composition. The activity of SCFAs derived from the microbiota that modulate (Treg) differentiation is based on HDAC inhibition, and PSA in *B. fragilis*, which promotes Treg induction, relies on TLR2 signaling (Geuking et al., 2014). Segmented filamentous bacteria induce IL-17-producing Th17 cells, which are the main elements of mucosal defense. It is known that the microbiota also affects systemic immune responses, thus contributing to the development of autoimmunity and allergic diseases. Studies carried out in germ-free mice show higher iNKT cell levels, which cause the mice to become more susceptible to experimental colitis and asthma. It has been discovered that gut microbiota composition in nonobese diabetic (NOD) mice can be influenced by gut microbiota availability for hormone-dependent regulation of autoimmunity (Geuking et al., 2014).

4.4 Microbiome-driven modulation of immunotherapy outcomes

The constitution of the gut microbiome is greatly important in the modulation of the effectiveness of ICIs, especially the ones acting on PD-1, PD-L1, and CTLA-4 (Kang et al., 2024; Li et al., 2019; Yousefi et al., 2024). Both preclinical and clinical studies have shown the support of the gut microbiome in environments where various responses to ICI therapy are being recorded. On the other hand, germ-free or antibiotic-treated mice reveal their low expression after the checkpoint blockade (Kang et al., 2024).

Specifically, bacterial colonies have been found to be an ICI therapy supporter or inhibitor. The bacteria that have been characterized to elicit a response are *A. muciniphila, Bifidobacterium* species (e.g., *B. pseudolongum, B. longum*), *F. prausnitzii, Ruminococcaceae, Lachnospiraceae,* and *Clostridium butyricum (C. butyricum)*, which release the immune cells of the CD8+ memory subtype to the site of the tumor, produce the cytokines IFN-γ and IL-12, and induce the maturation of the dendritic cells (Li et al., 2019; Kang et al., 2024; Yousefi et al., 2024). Conversely, facilitators and hindering elements are the proteobiotic bacteria such as *Fusobacterium nucleatum (F. nucleatum), Bacteroides ovatus,* and some strains of *Ruminococcus,* which inhibit T cells by increasing regulatory T cell populations and decreasing effector T cell function (Li et al., 2019; Yousefi et al., 2024).

The gut microbiota influences the immune system and ICI action through various mechanisms. Microbial metabolites, e.g., SCFAs, tryptophan derivatives, and inosine, induce the activation of CD8+ T cells and, as a result, are able to promote immune responses within the TME (Kang et al., 2024; Yousefi et al., 2024). Some specific SCFAs, such as butyrate and propionate, enhance anti-PD-1 therapy, while succinic acid, which comes from *F. nucleatum*, inhibits the immune system (Kang et al., 2024). *A. muciniphila* can attract CCR9+CXCR3+CD4+ T cells and modulate the CD4+ into a CD4+FoxP3+ Treg ratio, hence, it leads to the development of antitumor immunity (Fujimura et al., 2010). Furthermore, *Bifidobacterium* species can increase the activation of dendritic cells; as a result, the immune responses against tumors can be improved (Li et al., 2019).

The aim of investigations on the gut microbiota is to set it in the right way so that it would respond better to ICI through such interventions as FMT, probiotics, prebiotics, dietary modifications, and antibiotic avoidance. FMT, a procedure of transferring fecal matter from ICI responders to nonresponders, has been quite successful in the restoration of immunotherapy sensitivity, especially in melanoma and gastrointestinal cancers (Kang et al., 2024; Li et al., 2019; Yousefi et al., 2024). Probiotic strains that include *C. butyricum* (CBM588) and *B. longum* as part of the ingredients have been known to be associated with increases in cancer patients' subsequent progression-free survival (PFS) when they receive ICIs. Prebiotics such as inulin and resistant starch are seen to be the main supporters of the enhancement of beneficial gut bacteria (Kang et al., 2024). Interventional dietary programs that include high-fiber diets, fasting-mimicking diets, and ketogenic diets are the themes of current research on their potential in the reshaping of the gut microbiome and the subsequent creation of a more immune-friendly environment suitable for immunotherapy (Kang et al., 2024). The broad-spectrum antibiotic treatment is the agent that causes the gut microbiota to become disorganized and, consequently, reduces the effectiveness of ICI; thus, the outcomes are poor (Li et al., 2019).

Despite encouraging discoveries, a number of issues need to be addressed before the microbiome can become an efficient tool for cancer immunotherapy. The fact that the microbiome composition differs from one person to another is a stumbling block in the development of standardized microbiome-based treatments (Kang et al., 2024; Yousefi et al., 2024). In addition, the lack of standardized methodologies in microbiome analysis tests and treatment protocols is another major cause of low reproducibility in clinical studies (Yousefi et al., 2024). FMT and probiotic administration needed to be put through strict safety evaluations in order to avoid unforeseen side effects (Kang et al., 2024).

4.4.1 Role of the gut microbiome in immune checkpoint inhibitor therapy outcomes

Gut microbiome composition variations are responsible for the different therapeutic outcomes seen in persons, and they are critical in enabling the ICI therapy for patients to be finely tuned and optimized (Jiang et al., 2024; Li et al., 2022; Yousefi et al., 2024). Among the beneficial bacteria species mentioned, there are *A. muciniphila, Bifidobacterium, Lactobacillus, F. prausnitzii*, as well as members of *Ruminococcaceae* and *Lachnospiraceae* that may have improved responses to anti-PD-1 and anti-CTLA-4 therapies (Jiang et al., 2024; Li et al., 2022; Yousefi et al., 2024). These bacteria facilitate the development of advantageous immune responses by enhancing the activation of T cells, promoting the infiltration of effector T cells into tumors, and modulating cytokine production, including IFN-γ and IL-12 (Jiang et al., 2024; Yousefi et al., 2024). Also, the gut microbiome dysbiosis may be intertwined with the progression of immunosuppression and the reduced efficacy of ICI, reaching as high as an important issue not to be overlooked. To the contrary, the presence of a balanced microbiome is a significant issue to deal with for the most wanted immunotherapy outcomes, the balance of the immune responses to be maintained, and the undesired ones in tumors being suppressed (Li et al., 2022; Yousefi et al., 2024). Research indicates that nonresponders often have a higher abundance of species like *Bacteroides thetaiotaomicron* and *Bifidobacterium dentium*, which may contribute to immunosuppression (Jiang et al., 2024).

Microbiota transfer is the process of importing gut microbiota of ICI-responsive patients into nonresponders as a method that has been successful in averting resistance to PD-1 blockade in melanoma and gastrointestinal cancers (Jiang et al., 2024; Li et al., 2022; Yousefi et al., 2024). The clinical studies have revealed that FMT leads to a recognizable change in gut microbiota composition and associated improvement in the response of these patients to ICI therapy (Jiang et al., 2024; Li et al., 2022). Experimental findings that have been obtained from MCA205 mice with transplants show that FMT reinstates sensitivity to ICIs, thus enhancing treatment outcomes (Bredon et al., 2024). Strains like *B. longum, L. reuteri,* and *A. mucinophila* have been researched as potential adjunct therapies for the improvement of ICI efficacy. The given probiotics exert immune-supportive functions, including the enhancement of immune-promoting gut bacteria, inflammation reduction, and the activation of T cells, which are required for a good anticancer immune response (Jiang et al., 2024; Li et al., 2022).

Prebiotics, just like resistant starch, inulin, and oligofructose, are identified as the major supporters of the beneficial microbe's growth, leading to an immunologically favored gut environment (Li et al., 2022). These prebiotics render the synthesis of SCFAs, important metabolites which not only control immune cells' function but also improve immune responses during the use of ICIs (Jiang et al., 2024; Li et al., 2022; Yousefi et al., 2024). Furthermore, results from clinical trials have shown that a high-fiber diet is better related to PD-1 inhibitors compared to low-fiber intake, indicating that dietary changes can significantly affect immunotherapy's success (Jiang et al., 2024; Li et al., 2022).

SCFAs, the metabolic products of gut bacteria, are supposed to improve the sensitivity of checkpoint inhibitors by making TME immune-permissive and increasing T cell functions (Jiang et al., 2024; Li et al., 2022; Yousefi et al., 2024). For instance, *F. prausnitzii* has been found to be the most important in controlling immune function, which before this was not known. The scientists in the study that mentioned *F. prausnitzii* reaffirm that the gavage administration of this strain can replenish the potentially decreased antineoplastic effect of ICIs, even in the absence of antibiotic-driven gut flora perturbations (Bredon et al., 2024). RNA sequencing analysis done in a Petri dish model suggests that this strain of bacteria contributes to its positive effect through the production of an interleukin-17 cytokine in the vicinity of the T cells in the intestines, thus making the T cells stronger (Bredon et al., 2024).

The use of antibiotics has been shown to disrupt the gut microbiome, depleting beneficial bacterial species and leading to reduced efficacy of ICI therapy in multiple cancer types, including NSCLC and melanoma (Jiang et al., 2024; Yousefi et al., 2024). Antibiotic-induced microbiome disruption negatively impacts immune-permissive tumor environments, emphasizing the need for caution in their use during immunotherapy.

Several studies indicate that the composition of gut microbiota may serve as a predictive biomarker for the success of immunotherapy. Greater levels of beneficial bacteria, such as *A. muciniphila* and *F. prausnitzii,* have been linked to better PFS and OS in patients undergoing ICI treatment (Bredon et al., 2024; Jiang et al., 2024; Yousefi et al., 2024). Additionally, *A. muciniphila* has been linked to better clinical outcomes in NSCLC patients undergoing checkpoint inhibitor therapy, further reinforcing the potential of microbiome-based predictive models (Bredon et al., 2024).

4.5 Challenges and future directions

High soluble fiber consumption has been associated with an improvement in the response to anti-PD-1 therapy in mouse models, adding *A. muciniphila,* a mucosal-affecting who will influence the condition of the immune system (Newsome et al., 2022). The diet intake of pectin, which is a soluble fiber in fruits and veggies, leads to the growth of SCFA-makers of bacteria such as *Erysipelotrichaceae, Ruminococcaceae,* and *Bifidobacteriaceae,* and the increased suppression of anti-PD-1 therapy response in colorectal cancer models as one of the outcomes (Newsome et al., 2022). The Mediterranean diet brings in good microbial species like *F. prausnitzii* and *A. muciniphila,* which in turn are at higher levels with better immune reactions to immune checkpoint blockade (ICB) therapy, whereas a diet on processed foods, supplemented by red meat and sugar, contributes to gut dysbiosis; thus, immunotherapy effectiveness is reduced (David & Lev-Ari, 2024). These are concepts developed in this paragraph. Fasting and intermittent fasting raise microbiome diversity, which is tied, in a way, to better immunotherapy responses, whereas a high-sugar diet becomes the soil where deleterious bacteria like *Clostridium difficile* and *Clostridium perfringens* flourish in digesting track, leading to the possibility of immune suppression (Szczyrek et al., 2021). Polyunsaturated fatty acids (PUFAs) would reverse the immunotherapy outcomes by the mediation of myeloid-derived suppressor cells (MDSCs) and by the reduction of immunosuppression, while vitamin D through T cell activity and immune tolerance, and vitamin B1 in the synthesis role of IgA and mucosal immunity. High salt load induces Th17 cell activation and M1 macrophage polarization; these conditions are then utilized for the promotion of antitumor immunity and for needful changes in the flora of the gut (Szczyrek et al., 2021).

Environmental factors are of great importance when it comes to the composition of the microbiome as well as the success of immunotherapy. A person who takes antibiotics in the 30 days before the immune control point detection therapy has a bond association with less effectiveness of the treatment and worse survival because the bacteria are disrupted (Szczyrek et al., 2021). Because the microbiota diversity of the gut is reduced by the application of a broad-spectrum antibiotic, immune regulatory and antigen presentation processes are affected; thus, good clinical outcomes are not achieved (Oli et al., 2024). The immune system and the effectiveness of the treatments will also be affected by the types of bacterial disruption due to infections, pollution, and the location of the patients (David & Lev-Ari, 2024). Environmental immigration of gut flora in the context of a situation where patients receive FMT and probiotics, and the cells are increased in the immunotherapy subjects (Szczyrek et al., 2021). Various infection or lifestyle-related factors lead to distinct irAEs during immunotherapy therapy, one of the protective features of these events being the presence of certain bacterial taxa (Oli et al., 2024).

Perhaps, the weight gain perpetrated by poor health habits is another parameter to be thought about, which creates damage to the environment and the convoys of microbiota constructed in the gut and the immune system (Szczyrek et al., 2021). Obesity is one of the environmental factors, in addition to microbiota and the immune system, which interact by generating chronic inflammation through the production of increased cytokines, such as TNF-α, IL-6, and IFN-γ, that also have an effect on the efficacy of immunotherapy. In some cases, obesity can be a factor that enhances checkpoint inhibitor therapy responses because it will make the T cells stop being tired; however, it can lead to problems when excessive fat accumulates, namely impaired function of the cells that help to fight tumors (Szczyrek et al., 2021). High levels of glucose can increase the rates of poor immunotherapy responses by increasing the tumor metabolic processes, whereas ketogenic and calorie-restricted diets may enhance immune function by changing cellular metabolism to predominantly lipid oxidation and thus reducing the growth of tumors (Szczyrek et al., 2021).

The interaction between the genetic make-up of the host and the composition of the microbiota directly influences the immune response and thus the efficiency of the immune therapies. Although genetic factors have not yet been fully discovered, the interactions between the microbiota and host differ from one person to another, and thus, the immunotherapy response is affected (Newsome et al., 2022). The closely parallel evolution of the gut microbiota with the human population implies that the genetic factors inherited by individuals may be the underlying cause of the variance in the microbiota composition and the immune system synergies (Oli et al., 2024; Xie et al., 2024).

It is indicated that some microbial species are connected to distinct immunotherapy responses in patients with colorectal and hepatocellular carcinoma, bringing forth the idea of the genetic and microbial interplay as possibly crucial in influencing the treatment outcomes (Newsome et al., 2022). The interaction between the gut microbiome and the immune system happens in both ways, modulated by molecular mimicry, microbial metabolites, and antigen presentation, which in turn are both modulated by genetic, dietary, and environmental factors (David & Lev-Ari, 2024).

The diversity and composition of gut microbiota greatly influence immune responsiveness and thus determine whether or not the treatment with ICIs, especially like PD-1/PD-L1 inhibitors, will be effective. Patients with higher microbial species diversity and, in particular, higher health-promoting gut flora like Bifidobacterium and *A. muciniphila* have improved response rates to immunotherapy treatments, whereas those with lower microbial diversity display lower rates of success and are more likely to develop irAEs (Sang et al., 2024; Xie et al., 2024). The use of FMT has been explored as a possible treatment to change the gut flora and consequently boost the effect of immunotherapy. FMT clinical trials have shown evidence that healthy donor FMT enables the immune activity in tumor patients and, therefore, patients respond better to an anti-PD-1 therapy, as well as have longer PFS. In one study, 3 of 10 patients with anti-PD-1-refractory metastatic melanoma responded to FMT treatment without experiencing severe irAEs, emphasizing its potential for efficacy augmentation and safety affirmation, respectively. Nevertheless, the risks related to FMT include the transmission of pathogens, immune system dysregulation, and the microbiota heterogeneity between donors, which, in turn, leads to different therapeutic effects in the recipients. The unifying use of FMT is still a big hurdle, and differences in the delivery methods affect the outcomes of the treatment. Colonoscopy and enema-based means show the most efficacy and safety, respectively, while nasoduodenal tube delivery is potentially not as effective (Sang et al., 2024; Xie et al., 2024; Zhang et al., 2025).

Probiotics are used as a means to modulate the gut microbiota to increase the effectiveness of the immunotherapy. Some probiotic strains, such as *Lactobacillus* and *Bifidobacterium*, have been proven to stimulate the immune system by causing the activation of CD8+ T cells and increasing the production of IFN-γ, and this is how they work in promoting the process of tumor suppression. As expected, the commensal strains like *B. pseudolongum* were also able to stimulate new corresponding beneficial products involved in the tumor suppressor pathways. Inosine was the one that increased the most in the MTE with this strain; therefore, the observed ICI therapy was more effective. On the other hand, in a mouse model, microbial therapy associated with an 11-bacteria-based consortium was able to induce the production of IFN-γ by CD8+ T cells in the neighboring tumor tissue without causing colon inflammation. Conversely, the helpful supplement of probiotics in all cancer patients might pose some side effects, such as a disrupted microbial homeostasis or the emergence of resistance to antibiotics, which could result in the unsuccessful outcome of the therapy. A cocktail of probiotics with multiple strains, referred to as multistrain probiotics, have improved results in ulcerative colitis (UC); however, there was no microbiome-targeted therapy (MTT), which was significantly better than placebo in Crohn's disease (CD), indicating the necessity of different medication strategies based on disease subtypes and severity (Sang et al., 2024; Xie et al., 2024; Zhang et al., 2025).

Dietary modifications have also been investigated as a means to improve microbiota diversity and immunotherapy efficacy. High-fiber and high-salt diets have been associated with increased microbial diversity and enhanced immune responses, leading to better clinical outcomes in patients receiving ICIs. Microbial fermentation of dietary fibers produces SCFAs, which help maintain intestinal immune homeostasis and contribute to the therapeutic success of immunotherapy (Xie et al., 2024). Antibiotic use is another critical factor influencing the efficacy of microbiome-targeted immunotherapy. Broad-spectrum antibiotics disrupt gut microbiota homeostasis and eliminate beneficial bacteria essential for immune modulation, reducing treatment efficacy. Retrospective studies have shown that patients who received antibiotics had shorter OS and PFS compared to those who did not, indicating that indiscriminate antibiotic use could compromise immunotherapy success. However, some conflicting findings suggest that in specific cases, antibiotic administration does not significantly alter major microbial compositions affecting treatment efficacy, highlighting the complexity of microbiota-immune interactions (Sang et al., 2024; Xie et al., 2024).

Microbial ecosystem therapeutics, such as MET4, have been developed to provide an alternative to FMT while maintaining a balanced microbial environment. MET4 is designed to include key bacterial strains associated with improved immunotherapy responses, allowing for controlled and reproducible microbiota modulation without the risks associated with donor-dependent FMT. Early clinical trials have shown promising safety and tolerability results, suggesting that microbial therapeutics could be a viable strategy for enhancing immunotherapy while minimizing risks (Sang et al., 2024). The role of gut microbiota in modulating immune-related toxicities has also been investigated, with findings indicating that certain bacterial taxa, such as *Blautia* and *Bacteroidetes*, may help reduce the severity of irAEs by inducing Tregs and maintaining gut barrier integrity (Xie et al., 2024).

Despite these promising findings, the complexity of microbiome-immunotherapy interactions necessitates further research to establish causal relationships and refine therapeutic strategies. Personalized approaches that consider patient-specific microbiome profiles, lifestyle factors, and genetic predispositions will be essential in developing microbiome-based adjunctive therapies that maximize immunotherapy efficacy while mitigating risks. High-quality randomized controlled trials (RCTs) are needed to further refine microbiome-targeted therapies and establish standardized protocols that maximize benefits while minimizing potential complications (Xie et al., 2024; Zhang et al., 2025).

4.6 Conclusion

The intricate interplay between the microbiome and the immune system has emerged as a pivotal factor in the success of immunotherapy, particularly in cancer treatment. Research has demonstrated that gut microbiota plays a crucial role in shaping immune responses, modulating the efficacy of ICIs, adoptive T cell therapies, and cancer vaccines. The microbiome influences tumor progression and therapeutic outcomes by regulating immune cell activation, antigen presentation, and the inflammatory landscape within the TME. The presence of beneficial bacterial species, such as *A. muciniphila*, Bifidobacterium, and *F. prausnitzii*, has been associated with enhanced responses to immunotherapy, while microbial dysbiosis can impair immune surveillance and promote tumor immune evasion. These findings underscore the importance of a balanced and diverse microbiota in optimizing immunotherapy outcomes.

One of the most significant contributions of microbiome research to immunotherapy is the identification of specific microbial metabolites that influence immune responses. SCFAs, including butyrate and propionate, regulate immune cell differentiation and cytokine production, creating a more favorable immune environment for cancer treatment. Similarly, microbial-derived tryptophan metabolites interact with immune signaling pathways, modulating the activity of regulatory T cells and effector T cells. The presence or absence of these metabolites can determine the effectiveness of ICB therapies, highlighting the microbiome's role as a key determinant of treatment success. Moreover, the gut microbiota produces molecular mimics of tumor antigens, enhancing cross-reactive immune responses and further influencing the efficacy of immunotherapy.

Recent advances in microbiome-based interventions have opened new avenues for enhancing cancer treatment efficacy. FMT has demonstrated potential in restoring beneficial microbial communities in immunotherapy-resistant patients, improving treatment responses by modulating immune activation and inflammation. Probiotic supplementation with specific bacterial strains has also been explored as an adjunct therapy to boost antitumor immunity. Furthermore, engineered microbial therapies, including synthetic bacterial consortia and live biotherapeutics, are being developed to precisely modulate immune responses, offering a promising direction for personalized medicine. These interventions highlight the growing potential of microbiome-targeted strategies in optimizing cancer immunotherapy.

Despite its transformative potential, the integration of microbiome research into clinical practice faces several challenges. The inter-individual variability in microbiome composition poses a significant hurdle in developing standardized microbiome-based therapies. Factors such as genetics, diet, antibiotic use, and environmental exposures influence microbial diversity, making it difficult to establish universally effective microbiota-targeted interventions.

Additionally, concerns regarding the safety and regulatory oversight of microbiome-modulating therapies remain critical issues that must be addressed before widespread clinical application. FMT, for instance, carries risks related to pathogen transmission and immune dysregulation, necessitating stringent screening and quality control measures. Probiotics and prebiotics, while promising, require further validation in large-scale clinical trials to confirm their efficacy and safety in cancer patients undergoing immunotherapy.

The impact of microbiome composition on irAEs further underscores its clinical significance. Studies have shown that certain bacterial taxa are protective against severe immune-mediated toxicities associated with checkpoint inhibitor therapy, suggesting that microbiome modulation could be employed to reduce treatment-associated side effects. Understanding these microbial interactions may lead to novel strategies for mitigating irAEs while maintaining therapeutic efficacy. Furthermore, the influence of diet on microbiome diversity and immunotherapy outcomes has gained considerable attention. High-fiber diets, fasting-mimicking regimens, and ketogenic diets have been associated with improved responses to ICB, reinforcing the idea that dietary interventions can serve as a practical and noninvasive means of optimizing immunotherapy.

The field of microbiome research is evolving rapidly, with emerging technologies enabling deeper insights into host-microbe interactions. Metagenomics, metabolomics, and single-cell sequencing techniques have revolutionized our understanding of microbial diversity and function, facilitating the identification of key microbial biomarkers associated with immunotherapy response. Artificial intelligence and machine learning are being increasingly applied to analyze complex microbiome datasets, allowing for more precise predictions of treatment outcomes and personalized therapeutic strategies. The integration of these cutting-edge approaches with immunotherapy holds the potential to refine patient selection, improve treatment efficacy, and pave the way for microbiome-driven precision medicine.

While the promise of microbiome modulation in immunotherapy is undeniable, translating these insights into tangible clinical applications requires a concerted effort from researchers, clinicians, and regulatory bodies. Standardized methodologies for microbiome analysis, reproducibility in clinical trials, and well-defined therapeutic protocols must be established to ensure the reliable implementation of microbiome-targeted interventions. Collaboration between multidisciplinary teams, including microbiologists, immunologists, oncologists, and bioinformaticians, will be essential in overcoming existing challenges and unlocking the full potential of microbiome-based therapies.

Future research should aim to uncover the underlying mechanisms behind the interactions between the microbiome and immunotherapy. Although links between certain microbial species and treatment outcomes have been identified, more studies are needed to explore the specific roles these bacteria play in immune modulation. Gaining a deeper understanding of the bidirectional relationship between the gut microbiota and the immune system will help in developing targeted microbial therapies that can boost immunotherapy effectiveness while reducing potential risks. Furthermore, investigating the microbiome's influence beyond the gut, including its interactions with other mucosal surfaces like the lungs and skin, could provide valuable insights into broader immune regulation.

The intersection of microbiome science and immunotherapy represents a paradigm shift in cancer treatment, offering new opportunities for enhancing patient outcomes through precision medicine. The ability to harness the microbiome's immunomodulatory properties opens the door to novel therapeutic strategies that go beyond traditional pharmacological interventions. As research in this field advances, microbiome-based approaches will likely become an integral component of future immunotherapy regimens, transforming the landscape of cancer treatment and immune-based therapies. While significant challenges remain, the continued exploration of microbiome-driven immunomodulation holds the promise of revolutionizing oncology and reshaping the future of medicine.

References

Bassiony, M., Aluko, A. V., & Radosevich, J. A. (2020). *Immunotherapy and cancer precision medicine in oncology* (pp. 133–156). Wiley. https://doi.org/10.1002/9781119432487.ch5.

Bibbò, S., Porcari, S., Del Vecchio, L. E., Severino, A., Mullish, B. H., Ianiro, G., Gasbarrini, A., & Cammarota, G. (2023). Gut microbiota and immunotherapy of renal cell carcinoma. *Human Vaccines and Immunotherapeutics, 19*(3). https://doi.org/10.1080/21645515.2023.2268982.

Bredon, M., Danne, C., Pham, H. P., Ruffié, P., Bessede, A., Rolhion, N., Creusot, L., Brot, L., Alonso, I., Langella, P., Derosa, L., Cortot, A. B., Routy, B., Zitvogel, L., Segata, N., & Sokol, H. (2024). *Faecalibaterium prausnitzii* strain EXL01 boosts efficacy of immune checkpoint inhibitors. *OncoImmunology, 13*(1). https://doi.org/10.1080/2162402X.2024.2374954.

Brown, J. A., Bashir, H., & Zeng, M. Y. (2025). Lifelong partners: Gut microbiota-immune cell interactions from infancy to old age. *Mucosal Immunology, 18*(3), 509–523. https://doi.org/10.1016/j.mucimm.2025.01.006.

David, A., & Lev-Ari, S. (2024). Targeting the gut microbiome to improve immunotherapy outcomes: A review. *Integrative Cancer Therapies, 23*. https://doi.org/10.1177/15347354241269870.

Falony, G., Vandeputte, D., Caenepeel, C., Vieira-Silva, S., Daryoush, T., Vermeire, S., & Raes, J. (2019). The human microbiome in health and disease: Hype or hope. *Acta Clinica Belgica: International Journal of Clinical and Laboratory Medicine, 74*(2), 53–64. https://doi.org/10.1080/17843286.2019.1583782.

Fujimura, K. E., Slusher, N. A., Cabana, M. D., & Lynch, S. V. (2010). Role of the gut microbiota in defining human health. *Expert Review of Anti-Infective Therapy, 8*(4), 435–454. https://doi.org/10.1586/eri.10.14.

Geuking, M. B., Köller, Y., Rupp, S., & McCoy, K. D. (2014). The interplay between the gut microbiota and the immune system. *Gut Microbes, 5*(3). https://doi.org/10.4161/gmic.29330.

Graham, D. B., & Xavier, R. J. (2023). Conditioning of the immune system by the microbiome. *Trends in Immunology, 44*(7), 499–511. https://doi.org/10.1016/j.it.2023.05.002.

Hosseinkhani, F., Heinken, A., Thiele, I., Lindenburg, P. W., Harms, A. C., & Hankemeier, T. (2021). The contribution of gut bacterial metabolites in the human immune signaling pathway of non-communicable diseases. *Gut Microbes, 13*(1), 1–22. https://doi.org/10.1080/19490976.2021.1882927.

Humphries, A., & Daud, A. (2018). The gut microbiota and immune checkpoint inhibitors. *Human Vaccines and Immunotherapeutics, 14*(9), 2178–2182. https://doi.org/10.1080/21645515.2018.1442970.

Inamura, K. (2020). Roles of microbiota in response to cancer immunotherapy. *Seminars in Cancer Biology, 65*, 164–175. https://doi.org/10.1016/j.semcancer.2019.12.026.

Jia, D., Kuang, Z., & Wang, L. (2024). The role of microbial indole metabolites in tumor. *Gut Microbes, 16*(1). https://doi.org/10.1080/19490976.2024.2409209.

Jiang, S., Ma, W., Ma, C., Zhang, Z., Zhang, W., & Zhang, J. (2024). An emerging strategy: Probiotics enhance the effectiveness of tumor immunotherapy via mediating the gut microbiome. *Gut Microbes, 16*(1). https://doi.org/10.1080/19490976.2024.2341717.

Jiang, Y., Jia, D., Sun, Y., Ding, N., & Wang, L. (2023). Microbiota: A key factor affecting and regulating the efficacy of immunotherapy. *Clinical and Translational Medicine, 13*(12). https://doi.org/10.1002/ctm2.1508.

Jones, M. L., Ganopolsky, J. G., Martoni, C. J., Labbé, A., & Prakash, S. (2014). Emerging science of the human microbiome. *Gut Microbes, 5*(4), 446–457. https://doi.org/10.4161/gmic.29810.

Kang, X., Lau, H. C. H., & Yu, J. (2024). Modulating gut microbiome in cancer immunotherapy: Harnessing microbes to enhance treatment efficacy. *Cell Reports Medicine, 5*(4). https://doi.org/10.1016/j.xcrm.2024.101478.

Kedia, S., & Ahuja, V. (2023). Human gut microbiome: A primer for the clinician. *JGH Open, 7*(5), 337–350. https://doi.org/10.1002/jgh3.12902.

Keely, S. J., Cotter, P. D., Wahlstrom, A., Schellekens, H., Weinkove, D., & Barrett, K. E. (2025). From human to superhuman: The impact of the microbiome on physiology. *Journal of Physiology, 603*(4), 797–807. https://doi.org/10.1113/JP287883.

Kim, C. H. (2025). Functional regulation of cytotoxic T cells by gut microbial metabolites. *Gut Microbes Reports, 2*(1). https://doi.org/10.1080/29933935.2025.2454002.

Kogut, M. H., Lee, A., & Santin, E. (2020). Microbiome and pathogen interaction with the immune system. *Poultry Science, 99*(4), 1906–1913. https://doi.org/10.1016/j.psj.2019.12.011.

Li, W., Deng, Y., Chu, Q., & Zhang, P. (2019). Gut microbiome and cancer immunotherapy. *Cancer Letters, 447*, 41–47. https://doi.org/10.1016/j.canlet.2019.01.015.

Li, X., Zhang, S., Guo, G., Han, J., & Yu, J. (2022). Gut microbiome in modulating immune checkpoint inhibitors. *eBioMedicine, 82*, 104163. https://doi.org/10.1016/j.ebiom.2022.104163.

Lin, A., Jiang, A., Huang, L., Li, Y., Zhang, C., Zhu, L., Mou, W., Liu, Z., Zhang, J., Cheng, Q., Wei, T., & Luo, P. (2025). From chaos to order: Optimizing fecal microbiota transplantation for enhanced immune checkpoint inhibitors efficacy. *Gut Microbes, 17*(1). https://doi.org/10.1080/19490976.2025.2452277.

Moges, B., & Mengistu, D. Y. (2024). Metagenomics approaches for studying the human microbiome. *All Life, 17*(1). https://doi.org/10.1080/26895293.2024.2350166.

Newsome, R. C., Yang, Y., & Jobin, C. (2022). The microbiome, gastrointestinal cancer, and immunotherapy. *Journal of Gastroenterology and Hepatology (Australia), 37*(2), 263–272. https://doi.org/10.1111/jgh.15742.

Oli, A. N., Adejumo, S. A., Rowaiye, A. B., Ogidigo, J. O., Hampton-Marcell, J., & Ibeanu, G. C. (2024). Tumour immunotherapy and applications of immunological products: A review of literature. *Journal of Immunology Research, 2024*(1). https://doi.org/10.1155/2024/8481761.

Pham, F., Moinard-Butot, F., Coutzac, C., & Chaput, N. (2021). Cancer and immunotherapy: A role for microbiota composition. *European Journal of Cancer, 155*, 145–154. https://doi.org/10.1016/j.ejca.2021.06.051.

Rezasoltani, S., Yadegar, A., Aghdaei, H. A., & Zali, M. A. (2021). Modulatory effects of gut microbiome in cancer immunotherapy: A novel paradigm for blockade of immune checkpoint inhibitors. *Cancer Medicine, 10*(3), 1141–1154. https://doi.org/10.1002/cam4.3694.

Said, S. S., & Ibrahim, W. N. (2025). Gut microbiota–tumor microenvironment interactions: Mechanisms and clinical implications for immune checkpoint inhibitor efficacy in cancer. *Cancer Management and Research, 17*, 171–192. https://doi.org/10.2147/CMAR.S405590.

Sang, Y., Zheng, K., Zhao, Y., Liu, Y., Zhu, S., Xie, X., Shang, L., Liu, J., & Li, L. (2024). Efficacy and regulatory strategies of gut microbiota in immunotherapy: A narrative review. *Translational Cancer Research, 13*(4), 2043–2063. https://doi.org/10.21037/tcr-24-316.

Strouse, C., Mangalam, A., & Zhang, J. (2019). Bugs in the system: Bringing the human microbiome to bear in cancer immunotherapy. *Gut Microbes, 10*(2), 109–112. https://doi.org/10.1080/19490976.2018.1511665.

Szczyrek, M., Bitkowska, P., Chunowski, P., Czuchryta, P., Krawczyk, P., & Milanowski, J. (2021). Diet, microbiome, and cancer immunotherapy—A comprehensive review. *Nutrients, 13*(7), 2217. https://doi.org/10.3390/nu13072217.

Tannock, G. W. (2024). Scoring microbiota function: A proposal to use features of evolutionary, symbiotic innovation to recognize a "Healthy" human gut microbiota. *Gut Microbes Reports, 1*(1). https://doi.org/10.1080/29933935.2024.2376543.

Villemin, C., Six, A., Neville, B. A., Lawley, T. D., Robinson, M. J., & Bakdash, G. (2023). The heightened importance of the microbiome in cancer immunotherapy. *Trends in Immunology, 44*(1), 44–59. https://doi.org/10.1016/j.it.2022.11.002.

Xie, J., Liu, M., Deng, X., Tang, Y., Zheng, S., Ou, X., Tang, H., Xie, X., Wu, M., & Zou, Y. (2024). Gut microbiota reshapes cancer immunotherapy efficacy: Mechanisms and therapeutic strategies. *iMeta, 3*(1). https://doi.org/10.1002/imt2.156.

Yang, L., Ning, Q., & Tang, S. S. (2022). Recent advances and next breakthrough in immunotherapy for cancer treatment. *Journal of Immunology Research, 2022.* https://doi.org/10.1155/2022/8052212.

Yang, L., Wang, Q., He, L., & Sun, X. (2024). The critical role of tumor microbiome in cancer immunotherapy. *Cancer Biology and Therapy, 25*(1). https://doi.org/10.1080/15384047.2024.2301801.

Yin, Q., Ni, J., & Ying, J. (2024). Potential mechanisms and targeting strategies of the gut microbiota in antitumor immunity and immunotherapy. *Immunity, Inflammation and Disease, 12*(7). https://doi.org/10.1002/iid3.1263.

Yousefi, Y., Baines, K. J., & Vareki, S. M. (2024). Microbiome bacterial influencers of host immunity and response to immunotherapy. *Cell Reports Medicine, 5*(4). https://doi.org/10.1016/j.xcrm.2024.101487.

Zhang, H., Xie, Y., Cao, F., & Song, X. (2024). Gut microbiota-derived fatty acid and sterol metabolites: Biotransformation and immunomodulatory functions. *Gut Microbes, 16*(1). https://doi.org/10.1080/19490976.2024.2382336.

Zhang, T., Li, X., Li, J., Sun, F., & Duan, L. (2025). Gut microbiome-targeted therapies as adjuvant treatments in inflammatory bowel diseases: A systematic review and network meta-analysis. *Journal of Gastroenterology and Hepatology (Australia), 40*(1), 78–88. https://doi.org/10.1111/jgh.16795.

5

Microbiome-based strategies to overcome chemoresistance: Probiotics and prebiotics in cancer therapy

Prashanth Kotthapalli, Deepthi Joji and Ann Catherine Archer

DEPARTMENT OF MICROBIOLOGY, JSS ACADEMY OF HIGHER EDUCATION AND RESEARCH, MYSURU, KARNATAKA, INDIA

5.1 Introduction

Cancer remains one of the foremost causes of mortality and morbidity worldwide, responsible for more than 10 million deaths annually (Sung, 2021). Despite significant advances in cancer detection, diagnosis, and targeted therapies, chemotherapy remains the gold standard of treatment for both solid tumors and hematological malignancies. Conventional drugs such as antimetabolites, platinum compounds, taxanes, and anthracyclines work primarily by causing DNA damage, triggering apoptosis, and inhibiting cell division. However, clinical success is often restricted due to the development of chemoresistance, a phenomenon that significantly affects treatment, tumor relapse, and poor overall survival (Longley & Johnston, 2005). Chemoresistance may be intrinsic, meaning tumor cells possess innate resistance mechanisms, or acquired, where resistance develops due to repeated exposure to drugs via clonal selection and adaptive cellular reprogramming (Holohan et al., 2013). Classical mechanisms include drug efflux, mutations in drug targets, enhanced DNA repair pathways, activation of survival signaling, evasion of apoptosis, and metabolic reprogramming (Dongre & Weinberg, 2019; Gottesman, 2016; Vasan et al., 2019).

In recent years, the human microbiome has emerged as an important factor in cancer research. The term, “microbiome” refers to the collective genome of microbial communities that harbor the different body sites, particularly the gastrointestinal tract (Turnbaugh et al., 2007). The gut microbiota is made up of trillions of microorganisms that perform essential physiological functions, including digestion, bile acid transformation, vitamin synthesis, short-chain fatty acid production (SCFA), bacteriocin production, and educating the immune system (Flint et al., 2012). Advances in metagenomics and systems biology have enabled us to understand the microbiome

The Microbiome and Cancer Treatment: Overcoming Resistance and Enhancing Efficacy.
DOI: https://doi.org/10.1016/B978-0-443-33206-7.00003-0

and its critical role in regulating health and disease. The relationship between cancer and the microbiome is complex and bidirectional. While dysbiosis (alteration in microbial composition and diversity) is implicated in carcinogenesis involving mechanisms like chronic inflammation, genotoxic metabolite production, metabolic perturbations, and immune dysregulation (Garrett, 2015). Commensal microorganisms exert protective, anti-inflammatory, and immune-stimulatory effects that suppress carcinogenesis and improve antitumor immunity. Bacteria such as *Fusobacterium nucleatum* are directly implicated in the development of tumors and adverse outcomes in colorectal cancer (CRC) (Yu et al., 2017). Accumulating evidence shows that the microbiome can modulate responses to anticancer therapies. Landmark studies have shown that gut microbiota dysbiosis induced by antibiotics reduces the efficacy of platinum-based chemotherapy and cyclophosphamide in preclinical models (Iida et al., 2013; Viaud et al., 2013). Moreover, intratumor bacteria have been shown to metabolize chemotherapeutic drugs, inactivating them, while microbial enzymes can exacerbate toxicity and limit dosing due to reactivation of specific drugs in the gut (Geller, 2017). Thus, microbiome can influence both therapeutic efficacy and adverse outcomes.

The microbiome is also known to shape and tailor systemic immune responses that are essential for chemotherapy and immunotherapy outcomes. Certain gut microorganisms are associated with stimulating the immune response to inhibitors in lung cancer and melanoma patients (Gopalakrishnan et al., 2018; Routy et al., 2018). In addition, host genetics, diet, antibiotic exposure, etc., can contribute to interindividual variability in the microbiome, leading to varied treatment responses. These insights have thus led to the concept of the "microbiome-cancer-drug interaction axis," where microbiota mediates between host biology and therapeutic interventions.

Given the growing evidence of the role of the microbiome in cancer, microbiome-targeted interventions have gained increased attention as adjunctive strategies to overcome chemoresistance and improve efficacy. Probiotics and prebiotic supplementation are among the approaches widely studied to modulate gut microbiota balance, reduce toxicity, and enhance treatment efficacy. Other approaches include fecal microbiota transplantation (FMT), postbiotic metabolites, and engineered live biotherapeutics. Studies have shown that modulation of SCFA production, attenuation of inflammation, and regulation of immune responses may improve the sensitivity and responsiveness of tumors to chemotherapy. However, many mechanistic studies, randomized controlled trials, and regulatory frameworks are needed for widespread implementation of microbiome-based therapeutic strategies.

This chapter gives an overview of current knowledge on microbiome-based strategies to overcome chemoresistance with emphasis on probiotics and prebiotics as modulators of cancer therapy outcomes. We have attempted to provide an understanding of how microbiota-targeted interventions can improve therapeutic efficacy in cancer by delving into the mechanistic pathways of chemoresistance, the role of the microbiome in drug metabolism, immune signaling, and recent translational approaches. Ultimately, integrating microbiome science into cancer care provides an opportunity to develop personalized and more effective treatment regimens.

5.2 Mechanism of chemoresistance in cancer

Chemoresistance in cancer therapy presents a significant challenge that compromises the efficacy of chemotherapy, resulting in treatment failure, relapse, and suboptimal patient outcomes. This phenomenon refers to the resistance that cancer cells develop against chemotherapeutic agents and can be primarily categorized into intrinsic and acquired types. Several factors contribute to chemoresistance, including genetic mutations, drug efflux mechanisms, enhanced DNA repair, influences from the tumor microenvironment (TME), epigenetic modifications, and alterations in cell signaling pathways (Alfarouk et al., 2015). Mechanistically, cancer cells develop resistance by increasing drug efflux and reducing drug accumulation via upregulation of ATP-binding cassette (ABC) transporters (Gottesman, 2016). Mechanisms such as enhanced DNA repair, mutations in drug targets, activation of prosurvival signaling pathways such as PI3K/AKT and NF-κB, induction of epithelial-mesenchymal transition (EMT), and inhibition of apoptosis also contribute to chemoresistance (Dongre & Weinberg, 2019; Vasan et al., 2019).

Intrinsic chemoresistance is characterized by the presence of resistance mechanisms before chemotherapy exposure, with tumors exhibiting genetic or epigenetic traits that render them unresponsive to treatment (Zheng, 2017). Mutations in the *KEAP1* and *NFE2L2* genes, which are involved in the regulation of cellular defense, exemplify these characteristics. Mutations in the KEAP1/NFE2L2 pathway play a significant role in the chemotherapeutic response of nonsmall cell lung cancer (NSCLC) patients, often leading to poorer outcomes and chemoresistance. Specifically, these mutations are associated with increased tumor aggressiveness, resistance to platinum-based chemotherapy, and shorter time to treatment failure and overall survival. KEAP1 is a negative regulator of NFE2L2 (or NRF2), which controls cellular antioxidant responses. Mutations result in constitutive activation of NRF2, enhancing the cellular defense mechanism against oxidative stress, which in turn promotes cancer cell survival and chemoresistance (Jeong, 2020). TME, comprising elements such as blood vessels and immune cells, protects cancer cells by restricting drug penetration and creating hypoxic conditions. The TME, particularly tumor-associated stromal cells, plays a crucial role in chemoresistance by protecting tumor cells from cell death through multiple mechanisms. Tumor-associated stromal cells include fibroblasts, especially carcinoma-associated fibroblasts (CAFs), mesenchymal stem cells (MSCs), immune cells, endothelial cells, and adipocytes (Ni et al., 2021). These cells interact closely with tumor cells and influence their survival and response to chemotherapy. Stromal cells protect tumor cells by modulating cancer cell sensitivity to apoptosis via cell-to-cell and cell-matrix interactions and releasing soluble factors such as cytokines and chemokines that promote tumor growth, survival, and resistance signaling pathways. CAFs secrete factors like stromal cell-derived factor 1 (SDF-1), tumor growth factor-beta (TGF-b), and interleukins that activate survival pathways such as nuclear factor-kappa B (NF-kB) and B-cell lymphoma-extra-large (Bcl-xL) in tumor cells, promoting chemoresistance. MSCs and CAFs can promote tumor cell quiescence, enhance cancer stem cell populations, and supply metabolic support, shielding tumor cells from cytotoxic drugs (Castells et al., 2012; Wu et al., 2021).

5.3 Human microbiome and cancer development

The human gastrointestinal tract is colonized by a dense and metabolically active microbial ecosystem comprised of bacteria, archaea, fungi, viruses, and protozoa. The bacterial load alone amounts to 10^{14}, collectively exceeding that of the host genome (Turnbaugh et al., 2007). *Firmicutes, Actinobacteria, Proteobacteria,* and *Bacteroidetes* are the dominant bacterial phyla found varying with individuals and affected by geography, diet, host genetics, and environmental exposure. Apart from the taxonomic composition, the functional and metabolic functions of the microbiota, namely the metabolites, structural components, and enzymatic activities, play an important role in host physiology. SCFA production, bile acid transformation, vitamin synthesis, and immune system training are some of the functions attributed to the gut microbiota (Flint et al., 2012). This dynamic ecosystem thus maintains immune tolerance and intestinal barrier integrity in homoeostatic conditions. Reduction in microbial diversity and increase in inflammatory taxa are observed in cancers including colorectal, gastric, breast, lung, and pancreatic (Garrett, 2015). The human microbiome significantly influences cancer development, presenting both potential risks and opportunities for its diagnosis and treatment. The microbiome plays a crucial role in modulating the effectiveness and adverse effects of chemotherapy and immunotherapy. Microbial communities can impact cancer by producing carcinogenic compounds or genotoxins, which may lead to chronic inflammation and create a tumor-promoting environment. Furthermore, these communities can modulate the immune response, sometimes suppressing antitumor immunity or, under certain conditions, enhancing it (Kandalai et al., 2023; Xia et al., 2023). The modification of metabolic pathways, particularly those involved in bile acid metabolism, can result in the synthesis of metabolites that promote tumor growth, such as deoxycholic acid (DCA). Studies in germ-free animals and antibiotic-treated mice have shown that removing or altering the microbiome can reduce tumor formation in organs such as the colon, liver, and stomach (Kennedy et al., 2018; Ma et al., 2024; Manca, 2020). In humans, eradication of specific pathogens (e.g., *Helicobacter pylori* in gastric cancer) lowers cancer risk or leads to regression of certain lymphomas. The microbiome can modulate the efficacy and toxicity of chemotherapy and immunotherapy (Marashi et al., 2024; Pappas-Gogos, 2022). Certain microbial compositions enhance responses to immune checkpoint inhibitors (ICIs), while others may increase side effects or resistance to treatment. Research increasingly demonstrates that the communities of microbes residing in and on the body, especially in the gut, can both promote and inhibit tumorigenesis, influencing cancer risk, tumor risk, tumor growth, metastasis, and even responses to treatment. The disruption of the normal microbial equilibrium is closely associated with an elevated risk of cancer. Dysbiosis can result in an overrepresentation of potentially harmful bacteria, such as *F. nucleatum*, in CRC, while simultaneously reducing beneficial microbes, thereby contributing to a protumorigenic environment (Kang et al., 2025; Ranjbar et al., 2021).

F. nucleatum is overabundant in colorectal, esophageal, pancreatic, and breast cancers. It promotes tumor growth by inhibiting antitumor immune responses, reducing tumor-infiltrating lymphocytes (TILs), and activating immune checkpoints (TIGT, CEACAM1), which facilitate immune evasion and metastasis (Alon-Maimon et al., 2022;Gur et al., 2019; Ou et al., 2022).

Specific gut microbiota, such as *Escherichia coli* strains that produce the genotoxin colibactin, have been shown to directly damage DNA and initiate CRC. Additionally, *F. nucleatum* is associated with both colorectal and breast cancer through its role in promoting inflammation and tumor growth. In skin cancer, an increased presence of *Staphylococcus aureus* has been observed on the skin of patients with squamous cell carcinoma, suggesting that even the local microbiome can contribute to carcinogenesis. Furthermore, the microbiome of the urinary and reproductive tracts, exemplified by the presence of *H. hepaticus* in mouse models, has been demonstrated to drive prostate cancer through chronic inflammation (Poutahidis et al., 2013). Clinical studies have demonstrated that a favorable gut microbiome profile, characterized by an abundance of *A. muciniphila*, can enhance patient responses to ICIs, which are employed in the treatment of cancers such as melanoma and NSCLC. Conversely, disruptions to the microbiome caused by antibiotics are associated with poorer outcomes and reduced survival rates (Grenda et al., 2022; Jin et al., 2025; Zhao et al., 2023).

Recent research has identified *Morganella morganii* as a significant producer of a novel class of small-molecule genotoxins known as indolimines. These compounds have been demonstrated to induce DNA damage and abnormal cell proliferation, thereby exacerbating tumor growth in CRC models. Through the application of integrated untargeted metabolomics and electrophoresis-based bioactivity-guided fractionation, Cao et al. (2022) identified indolimines as genotoxic metabolites produced by *M. morganii*, a bacterium prevalent in the gut microbiota of patients with CRC and inflammatory bowel disease (IBD) (Cao et al., 2022). In murine models of CRC, strains of *M. morganii* capable of producing indolimines were observed to significantly increase tumor burden and intestinal permeability. Conversely, *M. morganii* mutants deficient in indolimine synthesis did not induce DNA damage or promote tumor growth, thereby demonstrating the direct involvement of these metabolites in tumorigenesis (Dougherty & Jobin, 2023; Sun et al., 2023). Indolimines were found to upregulate genes involved in cell cycle regulation, chromosome segregation, and DNA biosynthesis in intestinal epithelial cells, suggesting that these metabolites promote abnormal cell proliferation in addition to causing DNA damage. The production of indolimines requires a specific bacterial enzyme, aspartate aminotransferases (AAT), and deletion of the corresponding gene abolishes genotoxicity and tumor-promoting effects (Allen & Sears, 2019; Pérez Escriva et al., 2025; Leake, 2022). On the other hand, *Clostridium difficile* and *Pseudomonas aeruginosa* exotoxin A (ETA) induce apoptosis and disrupt cell cycle progression, which can either suppress or promote tumor growth. Certain bacteria produce nucleomodulins, which are proteins capable of entering the host cell nucleus to modulate gene expression. These bacterial nucleomodulins can infiltrate the host nucleus and influence critical regulators such as p53, potentially disrupting processes like apoptosis and DNA repair. However, their exact role in human cancer is still under investigation (Hirakata et al., 1999; Nottrott et al., 2007). The findings underscore the dual role of microbial communities in either promoting carcinogenesis or enhancing anticancer immune responses, thereby positioning the microbiome as a promising target for innovative strategies in cancer prevention, diagnosis, and personalized therapy. The elucidation of the role of the microbiome in cancer has spurred interest in its modulation through antibiotics, probiotics, dietary interventions, or fecal

Table 5.1 Molecular and pathophysiological roles of critical bacteria in tumorigenesis.

Bacteria	Molecular features	Clinicopathological links	Mechanistic role	References
pks^{+} *Escherichia coli*	Carries 54 kb pks genomic island encoding colibactin, a genotoxin causing DNA double-strand breaks	Associated with colorectal cancer (CRC), contributes to DNA damage and mutational signatures	Colibactin induces DNA cross-links and breaks, causing cell cycle arrest and genomic instability, promoting carcinogenesis	Chen et al. (2023), Chu et al. (2025), He et al. (2024), Iyadorai et al. (2020), Joo et al. (2024)
Enterotoxigenic *Bacteroides fragilis* (ETBF)	Produces *Bacteroides fragilis* toxin (BFT) that cleaves E-cadherin, induces IL-8 secretion	Linked with inflammatory bowel disease, diarrhea, and CRC, especially serrated lesions and adenomas	BFT disrupts epithelial integrity, promotes inflammation and epithelial proliferation, leading to colon carcinogenesis	Dadgar-Zankbar et al. (2023), Purcell et al. (2017), Voutsadakis (2025), Yang et al. 2024)
Fusobacterium nucleatum	Adhesin FadA binds E-cadherin, activates the Î^{2}-catenin/Wnt pathway	Enriched in CRC; promotes tumor growth and inflammation	FadA invasion stabilizes β-catenin, activates oncogenes (Myc, Cyclin D1), and induces NF-κB-dependent inflammation	Kulmambetova et al. (2024), Phipps et al. (2025), Rubinstein et al. (2013), Dewan et al. (2025), Wang (2024)
Streptococcus gallolyticus	Pil1 collagen-binding protein binds host factors, activates contact system, releasing bradykinin	Associated with colorectal cancer and infective endocarditis in elderly	Activates human contact system and coagulation pathways, promoting inflammation and bacterial colonization of colon tissues	Kumar et al. (2022), Pasquereau-Kotula et al. (2018), Taylor et al. (2023), Aymeric (2018), Isenring (2018)

(*continued on next page*)

Parvimonas micra	Two phylotypes with different adhesion abilities, epigenetically reprogram colonocytes	Enriched in CRC tissues and feces, associated with poor survival	Induces colonocyte proliferation, modulates the Th17 immune response, promotes Wnt signaling, and colorectal tumorigenesis	Bergsten et al. (2022), Fukuoka et al. (2023), Lin et al. (2025), Löwenmark et al. (2024)
Peptostreptococcus stomatis	Surface protein FBA attaches to CRC cells, activates ERBB2-MAPK (MEK)-ERK signaling	Frequently isolated from CRC patients; promotes tumorigenesis	Activates ERBB2 signaling, suppresses apoptosis, impairs the gut barrier, and reduces responsiveness to targeted therapy	Huang et al. (2024), Sabour et al. (2025)
Gemella morbillorum	Contains manganese transport/adhesins, choline-binding proteins, surface proteins interacting with ECM components	Causes endocarditis, associated with colon adenomas and carcinoma	Involved in opportunistic infections; potential virulence through adhesion; epidemiology links it to CRC and immunocompromised conditions	López and Martín-Galiano (2020); Khan et al. (2004), Roche and Smyth (2005), Valipour et al. (2005)
Prevotella copri	Genome encodes superoxide reductase and phosphoadenosine phosphosulfate reductase, involved in sulfur metabolism	Increase in inflammatory diseases like rheumatoid arthritis; role in inflammation	Produces molecules that modulate host oxidative stress and inflammation, potentially contributing to mucosal barrier response and disease	Drago (2019), Guerreiro et al. (2018), Scher et al. (2013), Abdelsalam et al. (2023)

transplants as a potential strategy for cancer prevention and treatment. The role of some bacteria in tumorigenesis is listed in Table 5.1.

5.4 The microbiome-cancer-drug interaction axis

The microbiome-cancer-drug interaction axis is a communication network where the microbiota influences the development of cancer and affects therapeutic efficacy by modifying the immune and metabolic pathways. Pathogen recognition receptors (PRRs) such as Toll-like receptors 4 (TLR4) underlying the intestinal lumen are responsible for identifying microbe-associated membrane patterns (MAMPs) such as lipopolysaccharide of bacteria, thus driving the axis crosstalk. The detection of MAMPs subsequently activates neutrophils, followed by upregulation of CD38, an enzyme that breaks down NAD+, causing its depletion in the TME. NAD+ is an important coenzyme present in all living cells involved in energy metabolism via oxidative phosphorylation, DNA repair (via PARP enzymes), and regulates enzymes, namely sirtuins, which control inflammation and aging (Xie, 2025). The depletion of NAD+ triggers neuroinflammation and anxiety-like behavior in preclinical cancer models such as colitis-associated CRC mouse models. This triggered anxiety further aggravates tumor progression by augmenting the TLR4-CD38-NAD+ axis crosstalk through the release of stress-induced cortisol, creating a vicious feedback loop. Surprisingly, cancer cells are found to counteract the NAD+ scarcity by upregulating the biosynthesis enzymes like nicotinamide phosphoribosyltransferase (NAMPT), allowing rapid proliferation, ATP production, and redox balance through glycolysis, serine synthesis, and the Warburg effect. High levels of NAD+ cause biomass production and immune evasion, making the cells vulnerable to NAMPT inhibitors (NAMPTi), mainly FK866. The inhibitors act by reducing the NAD+ in the intratumoral environment, leading to enhanced antitumor immunity and subsequently limiting the immunosuppressive myeloid-derived suppressor cells (MDSCs) and tumor-associated neutrophils (TANs). These inhibitors work synergistically with immunotherapies, including antiprogrammed cell death protein-1 (anti-PD1), poly (ADP-ribose) polymerase (PARP) inhibitors, or metformin. On the other hand, in ovarian cancer models, NAD+ precursors like nicotinamide can enhance T-cell function via activation of the STING pathway, countering the competition between tumor and NAD+, thereby improving effector T-cell infiltration. Microbiome modulation (by probiotics of fecal microbiota transplantation) stimulated NAD+ signaling is thus an efficient strategy to optimize NAMPTi efficacy by reducing dysbiosis and suppressing TLR4 signaling.

It was observed that dysbiosis due to chemotherapy or stress results in comorbid anxiety in cancer patients. It was found that the TLR4-CD38-NAD+ signaling pathway in neutrophils acts as a bridge between peripheral metabolic imbalance and effects on the central nervous system, thus contributing to the poor outcomes seen in anxiety patients. Interventions like NAD+ boosters, including microbiota modulation strategies or nicotinamide riboside (NR), could disrupt this pathway. Additionally, niacin, which restores NAD+ in cachectic tissues, is known to improve mitochondrial function and reduce cancer-related muscle wasting. Another molecule, nicotinamide mononucleotide (NMN), rapidly raises systemic NAD+ levels, supporting sirtuin activity and alleviating dysbiosis-related anxiety. However, high doses can have a risk of feedback inhibition of NAD+ synthesis (Lai et al., 2026).

Oral and gut microbiota engage in bidirectional communication that influences head and neck cancer progression through microbial translocation, metabolite exchange, and immune modulation. This "oral-gut axis" involves oral pathogens like Porphyromonas gingivalis migrating to the gut via swallowed saliva, altering gut ecology and promoting a protumorigenic environment via pathways such as MAPK/ERK signaling. Gut-derived metabolites, including SCFAs and bile acids, in turn systematically affect oral inflammation and antitumor immunity in head and neck cancer (Shetty & Shetty, 2024). Dysbiosis in head and neck cancer patients shows oral enrichment of pathogens linked to human papillomavirus (HPV) status, tumor staging, and poor prognosis, while gut shifts influence radiotherapy and immunotherapy responses. Pathogens like Porphyromonas gingivalis and *F. nucleatum* correlate with HPV-positive tumors, potentially exacerbating chronic inflammation that modulates HPV persistence and oncogenesis (Constantin et al., 2023). About one-third of gut microbiota originates from oral mucosa in healthy individuals, amplifying crosstalk during disease when barriers fail. This axis fosters sustained inflammation and tumor invasion, with specific taxa like *Clostridium* potentially improving outcomes in oral squamous cell carcinoma. Probiotics and antimicrobial peptides like nisin target the oral-gut axis to restore microbial balance, reduce mucosal injury, and enhance treatment efficacy (Al-Qadami et al., 2022).

Pancreatic ductal adenocarcinoma (PDAC) is characterized by intricate interactions wherein the gut microbiome exerts influence on stemness and the TME through the gut-pancreas axis. Recent studies underscore the role of microbial dysbiosis in promoting cancer stem cell properties, inflammation, and resistance to therapy. The gut microbiome impacts systemic health and the progression of PDAC via metabolites and signals that reach the pancreas. Dysbiotic microbes, such as *F. nucleatum* and *Porphyromonas gingivalis*, increase protumor cytokines like CXCL1 and interleukin-8 (IL-8), thereby facilitating EMT and metastasis (Arikath et al., 2026). This axis modulates pathways, including NF-kB and STAT3, thereby enhancing cellular plasticity within the TME. The composition of the tumor microbiome drives stem-like traits in PDAC cells by altering TME dynamics, such as fibrosis and immune evasion. Metabolites, such as SCFAs from bacteria like *Lactobacillus reuteri*, can inhibit growth through TLR2 signaling and natural killer (NK) cell activation, whereas others, like Trimethylamine N-oxide (TMAO), enhance T-cell responses under hypoxic conditions. Bacterial extracellular vesicles further support stem cell maintenance and metabolic reprogramming (Daniel et al., 2025).

Traditional Chinese medicinal plants, such as *Dioscorea bulbifera*, present potent anticancer properties but also pose significant risks of drug-induced liver injury, a primary cause of the discontinuation of herbal therapies globally. The rhizome of *D. bulbifera*, traditionally employed in Asian folk medicine for the treatment of abscesses and tumors, contains diterpenoids like Diosbulbin B, which inhibit sarcoma growth through the induction of oxidative stress in cancer cells. However, the reactive metabolites of Diosbulbin B are associated with severe hepatotoxicity, as evidenced by elevated ALT/AST levels and idiosyncratic liver failure, as documented in clinical cases and preclinical models (Zhao et al., 2017). Diosbulbin B, a compound derived from *D. bulbifera*, demonstrates potential in mitigating thyromegaly induced by propylthiouracil (PTU) in murine models. This effect is mediated through the modulation of gut microbiota, enhancement of SCFA production, and influence on thyroid function. Diosbulbin B was observed to reduce thyroid function markers, alleviate pathological changes, and diminish inflammation and oxidative damage in thyroid tissue. It also normalized disrupted fatty acid metabolism, restored fecal SCFAs such as propionic acid, butyric acid, and acetic acid, and rebalanced gut microbiota by increasing beneficial bacteria, including *Firmicutes, Bacteroidota*, and *Verrucomicrobia*, while reducing harmful microbes (Ji et al., 2021). Diosbulbin C, another bioactive compound isolated from the extract of *D. bulbifera* L., a traditional medicinal plant, has been shown to effectively inhibit the proliferation of NSCLC cells, such as A549 and H1299 lines, primarily by inducing cell cycle arrest in the G0/G1 phase. Diosbulbin C downregulates key proteins, including p-AKT, DHFR, TYMS, and CDK4, thereby disrupting cell cycle progression and preventing entry into the S phase (Zhu et al., 2023).

Conventional treatments like resection and targeted therapies often fail to address the gut-liver axis, where microbial dysbiosis exacerbates oncogenesis through impaired metabolite production and weakened immunity. Fungal-derived agents that modulate the gut microbiota to generate antitumor compounds represent a promising adjunctive strategy. Huaier granule (HEG), derived from the medicinal fungus *Trametes robiniophila*, enriches beneficial gut bacteria like *Adlercreutzia equolifaciens*, boosting production of the metabolite equol, which directly suppresses hepatocellular carcinoma progression. This occurs through cell cycle arrest in the G0/G1 phase via inhibition of cyclin E1-CDK2/Rb signaling and blockade of MAPK pathways, enhancing liver immunity in orthotopic mouse models. Equol strengthens intestinal barriers and colon immunity, linking microbial shifts to reduced tumor burden and improved immune microenvironments. Clinical evidence supports the adjunctive role of HEG in improving survival and lowering HCC recurrence postresection (Wei et al., 2026).

5.4.1 Microbial biotransformation of chemotherapeutic drugs

Microorganisms are known to directly metabolize drugs, alter their pharmacokinetics, or modulate host metabolic pathways. Irinotecan, a topoisomerase I inhibitor used in the treatment of colon cancer, is metabolized in the liver to an inactive glucuronide form. However, intestinal bacterial β-glucuronidases can reconvert this inactive form back to its active state, leading to severe diarrhea and mucositis (Wallace et al., 2010). Inhibition of microbial β-glucuronidases has been shown to decrease gastrointestinal symptoms without affecting antitumor efficacy (Roberts et al., 2013). Similarly, gemcitabine is metabolized into its inactive form by certain gut bacteria, leading to chemoresistance in PDAC (Geller, 2017). *Gammaproteobacteria* associated with tumors are reported to contribute to resistance mechanisms, underscoring the significance of intratumoral microbiota in influencing drug response. Additionally, the drug cyclophosphamide modifies intestinal permeability, leading to bacterial endotoxemia in secondary lymphoid organs. This process stimulates Th17 and memory Th1 immune responses, thereby enhancing anticancer efficacy (Viaud et al., 2013). Nevertheless, the depletion of gut microbiota through antibiotic intervention diminishes these immune-mediated effects. These studies suggest that the microbiome can affect chemotherapy outcomes and resistance through

Table 5.2 Key bacterial cyclomodulins and their producers.

Cyclomodulins type	Bacterial producers	Mechanism of action	References
Cytotoxic necrotizing factors (CNFs)	*Escherichia coli, Yersinia pseudotuberculosis, Shigella spp., Salmonella enterica*	Activate Rho GTPases, disrupt the actin cytoskeleton, stimulate cell cycle and DNA replication, block cytokinesis, and modulate apoptosis	Chaoprasid et al. (2021), Markelova et al. (2022)
Cycle inhibiting factors (CIFs)	Enteropathogenic *E. coli (EPEC),* Enterohemorrhagic *E. coli (EHEC), Burkholderia pseudomallei, Yersinia pseudotuberculosis, Photorhabdus luminescens, Photorhabdus asymbiotica*	Arrest the cell cycle at G1/S and G2/M phases, and slow apoptosis by inhibiting proteasomal degradation	El-Aouar Filho et al. (2017), Taieb et al. (2011)
Cytolethal distending toxins (CDTs)	*E. coli, Campylobacter jejuni, Aggregatibacter actinomycetemcomitans, Haemophilus ducreyi, Helicobacter hepaticus, Shigella dysenteriae*	Induce DNA damage, cause cell cycle arrest (often at G2/M phase), promote genomic instability	Lai et al. (2016), Gargi et al. (2012)
Bacteroides fragilis toxin (BFT)	*Bacteroides fragilis*	Disrupts E-cadherin/b-catenin complex, promotes c-Myc expression and cell proliferation	Lee et al. (2022), Wu (2021)
Mycolactone	*Mycobacterium ulcerans*	Induces G0/g1 cell cycle arrest, triggers apoptosis via actin cytoskeleton remodeling	George et al. (2000), Sarfo et al. (2016)
Phenol-soluble modulins (PSMs)	*Staphylococcus aureus*	Delay G2/M transition, decrease host cell proliferation, and alter defensin gene expression	Deplanche (2016)

mechanisms such as metabolic activation or inactivation, immunomodulation, and altered drug distribution within the host.

5.4.2 Dysbiosis and variability in chemotherapy response

The disruption of the gut microbiota by cytotoxic agents can lead to increased intestinal permeability, systemic inflammation, and susceptibility to infections, complicating the therapeutic course. Variability in the response to chemotherapy and immunotherapy cannot be solely attributed to tumor genomics. Recent evidence has identified the composition of the microbiome as a crucial determinant of therapeutic efficacy. Previous studies have demonstrated an association between specific bacterial taxa and the response to ICIs. Patients with melanoma and lung cancer receiving anti-PD1 therapy exhibited improved progression-free survival, which correlated with an enrichment of *Akkermansia muciniphila, Faecalibacterium*, and *Bifidobacterium* species. Conversely, the administration of broad-spectrum antibiotics either during or before treatment has been correlated with reduced survival rates, likely due to the disruption of the microbiome (Pinato et al., 2019). Elevated levels of *F. nucleatum* have been linked to resistance against 5-fluorouracil and oxaliplatin, mediated through the induction of autophagy and the activation of TLR4-MyD88 signaling pathways (Yu et al., 2017).

5.4.3 Genotoxicity and microbial cyclomodulins in cancer

Genotoxicity describes the capacity of certain agents, such as chemicals, radiation, and microbial products, to inflict damage on the genetic material of cells, resulting in mutations, genomic instability, and potentially cancer. Among these microbial products, cyclomodulins are particularly significant in the context of cancer pathogenesis (Table 5.2). These bacterial toxins are known to cause DNA damage, alter the cell cycle, and disrupt the homeostasis of host cells, thereby heightening the risk of malignant transformation. Cyclomodulins, including toxins like colibactin (produced by *Escherichia coli*), CagA (from *H. pylori*), and BFT (from *Bacteroides fragilis*), modulate the host cell cycle, disrupt DNA integrity, and interfere with regulatory pathways central to cellular homeostasis. Their activity assists bacterial survival and adaptation but also creates conditions that may predispose to tumorigenesis within the host (Nougayrède et al., 2005; Oswald et al., 2005). Cyclomodulins can induce DNA strand breaks, interfere with repair mechanisms, and cause genomic instability, a hallmark of cancer initiation. These toxins arrest the host cell cycle, often at the G2/M checkpoint, leading to abnormal cell proliferation or delayed apoptosis. This persistent disturbance may trigger malignant transformation. Cyclomodulins can block cytokinesis while stimulating DNA replication, which leads to polyploidization and genomic instability, a potential step toward malignant transformation. Genotoxins like colibactin induce DNA damage and mutations in intestinal epithelial cells, promoting CRC, with evidence of mutational signature enrichment in CRC genomes from colibactin exposure (El-Aouar Filho et al., 2017). Cyclomodulins impair apoptosis and cell cycle regulation, prolonging bacterial colonization and potentially contributing to tumor growth and resistance to therapies such as radiation. Some cyclomodulins are linked to precancerous lesions and tumor progression via modulating the TME and host cell signaling pathways involved in proliferation, metastasis, and immune evasion. Cyclomodulins contribute to changes in epithelial layer turnover, favoring prolonged colonization by pathogenic bacteria, which may disrupt tissue homeostasis and contribute to carcinogenesis. Other bacterial effectors associated with cancer progression include those impacting angiogenesis, metastasis and immune modulation (Morgan et al., 2022). The carcinogenic effect of cyclomodulins depends on factors such as host genetic predisposition, chronic inflammation, the composition of the microbial environment, and the biochemical diversity of host cells. Bacterial metabolites like butyrate and secondary bile acids also interact with cyclomodulins in modulating cancer risk (Markelova et al., 2022). A study by Kristyna et al. (n.d.) examined the frequent occurrence of *E. coli* strains positive for cyclomodulin genes in CRC and assessed a cost-effective screening method utilizing culture and other molecular-based techniques. The findings revealed a significant association between CRC and *E. coli* isolates containing colibactin genes (*clbB, clbN*), the *cnf* gene, and, notably, a hemolytic phenotype of *E. coli*. The assay employed in this study was most effective as an auxiliary marker when used in conjunction with established fecal immunochemical tests, rather than as a standalone screening tool (Mezerová et al., 2021).

5.5 Probiotics in cancer: Mechanisms and applications

Probiotics, defined as live microorganisms, confer health benefits to the host when administered in sufficient quantities. In the realm of cancer therapy, probiotics of significant interest predominantly include strains from the *Lactobacillus* genus (such as *L. rhamnosus* GG, *L. plantarum, L. acidophilus, L. casei*) and the *Bifidobacterium* genus (such as *B. lactis, B. bifidum*). These probiotics exert anticancer effects through a variety of mechanisms, including modulation of the immune system, reduction of inflammation, induction of apoptosis, and enhancement of therapeutic outcomes when used alongside chemotherapy (Fijan, 2014; Plaza-Diaz et al., 2019). Probiotics enhance innate and adaptive immunity by stimulating pattern recognition receptors such as TLRs and NOD-like receptors (NLRs), which promote antitumor immune responses. They increase cytotoxic T cell and NK cell infiltration in tumors, enhance production of antitumor cytokines like interferon-gamma and IL-12, and reduce regulatory T (T-reg) cell functions that suppress immunity. Probiotics can decrease proinflammatory cytokines such as TNF-alpha and IL-6 and increase anti-inflammatory cytokines like IL-10, which helps to modulate the TME and reduce cancer progression (Li et al., 2024; Mazziotta et al., 2023). Certain probiotic strains promote cancer cell apoptosis by activating intrinsic pathways involving caspases and cytochrome C release. They can also induce cell cycle arrest and inhibit tumor cell proliferation. Probiotics such as *L. rhamnosus* and *L. plantarum* increase intracellular reactive oxygen species (ROS), which trigger the mitochondrial intrinsic pathway leading to cytochrome C release, activation of caspase-9 and caspase-3, and ultimately apoptosis. They also modulate the expression of proapoptotic proteins (e.g., Bax) and downregulate antiapoptotic proteins (e.g., Bcl-2), increasing the Bax/Bcl-2 ratio that favors apoptosis induction. Probiotics increase beneficial metabolites (e.g., butyrate) that have anticancer and immunomodulatory effects (Abolhassani et al., 2025;

Amin et al., 2023). The supernatant of *L. rhamnosus* has been demonstrated to enhance the expression of proapoptotic genes, diminish the expression of genes associated with cell cycle progression, such as cyclin D1 and cyclin E, and reduce the expression of proliferation-related oncogenes, including ERBB2. These combined effects of apoptosis induction and cell cycle arrest contribute to the anticancer potential of probiotics (Dehghani et al., 2021). *L. acidophilus* CICC 6074 has been shown to inhibit growth and induce apoptosis in CRC cells both in vitro and in an HT-29 cell-induced mouse model. Specifically, the S-layer protein from *L. acidophilus* CICC 6074 significantly suppressed the proliferation of HT-29 CRC cells by causing cell cycle arrest in the G1 phase. This was achieved through upregulation of tumor suppressor proteins p53, p21, and p16 and downregulation of cell cycle regulators CDK1 and cyclin B. The apoptosis in these cancer cells was evidenced morphologically by chromatin condensation and nuclear fragmentation and mechanistically linked to activation of both death receptor and mitochondrial apoptotic pathways. The bacteria also inhibited the PI3K/AKT cell survival signaling pathway and Fas ligand synthesis, contributing to reduced cancer cell invasion and survival (Guo et al., 2020; Zhang et al., 2020)

Probiotic strains can metabolize immunosuppressive molecules, notably adenosine, within the TME. Engineered probiotics have shown the ability to convert adenosine into inosine, which curbs immune suppression and enhances cytotoxic immune activity against tumors (Akbariqomi et al., 2025). Probiotics exert anticancer effects by producing anticarcinogenic metabolites such as SCFAs and conjugated linolenic acid, which induce apoptosis and inhibit cell proliferation in cancer cells. SCFAs, especially butyrate, induce apoptosis in cancer cells by inhibiting histone deacetylase (HDAC) activity, raising the expression of proapoptotic genes, generating ROS that trigger DNA damage, and reducing cell viability through changes in gene expression related to survival and proliferation. Strains such as *L. casei, L. rhamnosus* GG disrupt cancer-promoting signaling pathways such as IL-6/STAT3, reduce the production of angiogenic and prometastatic factors such as IL-1b, vascular endothelial growth factor (VEGF). *L. rhamnosus* GG decreases proangiogenic mediators such as VEGF-C and VEGF-D, playing a role in inhibiting the formation of new blood vessels necessary for tumor growth and metastasis (Liotti et al., 2022; Thapa et al., 2024; Tsvetikova & Koshel, 2020; Wang et al., 2025).

Probiotics are known to produce antibacterial substances, lower intestinal pH, and reduce the activity of procarcinogenic enzymes such as β-glucuronidase and nitroreductase. These enzymes are recognized for their role in converting procarcinogens into carcinogens, thereby mitigating cancer risks. Additionally, probiotics enhance the intestinal barrier and immune responses, further limiting inflammation and the translocation of pathogens (Yang et al., 2025). Clinical studies show probiotics can improve immune function, reduce inflammation, and alleviate chemotherapy side effects such as diarrhea and abdominal pain. They may also enhance tumor regression when combined with treatments like radiation therapy and immunotherapy (Deleemans et al., 2021; Rodriguez-Arrastia et al., 2021; Sevcikova et al., 2022). Oral probiotics have been shown to mitigate diarrhea, which is induced by chemotherapy, oral mucositis, and gastrointestinal toxicities, thereby enhancing the quality of life for patients. Research indicates that probiotics can reduce postoperative infections, radiation-induced diarrhea, and chemotherapy-related gastrointestinal complications in patients with CRC (Agraib et al., 2020; Lin & Shen, 2020). Ongoing clinical investigations are examining the use of probiotics in conjunction with chemotherapy for canine bladder cancer and lymphoma. The canine subjects were treated with a standard chemotherapy regimen, which included cyclophosphamide, doxorubicin, vincristine, and prednisone (CHOP). These canines exhibited signs of gastrointestinal microbiome dysbiosis, such as altered levels of *C. hiranonis* and *Fusobacterium*. Administration of probiotics resulted in increased fecal concentrations of *Streptococcus* and *E. coli*, with no adverse side effects observed (Tsvetikova & Koshel, 2020). Additional benefits associated with probiotic use include a reduction in pain index, dyspnea, and insomnia during treatment, although their effects on fatigue, appetite loss, and abdominal distension were not significant. Some studies suggest that the effectiveness of probiotics may be influenced by population characteristics, and findings related to other cancer-related side effects or the prevention of CRC are less consistent or necessitate further investigation (Belloni et al., 2025; Kechagia et al., 2013; Umeano et al., 2024). Some in vivo and clinical studies related to probiotics used to mitigate cancer have been outlined in Table 5.3 .

5.6 Prebiotics and synbiotics in cancer therapy

Prebiotics are nondigestible substrates selectively fermented by gut microorganisms that confer a health benefit on the host by modulation of gut microbiota (Gibson et al., 2017). Traditionally, nondigestible fibers such as inulin, fructooligosaccharides (FOS), galactooligosaccharides (GOS), resistant starch, etc., have been known to act as prebiotics (Slavin, 2013). While probiotics are live microorganisms, prebiotics function by enriching beneficial gut microorganisms such as *Lactobacillus* and *Bifidobacterium* species. In cancer treatment, prebiotics have been recognized for their ability to modulate tumor-associated dysbiosis, affect chemotherapy outcomes, and reduce treatment-related toxicities. They may enhance digestive health, relieve constipation, improve mineral absorption, and bolster immune function. Regular consumption of prebiotics can result in increased gas, bloating, and occasionally mild gastrointestinal discomfort, particularly at higher doses; however, these effects are generally temporary. Microbial dysbiosis can compromise therapeutic effectiveness and worsen conditions such as diarrhea, mucositis, and systemic inflammation (Alexander et al., 2017). Prebiotics can improve host resilience during chemotherapy by restoring the microbial gut balance and metabolic capacity. Current evidence regarding the efficacy of prebiotics in alleviating symptoms of depression is limited, with the majority of studies indicating nonsignificant effects. However, there are indications that prebiotics may be beneficial in addressing certain symptoms of anxiety (Brownawell et al., 2012; Davani-Davari et al., 2019; Deehan et al., 2024). Prebiotics and related supplements serve as adjunctive therapies that may reduce the incidence and severity of gastrointestinal side effects, such as diarrhea, commonly induced by chemotherapy and radiotherapy. Prebiotics contribute to maintaining the integrity of the gut barrier and regulating immune responses. They have the potential to modulate inflammatory pathways and decrease the activity of harmful gut enzymes that facilitate carcinogen activation. Through the modulation of microbiota, prebiotics may also lower the risk of infection and enhance recovery following cancer therapy (Khorashadizadeh et al., 2024; Rau et al., 2024; Siritientong et al., 2025). Scientific evidence indicates that prebiotics, including

Table 5.3 Studies listing the use of probiotics in different cancer models and their mechanism of action.

Bacteria	Product	Cancer type	Mechanism of action	References	Clinical trial status
Firmicutes, *Actinobacteria*, *Bacteroidetes*, and *Proteobacteria*	Butyrate	Colorectal cancer (CRC)	Inhibition of HDACs (Histone deacetylase), activation of cell surface receptors such as GPR41, GPR43, and GPR109A	Sun et al. (2024), Kang et al. (2023)	Preclinical
Lactobacillus reuteri	Reuterin	CRC, hepatocellular carcinoma (HCC)	Induction of oxidative stress, selective protein oxidation, inhibition of ribosomal biogenesis, and protein translation	Cui et al. (2024), Bell et al. (2022)	Preclinical
Pseudomonas aeruginosa	Azurin-p28	Melanoma, CRC, fibrosarcoma, HCC, breast cancer	Binding to the DNA-binding domain of the p53 tumor suppressor protein, proapoptotic activity, and antiproliferative activity	Wang et al., (2024), Yaghoubi et al. (2020)	Phase I (Completed) NCT00914914
Lactococcus lactis	Nisin ZP	Oral squamous cell carcinoma (OSCC), Lung cancer	Induction of apoptosis, cell cycle arrest, mitochondrial membrane depolarization, and generation of ROS (reactive oxygen species)	Wang et al. (2024), Patil et al. (2022)	Phase I/II (Ongoing) NCT06097468

(*continued on next page*)

Lactobacillus gallinarum	Indole-3-lactic acid (ILA)	CRC	ILA binds to AhR (Aryl hydrocarbon receptor) of tumor cells and inhibits the proliferation of tumor cells and promotes apoptosis	Jia et al. (2024)	Preclinical
Lactobacillus plantarum	Plantaricin BM-1	CRC	Induction of apoptosis by the induction of the caspase-3 pathway	Wang et al. (2023)	Preclinical
Enterococcus faecium	Enterocin 12a	Osteosarcoma, lung cancer, cervical cancer, and colon cancer	Dose-dependent inhibition of proliferation of the cancer cell lines, apoptosis-like morphological changes, permeabilising the cell membrane	Sharma et al. (2021)	Preclinical
Enterococcus faecium Por1	Enterocin A	Colon, gastric, and cervical cancer	Induction of sub-G and G1 phase arrest of the cell cycle, induction of apoptosis	Ankaiah et al. (2017)	Preclinical

inulin, FOS, β-glucan, pectin, and xylooligosaccharide (XOS), contribute to the maintenance of gut microbiome health, enhance immune system function, and may inhibit tumor growth. FOS, pectin, and polyphenols have also been shown to reduce tumor volume, promote apoptosis in cancer cells, and suppress cancer-related biomarkers in various cancer models, including those of colon, breast, prostate, and CRCs (Mishra et al., 2023; Kumari et al., 2024). Modified citrus pectin (MCP), a form of pectin and a soluble polysaccharide derived from citrus fruit peels and pulp, has demonstrated the ability to reduce cancer cell invasiveness and induce apoptosis in prostate cancer studies. MCP works primarily by antagonizing galectin-3, a carbohydrate-binding protein that facilitates cancer progression and metastasis. By disrupting galectin-3-mediated cell interactions, MCP impairs the ability of cancer cells to adhere, migrate, and survive, thereby increasing their susceptibility to apoptosis (Glinsky & Raz, 2009; Leclere et al., 2013; Yan & Katz, 2010). Resistant starch has been shown to provide protective effects against colon cancer and may affect drug response through enhanced butyrate production (Clarke, Young, & Topping, 2012). Similarly, preclinical studies with inulin-type fructans reported reduced tumor burden and improved immune function. These findings suggest that dietary interventions could be used as adjuvant strategies to optimize chemotherapeutic regimens. The scope of clinical research concerning prebiotic supplementation in cancer patients is currently limited (Urbancsek et al., 2001). Nonetheless, certain studies suggest that prebiotics may mitigate toxicity induced by chemotherapy and enhance quality of life. However, the diversity in microbiome analysis methodologies, dosing strategies, and study designs presents challenges in formulating universal recommendations. Synbiotics are combinations of probiotics and prebiotics that offer synergistic benefits of simultaneously introducing beneficial microorganisms and promoting their colonization. Postoperative infection and inflammation were notably reduced in CRC patients administered with synbiotics(Liu et al., 2025). Synbiotics enhance SCFA production, modulate the immune system, and reduce systemic endotoxemia. Diet-based modulation, including high-fiber and fermented foods, correlated with better microbiome diversity and better responses to immunotherapy in patients (Spencer et al., 2021).

5.7 Synergistic or combination effects of probiotics in cancer therapy

Probiotics and probiotic metabolites have demonstrated anticancer effects as previously described. Coadministration of butyrate and immune boosters substantially reduced carcinogenesis in vitro by inducing apoptosis (Jaye et al., 2022). Several probiotics have been studied in combination therapies. For example, probiotics with ICIs, probiotics with cisplatin (Miyake, 2023; Takada et al., 2022; Wang et al., 2019). Administration of *Bifidobacterium* and *Lactobacillus* showed synergistic effects with cisplatin and gemcitabine in in vivo urothelial cancer (Dadgar-Zankbar et al., 2023). Probiotic *L. rhamnosus* combined with cisplatin led to targeted delivery of cisplatin and reduced oxidative stress (Negi et al., 2020). Eight probiotic strains showed a synergistic effect with 5-FU in vitro in different intestinal, breast and lung cancer cells (Abd Ellatif et al., 2022). Coadministration of nivolumab and ipilimumab with CBM588 enhanced progression-free survival when compared to the control group (Dizman et al., 2022). *L. brevis* and tamoxifen, when administered in MCF-7 breast cancer cells, induced apoptosis by modulating the expression of the bax-bcl2 gene balance (Nasiri et al., 2021). A decrease in CRC cells' resistance markers (CD44, 133, 166, and ALDH1) was suppressed upon administration of *L. plantarum* ATCC 10241 and 5-FU (Kaźmierczak-Siedlecka et al., 2020).

5.8 Emerging microbiome-based strategies

5.8.1 Engineered probiotics and live biotherapeutics

Engineered probiotics are probiotic bacteria genetically modified to deliver therapeutic molecules to the targeted site using synthetic biology approaches. Genetically engineered *E. coli* Nissle 1917 have been developed to produce cytokines or cytotoxic agents in situ (Chowdhury et al., 2019). The live biotherapeutics can selectively target cancer cells harbored in hypoxic tumor environments, providing targeted drug delivery with reduced systemic toxicity. Engineered strains can be programmed to modulate immune response or produce enzymes that convert prodrugs into active components locally (Isabella et al., 2018). However, pharmacokinetics, biosafety containment, and regulatory concerns remain a challenge in this area.

5.8.2 Microbial metabolites and postbiotics

Postbiotics are bioactive metabolites obtained from microbial metabolism, including SCFAs, bacteriocins, exopolysaccharides, and peptidoglycan derivatives, which act as safer alternatives to live microorganisms like probiotics (Aguilar-Toalá et al., 2018). Bacteriocins such as nisin have demonstrated anticancer properties by inducing apoptosis and membrane destabilization in tumor cells (Joo, 2024). The small peptidic nature of nisin ensures that it selectively binds to the cancer cells and can be internalized easily, enhancing targeted delivery and effect. Nisin A reduced the viability and induced apoptosis in head and neck squamous cell carcinoma cell lines through mechanisms involving oxidative stress and membrane pore formation (Cotter et al., 2013). Comparable outcomes have been documented in studies involving colon cancer cells in vitro. In vivo models have demonstrated that the administration of bacteriocin results in a reduction of tumor burden, either independently or in conjunction with chemotherapy. This suggests the presence of synergistic or additive effects, alongside the modulation of gut microbiota and immune response. Microbial metabolites are known to significantly modulate systemic immune response and influence immune checkpoint inhibitor efficacy (Routy et al., 2018). The anticancer properties of SCFAs have been investigated in various preclinical models. Notably, butyrate inhibits histone deacetylases, leading to the upregulation of tumor-suppressing genes and the induction of apoptosis in colon cancer cells (Donohoe et al., 2012). Butyrate has shown a reduction in tumor size and multiplication by epigenetic and immune modulation (Lupton, 2004). In contrast, propionate and acetate appear to affect systemic metabolism and immune cell infiltration by interacting with specific receptors, GPR43 and GPR41, which regulate T-cell function. Developing defined metabolite cocktails can help avoid the risks associated with live probiotic bacteria, especially in immunocompromised cancer patients. Microbial exopolysaccharides derived from *Lactobacillus* and *Bifidobacterium* species augment innate and adaptive immune responses, leading to increased dendritic cell activation and Th1 polarization (Wang et al., 2025). The immunomodulatory effects, in conjunction with immune blockade therapies, may counteract tumor-associated immunosuppression and improve cytotoxic T-cell function. Recent research explores the encapsulation of postbiotics to protect against degradation during gastrointestinal transit and achieve targeted release. In a mouse model of CRC, butyrate-loaded nanoparticles improved colonic bioavailability and boosted antitumor immunity (Chen et al., 2020).

5.8.3 Fecal microbiota transplantation

Fecal microbiota transplantation (FMT) is a strategy used to modulate gut dysbiosis by transferring a stable community of gut microorganisms from the feces of healthy donors to individuals with diseases associated with gut dysbiosis. FMT is a powerful tool to restore a healthy microbiome composition that is often disrupted in cancer patients, particularly those undergoing chemotherapy or immunotherapy. Several studies show that FMT can reshape the gut microbial community to enhance antitumor immunity, reduce tumor growth, and reverse resistance to ICIs such as anti-PD-1 therapy. Research has demonstrated that among immunotherapy responders following FMT, there is a notable increase in the abundance of the phyla *Firmicutes* and *Actinobacteria* within the gut microbiome, which closely resembles the composition observed in healthy donors (Clavijo-Salomon & Trinchieri, 2025). FMT helps in the increased infiltration of $CD8^{+}$, i.e., cytotoxic T cells, into tumor tissue with the heightened activation of T cells and an increase in the production of cytokines such as interferon-gamma, which helps to collectively strengthen antitumor immunity (Kim et al., 2024). FMT derived from responders undergoing immunotherapy showed improved treatment efficacy in resistant metastatic melanoma cases by activating and increasing immune cell infiltration within the TME (Liu et al., 2025; Novelle et al., 2025; Zikou et al., 2024). FMT as a therapeutic strategy was first used in the fourth century in China, where fecal suspensions were used to treat patients suffering from severe diarrhea. In the modern context, Eiseman et al used fecal suspensions to treat four cases of pseudomembranous colitis in 1958 (Eiseman et al., 1958). The initial clinical trials investigating the application of FMT for the treatment of *Clostridium difficile* infection (CDI) were conducted in the Netherlands in 2013. These trials demonstrated that FMT was significantly more effective than vancomycin, an antibiotic, in treating recurrent CDI (Baunwall et al., 2020; Nood et al., 2013). Beyond treating CDI, FMT is being explored as a potential treatment option for a wide range of other conditions like IBD, irritable bowel syndrome, obesity, certain liver diseases, cancers, and metabolic disorders. Across these disease states, FMT helps not just as a microbial replacement but as a microbial ecosystem reset by helping restore microbial metabolites and immune regulation. Evidence highlights that the gut microbiome helps in maintaining a balance by suppressing or promoting tumorigenesis via its metabolites. FMT, being a strategy to modify the gut microbiota, offers a promising avenue for restoring the microbial balance and potentially improving cancer treatment outcomes, including overcoming chemoresistance

(Goldenberg & Merrick, 2021; Hou et al., 2025; Mullish et al., 2023). It is well known that gut dysbiosis can be linked to autoimmune responses, tumor development, and resistance to therapy. Clinical trials conducted by Baruch et al. (2021) and Davar et al. (2021) have investigated the impact of FMT on patients with PD-1-refractory metastatic melanoma, specifically examining their response to anti-PD-1 immunotherapy. ICIs, such as anti-PD1, play a crucial role in reactivating the antitumor functions of immune cells. However, an unfavorable microbiome can impede the efficacy of this therapeutic approach in many patients. Clinical trials involving human subjects have demonstrated that FMT can alter the microbiome composition in patients, thereby enhancing the effectiveness of anti-PD1 immunotherapy in individuals with PD-1-refractory melanoma (Jiang & Zhang, 2024; Pei et al., 2023; Ryan et al., 2024). This finding underscores the broader influence of the gut microbiome in modulating not only immunotherapy responses but also the overall efficacy of cancer treatments. Conversely, it has been demonstrated that *Bacteroides* spp. can expedite the conversion of sorivudine, an antiviral agent and synthetic analog of thymidine, to BVU (bromovinyluracil). BVU serves as an intermediate capable of inhibiting the degradation of 5-FU, thereby counteracting chemoresistance. Notably, 5-FU can decrease the populations of *Bacteroides* and *Lactobacillus* while increasing the abundance of *Staphylococcus* and *Clostridium*, leading to dysbiosis. Consequently, an approach such as FMT, which allows for favorable modulation of the microbiome, may represent a promising strategy to enhance the efficacy of cancer treatment (Diasio, 1998). Even though FMT is safe and easy to implement, the safety could be compromised if donor screening and further testing are inadequate. The human stool is highly variable in composition and is highly difficult to standardize. Another concern is the entry of pathogenic species, including multidrug-resistant species, which could be present in the feces of the healthy donor; hence, identifying and excluding such pathogenic strains becomes critical. Moreover, the effect of FMT tends to vary across people, as the intestinal flora tends to vary from person to person, and hence, the effect becomes hard to predict. FMT as a treatment option should be used with caution, as there are not many studies done regarding its long-term impact (Hourigan et al., 2021; Sartelli et al., 2020). In a certain clinical trial regarding the safety of FMT, it was reported that 20% of the patients who received FMT exhibited adverse effects like cramping, diarrhea, and abdominal pain, in contrast to 2% in those in the placebo group. Researchers are actively seeking to address these challenges by developing innovative approaches, such as cultured FMT (cFMT). In this method, rather than utilizing the entire stool, the donor microbiota is cultured in vitro under controlled conditions. This process ensures that the transplanted microbiota possesses a predictable composition, in contrast to raw FMT (Singh et al., 2024). An alternative approach has been developed that involves selecting donors based on their microbiome profiles, rather than randomly choosing stools from individuals who appear healthy. A study utilizing a murine model of IBD demonstrated that FMT from donors with a high abundance of beneficial microbiota resulted in superior restoration of the microbiota and consequently exhibited stronger therapeutic effects compared to donors with less desirable profiles (Dai et al., 2025). However, the majority of these modified approaches in FMT remain in their nascent stages. Consequently, further research is required to explore the formulation, duration, safety, and combinations of FMT treatments to enhance their efficacy (Sbahi & Di Palma, 2016; Wang et al., 2024).

5.8.4 Personalized microbiome modulation

Precision oncology has increasingly incorporated microbiome profiling using metagenomics, metabolomics, and systems biology methodologies. Analyses driven by artificial intelligence may facilitate the customization of personalized dietary, probiotic, or symbiotic interventions based on patient-specific microbiome signatures. Emerging clinical studies indicate that high-fiber diets have enhanced the response to immunotherapy in patients with advanced cancer (Spencer et al., 2021). Microbial analysis showed that subjects who consumed a high-fiber diet had higher microbial diversity and higher SCFA-producing taxa, enhancing therapeutic efficacy. Integration of machine learning with metagenomic, metabolomic and host genomic data accurately distinguished responders from nonresponders to chemotherapy in a CRC cohort study (Feng et al., 2015). The integration of microbiome data with tumor genomics and host immunophenotyping represents a pioneering area in cancer therapeutics. Extensive studies and reproducibility data are essential for the future application of personalized medicine.

5.9 Challenges, regulatory concerns, and future perspectives

Although microbiome-based strategies have shown promising results in preclinical and clinical models, several challenges lie in adapting these as therapeutic strategies. Microbiome-based interventions are complex due to variability between individuals, thus requiring the need to define a standard baseline microbiome signature at least at the geographical or regional level. The strain-specific effects of probiotics necessitate accurate characterization, genomic sequencing, and reproducibility testing (Hill et al., 2014). Additionally, dosage, formulation, shelf-life, and mode of administration significantly impact efficacy and need to be optimized. In terms of clinical trials, many oncology trials focused on microbiome include sample size and heterogeneous endpoints. Standardization of microbiome analysis, integration of metabolomics and harmonized clinical outcomes are required to predict therapeutic outcomes (Knight et al., 2018). Randomized controlled trials incorporating microbiome data will improve translational reliability. Regulatory frameworks for live biotherapeutics differ globally. In the United States, the Food and Drug Administration (FDA) classifies some microbiome products as biologics needing approval from an Investigational New Drug (IND). Integrated guidelines for safety, quality, and long-term surveillance are vital before widespread clinical adoption. Future directions include exploration of next-generation probiotics, engineered microbial consortia, and metabolite-based therapeutics integrated into oncology treatment regimens. Large-scale longitudinal studies are needed to establish mechanistic causal relationships and optimize treatment outcomes.

5.10 Conclusion and future directions

Emerging research reveals the gut microbiome as a key modulator of cancer therapy success, particularly against chemoresistance. Probiotics and prebiotics, by remodelling gut microbial ecosystems, bolstering host immune responses, and altering drug pharmacokinetics, present viable adjunct therapies to prime tumors for chemotherapeutic efficacy. Importantly, microbiota modulation unlike conventional pharmacological approaches targets the TME. However, mechanistic pathways linking specific microbial taxa, metabolic profiles and chemotherapeutic responses need to be elucidated. Precision microbiome therapeutics will be largely driven by multiomics including metagenomics and metabolomics to categorize patients through prediction of microbial signatures and chemoresistance enhancing diagnosis to therapy outcomes. Machine learning algorithms trained with fecal microbiome data from cohorts could be useful to predict outcomes and tailor interventions. Moreover, novel delivery systems, including synbiotics and engineered live biotherapeutics, could expand the therapeutic potential by ensuring targeted modulation of microbial functions relevant to drug resistance mechanisms. Integrating microbiome-based therapies with ICIs, targeted therapies and nanomedicine offers a compelling frontier, potentially yielding synergistic effects against chemoresistant tumors. Large-scale randomized controlled trials focusing on endpoints like minimal residual disease (MRD) and immune correlates are critical to validate these microbiome-based interventions and integrate them effectively into standard cancer care.

Acknowledgments

The authors are grateful to JSS Academy of Higher Education and Research for providing the necessary support. ACA acknowledges DBT Wellcome Trust India Alliance for grant of Early Career Fellowship (IA/E/20/1/505689).

Conflict of interest

The authors have no conflict of interest.

References

Abd Ellatif, S. A., Bouqellah, N. A., Abu-Serie, M. M., Razik, E. S. A., AL-surhanee, A. A., Askary, A. E., Daigham, G. E., & Mahfouz, A. Y. (2022). Assessment of probiotic efficacy and anticancer activities of *Lactiplantibacillus plantarum* ESSG1 (MZ683194.1) and *Lactiplantibacillus pentosus* ESSG2 (MZ683195.1) isolated from dairy products. *Environmental Science and Pollution Research, 29*(26), 39684–39701. https://doi.org/10.1007/s11356-022-18537-z.

Abdelsalam, N. A., Hegazy, S. M., & Aziz, R. K. (2023). The curious case of *Prevotella copri*. *Gut Microbes, 15*(2). doi:10.1080/19490976.2023.2249152.

Abolhassani, A., Esmaili, H., Rahati, S., & Jafarnejad, S. (2025). The role of *Lactobacillus* strain probiotics in breast cancer: Strain-specific mechanisms and therapeutic potential beyond probiotics. *Probiotics and Antimicrobial Proteins*. https://doi.org/10.1007/s12602-025-10741-w.

Agraib, L. M., Al-Shorman, A., Salah, S., Abu-hijlih, R., & Abuhijla, F. (2020). The effect of probiotics supplementation on the side effects of chemo radiotherapy for colorectal cancer: A literature review. *Oncology and Radiotherapy, 14*, 043–051.

Aguilar-Toalá, J. E., Garcia-Varela, R., Garcia, H. S., Mata-Haro, V., González-Córdova, A. F., Vallejo-Cordoba, B., & Hernández-Mendoza, A. (2018). Postbiotics: An evolving term within the functional foods field. *Trends in Food Science & Technology, 75*, 105–114. https://doi.org/10.1016/j.tifs.2018.03.009.

Akbariqomi, M., Kheirandish Zarandi, P., Abedi, A., Moghaddam, M. M., & Fooladi, A. A. I. (2025). Bacteria-based immunosuppressive tumor microenvironment reprogramming: A promising dawn in cancer therapy. *Microbial Cell Factories, 24*(1). https://doi.org/10.1186/s12934-025-02838-2.

Alexander, J. L., Wilson, I. D., Teare, J., Marchesi, J. R., Nicholson, J. K., & Kinross, J. M. (2017). Gut microbiota modulation of chemotherapy efficacy and toxicity. *Nature Reviews Gastroenterology and Hepatology, 14*(6), 356–365. https://doi.org/10.1038/nrgastro.2017.20.

Alfarouk, K. O., Stock, C. M., Taylor, S., Walsh, M., Muddathir, A. K., Verduzco, D., Bashir, A. H. H., Mohammed, O. Y., Elhassan, G. O., Harguindey, S., Reshkin, S. J., Ibrahim, M. E., & Rauch, C. (2015). Resistance to cancer chemotherapy: Failure in drug response from ADME to P-gp. *Cancer Cell International, 15*(1). https://doi.org/10.1186/s12935-015-0221-1.

Allen, J., & Sears, C. L. (2019). Impact of the gut microbiome on the genome and epigenome of colon epithelial cells: Contributions to colorectal cancer development. *Genome Medicine, 11*(1). https://doi.org/10.1186/s13073-019-0621-2.

Al-Qadami, G., Van Sebille, Y., Bowen, J., & Wardill, H. (2022). Oral-gut microbiome axis in the pathogenesis of cancer treatment-induced oral mucositis. *Frontiers in Oral Health, 3*, 881949. https://doi.org/10.3389/froh.2022.881949.

Amin, M., Navidifar, T., Saeb, S., Barzegari, E., & Jamalan, M. (2023). Tumor-targeted induction of intrinsic apoptosis in colon cancer cells by *Lactobacillus plantarum* and *Lactobacillus rhamnosus* strains. *Molecular Biology Reports, 50*(6), 5345–5354. https://doi.org/10.1007/s11033-023-08445-x.

Alon-Maimon, T., Mandelboim, O., & Bachrach, G. (2022). Fusobacterium nucleatum and cancer. Periodontology 2000, 89(1), 166–180. https://doi.org/10.1111/prd.12426

Ankaiah, D., Esakkiraj, P., Perumal, V., Ayyanna, R., & Venkatesan, A. (2017). Probiotic characterization of Enterococcus faecium por1: Cloning, over expression of Enterocin-A and evaluation of antibacterial, anti-cancer properties. *Journal of Functional Foods, 38*, 280–292. https://doi.org/10.1016/j.jff.2017.09.034.

Arikath, K., Batra, S. K., & Ponnusamy, M. P. (2026). Unveiling the gut-pancreas axis: Microbial influence on stemness and tumor microenvironment of PDAC. *Stem Cells, 44*(2), sxaf064. https://doi.org/10.1093/stmcls/sxaf064.

Aymeric, L., et al. (2018). Colorectal cancer specific conditions promote *Streptococcus gallolyticus* gut colonization. *Proceedings of the National Academy of Sciences, 115*(2). doi:10.1073/pnas.1715112115.

Baruch, E. N., Youngster, I., Ben-Betzalel, G., Ortenberg, R., Lahat, A., Katz, L., Adler, K., Dick-Necula, D., Raskin, S., Bloch, N., Rotin, D., Anafi, L., Avivi, C., Melnichenko, J., Steinberg-Silman, Y., Mamtani, R., Harati, H., Asher, N., Shapira-Frommer, R., … Boursi, B. (2021). Fecal microbiota transplant promotes response in immunotherapy-refractory melanoma patients. *Science, 371*(6529), 602–609. https://doi.org/10.1126/science.abb5920.

Baunwall, S. M. D., Lee, M. M., Eriksen, M. K. jæ, Mullish, B. H., Marchesi, J. R., Dahlerup, J. F., & Hvas, C. L. (2020). Faecal microbiota transplantation for recurrent Clostridioides difficile infection: An updated systematic review and meta-analysis. *EClinicalMedicine, 29-30*, 100642. https://doi.org/10.1016/j.eclinm.2020.100642.

Bell, H. N., Rebernick, R. J., Goyert, J., Singhal, R., Kuljanin, M., Kerk, S. A., Huang, W., Das, N. K., Andren, A., Solanki, S., Miller, S. L., Todd, P. K., Fearon, E. R., Lyssiotis, C. A., Gygi, S. P., Mancias, J. D., & Shah, Y. M. (2022). Reuterin in the healthy gut microbiome suppresses colorectal cancer growth through altering redox balance. *Cancer Cell, 40*(2), 185. https://doi.org/10.1016/j.ccell.2021.12.001.

Belloni, S., Arrigoni, C., Magon, A., Giacon, C., Ceruso, M. H., Alfredo Arcidiacono, M., Conte, G., & Caruso, R. (2025). Symptomatologic outcomes of gut microbiota modifiers (probiotics, prebiotics and synbiotics) in cancer care: A scoping review of randomized controlled trials. *Critical Reviews in Oncology/Hematology, 212*, 104779. https://doi.org/10.1016/j.critrevonc.2025.104779.

Bergsten, E., Mestivier, D., Donnadieu, F., Pedron, T., Barau, C., Meda, L. T., Mettouchi, A., Lemichez, E., Gorgette, O., Chamaillard, M., Vaysse, A., Volant, S., Doukani, A., Sansonetti, P. J., Sobhani, I., Nigro, G.,

(2022). Parvimonas micra, an oral pathobiont associated with colorectal cancer, epigenetically reprograms human primary intestinal epithelial cells. bioRxiv., https://doi.org/10.1101/2022.05.14.491935.

Brownawell, A. M., Caers, W., Gibson, G. R., Kendall, C. W. C., Lewis, K. D., Ringel, Y., & Slavin, J. L. (2012). Prebiotics and the health benefits of fiber: Current regulatory status, future research, and goals. *The Journal of Nutrition, 142*(5), 962–974. https://doi.org/10.3945/jn.112.158147.

Cao, Y., Oh, J., Xue, M., Huh, W. J., Wang, J., Gonzalez-Hernandez, J. A., Rice, T. A., Martin, A. L., Song, D., Crawford, J. M., Herzon, S. B., & Palm, N. W. (2022). Commensal microbiota from patients with inflammatory bowel disease produce genotoxic metabolites. *Science, 378*(6618). https://doi.org/10.1126/science.abm3233.

Castells, M., Thibault, B. ît, Delord, J.-P., & Couderc, B. (2012). Implication of tumor microenvironment in chemoresistance: Tumor-associated stromal cells protect tumor cells from cell death. *International Journal of Molecular Sciences, 13*(8), 9545–9571. https://doi.org/10.3390/ijms13089545.

Chaoprasid, P., Lukat, P., Mühlen, S., Heidler, T., Gazdag, E.-M., Dong, S., Bi, W., Rüter, C., Kirchenwitz, M., Steffen, A., Jänsch, L., Stradal, T. E. B., Dersch, P., & Blankenfeldt, W. (2021). Crystal structure of bacterial cytotoxic necrotizing factor CNF Y reveals molecular building blocks for intoxication. *The EMBO Journal, 40*(4). https://doi.org/10.15252/embj.2020105202.

Chen, B., Ramazzotti, D., Heide, T., Spiteri, I., Fernandez-Mateos, J., James, C., Magnani, L., Graham, T. A., & Sottoriva, A. (2023). Contribution of pks+*E. coli* mutations to colorectal carcinogenesis. *Nature Communications, 14*(1). https://doi.org/10.1038/s41467-023-43329-5.

Chen, D., Jin, D., Huang, S., et al. (2020). Clostridium butyricum, a butyrate-producing probiotic, inhibits intestinal tumor development through modulating Wnt signaling and gut microbiota. *Cancer Letters, 469*, 456–467. https://doi.org/10.1016/j.canlet.2019.11.019.

Chowdhury, S., Castro, S., Coker, C., Hinchliffe, T. E., Arpaia, N., & Danino, T. (2019). Programmable bacteria induce durable tumor regression and systemic antitumor immunity. *Nature Medicine, 25*(7), 1057–1063. https://doi.org/10.1038/s41591-019-0498-z.

Chu, Y. L., Georgeson, P., Clendenning, M., Mahmood, K., Walker, R., Como, J., Joseland, S., Preston, S. G., Rice, T., Lynch, B. M., Milne, R. L., Southey, M. C., Giles, G. G., Phipps, A. I., Hopper, J. L., Win, A. K., Rosty, C., Macrae, F. A., Winship, I., … Joo, J. E. (2025). Intratumoural pks Escherichia coli is associated with risk of metachronous colorectal cancer and adenoma development in people with Lynch syndrome. *eBioMedicine, 114*, 105661. https://doi.org/10.1016/j.ebiom.2025.105661.

Clarke, J. M., Young, G. P., Topping, D. L., et al. (2012). Butyrate delivered by butyrylated starch increases distal colonic epithelial apoptosis in carcinogen-treated rats. *Carcinogenesis, 33*(1), 197–202. https://doi.org/10.1093/carcin/bgr254.

Constantin, M., Chifiriuc, M. C., Mihaescu, G., et al. (2023). Implications of oral dysbiosis and HPV infection in head and neck cancer: From molecular and cellular mechanisms to early diagnosis and therapy. *Frontiers in Oncology, 13*, 1273516. https://doi.org/10.3389/fonc.2023.1273516.

Cotter, P. D., Ross, R. P., & Hill, C. (2013). Bacteriocins — a viable alternative to antibiotics? *Nature Reviews Microbiology, 11*(2), 95–105. doi:10.1038/nrmicro2937.

Cui, L., Xu, X., Fan, H., Wan, X., Chen, Q., Zhang, J., Tao, C., Du, Z., Wang, Y., Zhang, J., Zeng, J., Zhang, Y., Zhang, C., Li, L., Bu, Y., & Lei, Y. (2024). Reuterin promotes pyroptosis in hepatocellular cancer cells through mtDNA-mediated STING activation and caspase 8 expression. *Cancer Letters, 601*, 217183. https://doi.org/10.1016/j.canlet.2024.217183.

Dadgar-Zankbar, L., Shariati, A., Bostanghadiri, N., Elahi, Z., Mirkalantari, S., Razavi, S., Kamali, F., & Darban-Sarokhalil, D. (2023). Evaluation of enterotoxigenic *Bacteroides fragilis* correlation with the expression of cellular signaling pathway genes in Iranian patients with colorectal cancer. *Infectious Agents and Cancer, 18*(1). https://doi.org/10.1186/s13027-023-00523-w.

Dai, Z., Cheng, W., Peng, H., Qiu, X., Sun, J., Liu, X., Sun, X., Cai, J., Wang, J., Li, G., Lv, Y., Chen, S., & Zhong, Z. (2025). Microbiota composition-based donor selection affects FMT efficacy in a murine colitis model. *Frontiers in Immunology, 16*. https://doi.org/10.3389/fimmu.2025.1635244.

Daniel, N., Farinella, R., Belluomini, F., et al. (2025). The relationship of the microbiome, associated metabolites and the gut barrier with pancreatic cancer. *Seminars in Cancer Biology, 112*, 43–57. https://doi.org/10.1016/j.semcancer.2025.03.002.

Davani-Davari, D., Negahdaripour, M., Karimzadeh, I., Seifan, M., Mohkam, M., Masoumi, S., Berenjian, A., & Ghasemi, Y. (2019). Prebiotics: Definition, types, sources, mechanisms, and clinical applications. *Foods, 8*(3), 92. https://doi.org/10.3390/foods8030092.

Davar, D., Dzutsev, A. K., McCulloch, J. A., Rodrigues, R. R., Chauvin, J.-M., Morrison, R. M., Deblasio, R. N., Menna, C., Ding, Q., Pagliano, O., Zidi, B., Zhang, S., Badger, J. H., Vetizou, M., Cole, A. M., Fernandes, M. R., Prescott, S., Costa, R. G. F., Balaji, A. K., ... Zarour, H. M. (2021). Fecal microbiota transplant overcomes resistance to anti–PD-1 therapy in melanoma patients.. *Science, 371*(6529), 595–602. https://doi.org/10.1126/science.abf3363.

Deehan, E. C., Antwan, S. A. l, Witwer, R. S., Guerra, P., John, T., & Monheit, L. (2024). Revisiting the concepts of prebiotic and prebiotic effect in light of scientific and regulatory progress—A consensus paper from the Global Prebiotic Association. *Advances in Nutrition, 15*(12), 100329. https://doi.org/10.1016/j.advnut.2024.100329.

Dehghani, N., Tafvizi, F., & Jafari, P. (2021). Cell cycle arrest and anti-cancer potential of probiotic Lactobacillus rhamnosus against HT-29 cancer cells. *BioImpacts, 11*(4), 245–252. https://doi.org/10.34172/bi.2021.32.

Deleemans, J. M., Gajtani, Z., Baydoun, M., Reimer, R. A., Piedalue, K. A., & Carlson, L. E. (2021). The use of prebiotic and probiotic interventions for treating gastrointestinal and psychosocial health symptoms in cancer patients and survivors: A systematic review. *Integrative Cancer Therapies, 20*. https://doi.org/10.1177/15347354211061733.

Deplanche, M., et al. (2016). Staphylococcus aureus Phenol-Soluble Modulins Impair Interleukin Expression in Bovine Mammary Epithelial Cells. *Infection and Immunity, 84*(6), 1682–1692. doi:10.1128/IAI.01330-15.

Dewan, A., Tattoli, I., & Mascellino, M. T. (2025). The Impact of Fusobacterium nucleatum and the Genotypic Biomarker KRAS on Colorectal Cancer Pathogenesis. *International Journal of Molecular Sciences, 26*(14), 6958. doi:10.3390/ijms26146958.

Diasio, R. B. (1998). Sorivudine and 5-fluorouracil; A clinically significant drug-drug interaction due to inhibition of dihydropyrimidine dehydrogenase. *British Journal of Clinical Pharmacology, 46*(1), 1–4. https://doi.org/10.1046/j.1365-2125.1998.00050.x.

Dizman, N., Meza, L., Bergerot, P., Alcantara, M., Dorff, T., Lyou, Y., Frankel, P., Cui, Y., Mira, V., Llamas, M., Hsu, J., Zengin, Z., Salgia, N., Salgia, S., Malhotra, J., Chawla, N., Chehrazi-Raffle, A., Muddasani, R., Gillece, J., ... Pal, S. K. (2022). Nivolumab plus ipilimumab with or without live bacterial supplementation in metastatic renal cell carcinoma: A randomized phase 1 trial. *Nature Medicine, 28*(4), 704–712. https://doi.org/10.1038/s41591-022-01694-6.

Dongre, A., & Weinberg, R. A. (2019). New insights into the mechanisms of epithelial–mesenchymal transition and implications for cancer. *Nature Reviews Molecular Cell Biology, 20*(2), 69–84. doi:10.1038/s41580-018-0080-4.

Donohoe, D. R., Collins, L. B., Wali, A., Bigler, R., Sun, W., & Bultman, S. J. (2012). The Warburg effect dictates the mechanism of butyrate-mediated histone acetylation and cell proliferation. *Molecular Cell, 48*(4), 612–626. https://doi.org/10.1016/j.molcel.2012.08.033.

Dougherty, M. W., & Jobin, C. (2023). Intestinal bacteria and colorectal cancer: Etiology and treatment. *Gut Microbes, 15*(1). https://doi.org/10.1080/19490976.2023.2185028.

Drago, L. (2019). *Prevotella copri* and microbiota in rheumatoid arthritis: Fully convincing evidence? *Journal of Clinical Medicine, 8*(11), 1837. https://doi.org/10.3390/jcm8111837.

Eiseman, B., Silen, W., Bascom, G. S., & Kauvar, A. J. (1958). Fecal enema as an adjunct in the treatment of pseudomembranous. *Surgery, 44*(5), 854–859.

El-Aouar Filho, R. A., Nicolas, A., De Paula Castro, T. L., Deplanche, M., De Carvalho Azevedo, V. A., Goossens, P. L., Taieb, F., Lina, G., Le Loir, Y., & Berkova, N. (2017). Heterogeneous family of cyclomodulins:

Smart weapons that allow bacteria to hijack the eukaryotic cell cycle and promote infections. *Frontiers in Cellular and Infection Microbiology, 7*(MAY). https://doi.org/10.3389/fcimb.2017.00208.

Feng, Q., Liang, S., Jia, H., Stadlmayr, A., Tang, L., Lan, Z., … Wang, J. (2015). Gut microbiome development along the colorectal adenoma-carcinoma sequence. *Nature Communications, 6*, 6528. https://doi.org/10.1038/ncomms7528.

Fijan, S. (2014). Microorganisms with claimed probiotic properties: An overview of recent literature. *International Journal of Environmental Research and Public Health, 11*(5), 4745–4767. https://doi.org/10.3390/ijerph110504745.

Flint, H. J., Scott, K. P., Duncan, S. H., Louis, P., & Forano, E. (2012). Microbial degradation of complex carbohydrates in the gut. *Gut Microbes, 3*(4), 289–306. https://doi.org/10.4161/gmic.19897.

Fukuoka, H., Tourlousse, D. M., Ohashi, A., Suzuki, S., Nakagawa, K., Ozawa, M., Ishibe, A., Endo, I., & Sekiguchi, Y. (2023). Elucidating colorectal cancer-associated bacteria through profiling of minimally perturbed tissue-associated microbiota. *Frontiers in Cellular and Infection Microbiology, 13*. https://doi.org/10.3389/fcimb.2023.1216024.

Gargi, A., Reno, M., & Blanke, S. R. (2012). Bacterial toxin modulation of the eukaryotic cell cycle: are all cytolethal distending toxins created equally? *Frontiers in Cellular and Infection Microbiology, 2*. doi:10.3389/fcimb.2012.00124.

Garrett, W. S. (2015). Cancer and the microbiota. *Science, 348*(6230), 80–86. https://doi.org/10.1126/science.aaa4972.

Geller, L. T., et al. (2017). Potential role of intratumor bacteria in mediating tumor resistance to the chemotherapeutic drug gemcitabine. *Science, 357*(6356), 1156–1160. doi:10.1126/science.aah5043.

George, K. M., Pascopella, L., Welty, D. M., & Small, P. L. C. (2000). A mycobacterium ulcerans toxin, mycolactone, causes apoptosis in guinea pig ulcers and tissue culture cells. *Infection and Immunity, 68*(2), 877–883. https://doi.org/10.1128/IAI.68.2.877-883.2000.

Gibson, G. R., Hutkins, R., Sanders, M. E., Prescott, S. L., Reimer, R. A., Salminen, S. J., Scott, K., Stanton, C., Swanson, K. S., Cani, P. D., Verbeke, K., & Reid, G. (2017). Expert consensus document: The International Scientific Association for Probiotics and Prebiotics (ISAPP) consensus statement on the definition and scope of prebiotics. *Nature Reviews Gastroenterology and Hepatology, 14*(8), 491–502. https://doi.org/10.1038/nrgastro.2017.75.

Glinsky, V. V., & Raz, A. (2009). Modified citrus pectin anti-metastatic properties: one bullet, multiple targets. *Carbohydrate Research, 344*(14), 1788–1791. doi:10.1016/j.carres.2008.08.038.

Goldenberg, S. D., & Merrick, B. (2021). The role of faecal microbiota transplantation: Looking beyond *Clostridioides difficile* infection. *Therapeutic Advances in Infectious Disease, 8*. https://doi.org/10.1177/2049936120981526.

Gopalakrishnan, V., Spencer, C. N., Nezi, L., Reuben, A., Andrews, M. C., Karpinets, T. V., Prieto, P. A., Vicente, D., Hoffman, K., Wei, S. C., Cogdill, A. P., Zhao, L., Hudgens, C. W., Hutchinson, D. S., Manzo, T., Petaccia De Macedo, M., Cotechini, T., Kumar, T., Chen, W. S., … Wargo, J. A. (2018). Gut microbiome modulates response to anti-PD-1 immunotherapy in melanoma patients. *Science, 359*(6371), 97–103. Available from https://doi.org/10.1126/science.aan4236 .

Gottesman, M. M., et al. (2016). Toward a Better Understanding of the Complexity of Cancer Drug Resistance. *Annual Review of Pharmacology and Toxicology, 56*(1), 85–102. doi:10.1146/annurev-pharmtox-010715-103111.

Grenda, A., Iwan, E., Chmielewska, I., Krawczyk, P. ł, Giza, A., Bomba, A., Frąk, M., Rolska, A., Szczyrek, M. ł, Kieszko, R., Kucharczyk, T., Jarosz, B. oż, Wasyl, D., & Milanowski, J. (2022). Presence of *Akkermansiaceae* in gut microbiome and immunotherapy effectiveness in patients with advanced non-small cell lung cancer. *AMB Express, 12*(1). https://doi.org/10.1186/s13568-022-01428-4.

Guerreiro, C. S., Calado, Â., Sousa, J., & Fonseca, J. E. (2018). Diet, microbiota, and gut permeability-the unknown triad in rheumatoid arthritis. *Frontiers in Medicine, 5*. Available from https://doi.org/10.3389/fmed.2018.00349 .

Guo, Y., Zhang, T., Gao, J., Jiang, X., Tao, M., Zeng, X., Wu, Z., & Pan, D. (2020). *Lactobacillus acidophilus* CICC 6074 inhibits growth and induces apoptosis in colorectal cancer cells in vitro and in HT-29 cells induced-mouse model. *Journal of Functional Foods, 75*, 104290. https://doi.org/10.1016/j.jff.2020.104290.

Gur, C., Maalouf, N., Shhadeh, A., Berhani, O., Singer, B. B., Bachrach, G., & Mandelboim, O. (2019). *Fusobacterium nucleatum* supresses anti-tumor immunity by activating CEACAM1. *OncoImmunology, 8*(6), e1581531. https://doi.org/10.1080/2162402x.2019.1581531.

He, X., Ren, E., Dong, L., Yuan, P., Zhu, J., Liu, D., & Wang, J. (2024). Contribution of PKS+*Escherichia coli* to colon carcinogenesis through the inhibition of exosomal miR-885-5p. *Heliyon, 10*(18), e37346. https://doi.org/10.1016/j.heliyon.2024.e37346.

Hill, C., Guarner, F., Reid, G., Gibson, G. R., Merenstein, D. J., Pot, B., Morelli, L., Berni Canani, R., Flint, H. J., Salminen, S., Calder, P. C., & Sanders, M. E. (2014). The International Scientific Association for Probiotics and Prebiotics consensus statement on the scope and appropriate use of the term probiotic. *Nature Reviews Gastroenterology & Hepatology, 11*(8), 506–514. https://doi.org/10.1038/nrgastro.2014.66.

Hirakata, Y., Kirikae, T., Kirikae, F., Yamaguchi, T., Izumikawa, K., Takemura, H., Maesaki, S., Tomono, K., Yamada, Y., Kamihira, S., Nakano, M., Kitamura, S., & Kohno, S. (1999). Effect of *Pseudomonas aeruginosa* exotoxin A on endotoxin-induced tumour necrosis factor production in murine lung. *Journal of Medical Microbiology, 48*(5), 471–477. https://doi.org/10.1099/00222615-48-5-471.

Holohan, C., Van Schaeybroeck, S., Longley, D. B., & Johnston, P. G. (2013). Cancer drug resistance: An evolving paradigm. *Nature Reviews Cancer, 13*(10), 714–726. https://doi.org/10.1038/nrc3599.

Hou, S., Yu, J., Li, Y., Zhao, D., & Zhang, Z. (2025). Advances in fecal microbiota transplantation for gut dysbiosis-related diseases. *Advanced Science, 12*(13). https://doi.org/10.1002/advs.202413197.

Hourigan, S. K., Nicholson, M. R., Kahn, S. A., & Kellermayer, R. (2021). Updates and challenges in fecal microbiota transplantation for *Clostridioides difficile* infection in children. *Journal of Pediatric Gastroenterology and Nutrition, 73*(4), 430–432. https://doi.org/10.1097/MPG.0000000000003229.

Huang, P., Ji, F., Cheung, A. H. o-K., Fu, K., Zhou, Q., Ding, X., Chen, D., Lin, Y., Wang, L., Jiao, Y., Chu, E. S. H., Kang, W., To, K. F., Yu, J., & Wong, C. C. (2024). *Peptostreptococcus stomatis* promotes colonic tumorigenesis and receptor tyrosine kinase inhibitor resistance by activating ERBB2-MAPK. *Cell Host & Microbe, 32*(8), 1365. https://doi.org/10.1016/j.chom.2024.07.001.

Iida, N., Dzutsev, A., Stewart, C. A., Smith, L., Bouladoux, N., Weingarten, R. A., Molina, D. A., Salcedo, R., Back, T., Cramer, S., Dai, R.-M., Kiu, H., Cardone, M., Naik, S., Patri, A. K., Wang, E., Marincola, F. M., Frank, K. M., Belkaid, Y., … Goldszmid, R. S. (2013). Commensal bacteria control cancer response to therapy by modulating the tumor microenvironment. *Science, 342*(6161), 967–970. https://doi.org/10.1126/science.1240527.

Isabella, V. M., Ha, B. N., Castillo, M. J., Lubkowicz, D. J., Rowe, S. E., Millet, Y. A., Anderson, C. L., Li, N., Fisher, A. B., West, K. A., Reeder, P. J., Momin, M. M., Bergeron, C. G., Guilmain, S. E., Miller, P. F., Kurtz, C. B., & Falb, D. (2018). Development of a synthetic live bacterial therapeutic for the human metabolic disease phenylketonuria. *Nature Biotechnology, 36*(9), 857–864. https://doi.org/10.1038/nbt.4222.

Isenring, J., et al. (2018). Streptococcus gallolyticus subsp. gallolyticus endocarditis isolate interferes with coagulation and activates the contact system. *Virulence, 9*(1), 248–261. doi:10.1080/21505594.2017.1393600.

Iyadorai, T., Mariappan, V., Vellasamy, K. M., Wanyiri, J. W., Roslani, A. C., Lee, G. K., Sears, C., Vadivelu, J., & Mizoguchi, E. (2020). Prevalence and association of pks+*Escherichia coli* with colorectal cancer in patients at the University Malaya Medical Centre, Malaysia. *PLoS One, 15*(1), e0228217. https://doi.org/10.1371/journal.pone.0228217.

Jaye, K., Chang, D., Li, C. G., & Bhuyan, D. J. (2022). Gut metabolites and breast cancer: The continuum of dysbiosis, breast cancer risk, and potential breast cancer therapy. *International Journal of Molecular Sciences, 23*(16), 9490. https://doi.org/10.3390/ijms23169490.

Jeong, Y., et al. (2020). Role of KEAP1/NFE2L2 Mutations in the Chemotherapeutic Response of Patients with Non-Small Cell Lung Cancer. *Clinical Cancer Research, 26*(1), 274–281. doi:10.1158/1078-0432.CCR-19-1237.

Ji, H., Liu, C., Tong, N., et al. (2021). Metabonomic approaches investigate diosbulbin B-induced pulmonary toxicity and elucidate its underlying mechanism in male mice. *Toxicology Research, 10*(2), 272–276. https://doi.org/10.1093/toxres/tfab014.

Jia, D., Kuang, Z., & Wang, L. (2024). The role of microbial indole metabolites in tumor. *Gut Microbes, 16*(1). https://doi.org/10.1080/19490976.2024.2409209.

Jiang, H., & Zhang, Q. (2024). Gut microbiota influences the efficiency of immune checkpoint inhibitors by modulating the immune system (Review). *Oncology Letters, 27*(2). https://doi.org/10.3892/ol.2024.14221.

Jin, Y., Jie, Z., & Fan, X. (2025). Gut microbes and immunotherapy for non-small cell lung cancer: a systematic review. *Frontiers in Oncology*, (15.). doi:10.3389/fonc.2025.1518474.

Joo, J. E., et al. (2024). Intratumoral presence of the genotoxic gut bacteria pks+ E. coli, Enterotoxigenic Bacteroides fragilis, and Fusobacterium nucleatum and their association with clinicopathological and molecular features of colorectal cancer. *British Journal of Cancer, 130*(5), 728–740. doi:10.1038/s41416-023-02554-x.

Joo, J. E., Chu, Y. L., Georgeson, P., Walker, R., Mahmood, K., Clendenning, M., Meyers, A. L., Como, J., Joseland, S., Preston, S. G., Diepenhorst, N., Toner, J., Ingle, D. J., Sherry, N. L., Metz, A., Lynch, B. M., Milne, R. L., Southey, M. C., Hopper, J. L., … Buchanan, D. D. (2024). Intratumoral presence of the genotoxic gut bacteria pks + *E. coli, Enterotoxigenic Bacteroides fragilis*, and *Fusobacterium nucleatum* and their association with clinicopathological and molecular features of colorectal cancer. *British Journal of Cancer, 130*(5), 728–740. https://doi.org/10.1038/s41416-023-02554-x.

Kandalai, S., Li, H., Zhang, N., Peng, H., & Zheng, Q. (2023). The human microbiome and cancer: A diagnostic and therapeutic perspective. *Cancer Biology & Therapy, 24*(1). https://doi.org/10.1080/15384047.2023.2240084.

Kang, J., Sun, M., Chang, Y. i, Chen, H., Zhang, J., Liang, X., & Xiao, T. (2023). Butyrate ameliorates colorectal cancer through regulating intestinal microecological disorders. *Anti-Cancer Drugs, 34*(2), 227–237. https://doi.org/10.1097/cad.0000000000001413.

Kang, Z., Jiang, S., Fang, J.-Y., & Chen, H. (2025). Intestinal dysbiosis and colorectal cancer. *Chinese Medical Journal, 138*(11), 1266–1287. https://doi.org/10.1097/cm9.0000000000003617.

Kaźmierczak-Siedlecka, K., Ruszkowski, J., Skonieczna-Żydecka, K., Jędrzejczak, J., Folwarski, M., & Makarewicz, W. (2020). Gastrointestinal cancers: The role of microbiota in carcinogenesis and the role of probiotics and microbiota in anti-cancer therapy efficacy. *Central European Journal of Immunology, 45*(4), 476–487. https://doi.org/10.5114/ceji.2020.103353.

Kechagia, M., Basoulis, D., Konstantopoulou, S., Dimitriadi, D., Gyftopoulou, K., Skarmoutsou, N., & Fakiri, E. M. (2013). Health benefits of probiotics: A review. *ISRN Nutrition., 2013*, 1–7. https://doi.org/10.5402/2013/481651.

Kennedy, E. A., King, K. Y., & Baldridge, M. T. (2018). Mouse Microbiota Models: Comparing Germ-Free Mice and Antibiotics Treatment as Tools for Modifying Gut Bacteria. *Frontiers in Physiology, 9*. doi:10.3389/fphys.2018.01534.

Khan, R., Urban, C., Rubin, D., & Segal-Maurer, S. (2004). Subacute endocarditis caused by *Gemella haemolysans* and a review of the literature. *Scandinavian Journal of Infectious Diseases, 36*(11-12), 885–888. https://doi.org/10.1080/00365540410024916.

Khorashadizadeh, S., Abbasifar, S., Yousefi, M., Fayedeh, F., & Ghalibaf, A. A. M. (2024). The role of microbiome and probiotics in chemo-radiotherapy-induced diarrhea: A narrative review of the current evidence. *Cancer Reports, 7*(10). https://doi.org/10.1002/cnr2.70029.

Kim, Y., Kim, G., Kim, S., Cho, B., Kim, S.-Y., Do, E.-J., Bae, D.-J., Kim, S., Kweon, M.-N., Song, J. S., Park, S. H., Hwang, S. W., Kim, M.-N., Kim, Y., Min, K., Kim, S.-H., Adams, M. D., Lee, C., Park, H., & Park, S. Y. (2024). Fecal microbiota transplantation improves anti-PD-1 inhibitor efficacy in unresectable or metastatic solid cancers refractory to anti-PD-1 inhibitor. *Cell Host & Microbe, 32*(8), 1380. https://doi.org/10.1016/j.chom.2024.06.010.

Knight, R., Vrbanac, A., Taylor, B. C., Aksenov, A., Callewaert, C., Debelius, J., Gonzalez, A., Kosciolek, T., McCall, L.-I., McDonald, D., Melnik, A. V., Morton, J. T., Navas, J., Quinn, R. A., Sanders, J. G., Swafford, A. D., Thompson, L. R., Tripathi, A., Xu, Z. Z., … Dorrestein, P. C. (2018). Best practices for analysing microbiomes. *Nature Reviews Microbiology, 16*(7), 410–422. https://doi.org/10.1038/s41579-018-0029-9.

Kulmambetova, G., Kurentay, B., Gusmaulemova, A., Utupov, T., Auganova, D., Tarlykov, P., Mamlin, M., Khamzina, S., Shalekenov, S., & Kozhakhmetov, A. (2024). Association of *Fusobacterium nucleatum* infection with colorectal cancer in Kazakhstani patients. *Frontiers in Oncology, 14.* https://doi.org/10.3389/fonc.2024.1473575.

Kumar, R., Culver Taylor, J., Jain, A., Jung, S. Y., Garza, V., Xu, Y. i, & Hakansson, A. P. (2022). Modulation of the extracellular matrix by *Streptococcus gallolyticus* subsp. *Gallolyticus* and importance in cell proliferation. *PLoS Pathogens, 18*(10), e1010894. https://doi.org/10.1371/journal.ppat.1010894.

Kumari, T., Kumar Bag, K., Baran Das, A., & Chandra Deka, S. (2024). Synergistic role of prebiotics and probiotics in gut microbiome health: Mechanisms and clinical applications. *Food Bioengineering, 3*(4), 407–424. https://doi.org/10.1002/fbe2.12107.

Lai, C. K., Chen, Y. A., Lin, C. J., Lin, H. J., Kao, M. C., Huang, M. Z., Lin, Y. H., Chiang-Ni, C., Chen, C. J., Lo, U. G., Lin, L. C., Lin, H., Hsieh, J. T., & Lai, C. H. (2016). Molecular mechanisms and potential clinical applications of *Campylobacter jejuni* cytolethal distending toxin. *Frontiers in Cellular and Infection Microbiology, 6.* https://doi.org/10.3389/fcimb.2016.00009.

Lai, F., Yuan, Y., Dong, H., Guo, D., Yang, Z., & Tian, L. (2026). Chemotherapy-induced gut microbiota dysbiosis exacerbates cancer-related fatigue in breast cancer patients via neuroimmune-endocrine indicators. *Frontiers in Oncology, 16,* 1710457. https://doi.org/10.3389/fonc.2026.1710457.

Leake, I. (2022). Genotoxins from gut bacteria. *Nature Biotechnology, 40*(12), 1765. https://doi.org/10.1038/s41587-022-01605-7.

Leclere, L., Cutsem, P. van and Michiels, C. (2013) Anti-cancer activities of pH- or heat-modified pectin. *Frontiers in Pharmacology*, 4. doi:10.3389/fphar.2013.00128.

Lee, C.-G., Hwang, S., Gwon, S.-Y., Park, C., Jo, M., Hong, J.-E., & Rhee, K. i-J. (2022). *Bacteroides fragilis* toxin induces intestinal epithelial cell secretion of interleukin-8 by the E-cadherin/β-catenin/NF-κB dependent pathway. *Biomedicines, 10*(4), 827. https://doi.org/10.3390/biomedicines10040827.

Li, Z., Xiong, W., Liang, Z., Wang, J., Zeng, Z., Kołat, D., Li, X. i, Zhou, D., Xu, X., & Zhao, L. (2024). Critical role of the gut microbiota in immune responses and cancer immunotherapy. *Journal of Hematology & Oncology, 17*(1). https://doi.org/10.1186/s13045-024-01541-w.

Lin, S., & Shen, Y. (2020). The efficacy and safety of probiotics for prevention of chemoradiotherapy-induced diarrhea in people with abdominal and pelvic cancer: A systematic review and meta-analysis based on 23 randomized studies. *International Journal of Surgery, 84,* 69–77. https://doi.org/10.1016/j.ijsu.2020.10.012.

Lin, Y., Lau, H. C.-H., Liu, C., Ding, X., Sun, Y., Rong, J., Zhang, X., Wang, L., Yuan, K., Miao, Y., Wu, W. K. a-K., Wong, S. H., Sung, J. J.-Y., & Yu, J. (2025). Multi-cohort analysis reveals colorectal cancer tumor location-associated fecal microbiota and their clinical impact. *Cell Host & Microbe, 33*(4), 589. https://doi.org/10.1016/j.chom.2025.03.012.

Liotti, F., Marotta, M., Sorriento, D., Pagliuca, C., Caturano, V., Mantova, G., Scaglione, E., Salvatore, P., Melillo, R. M., & Prevete, N. (2022). Probiotic *Lactobacillus rhamnosus* GG (LGG) restrains the angiogenic potential of colorectal carcinoma cells by activating a proresolving program via formyl peptide receptor 1. *Molecular Oncology, 16*(16), 2959–2980. https://doi.org/10.1002/1878-0261.13280.

Liu, Y., Li, X., Chen, Y., Yao, Q., Zhou, J., Wang, X., Meng, Q., Ji, J., Yu, Z., & Chen, X. (2025). Fecal microbiota transplantation: Application scenarios, efficacy prediction, and factors impacting donor-recipient interplay. *Frontiers in Microbiology, 16*. https://doi.org/10.3389/fmicb.2025.1556827.

Longley, D. B., & Johnston, P. G. (2005). Molecular mechanisms of drug resistance. *The Journal of Pathology, 205*(2), 275–292. https://doi.org/10.1002/path.1706.

López, E. G., & Martín-Galiano, A. J. (2020). The versatility of opportunistic infections caused by Gemella isolates is supported by the carriage of virulence factors from multiple origins. *Frontiers in Microbiology, 11*. https://doi.org/10.3389/fmicb.2020.00524.

Löwenmark, T., Köhn, L., Kellgren, T., Rosenbaum, W., Bronnec, V., Löfgren-Burström, A., Zingmark, C., Larsson, P., Dahlberg, M., Schroeder, B. O., Wai, S. N., Ljuslinder, I., Edin, S., & Palmqvist, R. (2024). Parvimonas micra forms a distinct bacterial network with oral pathobionts in colorectal cancer patients. *Journal of Translational Medicine, 22*(1). https://doi.org/10.1186/s12967-024-05720-8.

Lupton, J. R. (2004). Microbial degradation products influence colon cancer risk: The butyrate controversy. *Journal of Nutrition, 134*, 479–482. https://doi.org/10.1093/jn/134.2.47900223166-2.

Ma, Z., Zuo, T., Frey, N., & Rangrez, A. Y. (2024). A systematic framework for understanding the microbiome in human health and disease: From basic principles to clinical translation. *Signal Transduction and Targeted Therapy, 9*(1). https://doi.org/10.1038/s41392-024-01946-6.

Manca, C., et al. (2020). Germ-free mice exhibit profound gut microbiota-dependent alterations of intestinal endocannabinoidome signaling. *Journal of Lipid Research, 61*(1), 70–85. doi:10.1194/jlr.RA119000424.

Marashi, A., Hasany, S., Moghimi, S., Kiani, R., Asl, S. M., Alavi Dareghlou, Y., Lorestani, P., Varmazyar, S., Jafari, F., Ataeian, S., Naghavi, K., Mohammad Sajjadi, S., Haratian, N., Alinezhad, A., Azhdarimoghaddam, A., Rafiei, S. K. S., & Asadi Anar, M. (2024). Targeting gut-microbiota for gastric cancer treatment: A systematic review. *Frontiers in Medicine, 11*. https://doi.org/10.3389/fmed.2024.1412709.

Markelova, N. N., Semenova, E. F., Sineva, O. N., & Sadykova, V. S. (2022). The role of cyclomodulins and some microbial metabolites in bacterial microecology and macroorganism carcinogenesis. *International Journal of Molecular Sciences, 23*(19), 11706. https://doi.org/10.3390/ijms231911706.

Mazziotta, C., Tognon, M., Martini, F., Torreggiani, E., & Rotondo, J. C. (2023). Probiotics mechanism of action on immune cells and beneficial effects on human health. *Cells, 12*(1), 184. https://doi.org/10.3390/cells12010184.

Mezerová, K. ý, Starý, L. ír, Zbořil, P., Klementa, I., Stašek, M., Špička, P., Skalický, P., & Raclavský, V. (2021). Cyclomodulins and hemolysis in *E. coli* as potential low-cost non-invasive biomarkers for colorectal cancer screening. *Life, 11*(11), 1165. https://doi.org/10.3390/life11111165.

Mishra, P., Badiyani, V. M., Jain, S., et al. (2023). Prebiotics: Ignored player in the fight against cancer. *Cancer Reports, 6*(11), e1870. https://doi.org/10.1002/cnr2.1870.

Miyake, M., et al. (2023). Probiotics enhances anti-tumor immune response induced by gemcitabine plus cisplatin chemotherapy for urothelial cancer. *Cancer Science, 114*(3), 1118–1130. doi:10.1111/cas.15666.

Morgan, R. N., Saleh, S. E., Farrag, H. A., & Aboulwafa, M. M. (2022). Bacterial cyclomodulins: Types and roles in carcinogenesis. *Critical Reviews in Microbiology, 48*(1), 42–66. https://doi.org/10.1080/1040841X.2021.1944052.

Mullish, B. H., Tohumcu, E., Porcari, S., Fiorani, M., Tommaso, N. D., Gasbarrini, A., Cammarota, G., Ponziani, F. R., & Ianiro, G. (2023). The role of faecal microbiota transplantation in chronic noncommunicable disorders. *Journal of Autoimmunity, 141*, 103034. https://doi.org/10.1016/j.jaut.2023.103034.

Nasiri, Z., Montazeri, H., Akbari, N., Mirfazli, S. S., & Tarighi, P. (2021). Synergistic cytotoxic and apoptotic effects of local probiotic *Lactobacillus brevis* isolated from regional dairy products in combination with tamoxifen. *Nutrition and Cancer, 73*(2), 290–299. https://doi.org/10.1080/01635581.2020.1743871.

Negi, D., Singh, A., Joshi, N., & Mishra, N. (2020). Cisplatin and probiotic biomass loaded pessaries for the management of cervical cancer. *Anti-Cancer Agents in Medicinal Chemistry, 20*(5), 589–598. https://doi.org/10.2174/1871520619666191211110640.

Ni, Y., Zhou, X., Yang, J., Shi, H., Li, H., Zhao, X., & Ma, X. (2021). The role of tumor-stroma interactions in drug resistance within tumor microenvironment. *Frontiers in Cell and Developmental Biology, 9*. https://doi.org/10.3389/fcell.2021.637675.

Nood, E., Vrieze, A., Nieuwdorp, M., Fuentes, S., Zoetendal, E. G., Vos, W. M., Visser, C. E., Kuijper, E. dJ., Bartelsman, J. F. W. M., Tijssen, J. G. P., Speelman, P., Dijkgraaf, M. G. W., & Keller, J. J. (2013). Duodenal infusion of donor feces for recurrent *Clostridium difficile*. *New England Journal of Medicine, 368*(5), 407–415. https://doi.org/10.1056/nejmoa1205037.

Nottrott, S., Schoentaube, J., Genth, H., Just, I., & Gerhard, R. (2007). *Clostridium difficile* toxin A-induced apoptosis is p53-independent but depends on glucosylation of Rho GTPases. *Apoptosis, 12*(8), 1443–1453. https://doi.org/10.1007/s10495-007-0074-8.

Nougayrède, J. P., Taieb, F., De Rycke, J., & Oswald, E. (2005). Cyclomodulins: Bacterial effectors that modulate the eukaryotic cell cycle. *Trends in Microbiology, 13*(3), 103–110. https://doi.org/10.1016/j.tim.2005.01.002.

Novelle, M. G., Naranjo-Martínez, B., López-Cánovas, J. L., & Díaz-Ruiz, A. (2025). Fecal microbiota transplantation, a tool to transfer healthy longevity. *Ageing Research Reviews, 103*, 102585. https://doi.org/10.1016/j.arr.2024.102585.

Oswald, E., Nougayrède, J.-P., Taieb, F. rédé, & Sugai, M. (2005). Bacterial toxins that modulate host cell-cycle progression. *Current Opinion in Microbiology, 8*(1), 83–91. https://doi.org/10.1016/j.mib.2004.12.011.

Ou, S., Wang, H., Tao, Y., Luo, K., Ye, J., Ran, S., Guan, Z., Wang, Y., Hu, H., & Huang, R. (2022). *Fusobacterium nucleatum* and colorectal cancer: From phenomenon to mechanism. *Frontiers in Cellular and Infection Microbiology, 12*. https://doi.org/10.3389/fcimb.2022.1020583.

Pappas-Gogos, G., et al. (2022). The Implication of Gastric Microbiome in the Treatment of Gastric Cancer. *Cancers, 14*(8), 2039. doi:10.3390/cancers14082039.

Pasquereau-Kotula, E., Martins, M., Aymeric, L., & Dramsi, S. (2018). Significance of *Streptococcus gallolyticus* subsp. *Gallolyticus* association with colorectal cancer. *Frontiers in Microbiology, 9*. https://doi.org/10.3389/fmicb.2018.00614.

Patil, S. M., & Kunda, N. K. (2022). Nisin ZP, an Antimicrobial Peptide, Induces Cell Death and Inhibits Non-Small Cell Lung Cancer (NSCLC) Progression in vitro in 2D and 3D Cell Culture. *Pharmaceutical Research, 39*(11), 2859–2870. https://doi.org/10.1007/s11095-022-03220-2.

Pei, B., Ma, X., Wu, N., Wang, C., & Yang, W. (2023). Effect of microbiome group on immune checkpoint inhibitors in treatment of gastrointestinal tumors. *Chinese Journal of Cancer Research, 35*(3), 252–265. https://doi.org/10.21147/j.issn.1000-9604.2023.03.05.

Pérez Escriva, P., Correia Tavares Bernardino, & Letellier, E. (2025). De-coding the complex role of microbial metabolites in cancer. *Cell Reports, 44*(3), 115358. https://doi.org/10.1016/j.celrep.2025.115358.

Phipps, A. I., Hill, C. M., Lin, G., Malen, R. C., Reedy, A. M., Kahsai, O., Ammar, H., Curtis, K., Ma, N., Randolph, T. W., Ma, J., Ogino, S., Newcomb, P. A., & Hullar, M. A. J. (2025). *Fusobacterium nucleatum* enrichment in colorectal tumor tissue: Associations with tumor characteristics and survival outcomes. *Gastro Hep Advances, 4*(6), 100644. https://doi.org/10.1016/j.gastha.2025.100644.

Pinato, D. J., Howlett, S., Ottaviani, D., Urus, H., Patel, A., Mineo, T., Brock, C., Power, D., Hatcher, O., Falconer, A., Ingle, M., Brown, A., Gujral, D., Partridge, S., Sarwar, N., Gonzalez, M., Bendle, M., Lewanski, C., Newsom-Davis, T., … Bower, M. (2019). Association of prior antibiotic treatment with survival and response to immune checkpoint inhibitor therapy in patients with cancer. *JAMA Oncology, 5*(12), 1774. https://doi.org/10.1001/jamaoncol.2019.2785.

Plaza-Diaz, J., Ruiz-Ojeda, F. J., Gil-Campos, M., & Gil, A. (2019). Mechanisms of action of probiotics. *Advances in Nutrition, 10*(suppl_1), S49. https://doi.org/10.1093/advances/nmy063.

Poutahidis, T., Cappelle, K., Levkovich, T., Lee, C.-W., Doulberis, M., Ge, Z., Fox, J. G., Horwitz, B. H., Erdman, S. E., & Fang, D. (2013). Pathogenic intestinal bacteria enhance prostate cancer development via systemic activation of immune cells in mice. *PLoS One, 8*(8), e73933. https://doi.org/10.1371/journal.pone.0073933.

Purcell, R. V., Pearson, J., Aitchison, A., Dixon, L., Frizelle, F. A., Keenan, J. I., & Brim, H. (2017). Colonization with enterotoxigenic Bacteroides fragilis is associated with early-stage colorectal neoplasia. *PLOS One, 12*(2), e0171602. https://doi.org/10.1371/journal.pone.0171602.

Ranjbar, M., Salehi, R., Haghjooy Javanmard, S., Rafiee, L., Faraji, H., jafarpor, S., Ferns, G. A., Ghayour-Mobarhan, M., Manian, M., & Nedaeinia, R. (2021). The dysbiosis signature of *Fusobacterium nucleatum* in colorectal cancer-cause or consequences? A systematic review. *Cancer Cell International, 21*(1). https://doi.org/10.1186/s12935-021-01886-z.

Rau, S., Gregg, A., Yaceczko, S., & Limketkai, B. (2024). Prebiotics and probiotics for gastrointestinal disorders. *Nutrients, 16*(6), 778. https://doi.org/10.3390/nu16060778.

Roberts, A. B., Wallace, B. D., Venkatesh, M. K., Mani, S., & Redinbo, M. R. (2013). Molecular insights into microbial β-glucuronidase inhibition to abrogate CPT-11 toxicity. *Molecular Pharmacology, 84*(2), 208–217. https://doi.org/10.1124/mol.113.085852.

Roche, M., & Smyth, E. (2005). A case of septic arthritis due to infection with *Gemella morbillorum. Journal of Infection, 51*(3), e187. https://doi.org/10.1016/j.jinf.2005.01.009.

Rodriguez-Arrastia, M., Martinez-Ortigosa, A., Rueda-Ruzafa, L., Ayora, A. F., & Ropero-Padilla, C. (2021). Probiotic supplements on oncology patients' treatment-related side effects: A systematic review of randomized controlled trials. *International Journal of Environmental Research and Public Health, 18*(8), 4265. https://doi.org/10.3390/ijerph18084265.

Routy, B., Le Chatelier, E., Derosa, L., Duong, C. P. M., Alou, M. T., Daillère, R., Fluckiger, A. é, Messaoudene, M., Rauber, C., Roberti, M. P., Fidelle, M., Flament, C., Poirier-Colame, V., Opolon, P., Klein, C., Iribarren, K., Mondragón, L., Jacquelot, N., Qu, B. o, … Zitvogel, L. (2018). Gut microbiome influences efficacy of PD-1-based immunotherapy against epithelial tumors. *Science, 359*(6371), 91–97. https://doi.org/10.1126/science.aan3706.

Rubinstein, M. R., Wang, X., Liu, W., Hao, Y., Cai, G., & Han, Y. W. (2013). *Fusobacterium nucleatum* promotes colorectal carcinogenesis by modulating E-cadherin/β-catenin signaling via its FadA adhesin. *Cell Host and Microbe, 14*(2), 195–206. https://doi.org/10.1016/j.chom.2013.07.012.

Ryan, T., Ling, S., Trinh, A., & Segal, J. P. (2024). The role of the microbiome in immune checkpoint inhibitor colitis and hepatitis. *Best Practice & Research Clinical Gastroenterology, 72*, 101945. https://doi.org/10.1016/j.bpg.2024.101945.

Sabour, S., Sadeghi Koupaei, H., Ghasemi, H., Amin, M., & Azimi, T. (2025). Anaerobic gut bacteria and their potential role in the initiation, exacerbation, and development of human colorectal cancer: A narrative review. *Frontiers in Cellular and Infection Microbiology, 15*. https://doi.org/10.3389/fcimb.2025.1559001.

Sarfo, F. S., Phillips, R., Wansbrough-Jones, M., & Simmonds, R. E. (2016). Recent advances: Role of mycolactone in the pathogenesis and monitoring of *Mycobacterium ulcerans* infection/Buruli ulcer disease. *Cellular Microbiology, 18*(1), 17–29. Available from https://doi.org/10.1111/cmi.12547 .

Sartelli, M., Pagani, L., Iannazzo, S., Moro, M. L., Viale, P., Pan, A., Ansaloni, L., Coccolini, F., D'Errico, M. M., Agreiter, I., Nespola, G. A., Barchiesi, F., Benigni, V., Binazzi, R., Cappanera, S., Chiodera, A., Cola, V., Corsi, D., Cortese, F., … Catena, F. (2020). A proposal for a comprehensive approach to infections across the surgical pathway. *World Journal of Emergency Surgery, 15*(1). https://doi.org/10.1186/s13017-020-00295-3.

Sbahi, H., & Di Palma, J. A. (2016). Faecal microbiota transplantation: Applications and limitations in treating gastrointestinal disorders. *BMJ Open Gastroenterology, 3*(1), e000087. https://doi.org/10.1136/bmjgast-2016-000087.

Scher, J. U., Sczesnak, A., Longman, R. S., Segata, N., Ubeda, C., Bielski, C., Rostron, T., Cerundolo, V., Pamer, E. G., Abramson, S. B., Huttenhower, C., & Littman, D. R. (2013). Expansion of intestinal *Prevotella copri* correlates with enhanced susceptibility to arthritis. *eLife, 2*(2). https://doi.org/10.7554/elife.01202.

Sevcikova, A., Izoldova, N., Stevurkova, V., Kasperova, B., Chovanec, M., Ciernikova, S., & Mego, M. (2022). The impact of the microbiome on resistance to cancer treatment with chemotherapeutic agents and immunotherapy. *International Journal of Molecular Sciences, 23*(1), 488. https://doi.org/10.3390/ijms23010488.

Sharma, P., Kaur, S., Singh Chadha, B., Kaur, R., Kaur, M., & Kaur, S. (2021). Anticancer and antimicrobial potential of enterocin 12a from *Enterococcus faecium. BMC Microbiology, 21*(1). https://doi.org/10.1186/s12866-021-02086-5.

Shetty, V. V., & Shetty, S. S. (2024). Exploring the gut microbiome and head and neck cancer interplay. *Pathology - Research and Practice, 263*, 155603. https://doi.org/10.1016/j.prp.2024.155603.

Singh, V., Choi, S.-D., Mahra, K., Son, H. W., Lee, H., Lee, Y.-J., Kim, E. S., & Shin, J.-H (2024). Cultured fecal microbial community and its impact as fecal microbiota transplantation treatment in mice gut inflammation. *Applied Microbiology and Biotechnology, 108*(1). https://doi.org/10.1007/s00253-024-13295-z.

Siritientong, T., Thet, D., Leelakanok, N., & Areepium, N. (2025). Oral probiotic supplementation to alleviate diarrhea induced by fluoropyrimidines or irinotecan-based chemotherapy: A systematic review and meta-analysis. *Complementary Therapies in Medicine, 89*, 103151. https://doi.org/10.1016/j.ctim.2025.103151.

Slavin, J. (2013). Fiber and prebiotics: Mechanisms and health benefits. *Nutrients, 5*(4), 1417–1435. https://doi.org/10.3390/nu5041417.

Spencer, C. N., McQuade, J. L., Gopalakrishnan, V., McCulloch, J. A., Vetizou, M., Cogdill, A. P., Wadud Khan, M. A., Zhang, X., White, M. G., Peterson, C. B., Wong, M. C., Morad, G., Rodgers, T., Badger, J. H., Helmink, B. A., Andrews, M. C., Rodrigues, R. R., Morgun, A., Kim, Y. S., … Wargo, J. A. (2021). Dietary fiber and probiotics influence the gut microbiome and melanoma immunotherapy response. *Science, 374*(6575), 1632–1640. https://doi.org/10.1126/science.aaz7015.

Sun, J., Chen, F., & Wu, G. (2023). Potential effects of gut microbiota on host cancers: focus on immunity, DNA damage, cellular pathways, and anticancer therapy. *The ISME Journal, 17*(10), 1535–1551. doi:10.1038/s41396-023-01483-0.

Sun, J., Chen, S., Zang, D., Sun, H., Sun, Y., & Chen, J. (2024). Butyrate as a promising therapeutic target in cancer: From pathogenesis to clinic (Review). *International Journal of Oncology, 64*(4). https://doi.org/10.3892/ijo.2024.5632.

Sung, H., et al. (2021). Global Cancer Statistics 2020: GLOBOCAN Estimates of Incidence and Mortality Worldwide for 36 Cancers in 185 Countries. *CA: A Cancer Journal for Clinicians, 71*(3), 209–249doi. doi:10.3322/caac.21660.

Taieb, F., Nougayrède, J.-P., & Oswald, E. (2011). Cycle Inhibiting Factors (Cifs): Cyclomodulins That Usurp the Ubiquitin-Dependent Degradation Pathway of Host Cells. *Toxins, 3*(4), 356–368. doi:10.3390/toxins3040356.

Takada, K., Buti, S., Bersanelli, M., Shimokawa, M., Takamori, S., Matsubara, T., Takenaka, T., Okamoto, T., Hamatake, M., Tsuchiya-Kawano, Y., Otsubo, K., Nakanishi, Y., Okamoto, I., Pinato, D. J., Cortellini, A., & Yoshizumi, T. (2022). Antibiotic-dependent effect of probiotics in patients with non-small cell lung cancer treated with PD-1 checkpoint blockade. *European Journal of Cancer, 172*, 199–208. https://doi.org/10.1016/j.ejca.2022.06.002.

Taylor, J. C., Kumar, R., Xu, J., & Xu, Y. (2023). A pathogenicity locus of *Streptococcus gallolyticus* subspecies *gallolyticus. Scientific Reports, 13*(1). https://doi.org/10.1038/s41598-023-33178-z.

Thapa, D., Kumar, V., Naik, B., Kumar, V., Kumar Gupta, A., Kishore Mohanta, Y., Mishra, B., & Rustagi, S. (2024). Harnessing probiotic foods: Managing cancer through gut health. *Food Science and Biotechnology, 33*(9), 2141–2160. https://doi.org/10.1007/s10068-024-01638-5.

Tsvetikova, S. A., & Koshel, E. I. (2020). Microbiota and cancer: Host cellular mechanisms activated by gut microbial metabolites. *International Journal of Medical Microbiology, 310*(4), 151425. https://doi.org/10.1016/j.ijmm.2020.151425.

Turnbaugh, P. J., Ley, R. E., Hamady, M., Fraser-Liggett, C. M., Knight, R., & Gordon, J. I. (2007). The human microbiome project. *Nature, 449*(7164), 804–810. https://doi.org/10.1038/nature06244.

Umeano, L., Iftikhar, S., Alhaddad, S. F., Paulsingh, C. N., Faisal Riaz, M., Garg, G., & Mohammed, L. (2024). Effectiveness of probiotic use in alleviating symptoms of irritable bowel syndrome: A systematic review. *Cureus, 16*(4). https://doi.org/10.7759/cureus.58306.

Urbancsek, H., Kazar, T., Mezes, I., & Neumann, K. (2001). Results of a double-blind, randomized study to evaluate the efficacy and safety of Antibiophilus® in patients with radiation-induced diarrhoea. *European Journal of Gastroenterology & Hepatology, 13*(4), 391–396. https://doi.org/10.1097/00042737-200104000-00015.

Valipour, A., Koller, H., Setinek, U., & Burghuber, O. C. (2005). Pleural empyema associated with *Gemella morbillorum*: Report of a case and review of the literature. *Scandinavian Journal of Infectious Diseases, 37*(5), 378–381. https://doi.org/10.1080/00365540510035319.

Vasan, N., Baselga, J., & Hyman, D. M. (2019). A view on drug resistance in cancer. *Nature, 575*(7782), 299–309. doi:10.1038/s41586-019-1730-1.

Viaud, S., Saccheri, F., Mignot, G., Yamazaki, T., Daillère, R., Hannani, D., Enot, D. P., Pfirschke, C., Engblom, C., Pittet, M. J., Schlitzer, A., Ginhoux, F., Apetoh, L., Chachaty, E., Woerther, P.-L., Eberl, G. é, Bérard, M., Ecobichon, C., Clermont, D., … Zitvogel, L. (2013). The intestinal microbiota modulates the anticancer immune effects of cyclophosphamide. *Science, 342*(6161), 971–976. https://doi.org/10.1126/science.1240537.

Voutsadakis, I. A. (2025). Genomic alterations in the WNT/β-catenin pathway and resistance of colorectal cancer cells to pathway-targeting therapies. *Exploration of Targeted Anti-tumor Therapy, 6*. https://doi.org/10.37349/etat.2025.1002295.

Wallace, B. D., Wang, H., Lane, K. T., Scott, J. E., Orans, J., Koo, J. S., Venkatesh, M., Jobin, C., Yeh, L. A., Mani, S., & Redinbo, M. R. (2010). Alleviating cancer drug toxicity by inhibiting a bacterial enzyme. *Science, 330*(6005), 831–835. https://doi.org/10.1126/science.1191175.

Wang, H., Zheng, L., Yang, C., Jia, L., Zhou, R., Liu, H., Dong, Y., Xu, X., Shi, G., Yang, J., Li, Y., Yuan, H., Cen, J., Zhang, G., Yu, L. e, Guo, T., Jiang, H., Liu, Y., Wang, X., Li, Z., & Wang, J. (2025). Probiotic-mediated tumor microenvironment reprogramming with protease-sensitive interleukin-15 and photothermal therapy. *Cell Reports Medicine, 6*(6), 102191. https://doi.org/10.1016/j.xcrm.2025.102191.

Wang, H. e, Jin, J., Pang, X., Bian, Z., Zhu, J., Hao, Y., Zhang, H., & Xie, Y. (2023). Plantaricin BM-1 decreases viability of SW480 human colorectal cancer cells by inducing caspase-dependent apoptosis. *Frontiers in Microbiology, 13*. https://doi.org/10.3389/fmicb.2022.1103600.

Wang, N., et al. (2024). *Fusobacterium nucleatum* induces chemoresistance in colorectal cancer by inhibiting pyroptosis via the Hippo pathway. *Gut Microbes, 16*(1). doi:10.1080/19490976.2024.2333790.

Wang, N. i, Zhang, L. u, Leng, X.-X. u, Xie, Y. i-L. e, Kang, Z. i-R., Zhao, L. i-C., Song, L.-H., Zhou, C.-B., & Fang, J.-Y. (2024). *Fusobacterium nucleatum* induces chemoresistance in colorectal cancer by inhibiting pyroptosis via the Hippo pathway. *Gut Microbes, 16*(1). https://doi.org/10.1080/19490976.2024.2333790.

Wang, T., Zheng, N., Luo, Q., Jiang, L. i, He, B., Yuan, X., & Shen, L. (2019). Probiotics *Lactobacillus reuteri* Abrogates immune checkpoint blockade-associated colitis by inhibiting group 3 innate lymphoid cells. *Frontiers in Immunology, 10*. https://doi.org/10.3389/fimmu.2019.01235.

Wang, W., Xu, Y., Chu, Y., Zhang, H., Zhou, L., Zhu, H., … Peng, H. (2025). Lactobacillus-based probiotic cocktail inhibits colitis-associated cancer by altering intestinal metabolism. *International Journal of Clinical and Experimental Pathology, 18*(7), 317–334. https://doi.org/10.62347/USLL6631.

Wei, X., Huang, H., Wang, F., et al. (2026). Modulation of gut microbiota and its metabolite equol by Huaier granule suppresses hepatocellular carcinoma via the gut-liver axis. *NPJ Biofilms and Microbiomes, 12*, 54. https://doi.org/10.1038/s41522-026-00919-7.

Wu, P., et al. (2021). Adaptive Mechanisms of Tumor Therapy Resistance Driven by Tumor Microenvironment. *Frontiers in Cell and Developmental Biology, 9.* doi:10.3389/fcell.2021.641469.

Wu, P., Gao, W., Su, M., Nice, E. C., Zhang, W., Lin, J., & Xie, N. (2021). Adaptive mechanisms of tumor therapy resistance driven by tumor microenvironment. *Frontiers in Cell and Developmental Biology, 9.* https://doi.org/10.3389/fcell.2021.641469.

Xia, C., Su, J., Liu, C., Mai, Z., Yin, S., Yang, C., & Fu, L. (2023). Human microbiomes in cancer development and therapy. *MedComm, 4*(2). https://doi.org/10.1002/mco2.221.

Xie, Q., et al. (2025). Unlocking the power of probiotics, postbiotics: targeting apoptosis for the treatment and prevention of digestive diseases. *Frontiers in Nutrition, 12.* doi:10.3389/fnut.2025.1570268.

Yaghoubi, A., Khazaei, M., Avan, A., Hasanian, S. M., Cho, W. C., & Soleimanpour, S. (2020). p28 bacterial peptide, as an anticancer agent. *Frontiers in Oncology, 10.* https://doi.org/10.3389/fonc.2020.01303.

Yan, J., & Katz, A. (2010). PectaSol-C modified citrus pectin induces apoptosis and inhibition of proliferation in human and mouse androgen-dependent and- independent prostate cancer cells. *Integrative Cancer Therapies, 9*(2), 197–203. https://doi.org/10.1177/1534735410369672.

Yang, J., Wang, X., Hu, T., Huang, H., Chen, G., Jin, B. o, Zeng, G., & Liu, J. (2024). Entero-toxigenic *Bacteroides fragilis* contributes to intestinal barrier injury and colorectal cancer progression by mediating the BFT/STAT3/ZEB2 pathway. *Cell Cycle, 23*(1), 70–82. https://doi.org/10.1080/15384101.2024.2309005.

Yang, R., Liu, W., Cai, S., Feng, X., Chen, Y., Cheng, X., Ma, J., Ma, W., Tian, Z., & Yang, W. (2025). Evaluation of the efficacy of probiotics in the chemoradiotherapy of colorectal cancer: A meta-analysis of randomized controlled trials. *BMC Gastroenterology, 25*(1). https://doi.org/10.1186/s12876-025-03914-y.

Yu, T. C., Guo, F., Yu, Y., Sun, T., Ma, D., Han, J., Qian, Y., Kryczek, I., Sun, D., Nagarsheth, N., Chen, Y., Chen, H., Hong, J., Zou, W., & Fang, J.- Y. (2017). *Fusobacterium nucleatum* promotes chemoresistance to colorectal cancer by modulating autophagy. *Cell, 170*(3), 548. https://doi.org/10.1016/j.cell.2017.07.008.

Zhang, T., Pan, D., Yang, Y., Jiang, X., Zhang, J., Zeng, X., Wu, Z., Sun, Y., & Guo, Y. (2020). Effect of *Lactobacillus acidophilus* CICC 6074 S-layer protein on colon cancer HT-29 cell proliferation and apoptosis. *Journal of Agricultural and Food Chemistry, 68*(9), 2639–2647. https://doi.org/10.1021/acs.jafc.9b06909.

Zhao, D.-S., Jiang, L.-L., Fan, Y.-X., et al. (2017). Investigation of Dioscorea bulbifera rhizome-induced hepatotoxicity in rats by a multisample integrated metabolomics approach. *Chemical Research in Toxicology, 30*(10), 1865–1873. https://doi.org/10.1021/acs.chemrestox.7b00176.

Zhao, X. u, Zhao, J., Li, D., Yang, H., Chen, C., Qin, M., Wen, Z., He, Z., & Xu, L. (2023). *Akkermansia muciniphila*: A potential target and pending issues for oncotherapy. *Pharmacological Research, 196*, 106916. https://doi.org/10.1016/j.phrs.2023.106916.

Zheng, H. C. (2017). The molecular mechanisms of chemoresistance in cancers. *Oncotarget, 8*(35), 59950–59964. https://doi.org/10.18632/oncotarget.19048.

Zhu, Z., Liu, Y., Zeng, J., et al. (2023). Diosbulbin C, a novel active ingredient in Dioscorea bulbifera L. extract, inhibits lung cancer cell proliferation by inducing G0/G1 phase cell cycle arrest. *BMC Complementary Medicine and Therapies, 23*, 436. https://doi.org/10.1186/s12906-023-04245-9.

Zikou, E., Koliaki, C., & Makrilakis, K (2024). The Role of Fecal Microbiota Transplantation (FMT) in the Management of Metabolic Diseases in Humans: A Narrative Review. *Biomedicines, 12*(8), 1871. https://doi.org/10.3390/biomedicines12081871.

6

Modulating gut microbiome in cancer immunotherapy: Harnessing microbes to enhance treatment efficacy

Ashish Mishra[a] and Sanjeev Kumar Sahu[b]

[a]APEX INSTITUTE OF PHARMACY, MIRZAPUR, UTTAR PRADESH, INDIA [b]SCHOOL OF PHARMACEUTICAL SCIENCES, LOVELY PROFESSIONAL UNIVERSITY, PHAGWARA, PUNJAB, INDIA

6.1 Introduction

The medical approach to cancer was reshaped by immunotherapy, which is utilized for treating an array of cancers and is growing in popularity. Immune checkpoint inhibitors (ICIs) have proven to be effective for the management of blood cancers as well as solid tumors. The mode of action of ICIs entails the suppression of the connection in T-lymphocytes to ligands for inhibitory receptors on cancerous or myeloid cells. This, consequently, results in the restimulation of the immune response, which is mediated by T-lymphocytes against tumor-associated antigens (Pardoll, 2015). Moreover, ICIs have recently been utilized in the therapeutic management of nonmetastatic malignancies in both neoadjuvant and adjuvant settings. Not only did ICI mobilize the immunological system to strike the tumor cells, but it additionally triggered a prolonged retention of T-lymphocytes, which is believed to reduce the possibility of persistent or recurring illness. This is a significant difference from the conventional chemotherapy that is frequently employed (Fridman et al., 2017). Minimal mutational load, minimal levels of antigens in the cancer cells (Rizvi et al., 2015). The absence of possible immunogenic pretreatment with radiation or chemotherapy (Carbone et al., 2017), and localized or systemic immunosuppression (Spranger et al., 2015). There are all possible pathways of action that might lead to resistance to immunotherapy using immunomodulatory drugs (Sivan et al., 2015). Host, tumor, and environmental variables are all included in the list of factors. The limit of the cancer prevention immune response, sometimes referred to as the cancer immune-set point, is determined by several parameters (Zitvogel et al., 2017). Recent research has shown that the gut microbiome serves as a crucial predictor of the cancer immunological set-point. Two studies that were published in 2015 clarified the relationship between the gastrointestinal microbiome and the effectiveness

The Microbiome and Cancer Treatment: Overcoming Resistance and Enhancing Efficacy.
DOI: https://doi.org/10.1016/B978-0-443-33206-7.00013-3

of ICIs in preclinical studies of mouse models. They demonstrated that cytotoxic T-lymphocyte-associated protein 4 (CTLA-4) and programmed death-1 (PD-1) inhibition only decreased tumor progression in mice that had *Bacteroides* and *Bifidobacterium* species as commensal intestinal flora (Vétizou et al., 2015). The gastrointestinal microbiome affects the effectiveness of both PD-1 and CTLA-4 inhibitors, along with significant clinical effects.

6.1.1 Historical perspective on microbiome research in oncology

Historical records associating cancer with germs extend back as far as 4000 years. Peregrine Laziosi, who lived throughout the 13th century, reported the spontaneous remission of his septic, ulcerative tibial bone cancer, which would have necessitated amputation (Cann et al., 2003). As a result of this, he was canonized in 1726. During the late 1800s, Busch and Fehleisen claimed that *Streptococcus* pyogenes illnesses were linked to spontaneous tumor regressions in several individuals. This was accomplished after the germ theory of infectious illness had been established (Fehleisen, 1882). Almost immediately after that, William Coley initiated the experimentation of a highly contentious and occasionally harmful vaccine that included live or heat-killed *Streptococcus* and *Serratia* species on terminal cancer individuals. It was subsequently proven that this vaccine led to a disease-free survival rate of over ten years in around thirty percent of the patients, and this represented 60 of a total of 220. This was considered the initial significant demonstration of immunotherapy (Starnes, 1992). At the same time, Thomas Glover and Virginia Livingston-Wheeler controversially asserted that bacteria could be grown from tumors and that bacterial vaccinations worked well against them. They also proposed that cancer was universally caused by bacteria (Glover, 1930; Taylor, 1993). The discipline deals with complex assertions that microorganisms may possess broad-spectrum roles in the pathophysiology, diagnosis, and therapy of cancer. The International Association for Cancer Registries (IACRs) has identified just eleven of the approximately 10^{12} different microbial species that exist on Earth (Locey & Lennon, 2016). These 11 microorganisms are classified as human carcinogens, also known as onco-microbes (International Agency for Research on Cancer, 2012). According to the findings of several experiments, extra microorganisms are accountable for the progression of cancer through the process of genotoxin-mediated mutagenesis. Microbiome-functional genomic connection is suggested by the fact that common alterations to p^{53} are only cancerous in the presence of microbially generated gallic acid, whereas they are beneficial in the gastrointestinal tract and organoids (Kadosh et al., 2020). A second aspect involves microbially produced secondary bile acids, which decrease hepatic sinusoidal CXCL16 levels (the exclusive ligand for CXCR6) and inhibit the clustering of CXCR6+ natural killer (NK) T cells, thereby impairing tumor immunosurveillance. This cancer-causing impact is mitigated by vancomycin therapy (Jia, 2019). These instances show how microorganisms or their activities might contribute to cancer rather than cause it directly.

6.1.2 Clinical significance and translational potential

Because of its substantial effect on both health and illness, the human gut microbiome is presently the subject of much investigation. The microbiome, especially the intestinal microbiome, is now a crucial aspect impacting the effectiveness and safety of cancer-specific immunotherapy, notably ICIs. It is quickly evolving, demonstrating considerable clinical importance and beneficial translational prospects (Gopalakrishnan et al., 2018a; Xavier et al., 2020).

The therapeutic significance of the microbiome in cancer immunotherapy is increasing, as data indicate a significant link between gut microbiota makeup and patient response to ICIs. Certain microbial taxa have been associated with improved treatment outcomes (Li et al., 2022). The microbiota can affect the metabolism of several pharmaceuticals, including chemotherapy and immunotherapy medicines, therefore influencing their effectiveness and toxicity (Alexander et al., 2017).

The translational potential of leveraging the microbiome in cancer immunotherapy is immense, offering several avenues for improving patient outcomes. Fecal material from healthy individuals or immunotherapy responders is transmitted to patients who are nonresponders or have dysbiosis in this highly promising approach. In melanoma and gastrointestinal malignancies, clinical trials have demonstrated that fecal microbiota transplantation (FMT) has the potential to transform nonresponders into responders, underscoring its potential to surmount immunotherapy resistance (Zhang et al., 2022). Dietary changes can drastically affect gut microbiota. Dietary habits that optimize the microbiota for immunotherapy responses are being studied (Zhang, 2022).

6.2 Fundamentals of gut microbiome in cancer biology

6.2.1 Composition and diversity of the gut microbiome

Numerous microorganisms, most of which are members of the bacterial domain, are found in the human gastrointestinal system. Due to several considering the implications on host physiology and health, there is an increasing interest in comprehending the role and function of gut microbial populations. The conditions that exist within the individual's gut are heterogeneous, with significant variation between the stomach and colon. Consequently, it is unsurprising that the microbes inhabiting the different regions of the digestive system vary in multiple dimensions, including the number of cells, composition, and metabolic rate.

After eating, stomach pH rises, impacting transit time. The research revealed that meal uniformity, osmolarity, nutritional content, and energy density affect the duration of transit. Normal people have a pH of 1–2, although diet can raise it. A culture-independent analysis of 23 stomach mucosa biopsy samples found 128 phylotypes, including *Firmicutes, Bacteroidetes, Proteobacteria, Actinobacteria, Fusobacteria,* and tiny components of other phyla (Bik et al., 2006). *Streptococcus salivarius, mitis, parasanguinis, Prevotella, Porphyromonas spp., Rothia dentocariosa, Atopobium parvulum, and Fusobacterium nucleatum* exist in the mouth. Nineteen of 23 subjects have *Helicobacter pylori.*

The small intestine, the longest section of the digestive system, alters and gains bacterial cell density. In ileostomy patients' ileal effluents, *Lactobacillus, Clostridiales, and Veillonella* species were found in significant numbers, while *Ruminococcus gnavus, R. obeum, and Bacteroides plebeius* species were at fewer dimensions (Booijink et al., 2010). A significant number of bacteria in the small intestine are facultative anaerobes; however, their prevalence diminishes from the

Table 6.1 Composition of microbes in gut (Blaut, 2018).

Stomach	Small intestine	Colon and feces
Streptococcus Gemella	*Streptococcus*	*Clostridium*
Porphyromonas prevotella	*Lactobacillus*	*Eubacterium*
Rothia Atopobium	*Caprococcus*	*Roseburia*
Fusobacterium	*Megasphaera*	*Caprococcus*
Helicobacter	*Brevibacillus*	*Dorea*
	Atopobium	*Blautia*
	Leptotrichia	*Bacteriodes*
	Neisseria	*Parabacteriodes*
		Porphyromonas
		Escherichia
		Citrobacter
		Bifidobacterium
		Atopobium
		Collinsella
		Slackia

duodenum to the terminal ileum due to the increasing limitation of oxygen and a drop in redox potential.

The colon is undoubtedly the most densely packed anatomical location. The colon harbors a diverse array of microbial species or phylotypes; nevertheless, estimations of these species in colonic contents or feces exhibit considerable variety. *Firmicutes, Bacteroidetes, Actinobacteria, and Proteobacteria* reside in the colonic content. The detailed numbers are represented through the tables given below (Table 6.1).

6.2.2 Mechanisms of microbiome-host interactions in health

The human microbiome, particularly the gut microbes, significantly influences the physiological functions of hosts through its connections with the body's immune system, metabolic processes and neurological system. Microbes such as these significantly influence the general well-being by facilitating the absorption of nutrients, digestion, and immune system regulation (Andoh, 2016). The production of metabolites by microbes, control of the defense system, and interactions within the gut-brain axis are among the many processes that govern how the gut microbiome influences human physiological processes. The production of metabolites, including neurotransmitters, bile acids, and short-chain fatty acids (SCFAs), is a primary mechanism by which the microbiome affects host health. The microbial digestion of dietary fibers generates SCFAs that include propionate, acetate and butyrate, which are crucial for preserving gut membrane integrity, regulating the level of energy, and promoting anti-inflammatory responses (Sajjad et al., 2024). Bile acids altered by intestinal microbiota govern the breakdown of lipids and affect host immunity (Noor et al., 2024).

Gut bacteria play a big role in how the immune system grows and works. Polysaccharide A, which is made by certain kinds of bacteria, such as *Bacteroides fragilis,* has been shown to facilitate the growth of regulatory T-cells (Treg), and this contributes to immune resistance. Also, gut microorganisms have an effect on pattern recognition receptors like toll-like receptors (TLRs). This sets off signaling pathways that change how inflammation is controlled and how the immune system responds (Sattar et al., 2024).

6.2.3 Dysbiosis in cancer patients: Patterns and implications

Having beneficial bacteria in our bodies is important for our health because they help with digestion, immunity, and metabolism. But this community of good bacteria is carefully balanced, and if it is dysregulated, that can lead to dysbiosis. It is related to an increased risk of cancers in the colon, stomach, esophagus, pancreas, larynx, breast, and liver. Indeed, gut bacteria may trigger or stop colorectal cancer. It accomplishes this through altering the process of inflammation because they are in intimate contact with the host intestinal epithelium (Jobin, 2013). The alpha-bug theory states that a main pathogen species like enterotoxigenic *Bacteroides fragilis* (ETBF) changes the microbiota in the gut to help cause colorectal cancer, likely by triggering inflammation via interleukin-17 (IL-17) and T-helper (TH) cells. Host-mediated, microbe-independent inflammation may initiate this process, whereas beneficial commensal bacteria can counteract and suppress it (Hajishengallis et al., 2012). After a tumor develops, ongoing inflammation in the intestines breaks the barrier, letting the bacteria get to the tumor tissue. These bacteria and their by-products cause more inflammatory signals, such as IL-17 cytokines, which promote the cancer spread (Grivennikov et al., 2012).

When bacteria get past weakened gut epithelial cells, the immune response of the host turns on several pattern recognition receptors. TLRs and NOD-like receptors (NLRs) are two pattern recognition receptors that are key to colon-rectal cancer (CRC) (Schwabe & Jobin, 2013). In addition, bacteria like *Escherichia Coli, Enterococcus faecalis,* and *B. fragilis* are being illustrated to "drive" the cancer initiation pathway via their genotoxic impacts (Fig. 6.1).

Studies on humans that compared the microbiota of the stomach of cancer patients with healthy controls indicate that bacteria other than *H. Pylori* must exist to help the mucosa move in a way that leads to the growth of stomach cancer (Aviles-Jimenez et al., 2014). In fact, a lot of people who have *H. Pylori* do not get stomach cancer (Dicksved et al., 2009). Salmonella infection is very important in the cancer of the gall bladder. Salmonella can live in the liver, which boosts the level of extracellular bile acid (Bibbò et al., 2022) in the body and is associated with the growth of tumors (Shukla et al., 1993). Viruses are also part of gut bacteria and can change the risk of getting cancer. Like, the human papillomavirus (HPV) can be found in almost all types of cervical cancer (Walboomers et al., 1999).

6.3 Microbiome-immune system crosstalk

6.3.1 Role of microbiota in immune development and function

Controlling immune cell growth and function at both mucosal and nonmucosal locations is a frequent way that microbiota regulates the immune system (Round & Mazmanian, 2009).

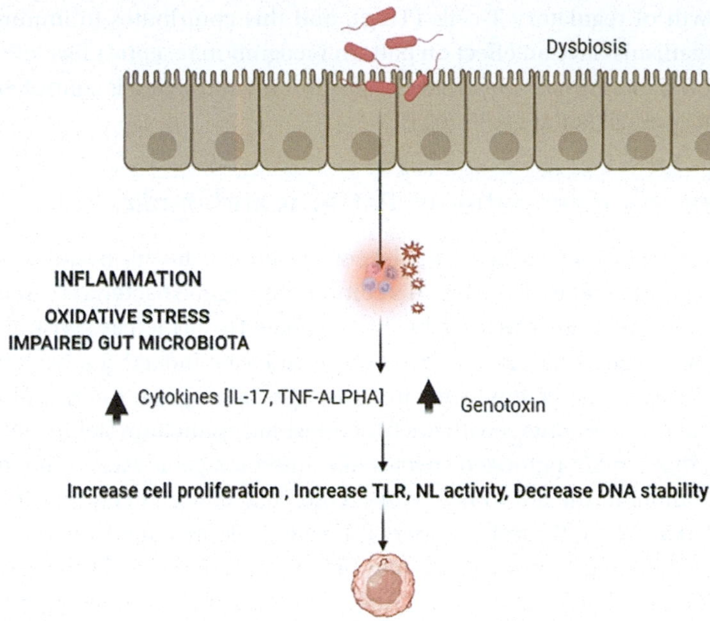

FIGURE 6.1 Dysbiosis in cancer.

Table 6.2 Role of microbiota in immune cells.

Mucosal sites	Nonmucosal sites
Promote cytokine production	*Neutrophil killing effects*
Regulate the functions of B-Cells	*Promote uveitis by activating retinal T lymphocytes*
Impact on IgA-producing B cell numbers	*Boost macrophages count*
Natural-killer cell cytolysis and IFN-γ responses	*To create a spleen germinal center, affect B cells*

The gut microbiota can affect the quantity of immune cells, implying that it may influence the development and operation of immune cells. Certain bacterial species can influence the maturation of certain immune cells at mucosal locations, including T helper 1 cells (Th1), Th17 cells, and colonic T regulatory (Treg) cells. Gut immune maturation depends on host-specific bacteria in mucosal locations. Restoration of the immune system via mouse microbiota colonization (Chung et al., 2012). Certain microbiota species mature dendritic cells, polarizing T cells toward regulatory Treg cells and boosting gut IL-10 production in mice (Eslami et al., 2016). Bone marrow, where myeloid and B cells grow, is heavily influenced by microbiota. Germ-free mice had fewer CD4+ T cells in their bone marrow, affecting bone density and immunological function (Sjögren et al., 2012). Since germ-free mice have the same amount of macrophages and dendritic cells, microbiota does not alter their growth (Mørland et al., 1979; Wilson et al., 2008). Microbiota enhances myeloid cell activation, cytokine release, and homeostasis. Summarized view of the role of microbiota in immune cells described below (Table 6.2).

Research suggests gut microbiota affects anticancer immune responses, which might improve immunotherapy for colorectal, gastric, liver, and lung cancer patients (Zitvogel et al., 2016). Commensal *Bifidobacterium* enhances anti-PD-L1 immunotherapy in JAX and TAC mice models for antitumor immunity (Sivan et al., 2015).

6.3.2 Key microbial metabolites affecting immune responses

The commensal microbiota bolsters the host immunological system via microbial chemicals that stimulate host cells, engaging with diverse receptors and molecular targets. Major microbial components such as RNA, DNA, proteins, and parts of cell walls are sensed by host receptors such as Toll-like, NLRs, C-type lectin, and RIG-1-like that detect microbial factors. Nonetheless, these microbial components represent just a small portion of what commensal bacteria generate to modulate the immunological system of the host. Microbial metabolites exert considerable influence on host metabolism. Specific metabolites modulate and enhance the immune system's functionality, while diminishing detrimental inflammatory reactions. A growing amount of research demonstrates that several microbial metabolites significantly modulate the immunological system via the receptors of the host as well as other target molecules. Immune cells exhibit receptors specific to metabolites, including P2 × 7, GPR41, GPR109A, aryl hydrocarbon receptor precursor (AhR), pregnane X receptor (PXR), farnesoid receptor X receptor (FXR), TGR5, and more molecular targets. Microbial metabolites and their receptors constitute a comprehensive network of signals that respond to variations in diet, health, and immunological conditions. Consequently, microbial metabolite signals facilitate nutrient extraction from the food and modulate host metabolism and the immune system. Microbial metabolites operate bidirectionally to enhance both tolerance and immunity, successfully combating infection while preventing inflammatory disorders. In pathogenic situations, detrimental effects of microbial metabolites have also been noted (Kim, 2018).

6.3.3 Barrier function and immune surveillance

The gastrointestinal tract has a well-organized mucosal barrier that inhibits unregulated translocation of microorganisms and antigens. It facilitates a controlled relationship between luminal constituents as well as the immune system, which are crucial for sustaining the immunity of the mucosa (Martini et al., 2017; Peterson & Artis, 2014). The mucosal immunity sustains immune tolerance to diverse antigens while eliciting immune responses to external pathogens. The intestinal mucosa harbors an assortment of immune cells, both innate and adaptive, that bolster barrier function through direct pathogen elimination, secretion of soluble mediators, formation of neutrophil extracellular traps, and protective immune responses. Anti-inflammatory cytokines, such as IL-10 and TGF-β, inhibit the effector capabilities of several immune cell types and enhance regulatory T cell responses (Neurath, 2014). Disruptions of the intestinal barrier modify the balance between the immune response and intestinal antigens. Facilitates the transfer of bacteria, germs, and antigens in the gut wall. Elicits a pronounced proinflammatory mucosal immune response (Neurath, 2014). The intestinal barrier and its role regulate the relationship between luminal components and the gut immune system. Delineates the boundary between the mucosal immune system and the external environment. Disruptions of intestinal epithelial cells or antimicrobial peptides may lead to heightened intestinal permeability. Inflammatory bowel disease, metabolic dysfunction-associated steatohepatitis, and colorectal cancer are indications of the etiology of this immune system activation (Neurath et al., 2025).

6.4 Impact of microbiome on cancer immunotherapy

Different species of bacteria make up the commensal microbiota, which is very important for both health and sickness. Changes in the normal microbiota have been linked to certain illnesses, including cancer, and they can also influence the efficacy of cancer therapies like immunotherapy. *Firmicutes* and *Bacteroides* are the two main types of phylum that make up the microbiota of adults. Different people and different parts of the body have different types of these phyla (Fessler et al., 2019).

6.4.1 Evidence from preclinical models

This section talks about how important it is to use big animal models to develop good onco-microbiotic medicines and keep an eye on them. Murine models have been useful for researching host-microbiome physiology because they include genetically similar mice and controlled lab settings. This helps scientists find microbiota that promote cancer and microbiota that increase therapy responses. Studies using mouse colon cancer models have shown how the gut microbiota affects the growth of colorectal tumors by changing the way inflammation works.

However, mouse models have certain problems. For example, their microbiomes are different from those of wild mice; mice that are kept in germ-free circumstances don't develop their immune system as well, and their microbiomes are more genetically influenced than those of people. Also, it's severely complicated to completely understand the complicated relationships between the microbiome, the immune response, and cancer in mice models.

Researchers examined how the microbiomes of humans and dogs are linked to inflammatory disorders, cancer, and how they respond to treatments. Environmental and genetic factors affect the hundreds of bacterial species that make up the microbiome of both humans and dogs. Things that happen early in life, such as being colonized by particular germs as a baby, might affect the likelihood of atopic diseases and being sick later in life. The types of bacteria that live in adults' bodies are affected by things including their food, medicines, and where they live. Genetics and the environment are the most important factors that shape the microbiome, yet both human and dog gut microbiomes show signs of being passed down from one generation to the next.

The gut microbiota of dogs is more like that of humans than that of other species that are often investigated, including mice. Dogs and people who live in the same places have microbiomes that are similar, which suggests that they affect each other in some way. Alterations in the variety and structure of microbes are associated with disease connections, which can affect health outcomes. Some bacteria have a distinct impact on people and dogs. For example, some bacteria are linked to colorectal cancer in people but are good for canine gut health.

There is also a discussion of how common surroundings affect the microbial makeup of different species (Kleber et al., 2022).

6.4.2 Clinical correlation studies

Numerous studies have examined how the microbiome affects the efficacy of immunotherapy and chemotherapy. Enteric alteration of bacteria has been associated with diminished therapeutic efficacy: antibiotic-treated animals had a reduced immune response to both immunotherapy and radiation therapy (Paulos et al., 2007). In murine models, *Bacteroides* and *Bifidobacterium* have been associated with the augmentation of anti-CTLA-4 activation and the responsiveness to anti-PD-L1 therapy (Pitt et al., 2016; Sivan et al., 2015; Vétizou et al., 2015). *Akkermansia* levels in human patients showed a positive correlation with partial response or stable illness, whereas in murine models, the repletion of *Akkermansia* by oral gavage successfully restored tumor responsiveness to CTLA-4 and PD-L1 therapies (Routy et al., 2018). Thirty-seven patients were recruited, and 34 patients were assessable for this report. To compare baseline gut flora, 32 healthy controls (HC) from the same region were included. In comparison to HC, LC gut microbiota demonstrated markedly reduced α-diversity. Patients who did not have immune-related adverse events had a relative abundance of *Bifidobacterium* ($P = .001$) and *Desulfovibrio* ($P = .0002$) in their gut microbiome. Patients who responded to combination chemo immunotherapy had an elevation in *Clostridiales* ($P = .018$) and a decrease in *Rikenellaceae* ($P = .016$). In response to chemoimmunotherapy, we noted an enrichment of *Finegoldia* in the nasal microbiome, alongside an increase in *Megasphaera* and a decrease in *Actinobacillus* in buccal samples. Longitudinal samples demonstrated a trend in alpha diversity and specific microbial alterations throughout the progression and resolution of immune-related adverse events (irAEs) (Chau et al., 2021).

6.4.3 Specific bacterial species of interest (e.g., *Akkermansia, Bifidobacterium*)

It has just come to light that immunotherapy for cancer is a revolutionary approach to the treatment of cancer. However, immunotherapy for cancer can only be beneficial to a limited number of patients, and the severe adverse effects that emerge during treatment might impair the effectiveness of the treatment or possibly put patients' lives in danger. Surprisingly, the gut microbiota known as *Akkermansia muciniphila* has the ability to greatly decrease carcinogenesis and boost antitumor effects. As a result, cancer immunotherapy can be more successful while also reducing the chance of adverse effects (Fan et al., 2023). An increasing amount of research indicates that gut bacteria may have a favorable effect on the clinical results of cancer treatment. The modulation of gut microbiota is a strategy to combat cancer, improving the effectiveness of cancer therapies, particularly immunotherapies. *Bifidobacterium*, frequently used as a probiotic

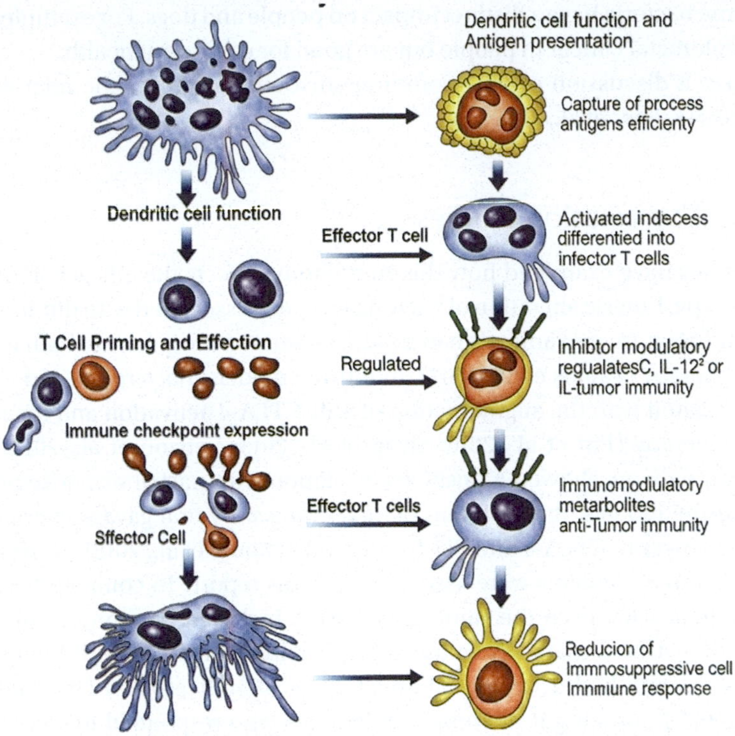

FIGURE 6.2 Immune system modulation.

for its health benefits, has demonstrated the capacity to enhance tumor management comparably to immune checkpoint blockade therapy, with combined treatment essentially eliminating tumor proliferation. Nonetheless, despite their recognized significance in promoting human health, the exact mechanisms by which Bifidobacteria confer positive effects in combating cancer remain little known. The significance of this expanding advantageous function regarding early diagnosis and therapeutic efficacy is noteworthy. The makeup of the microbiota serves as a predictor for illness presence or absence, potentially guiding the creation of innovative, less intrusive diagnostic procedures and facilitating the development of tailored therapies.

6.5 Mechanisms of microbiome influence on immunotherapy

The external surfaces of the human body host intricate ecosystems of bacteria, yeast, fungus, protozoa, archaea, and viruses. The assemblage of these bacteria constitutes the human microbiome, whereas the aggregate of their genes forms the human microbiome. The mechanisms encoded in the human microbiome significantly influence different facets of human physiology (Fig. 6.2). The intestinal microbiome is pivotal in controlling host metabolism and directing the proper growth and functioning of the immune system (Martin et al., 2019).

6.5.1 Enhancement of dendritic cell function and antigen presentation

The gut microbiota is essential in modulating the immune system, influencing both local and systemic responses. It interacts with the host immune system, facilitating effective responses to infections and tumors. The microbiome primarily regulates immune function by interacting in conjunction with the gut-associated lymphoid tissue (GALT), a crucial element of the immune system. The GALT possesses a significant concentration of immune cells, including dendritic cells, macrophages, and T-cells, and functions as a principal location for the initiation of immunological reactions. The growth of dendritic cells is affected by commensal bacteria in the gut. These cells are important for presenting antigens. This mechanism facilitates the initiation of activation of T-cells to elicit an adaptive immunological response, namely CD4+ helper T cells and CD8+ cytotoxic T cells (CTLs), which are crucial for an efficient antitumor immune system reaction. Certain microbial species have been demonstrated to facilitate the differentiation of CD4+ T cells into proinflammatory Th1 and Th17 subsets, both of which play a significant role in potent antitumor immunity (Bibbò et al., 2022).

6.5.2 Modulation of T cell priming and effector function

T cells are acknowledged as essential modulators of antitumor immune surveillance. The gut microbiome's metabolites have the ability to directly affect immunity inside the tumor microenvironment (TME), particularly SCFAs such as butyrate, acetate and propionate, which are crucial in regulating immunological processes. Proinflammatory interleukin-17-positive (IL-17+) γd T cells and inflammatory regulatory T cells can both have their differentiation and activation influenced by SCFAs (Xie and Liu, 2024). Other microbial metabolites, such as inosine derived from Bifidobacterium, augment T cell activation and antitumor immunity by boosting T cell-specific adenosine 2A receptor (A2AR) signaling. In addition to their beneficial effects, several microbial metabolites are seen to have detrimental effects on cancer. Gallic acid, a phenolic acid produced by gut microorganisms, can convert the tumor-suppressing function of mutant p53 into an oncogenic state (Kadosh et al., 2020). Additionally, it was demonstrated that succinic acid, which is generated from *Fusobacterium nucleatum*, inhibits the cyclic GMP-AMP synthase-interferon-beta (IFN-β) pathway. This results in a decrease in the amount of CD8+ cells trafficking to the TME and a reduction in antitumor immunity. It is important to highlight that although the effects of the gut microbiome on the TME are becoming more widely recognized, further study is required to completely comprehend the many processes that are involved and to create specific techniques for manipulating the gut microbiota to improve cancer immunotherapy.

6.5.3 Influence on immune checkpoint expression

Checkpoints in the immune system are mechanisms of regulation that prevent the immune system from attacking the body's own cells and tissues. This helps to ensure that the body can tolerate itself, and it also helps to minimize inflammation. By enabling the immune system to fight cancerous cells, ICIs have completely changed the way cancer is treated. A considerable percentage of patients either don't respond to these therapies or develop resistance. Emerging research points to a fascinating and crucial player in this equation: the host microbiota, particularly the gut microbiome. Far from being passive inhabitants, these vast communities of microorganisms exert a significant impact on the expression of immune checkpoints, thereby modulating the efficacy of immunotherapy.

Immune checkpoints like PD-1 and CTLA-4 act as "brakes" on the immune system, preventing excessive or autoimmune responses. These checkpoints are frequently used by cancerous tumor cells to avoid immune system recognition. The composition and function of the microbiota can directly impact the expression and activity of these critical immune regulators.

6.5.3.1 Modulating T-cell responses

Certain microbial species have been shown to augment antitumor immunity via enhancement of the activation and infiltration of CTLs, which are the primary effectors of ICI therapy. For instance, research has shown that species like *B. longum, Enterococcus faecium,* and *Collinsella aerofaciens* are more abundant in patients who respond well to PD-1 inhibitors. These bacteria can influence the immune microenvironment, leading to increased T-cell priming and proliferation. Conversely, disproportion in the gut microbiota or dysbiosis can counteract the effects of immunotherapy, potentially by promoting immunosuppressive cell types like regulatory T cells (Tregs) or by hindering the activation of effector T cells (Matson et al., 2018; Sivan et al., 2015).

6.5.3.2 Metabolite-mediated effects

The microbiota produces a diverse array of metabolites, including SCFAs, bile acids, and tryptophan derivatives, which can directly influence immune cell function and immune checkpoint expression. Butyrate, an SCFA produced by bacteria like *Faecalibacterium* and *Bifidobacterium,* has been shown to suppress the expression of PD-L1 (the ligand for PD-1) and IL-10 (an immunosuppressive cytokine) in tumor-associated macrophages, thereby enhancing antitumor immunity. Similarly, certain bacteria can produce inosine, which has been linked to improved efficacy of PD-1 blockade (Wang et al., 2023).

6.5.3.3 Direct interactions and signaling

While less understood, direct interactions between microbial components and host pattern recognition receptors on immune cells can also modulate immune checkpoint pathways. The specific microbial signatures present in the gut can influence the expression of costimulatory and coinhibitory molecules on various immune cell populations, ultimately shaping the overall immune landscape (Xie & Liu, 2024).

The growing understanding of the microbiota's influence on immune checkpoint expression has significant clinical implications, particularly for cancer immunotherapy.

6.5.4 Production of immunomodulatory metabolites

Significantly, one of the principal mechanisms by which the intestinal tract bacteria influence antitumor immunity is via metabolites. A variety of metabolites, which are microscopic molecules that may migrate from their original location in the gut and affect the local and systemic antitumor response, are produced or transformed by the gut microbiota to enhance the efficacy of ICIs (Davar et al., 2021). Consequently, we analyzed the processes of various intestinal bacteria metabolites and other characteristics of gut microbial signatures that facilitate antitumor response.

6.5.4.1 Inosine

B. pseudolongum and *A. muciniphila* produce Inosine, a purine metabolite that is essential for enhancing the effectiveness of ICIs (Mager et al., 2020). It has been previously demonstrated that inosine possesses immunosuppressive properties (He et al., 2017). Inosine enhances the immunogenic character of neoplastic cells. A study group discovered that Inosine can markedly improve the capacity of tumor cells to display tumor antigens, hence facilitating the recognition and destruction of tumor cells by cytotoxic immune cells, resulting in anticancer consequences (Bird, 2020). Subsequent mechanistic investigation revealed a considerable increase in the stimulation of the IFN-γ and tumor necrosis factor alpha (TNF-α) signaling pathways in tumor cells subjected to Inosine treatment. By promoting the synthesis of perforin and granzyme by tumor-specific T-cells and NK cells, IFN-γ can increase their cytotoxicity. This can also improve antigen presentation to promote inosine-mediated beneficial effects against cancer (Harjes, 2020). Inosine enhances the activation of immunological cells. The molecule inosine produced by intestinal metabolites may enhance the efficacy of ICIs by targeting the A2AR on T cells in models of intestinal cancer, bladder cancer, and melanoma (Mager et al., 2020). Inosine serves as an alternate carbon source for CD8+ T cells. Activation of oncogenic signaling pathways reprograms the metabolism of neoplastic cells.

6.5.4.2 Short-chain fatty acids

Colonic anaerobes generate SCFAs from undigested and ingested carbohydrates or glycoproteins produced by intestinal epithelial cells. The correlation between gut microbiota-derived SCFAs and nivolumab and pembrolizumab therapy in solid tumors has recently been validated (Nomura et al., 2020). SCFAs are integral to intricate intestinal microbial, immunological, and metabolic networks, influencing the functionality of immune and tumor cells. Histone deacetylase (HDAC) is inhibited by butyric acid, a metabolite of *Faecalibaculum rodentium* and *H. biformis*. It enhanced acetylation and impeded calcineurin-mediated activation of nuclear factor of activated cells, hence obstructing tumor cell proliferation (Zagato et al., 2020). SCFAs supply energy to immune cells. SCFAs produced by the gut microbiota can modulate glycolysis, the tricarboxylic acid (TCA) cycle, the pentose phosphate pathway (PPP), and fatty acid oxidation (FAO) in antitumor effector cells to enhance the efficacy of ICIs.

6.5.5 Reduction of immunosuppressive cell populations

Through the direct destruction of tumor cells and beneficial immunoregulatory effects, microorganisms not only encourage cancer but also prevent its onset and development. Certain bacteria can inhibit and mitigate cancer through immunological processes. The appropriate gut microbiota is essential for the development of the body's immune system; lack of it can lead to structural and functional impairments of the immune system as well as potentially contributing to cancer initiation. For example, the gut microbiota can facilitate the development of lymphocytes and the differentiation of immune cells, illustrating the impact of microbes on the structure and function of the immune system. Lymphoid tissue is categorized as core lymphoid organs and peripheral lymphoid organs. The centrally located lymphoid organs, comprising the bone marrow and thymus, are responsible for the generation of B and T lymphocytes. In contrast, the peripheral lymphoid organs, which include lymph nodes, spleen, and GALT, serve as sites where mature lymphocytes are activated by antigens to elicit immune system reactions. The gut microbiota is highly significant to both lymphoid organs, as evidenced by both early and modern research. In mouse models, 11 humans fecal bacterial strains improve immune checkpoint inhibitor activity, preventing and even curing cancer (Tanoue et al., 2019).

6.6 Therapeutic strategies for microbiome modulation

Microbiota modulation, a new field, promises improvements in the well-being of people, farming, and conservation of the environment through purposeful modifications in microbial community composition and functionality. This crucial topic encompasses several methods from dietary changes to advanced microbial engineering (Mutalub et al., 2022). Microbiota alteration affects not just gut health but also neurological illnesses, metabolic syndrome, infectious disease, and regulatory landscapes (Daly & Zarate-Lopez, 2021). There are numerous methods for modulating microbes, such as:

6.6.1 Dietary interventions and prebiotics

Diet may provide nourishment for some gut microbes by acting as a substrate through indigestible ingredients and digestive by-products, leading to exploitative competition. Because they cannot be broken down or absorbed in the upper gastrointestinal system, dietary fibers are essential. However, they can be fermented by gut bacteria in the large intestine. As per their function in the plant, fiber component, polysaccharide type, stimulated gastrointestinal solubility, digestion location, digestion products, and physical characteristics, dietary fibers can be categorized in a variety of ways (Staffolo et al., 2012). Their advantageous yields mostly rely on their physicochemical properties, including viscosity, solubility, and fermentability. Subsequent research indicates that the elevated levels of fermented dietary fiber augment satiety, even with reduced metabolizable calorie consumption, and that the pronounced satiety effect of resistant starch is due to its gradual fermentation rate and significant synthesis of SCFAs, especially butyrate (Silva et al., 2013). Prebiotics are a category of dietary fibers that withstand stomach acidity and mammalian digestive enzymes, providing several health benefits. The primary attribute of prebiotics is their selective enhancement of the proliferation and/or activity of gut bacteria linked to health and well-being. The most recognized prebiotics are inulin, fructooligosaccharides (FOS) (Zagato et al., 2020), lactulose, and galactooligosaccharides (GOS) (Roberfroid et al., 2010). Prebiotics have predominantly been evaluated for their ability to increase strains of

Bifidobacterium and *Lactobacillus* that generate lactate and acetate, therefore promoting host health through the process of fermentation of prebiotics (Adamberg et al., 2014).

6.6.2 Probiotics: Single and multistrain approaches

Known as the gut microbiota, the human gut is a complex ecosystem that is home to billions of bacteria. Keeping this microbial population in a healthy balance is essential for general health as it affects everything from immune system performance and mood to digestion and nutrient absorption. Probiotics, defined as live microorganisms that, when administered in adequate amounts, confer a health benefit on the host, have emerged as a popular dietary supplement to support gut health. However, a key question for consumers and clinicians alike remains: is a single-strain probiotic sufficient, or do multistrain formulations offer superior benefits?

6.6.3 Case for single-strain probiotics

Single-strain probiotics focus on the targeted delivery of a specific beneficial strain, such as *L. rhamnosus* GG or *B. lactis* Bp12. The rationale behind this approach is rooted in the concept of "strain-specificity," meaning the positive effects of a probiotic are often unique to the particular strain and the condition it aims to address. For instance, specific *Lactobacillus* strains have demonstrated potential in lowering the duration and severity of antibiotic-associated diarrhea (Fneish et al., 2025).

Research on single-strain probiotics allows for a clearer understanding of the mechanisms of action of a particular organism. This targeted approach can be highly effective when the specific probiotic strain has been rigorously studied and proven to be beneficial for a defined health outcome. Some studies suggest that in certain instances, a single strain may even be more effective than mixtures for specific conditions. For example, *L. rhamnosus* GG was found to be substantially more protective for necrotizing enterocolitis in preterm infants compared to some multistrain mixtures (McFarland, 2021).

6.6.4 Potential for multistrain probiotics

Multistrain probiotics, as their name suggests, combine several different bacterial strains, often from various genera like *Lactobacillus* and *Bifidobacterium*. The hypothesis here is that a diverse blend of probiotics might offer broader and more synergistic health benefits than a single strain. The combined action of multiple strains could lead to additive or even synergistic effects, where the overall benefits are greater than the sum of their individual parts.

Studies have explored the efficacy of multistrain probiotics across a range of conditions. For example, in managing irritable bowel syndrome, a meta-analysis of randomized clinical trials indicated that multistrain preparations improve IBS symptoms (Skrzydło-Radomańska et al., 2021). The varied mechanisms of action of different strains-such as competing with pathogens for nutrients and adhesion sites, producing antimicrobial compounds, and modulating the host immune system- could contribute to their enhanced efficacy in a multistrain formulation (Kwoji et al., 2021).

The choice between single and multistrain probiotics is not always straightforward, and the scientific literature presents a nuanced picture. While some studies favor multistrain products for their broader impact and potential synergy, others emphasize the significance of strain-specificity and the proven efficacy of certain single strains for targeted conditions. It's crucial to note that the effectiveness of any probiotic depends heavily on the specific strains included, their viability, dosage, and the individual's health status.

6.6.5 Fecal microbiota transplantation

FMT has arisen as a ground-breaking therapeutic methodology, aiming to restore a healthy microbial balance by transmission of feces from a healthy donor to a recipient. FMT entails the transfer of fecal matter, containing a diverse community of beneficial microorganisms, from a rigorously screened health donor into the gastrointestinal tract of a patient. The fundamental principle behind FMT is to replenish and reestablish a healthy microbial diversity in a dysbiotic gut, thereby outcompeting pathogenic bacteria and restoring normal physiological functions. The primary goal of FMT is to reinstate healthy and diverse gut microbiota in individuals suffering from dysbiosis, an imbalance in the microbial community that can contribute to various diseases. This therapeutic approach, though seemingly unconventional, has garnered significant scientific validation, particularly through rigorous studies published on platforms like PubMed.

The historical roots of FMT can be traced back centuries, but its modern scientific application gained prominence in the 21st century, primarily driven by its extraordinary effectiveness in treating recurrent *Clostridioides difficile* infection. *C. difficile* is a challenging pathogen that often thrives after antibiotic use, leading to severe and recurrent episodes of diarrhea and colitis. Numerous randomized controlled trials, extensively documented on PubMed, have demonstrated that FMT is vastly superior to conventional antibiotic treatments for rCDI, achieving cure rates often exceeding 85%–90%. The mechanism behind this success is believed to be the reestablishment of colonization resistance by the transplanted healthy microbiota, which outcompetes *C. difficile* and restores crucial metabolic functions that inhibit its growth (Gough et al., 2011).

The application of FMT is also being investigated for irritable bowel syndrome (IBS), metabolic syndrome (including obesity and type 2 diabetes), and even neurological conditions like Parkinson's disease and autism spectrum disorder. While these areas are still in earlier stages of research, PubMed houses a growing number of pilot studies, case reports, and even some small-scale clinical trials exploring these possibilities, indicating a broad scientific interest in the gut-brain axis and its therapeutic manipulation.

In conclusion, FMT has led to a significant fundamental transformation in our methodology for gut-related disease. Its proven efficacy in rCDI has paved the way for exploration into a broader spectrum of conditions where gut dysbiosis is a contributing factor. As our scientific understanding of the microbiome deepens, FMT and next-generation microbiome-based therapeutics hold immense promise for personalized medicine, offering innovative strategies to reestablish gut harmony and improve human health.

6.6.5.1 Antibiotics: Rational use and considerations

The history of antibiotics is thoroughly recorded, spanning from the discovery of penicillin in the 1940s to a prolific era of antibiotic development until the 1970s, since then, pharmaceutical companies have encouraged difficulties in discovering novel mechanism antibiotics, with the late-stage clinical pipeline and new introductions predominantly concentrating on minor incremental modifications to existing classes of antibiotics including quinolones, cephalosporin, carbapenam, tetracycline and aminoglycosides (Theuretzbacher et al., 2020). Investigations into the human microbiome have surged subsequent to the emergence of next-generation sequencing (Matson et al., 2018) technologies. This enhanced understanding reveals that broad-spectrum antibiotics induce considerable dysbiosis in the gut microbiota. Broad-spectrum antibiotics can change the natural human flora, particularly the gut flora, and cause dysbiosis as a side effect. Up to 30% of the bacteria in the gut can be impacted by the use of broad-spectrum antibiotics; clindamycin, for example, has been demonstrated to trigger microbial imbalance for up to 2 years after treatment ends, which can result in illnesses like *Clostridium difficile* infection (CDI) (Jernberg et al., 2010). The purported "Golden Age" of antibacterial discovery was the screening of natural materials, particularly fermentation broths and microbial extracts, only for their capacity to limit bacterial proliferation, irrespective of their mechanism of action. A dysbiotic microbiome may fail to execute essential processes, including nutrition provision, vitamin synthesis, and pathogen defense (Guarner & Malagelada, 2003). The impact of prenatal antibiotics on neonates is ambiguous; nonetheless, the bacteria that initially colonize an infant-postbirth significantly influence the formation of the microbiome. The method of birth for a newborn is a crucial element affecting the composition of their gut flora. Postnatal antibiotics can irrevocably disturb the normal succession of the microbiome, as a newborn is unlikely to be recolonized by a second dose of vaginal microorganisms. Prolonged antibiotic therapy (> 5 days) in preterm infants correlates with a heightened risk of late-onset sepsis (mainly due to group B *Streptococcus*), necrotizing enterocolitis, and high death rates (Kuppala et al., 2011; Verani & Schrag, 2010). Bactericidal agents diminish the total variety of newborns' gut microbiota and promote the emergence of drug-resistant microorganisms. Long after infancy, medications may continue to affect microbial diversity, succession, and resistance. The adult microbiome has been evaluated across many populations. It has been demonstrated that a wide variety of antibiotics can temporarily or permanently change the makeup of healthy adult microbiotas, often by depleting one or more taxa. The impact of an antibiotic on a microbial community in vivo is likely contingent upon the phylogenetic composition of that community and cannot be anticipated solely based on the susceptibilities of isolated individuals reported in vitro. The prediction of antibiotic effects is complicated by the diverse concentrations of the medication throughout the body and the varied phases of microbiological development (Wakomoto et al., 2013). Oral amoxicillin administration resulted in significant alterations in microbiome composition, persisting for an average of 30 days and seen for over 2 months in certain treated individuals (Cochetière et al., 2005).

6.6.5.2 Synbiotics and engineered bacteria

A symbiotic is the fusion of a bacterium, demonstrated or presumed to have good effects upon consumption (i.e., a probiotic), with a chemical that particularly promotes its proliferation (i.e., prebiotic), resulting in a synergistic impact when combined. Numerous probiotic pills are being advertised as synbiotics. These items often comprise a mixture of *Bifidobacterium, Lactobacillus,* or *Streptococcus* species, together with a carbon substrate (e.g., lactose, lactulose, or inulin) that facilitates the proliferation of these organisms. The term symbiotic denotes a synergistic interaction between the probiotic and prebiotic components. The formulation of synbiotics necessitates that the probiotic demonstrates enhanced efficacy in conjunction with a prebiotic compared to its absence, and conversely. Regrettably, limited experiments examine these aspects; prebiotics are seldom paired with a corresponding probiotic to demonstrate enhanced benefits to the host compared to the absence of either component, as evidenced in a recent synbiotic trial aimed at preventing sepsis in infants in rural India (Panigrahi et al., 2017). Notwithstanding that bacteria have been used as medicines for over a century, the clinical application of genetically modified bacteria as "smart" therapies and diagnostics is becoming a reality because of recent developments in synthetic biology. Bacteria engage closely with their environment in the human body, react to various diseases, and have been finely adapted by evolution to detect and synthesize physiological concentrations of relevant biomolecules. The integration of these characteristics with the capabilities of live organisms, such as chemotaxis and biomolecule secretion, may enable engineered bacterial systems to eventually surpass conventional diagnostics and therapies (Riglar & Silver, 2018).

6.6.5.3 *Postbiotics and microbial metabolites*

Postbiotics can help improve health in several ways. SCFAs are a very important type of metabolite that gut bacteria make by breaking down plant polysaccharides. These saturated aliphatic organic acids can reach concentrations close to mill molar levels in some places. Their carbon backbone can be anywhere from one to six.

Gut microbiota generate SCFAs from carbohydrates by intestinal microbial fermentation, predominantly in the colon, transforming nondigestible carbs into dietary fiber. You can also make SCFA from proteins or peptides that have not been broken down yet. SCFAs can also be used to make lipids or glucose. So, SCFAs made by gut microbes give host cells, like colonocytes, more energy. The fermentation of prebiotics like FOS and inulin produces the SCFA propionate, acetate, and butyrate. In the colon and feces, these are found in a ratio of about 60:20:20. Some other microorganisms use acetate to grow, and it also helps keep cholesterol levels in check. Propionate and butyrate are the main energy sources for epithelial cells and colonocytes. They help gluconeogenesis and cause colon cancer cells to die by promoting apoptosis. Using SCFAs in clinical studies and other more thorough methods can help researchers learn more about the connections between postbiotics, hosts, and gut microbiota. There are a lot of complicated enzymatic reactions that control how SCFAs are used in the body. These processes break down SCFAs and then use them in the body to make energy or to make important biomolecules. SCFAs' metabolic processes are very important for keeping energy levels stable and maintaining overall metabolic health. Bacteria are very important to the complex process of making and synthesizing many different peptides. Antimicrobial peptides use a variety of methods, such as stopping the synthesis of macromolecules and breaking down microbial membranes, to get rid

Table 6.3 Trials of gut microbiota on clinical outcomes of immunotherapy.

Year, country	Cancer type, sample size	Findings	References
2019, United States of America	Metastatic melanoma (n = 27)	Increased microbial diversity was associated with longer progression-free survival.	Peters et al. (2019)
2018, United States of America	Metastatic melanoma (n = 42)	The diversity of naturally occurring microbiota may serve as a biomarker for assessing the outcomes of checkpoint blockade therapy.	Matson et al. (2018)
2018, United States of America	Metastatic melanoma (n = 89)s	Increased diversity within the fecal microbiome was linked to a significant extension of progression-free survival when compared to individuals exhibiting intermediate or low diversity.	Gopalakrishnan et al. (2018b)
2018, France	Nonsmall cell lung carcinoma	*Akkermansia muciniphila* exhibited significant enrichment in responders compared to nonresponders.	Routy et al. (2018)

of bacteria synthesis and breaking down microbial membranes to get rid of bacterial pathogens (Prajapati et al., 2023).

6.7 Clinical applications and trials

The current analysis evaluated the influence of gut microbiota on clinical outcomes of immunotherapy and associated adverse events in cancer patients. Research (n = 10) consistently indicated that the gut microbiota before the administration of ICIs was correlated with improved effectiveness of ICIs and decreased adverse events (Table 6.3). Recent research on FMT has shown its modulatory effects on the composition and variety of the gut microbiome in patients with resistant malignancies as well as their potential to augment the effectiveness of ICIs.

6.8 Challenges and limitations

6.8.1 Technical challenges in microbiome analysis

Microbiome analysis faces significant technical hurdles across its workflow. A primary challenge lies in sample collection and handling, where contamination from the environment or host DNA can skew results, particularly in low-biomass samples. Variability between individuals and even within the same experimental design to discern meaningful biological signals.

DNA extraction methods introduce biases, as different techniques may favor certain microbial groups. During sequencing, choices like 16S rRNA gene primers influence detected diversity, and all methods contend with inherent sequencing errors. Host DNA contamination in samples often requires costly deep sequencing or specific enrichment.

Bioinformatic analysis presents its own complex landscape. Microbiome data is high-dimensional, sparse, and compositional, requiring specialized statistical approaches. Robust quality control for read trimming and chimera removal is crucial. Accurate taxonomic assignment depends on comprehensive databases. Finally, integrating microbiome data with host "omics" data and establishing causality remains a major analytical challenge, further complicated by a lack of standardization across studies, hindering reproducibility and comparability.

6.8.2 Interindividual variability and personalization

The gut microbiome significantly impacts cancer immunotherapy efficacy, but its high interindividual variability is a major hurdle. Each person's unique microbial composition, influenced by diet, genetics, and environment, means a beneficial microbiome for one patient may not be for another. This makes identifying universal microbial biomarkers challenging. Consequently, personalization is crucial. Strategies like baseline microbiome profiling to predict ICI response, followed by tailored interventions such as FMT, specific probiotics, or dietary changes, are being explored. The goal is to dynamically shape the gut microbiome to optimize individual patient outcomes and enhance immunotherapy's effectiveness.

6.8.3 Standardization of interventions

Achieving consistent and reproducible outcomes when modulating the gut microbiome for cancer immunotherapy hinges on the standardization of interventions. Currently, the lack of uniform protocols for approaches to FMT, probiotic administration, or dietary modifications poses a significant challenge. This includes standardizing donor selection for FMT, defining precise microbial consortia for probiotics, and establishing clear dietary guidelines. Without such standardization, comparing results across studies, conducting large-scale clinical trials, and ultimately integrating microbiome modulation into routine clinical practice remains difficult. Developing robust, evidence-based protocols is crucial for realizing the full therapeutic potential of the gut microbiome in cancer immunotherapy.

6.8.4 Regulatory considerations

Regulatory bodies like the FDA are grappling with how to classify and approve microbiome-based interventions for cancer. Challenges include defining these complex biological products, ensuring donor safety and product consistency for FMT, and establishing clear efficacy and safety guidelines. Robust clinical trials are essential to meet these evolving regulatory standards and enable widespread clinical adoption.

6.9 Future directions

Next-generation microbiome therapeutics aim for precision. Beyond broad interventions like FMT, they involve defined microbial consortia (specific bacterial strains) or engineered microbes designed to deliver therapeutic molecules. These advanced approaches leverage synthetic biology and a deeper understanding of host-microbe interactions to optimize treatment, potentially offering highly targeted and potent interventions with fewer side effects. Multiomics methodologies offer a comprehensive understanding of the microbiome by integrating data from various "omic" layers. This includes (1) metagenomics - who's there (composition) and what they can do (genetic potential); (2) metatranscriptomics - what genes are actively expressed (activity); (3) metaproteomics - what proteins are being produced (direct function); (4) metabolomics - what small molecules are being generated (functional outputs and host communication). By integrating these datasets, multiomics elucidates complex host-microbe interactions, identifies functional mechanisms, discovers novel biomarkers, and enables precise, personalized strategies for microbiome modulation.

A critical future direction involves developing robust predictive models that leverage gut microbiome data to forecast patient response to cancer immunotherapy. Utilizing advanced machine learning and artificial intelligence, these models will integrate baseline microbial composition, functional profiles (from multiomics data), and host characteristics. The goal is to identify specific microbial signatures or combinations that accurately distinguish responders from nonresponders, enabling personalized treatment stratification and guiding pretreatment microbiome modulation strategies to enhance therapeutic efficacy and minimize adverse effects.

Optimizing cancer immunotherapy outcomes will increasingly involve combining modalities that integrate modulation with existing treatments. This includes strategically pairing microbial interventions (e.g., specific probiotics, FMT, engineered bacteria) with ICIs, chemotherapy, or radiation therapy. The aim is to achieve synergistic effects, where the microbiome enhances antitumor immunity, mitigates treatment-related toxicities, or overcomes resistance mechanisms. Future research will focus on identifying optimal combinations and precise dosing strategies to maximize therapeutic efficacy and patient benefit.

6.10 Conclusion

This chapter concluded the role of gut microbiota in the immunotherapy of cancer. This shows the interindividual heterogeneity that exists in the makeup of microorganisms. Multiomics methods enhance comprehension of the functions of the microbiome. Probiotics have the potential to enhance immune responses related to cancer therapy. Particular strains have demonstrated the capacity to mitigate the adverse consequences. Modulating the microbiota can be beneficial to both the immune system and overall wellness. Intestinal bacteria have been shown to have an effect on the development of cancer and the effectiveness of therapy.

References

Adamberg, S., Sumeri, I., Uusna, R., Ambalam, P., Kondepudi, K. K., Adamberg, K., Wadstrom, T., & Asa, L. (2014). Survival and synergistic growth of mixed cultures of bifidobacteria and lactobacilli combined with prebiotic oligosaccharides in a gastrointestinal tract simulator. *Microbial Ecology in Health & Disease, 25*(0). https://doi.org/10.3402/mehd.v25.23062.

Alexander, J. L., Wilson, I. D., Teare, J., Marchesi, J. R., Nicholson, J. K., & Kinross, J. M. (2017). Gut microbiota modulation of chemotherapy efficacy and toxicity. *Nature Reviews Gastroenterology and Hepatology, 14*(6), 356–365. https://doi.org/10.1038/nrgastro.2017.20.

Andoh, A. (2016). Physiological role of gut microbiota for maintaining human health. *Digestion, 93*(3), 176–181. https://doi.org/10.1159/000444066.

Aviles-Jimenez, F., Vazquez-Jimenez, F., Medrano-Guzman, R., Mantilla, A., & Torres, J. (2014). Stomach microbiota composition varies between patients with non-atrophic gastritis and patients with intestinal type of gastric cancer. *Scientific Reports, 4*(1). https://doi.org/10.1038/srep04202.

Bibbò, S., Ianiro, G., Giambò, F., Settanni, C. R., Cammarota, G., & Gasbarrini, A. (2022). Role of gut microbiome on immunotherapy efficacy in melanoma. *Human Vaccines and Immunotherapeutics, 18*(3). https://doi.org/10.1080/21645515.2021.1926759.

Bik, E. M., Eckburg, P. B., Gill, S. R., Nelson, K. E., Purdom, E. A., Francois, F., Perez-Perez, G., Blaser, M. J., & Relman, D. A. (2006). Molecular analysis of the bacterial microbiota in the human stomach. *Proceedings of the National Academy of Sciences, 103*(3), 732–737. https://doi.org/10.1073/pnas.0506655103.

Bird, L. (2020). Microbial metabolite boosts immunotherapy. *Nature Reviews Immunology, 20*(11), 648–649. https://doi.org/10.1038/s41577-020-00465-z.

Blaut, M. (2018). *Composition and function of the gut microbiome: The gut microbiome in health and disease* (pp. 5–30). Springer International Publishing. https://doi.org/10.1007/978-3-319-90545-7_2.

Booijink, C. C. G. M., El-Aidy, S., Rajilić-Stojanović, M., Heilig, H. G. H. J., Troost, F. J., Smidt, H., Kleerebezem, M., De Vos, W. M., & Zoetendal, E. G. (2010). High temporal and inter-individual variation detected in the human ileal microbiota. *Environmental Microbiology, 12*(12), 3213–3227. https://doi.org/10.1111/j.1462-2920.2010.02294.x.

Cann, S. A. H., Netten, J. P. v, & Netten, C. v (2003). Dr William Coley and tumour regression: A place in history or in the future. *Postgraduate Medical Journal, 79*(938), 672–678.

Carbone, D. P., Reck, M., Paz-Ares, L., Creelan, B., Horn, L., Steins, M., Felip, E., Van Den Heuvel, M. M., Ciuleanu, T. E., Badin, F., Ready, N., Hiltermann, T. J. N., Nair, S., Juergens, R., Peters, S., Minenza, E., Wrangle, J. M., Rodriguez-Abreu, D., Borghaei, H., … Socinski, M. A. (2017). First-line nivolumab in stage IV or recurrent non-small-cell lung cancer. *New England Journal of Medicine, 376*(25), 2415–2426. https://doi.org/10.1056/NEJMoa1613493.

Chau, J., Yadav, M., Liu, B., Furqan, M., Dai, Q., Shahi, S., Gupta, A., Mercer, K. N., Eastman, E., Hejleh, T. A., Chan, C., Weiner, G. J., Cherwin, C., Lee, S. T. M., Zhong, C., Mangalam, A., & Zhang, J. (2021). Prospective correlation between the patient microbiome with response to and development of immune-mediated adverse effects to immunotherapy in lung cancer. *BMC Cancer, 21*(1). https://doi.org/10.1186/s12885-021-08530-z.

Chung, H., Pamp, S. J., Hill, J. A., Surana, N. K., Edelman, S. M., Troy, E. B., Reading, N. C., Villablanca, E. J., Wang, S., Mora, J. R., Umesaki, Y., Mathis, D., Benoist, C., Relman, D. A., & Kasper, D. L. (2012). Gut immune maturation depends on colonization with a host-specific microbiota. *Cell, 149*(7), 1578–1593. https://doi.org/10.1016/j.cell.2012.04.037.

Cochetière, M. F. D. e L. a, Lepage, T. D. P., Bourreille, A., Galmiche, J. P., & Dore, J. (2005). Resilience of the dominant human fecal microbiota upon short-course antibiotic challenge. *Journal of Clinical Microbiology, 43*(11).

Daly, M., & Zarate-Lopez, N. (2021). Functional gastrointestinal disorders: History taking skills in practice. *Clinical Medicine, 21*(5), e480. https://doi.org/10.7861/clinmed.2021-0189.

Davar, D., Dzutsev, A. K., McCulloch, J. A., Rodrigues, R. R., Chauvin, J. M., Morrison, R. M., Deblasio, R. N., Menna, C., Ding, Q., Pagliano, O., Zidi, B., Zhang, S., Badger, J. H., Vetizou, M., Cole, A. M., Fernandes, M. R., Prescott, S., Costa, R. G. F., Balaji, A. K., ... Zarour, H. M. (2021). Fecal microbiota transplant overcomes resistance to anti-PD-1 therapy in melanoma patients. *Science, 371*(6529), 595–602. https://doi.org/10.1126/science.abf3363.

Dicksved, J., Lindberg, M., Rosenquist, M., Enroth, H., Jansson, J. K., & Engstrand, L. (2009). Molecular characterization of the stomach microbiota in patients with gastric cancer and in controls. *Journal of Medical Microbiology, 58*(4), 509–516. https://doi.org/10.1099/jmm.0.007302-0Sweden.

Eslami, S., Hadjati, J., Motevaseli, E., Mirzaei, R., Bonab, S. F., Ansaripour, B., & Khoramizadeh, M. R. (2016). *Lactobacillus crispatus* strain SJ-3C-US induces human dendritic cells (DCs) maturation and confers an anti-inflammatory phenotype to DCs. *APMIS, 124*(8), 697–710. https://doi.org/10.1111/apm.12556.

Fan, S., Jiang, Z., Zhang, Z., Xing, J., Wang, D., & Tang, D. (2023). *Akkermansia muciniphila*: A potential booster to improve the effectiveness of cancer immunotherapy. *Journal of Cancer Research and Clinical Oncology, 149*(14), 13477–13494. https://doi.org/10.1007/s00432-023-05199-8.

Fehleisen, F. (1882). On the cultivation of erysipelas bacteria on artificial nutrient media and their transmissibility to humans. *German Medical Weekly, 8*(31), 553–554. https://doi.org/10.1055/s-0029-1196806.

Fessler, J., Matson, V., & Gajewski, T. F. (2019). Exploring the emerging role of the microbiome in cancer immunotherapy. *Journal for ImmunoTherapy of Cancer, 7*(1). https://doi.org/10.1186/s40425-019-0574-4.

Fneish, F. H., Abd El Galil, K. H., & Domiati, S. A. (2025). Evaluation of single and multi-strain probiotics with gentamicin against *E. coli* O157:H7: Insights from in vitro and in vivo studies. *Microorganisms, 13*(2). https://doi.org/10.3390/microorganisms13020460.

Fridman, W. H., Zitvogel, L., Sautès-Fridman, C., & Kroemer, G. (2017). The immune contexture in cancer prognosis and treatment. *Nature Reviews Clinical Oncology, 14*(12), 717–734. https://doi.org/10.1038/nrclinonc.2017.101.

Glover, T. (1930). The bacteriology of cancer. *Canada Lancet Practitioner, 75*, 92–111.

Gopalakrishnan, V., Helmink, B. A., Spencer, C. N., Reuben, A., & Wargo, J. A. (2018a). The influence of the gut microbiome on cancer, immunity, and cancer immunotherapy. *Cancer Cell, 33*(4), 570–580. https://doi.org/10.1016/j.ccell.2018.03.015.

Gopalakrishnan, V., Spencer, C. N., Nezi, L., Reuben, A., Andrews, M. C., Karpinets, T. V., Prieto, P. A., Vicente, D., Hoffman, K., Wei, S. C., Cogdill, A. P., Zhao, L., Hudgens, C. W., Hutchinson, D. S., Manzo, T., Petaccia De Macedo, M., Cotechini, T., Kumar, T., Chen, W. S., ... Wargo, J. A. (2018b). Gut microbiome modulates response to anti-PD-1 immunotherapy in melanoma patients. *Science, 359*(6371), 97–103. https://doi.org/10.1126/science.aan4236.

Gough, E., Shaikh, H., & Manges, A. R. (2011). Systematic review of intestinal microbiota transplantation (fecal bacteriotherapy) for recurrent *Clostridium difficile* infection. *Clinical Infectious Diseases, 53*(10), 994–1002. https://doi.org/10.1093/cid/cir632.

Grivennikov, S. I., Wang, K., Mucida, D., Stewart, C. A., Schnabl, B., Jauch, D., Taniguchi, K., Yu, G. Y., Österreicher, C. H., Hung, K. E., Datz, C., Feng, Y., Fearon, E. R., Oukka, M., Tessarollo, L., Coppola, V., Yarovinsky, F., Cheroutre, H., Eckmann, L., ... Karin, M. (2012). Adenoma-linked barrier defects and microbial products drive IL-23/IL-17-mediated tumour growth. *Nature, 491*(7423), 254–258. https://doi.org/10.1038/nature11465.

Guarner, F., & Malagelada, J. R. (2003). Gut flora in health and disease. *Lancet, 361*(9356), 512–519. https://doi.org/10.1016/S0140-6736(03)12489-0.

Hajishengallis, G., Darveau, R. P., & Curtis, M. A. (2012). The keystone-pathogen hypothesis. *Nature Reviews Microbiology, 10*(10), 717–725. https://doi.org/10.1038/nrmicro2873.

Harjes, U. (2020). Tumour-reactive T cells work remotely using IFNγ. *Nature Reviews Cancer, 20*(5), 261. https://doi.org/10.1038/s41568-020-0255-0.

He, B., Hoang, T. K., Wang, T., Ferris, M., Taylor, C. M., Tian, X., Luo, M., Tran, D. Q., Zhou, J., Tatevian, N., Luo, F., Molina, J. G., Blackburn, M. R., Gomez, T. H., Roos, S., Rhoads, J. M., & Liu, Y. (2017). Resetting microbiota by *Lactobacillus reuteri* inhibits T reg deficiency-induced autoimmunity via adenosine A2A receptors. *Journal of Experimental Medicine, 214*(1), 107–123. https://doi.org/10.1084/jem.20160961.

International Agency for Research on Cancer (2012). IARC monographs on the evaluation of carcinogenic risks to humans. Chemical agents and related occupations (100F). Lyon (France): International Agency for Research on Cancer.

Jernberg, C., Löfmark, S., Edlund, C., & Jansson, J. K. (2010). Long-term impacts of antibiotic exposure on the human intestinal microbiota. *Microbiology, 156*(11), 3216–3223. https://doi.org/10.1099/mic.0.040618-0Sweden.

Jia, B. (2019). Commentary: Gut microbiome-mediated bile acid metabolism regulates liver cancer via NKT cells. *Frontiers in Immunology, 10*. https://doi.org/10.3389/fimmu.2019.00282.

Jobin, C. (2013). Colorectal cancer: Looking for answers in the microbiota. *Cancer Discovery, 3*(4), 384–387. https://doi.org/10.1158/2159-8290.cd-13-0042.

Kadosh, E., Snir-Alkalay, I., Venkatachalam, A., May, S., Lasry, A., Elyada, E., Zinger, A., Shaham, M., Vaalani, G., Mernberger, M., Stiewe, T., Pikarsky, E., Oren, M., & Ben-Neriah, Y. (2020). The gut microbiome switches mutant p53 from tumour-suppressive to oncogenic. *Nature, 586*(7827), 133–138. https://doi.org/10.1038/s41586-020-2541-0.

Kim, C. H. (2018). Immune regulation by microbiome metabolites. *Immunology, 154*(2), 220–229. https://doi.org/10.1111/imm.12930.

Kleber, K. T., Iranpur, K. R., Perry, L. M., Cruz, S. M., Razmara, A. M., Culp, W. T. N., Kent, M. S., Eisen, J. A., Rebhun, R. B., & Canter, R. J. (2022). Using the canine microbiome to bridge translation of cancer immunotherapy from preclinical murine models to human clinical trials. *Frontiers in Immunology, 13*. https://doi.org/10.3389/fimmu.2022.983344.

Kuppala, V. S., Meinzen-Derr, J., Morrow, A. L., & Schibler, K. R. (2011). Prolonged initial empirical antibiotic treatment is associated with adverse outcomes in premature infants. *Journal of Pediatrics, 159*(5), 720–725. https://doi.org/10.1016/j.jpeds.2011.05.033.

Kwoji, I. D., Aiyegoro, O. A., Okpeku, M., & Adeleke, M. A. (2021). Multi-strain probiotics: Synergy among isolates enhances biological activities. *Biology, 10*(4). https://doi.org/10.3390/biology10040322.

Li, X., Zhang, S., Guo, G., Han, J., & Yu, J. (2022). Gut microbiome in modulating immune checkpoint inhibitors. *eBioMedicine, 82*, 104163. https://doi.org/10.1016/j.ebiom.2022.104163.

Locey, K. J., & Lennon, J. T. (2016). Scaling laws predict global microbial diversity. *Proceedings of the National Academy of Sciences, 113*(21), 5970–5975. https://doi.org/10.1073/pnas.1521291113.

Mager, L. F., Burkhard, R., Pett, N., Cooke, N. C. A., Brown, K., Ramay, H., Paik, S., Stagg, J., Groves, R. A., Gallo, M., Lewis, I. A., Geuking, M. B., & McCoy, K. D. (2020). Microbiome-derived inosine modulates response to checkpoint inhibitor immunotherapy. *Science, 369*(6510), 1481–1489. https://doi.org/10.1126/science.abc3421.

Martin, A. M., Sun, E. W., Rogers, G. B., & Keating, D. J. (2019). The influence of the gut microbiome on host metabolism through the regulation of gut hormone release. *Frontiers in Physiology, 10*. https://doi.org/10.3389/fphys.2019.00428.

Martini, E., Krug, S. M., Siegmund, B., Neurath, M. F., & Becker, C. (2017). Mend Your fences: The epithelial barrier and its relationship with mucosal immunity in inflammatory bowel disease. *Cellular and Molecular Gastroenterology and Hepatology, 4*(1), 33–46. https://doi.org/10.1016/j.jcmgh.2017.03.007.

Matson, V., Fessler, J., Bao, R., Chongsuwat, T., Zha, Y., Alegre, M. L., Luke, J. J., & Gajewski, T. F. (2018). The commensal microbiome is associated with anti-PD-1 efficacy in metastatic melanoma patients. *Science, 359*(6371), 104–108. https://doi.org/10.1126/science.aao3290.

McFarland, L. V. (2021). Efficacy of single-strain probiotics versus multi-strain mixtures: Systematic review of strain and disease specificity. *Digestive Diseases and Sciences, 66*(3), 694–704. https://doi.org/10.1007/s10620-020-06244-z.

Mørland, B., Smievoll, A. I., & Midtvedt, T. (1979). Comparison of peritoneal macrophages from germfree and conventional mice. *Infection and Immunity, 26*(3), 1129–1136. https://doi.org/10.1128/iai.26.3.1129-1136.1979.

Mutalub, Y. B., Abdulwahab, M., Mohammed, A., Yahkub, A. M., AL-Mhanna, S. B., Yusof, W., Tang, S. P., Rasool, A. H. G., & Mokhtar, S. S. (2022). Gut microbiota modulation as a novel therapeutic strategy in cardiometabolic diseases. *Foods, 11*(17). https://doi.org/10.3390/foods11172575.

Neurath, M. F. (2014). Cytokines in inflammatory bowel disease. *Nature Reviews Immunology, 14*(5), 329–342. https://doi.org/10.1038/nri3661.

Neurath, M. F., Artis, D., & Becker, C. (2025). The intestinal barrier: A pivotal role in health, inflammation, and cancer. *The Lancet Gastroenterology and Hepatology, 10*(6), 573–592. https://doi.org/10.1016/S2468-1253(24)00390-X.

Nomura, M., Nagatomo, R., Doi, K., Shimizu, J., Baba, K., Saito, T., Matsumoto, S., Inoue, K., & Muto, M. (2020). Association of short-chain fatty acids in the gut microbiome with clinical response to treatment with nivolumab or pembrolizumab in patients with solid cancer tumors. *JAMA Network Open, 3*(4), e202895. https://doi.org/10.1001/jamanetworkopen.2020.2895.

Noor, A., Bilal, A., & Ali, U. (2024). Towards personalized cancer care: A report of CRISPR-Cas9 applications in targeted therapies and precision medicine. *Journal of Health and Rehabilitation Research, 4*(2), 1375–1380.

Panigrahi, P., Parida, S., Nanda, N. C., Satpathy, R., Pradhan, L., Chandel, D. S., Baccaglini, L., Mohapatra, A., Mohapatra, S. S., Misra, P. R., Chaudhry, R., Chen, H. H., Johnson, J. A., Morris, J. G., Paneth, N., & Gewolb, I. H. (2017). A randomized synbiotic trial to prevent sepsis among infants in rural India. *Nature, 548*(7668), 407–412. https://doi.org/10.1038/nature23480.

Pardoll, D. (2015). Cancer and the immune system: Basic concepts and targets for intervention. *Seminars in Oncology, 42*, 523–538.

Paulos, C. M., Wrzesinski, C., Kaiser, A., Hinrichs, C. S., Chieppa, M., Cassard, L., Palmer, D. C., Boni, A., Muranski, P., Yu, Z., Gattinoni, L., Antony, P. A., Rosenberg, S. A., & Restifo, N. P. (2007). Microbial translocation augments the function of adoptively transferred self/tumor-specific CD8+ T cells via TLR4 signaling. *Journal of Clinical Investigation, 117*(8), 2197–2204. https://doi.org/10.1172/JCI32205.

Peters, B. A., Wilson, M., Moran, U., Pavlick, A., Izsak, A., Wechter, T., Weber, J. S., Osman, I., & Ahn, J. (2019). Relating the gut metagenome and metatranscriptome to immunotherapy responses in melanoma patients. *Genome Medicine, 11*(1). https://doi.org/10.1186/s13073-019-0672-4.

Peterson, L. W., & Artis, D. (2014). Intestinal epithelial cells: Regulators of barrier function and immune homeostasis. *Nature Reviews Immunology, 14*(3), 141–153. https://doi.org/10.1038/nri3608.

Pitt, J. M., Vétizou, M., Waldschmitt, N., Kroemer, G., Chamaillard, M., Boneca, I. G., & Zitvogel, L. (2016). Fine-tuning cancer immunotherapy: Optimizing the gut microbiome. *Cancer Research, 76*(16), 4602–4607. https://doi.org/10.1158/0008-5472.CAN-16-0448.

Prajapati, N., Patel, J., Singh, S., Yadav, V. K., Joshi, C., Patani, A., Prajapati, D., Sahoo, D. K., & Patel, A. (2023). Postbiotic production: Harnessing the power of microbial metabolites for health applications. *Frontiers in Microbiology, 14*. https://doi.org/10.3389/fmicb.2023.1306192.

Riglar, D. T., & Silver, P. A. (2018). Engineering bacteria for diagnostic and therapeutic applications. *Nature Reviews Microbiology, 16*(4), 214–225. https://doi.org/10.1038/nrmicro.2017.172.

Rizvi, N. A., Hellmann, M. D., Snyder, A., Kvistborg, P., Makarov, V., Havel, J. J., Lee, W., Yuan, J., Wong, P., Ho, T. S., Miller, M. L., Rekhtman, N., Moreira, A. L., Ibrahim, F., Bruggeman, C., Gasmi, B., Zappasodi, R., Maeda, Y., Sander, C., ... Chan, T. A. (2015). Mutational landscape determines sensitivity to PD-1 blockade in non-small cell lung cancer. *Science, 348*(6230), 124–128. https://doi.org/10.1126/science.aaa1348.

Roberfroid, M., Gibson, G. R., Hoyles, L., McCartney, A. L., Rastall, R., Rowland, I., Wolvers, D., Watzl, B., Szajewska, H., Stahl, B., Guarner, F., Respondek, F., Whelan, K., Coxam, V., Davicco, M.-J., Léotoing, L., Wittrant, Y., Delzenne, N. M., Cani, P. D., … Meheust, A. (2010). Prebiotic effects: Metabolic and health benefits. *British Journal of Nutrition, 104*(S2), S1. https://doi.org/10.1017/s0007114510003363.

Round, J. L., & Mazmanian, S. K. (2009). The gut microbiota shapes intestinal immune responses during health and disease. *Nature Reviews Immunology, 9*(5), 313–323. https://doi.org/10.1038/nri2515.

Routy, B., Le Chatelier, E., Derosa, L., Duong, C. P. M., Alou, M. T., Daillère, R., Fluckiger, A., Messaoudene, M., Rauber, C., Roberti, M. P., Fidelle, M., Flament, C., Poirier-Colame, V., Opolon, P., Klein, C., Iribarren, K., Mondragón, L., Jacquelot, N., Qu, B., … Zitvogel, L. (2018). Gut microbiome influences efficacy of PD-1-based immunotherapy against epithelial tumors. *Science, 359*(6371), 91–97. https://doi.org/10.1126/science.aan3706.

Sajjad, M. K., Bilal, A., Iftikhar, A., Awais, M., Asif, I., Shaheen, F., & Zahoor, G. (2024). Examining the association between pesticide exposures and chronic diseases in agricultural workers. *Remittances Review, 9*(2), 2153–2176.

Sattar, R. Z., Bilal, A., Bashir, S., Iftikhar, A., & Yaqoob, I. (2024). Embryotoxicity of fluconazole on developing chick embryos. *The Journal of Basic and Applied Zoology, 85*(1). https://doi.org/10.1186/s41936-024-00359-9.

Schwabe, R. F., & Jobin, C. (2013). The microbiome and cancer. *Nature Reviews Cancer, 13*(11), 800–812. https://doi.org/10.1038/nrc3610.

Shukla, V. K., Tiwari, S. C., & Roy, S. K. (1993). Biliary bile acids in cholelithiasis and carcinoma of the gall bladder. *European Journal of Cancer Prevention, 2*(2), 155–160. https://doi.org/10.1097/00008469-199303000-00008.

Silva, C. S., Bolhuis, J. E., Gerrits, W. J. J., Kemp, B., & Borne, J. J. G. C. (2013). Effects of dietary fibers with different fermentation characteristics on feeding motivation in adult female pigs. *Physiology & Behavior, 110–111*, 148–157. https://doi.org/10.1016/j.physbeh.2013.01.006.

Sivan, A., Corrales, L., Hubert, N., Williams, J. B., Aquino-Michaels, K., Earley, Z. M., Benyamin, F. W., Lei, Y. M., Jabri, B., Alegre, M. L., Chang, E. B., & Gajewski, T. F. (2015). Commensal *Bifidobacterium* promotes antitumor immunity and facilitates anti-PD-L1 efficacy. *Science, 350*(6264), 1084–1089. https://doi.org/10.1126/science.aac4255.

Sjögren, K., Engdahl, C., Henning, P., Lerner, U. H., Tremaroli, V., Lagerquist, M. K., Bäckhed, F., & Ohlsson, C. (2012). The gut microbiota regulates bone mass in mice. *Journal of Bone and Mineral Research, 27*(6), 1357–1367. https://doi.org/10.1002/jbmr.1588.

Skrzydło-Radomańska, B., Prozorow-Król, B., Cichoż-Lach, H., Majsiak, E., Bierła, J. B., Kanarek, E., Sowińska, A., & Cukrowska, B. (2021). The effectiveness and safety of multi-strain probiotic preparation in patients with diarrhea-predominant irritable bowel syndrome: A randomized controlled study. *Nutrients, 13*(3), 756. https://doi.org/10.3390/nu13030756.

Spranger, S., Bao, R., & Gajewski, T. F. (2015). Melanoma-intrinsic β-catenin signalling prevents anti-tumour immunity. *Nature, 523*(7559), 231–235. https://doi.org/10.1038/nature14404.

Staffolo, M. D., Bevilacqua, M. S. R. í, & Albertengo, L. (2012). Dietary fiber and availability of nutrients: A case study on yoghurt as a food model. In *The complex world of polysaccharides* (pp. 119–1497). InTech Open. https://doi.org/10.5772/54031.

Starnes, C. O. (1992). Coley's toxins in perspective. *Nature, 357*(6373), 11–12. https://doi.org/10.1038/357011a0.

Tanoue, T., Morita, S., Plichta, D. R., Skelly, A. N., Suda, W., Sugiura, Y., Narushima, S., Vlamakis, H., Motoo, I., Sugita, K., Shiota, A., Takeshita, K., Yasuma-Mitobe, K., Riethmacher, D., Kaisho, T., Norman, J. M., Mucida, D., Suematsu, M., Yaguchi, T., … Honda, K. (2019). A defined commensal consortium elicits CD8 T cells and anti-cancer immunity. *Nature, 565*(7741), 600–605. https://doi.org/10.1038/s41586-019-0878-z.

Taylor, G. (1993). Unconventional therapy. *Western Journal of Medicine, 158*(4), 428.

Theuretzbacher, U., Bush, K., Harbarth, S., Paul, M., Rex, J. H., Tacconelli, E., & Thwaites, G. E. (2020). Critical analysis of antibacterial agents in clinical development. *Nature Reviews Microbiology, 18*(5), 286–298. https://doi.org/10.1038/s41579-020-0340-0.

Verani, J. R., & Schrag, S. J. (2010). Group B streptococcal disease in infants: Progress in prevention and continued challenges. *Clinics in Perinatology, 37*(2), 375–392. https://doi.org/10.1016/j.clp.2010.02.002.

Vétizou, M., Pitt, J. M., Daillère, R., Lepage, P., Waldschmitt, N., Flament, C., Rusakiewicz, S., Routy, B., Roberti, M. P., Duong, C. P. M., Poirier-Colame, V., Roux, A., Becharef, S., Formenti, S., Golden, E., Cording, S., Eberl, G., Schlitzer, A., Ginhoux, F., … Zitvogel, L. (2015). Anticancer immunotherapy by CTLA-4 blockade relies on the gut microbiota. *Science, 350*(6264), 1079–1084. https://doi.org/10.1126/science.aad1329.

Wakamoto, Y., Dhar, N., Chait, R., Schneider, K., Signorino-Gelo, F., Leibler, S., & McKinney, J. D. (2013). Dynamic persistence of antibiotic-stressed mycobacteria. *Science, 339*(6115), 91–95.

Walboomers, J. M. M., Jacobs, M. V., Manos, M. M., Bosch, F. X., Kummer, J. A., Shah, K. V., Snijders, P. J. F., Peto, J., Meijer, C. J. L. M., & Muñoz, N. (1999). Human papillomavirus is a necessary cause of invasive cervical cancer worldwide. *Journal of Pathology, 189*(1), 12–19. https://doi.org/10.1002/(SICI)1096-9896(199909)189:1⟨12::AID-PATH431⟩3.0.CO;2-F.

Wang, J., Zhu, N., Su, X., Gao, Y., & Yang, R. (2023). Gut-microbiota-derived metabolites maintain gut and systemic immune homeostasis. *Cells, 12*(5), 793. https://doi.org/10.3390/cells12050793.

Wilson, N. S., Young, L. J., Kupresanin, F., Naik, S. H., Vremec, D., Heath, W. R., Akira, S., Shortman, K., Boyle, J., Maraskovsky, E., Belz, G. T., & Villadangos, J. A. (2008). Normal proportion and expression of maturation markers in migratory dendritic cells in the absence of germs or Toll-like receptor signaling. *Immunology and Cell Biology, 86*(2), 200–205. https://doi.org/10.1038/sj.icb.7100125.

Xavier, J. B., Young, V. B., Skufca, J., Ginty, F., Testerman, T., Pearson, A. T., Macklin, P., Mitchell, A., Shmulevich, I., Xie, L., Caporaso, J. G., Crandall, K. A., Simone, N. L., Godoy-Vitorino, F., Griffin, T. J., Whiteson, K. L., Gustafson, H. H., Slade, D. J., Schmidt, T. M., … Wargo, J. A. (2020). The cancer microbiome: Distinguishing direct and indirect effects requires a systemic view. *Trends in Cancer, 6*(3), 192–204. https://doi.org/10.1016/j.trecan.2020.01.004.

Xie, Y., & Liu, F. (2024). The role of the gut microbiota in tumor, immunity, and immunotherapy. *Frontiers in Immunology, 15*. https://doi.org/10.3389/fimmu.2024.1410928.

Zagato, E., Pozzi, C., Bertocchi, A., Schioppa, T., Saccheri, F., Guglietta, S., Fosso, B., Melocchi, L., Nizzoli, G., Troisi, J., Marzano, M., Oresta, B., Spadoni, I., Atarashi, K., Carloni, S., Arioli, S., Fornasa, G., Asnicar, F., Segata, N., … Rescigno, M. (2020). Endogenous murine microbiota member *Faecalibaculum rodentium* and its human homologue protect from intestinal tumour growth. *Nature Microbiology, 5*(3), 511–524. https://doi.org/10.1038/s41564-019-0649-5.

Zhang, J., Wu, K., Shi, C., & Li, G. (2022). Cancer immunotherapy: Fecal microbiota transplantation brings light. *Current Treatment Options in Oncology, 23*(12), 1777–1792. https://doi.org/10.1007/s11864-022-01027-2.

Zhang, P. (2022). Influence of foods and nutrition on the gut microbiome and implications for intestinal health. *International Journal of Molecular Sciences, 23*(17), 9588. https://doi.org/10.3390/ijms23179588.

Zitvogel, L., Ayyoub, M., Routy, B., & Kroemer, G. (2016). Microbiome and anticancer immunosurveillance. *Cell, 165*(2), 276–287. https://doi.org/10.1016/j.cell.2016.03.001.

Zitvogel, L., Pietrocola, F., & Kroemer, G. (2017). Nutrition, inflammation and cancer. *Nature Immunology, 18*(8), 843–850. https://doi.org/10.1038/ni.3754.

7

The impact of the microbiome on resistance to cancer treatment with chemotherapeutic agents and immunotherapy

Garima Malik[a], Shafia Bashir[b], Shazia Javeed[b], Meenakshi Dhanawat[c] and Jashan Girdhar[d]

[a]CHITKARA COLLEGE OF PHARMACY, CHITKARA UNIVERSITY, RAJPURA, PUNJAB, INDIA [b]DEPARTMENT OF PHARMACEUTICAL SCIENCES, UNIVERSITY OF KASHMIR, HAZRATBAL, SRINAGAR, INDIA [c]AMITY INSTITUTE OF PHARMACY, AMITY UNIVERSITY HARYANA, GURUGRAM, HARYANA, INDIA [d]TEERTHANKER MAHAVEER COLLEGE OF PHARMACY, TEERTHANKER MAHAVEER UNIVERSITY, MORADABAD, UTTAR PRADESH, INDIA

7.1 Introduction

Despite major advances in cancer treatment, therapy resistance remains the major cause of treatment failure and cancer deaths. Although cytotoxic chemotherapy, targeted therapies, and immunotherapeutic agents have revolutionized cancer treatment, significant clinical responses are observed in only a small proportion of cancer patients (Damodaran et al., 2025). Chemotherapeutic agents and other immunotherapeutic agents, such as immune checkpoint inhibitors (ICIs), exhibit considerable variability in treatment response among cancer patients, even when cancer cells are histopathologically and genetically similar in origin. While some cancer patients exhibit a dramatic response, with tumor remission, other patients exhibit a rapid progression of cancer, despite similar tumor mutational burden, programmed death-ligand 1 (PD-L1) expression, and driver gene mutations. These findings suggest that tumor genomics cannot fully explain the variability in treatment response in cancer patients (Birnboim-Perach & Benhar, 2024).

Resistance to cancer treatment has traditionally been attributed to tumor-intrinsic factors, including somatic mutations in drug targets, epigenetic changes in gene expression, overexpression of oncogenic signal transduction pathways, and overexpression of efflux transporters, such as ATP-binding cassette transporters (ABC) transporters, which decrease intracellular

The Microbiome and Cancer Treatment: Overcoming Resistance and Enhancing Efficacy.
DOI: https://doi.org/10.1016/B978-0-443-33206-7.00008-X

drug concentrations. Chemotherapeutic agents exhibit increased therapeutic resistance due to enhanced DNA repair, aberrant apoptosis, metabolic changes, and tumor-stroma interactions, which confer a survival advantage on cancer cells, thereby making them resistant to chemotherapy agents (Holohan et al., 2013). Immunotherapeutic agents, such as ICIs, exhibit increased therapy resistance due to decreased antigen presentation, decreased interferon-γ function, and tumor immune evasion due to increased expression of immune checkpoint molecules. While these models of cancer treatment failure and therapy resistance have offered significant insights into cancer treatment failure, they fail to explain the variability in clinical response and the unpredictability of cancer treatment outcomes (McMillin et al., 2013).

In recent years, the human microbiome has emerged as an important yet underinvestigated determinant of the outcomes of various forms of cancer treatment. The trillions of microbes that colonize the human gastrointestinal (GI) tract and have now been implicated in tumor tissues and systemic compartments represent a dynamic interface between human physiology and pharmacotherapy. The human microbiome is an active participant in the metabolism of xenobiotics and the regulation of human immune response and inflammatory cascades (Adlakha & Chhabra, 2025; Lei et al., 2025). The role of the gut microbiome in pharmacodynamics in the context of drug metabolism, modulation of drug availability, drug enzyme interaction, systemic cytokine profile modulation, and differentiation of immune cells in the tumor microenvironment is being increasingly well elucidated by various researchers. The cumulative evidence from this expanding body of work places the human microbiome as a critical determinant of the efficacy of various forms of cancer treatment and provides a new paradigm in the emerging field of microbiome oncology research (Chacon et al., 2025; Sevcikova et al., 2022).

Preclinical and clinical studies have provided compelling evidence for the role of the human microbiome as an important determinant of the outcomes of various forms of cancer treatment, especially in the context of chemotherapy and immunotherapy. Germ-free animal models and the use of antibiotics to deplete the microbiome have shown that there is a marked impairment in the response to chemotherapy and immunotherapy agents that can be completely restored by repopulating the gut with microbes. Such findings indicate that the signals from the human microbiome are essential to the optimal activation of the immune response in the tumor microenvironment to achieve therapeutic efficacy in the context of cancer treatment (Elkrief et al., 2025). In addition to preclinical evidence, various forms of human studies have provided compelling evidence to reinforce the relevance of the human microbiome in the context of various forms of cancer treatment. The use of antibiotics in the 30 to 60 days before the initiation of ICI treatment has been shown to be associated with reduced treatment efficacy and reduced survival in melanoma, nonsmall cell lung cancer (NSCLC), and urothelial cancers (Eiman et al., 2025).

Conversely, enrichment of specific microbial populations has also been associated with improved therapeutic outcomes. For instance, enrichment of *Akkermansia muciniphila, Bifidobacterium longum,* and other commensal microbes has been associated with improved dendritic cell activation, improved CD8+ T-cell priming, improved immune infiltration profiles in tumors, and improved progression-free survival (PFS) in ICI-treated patients. These microbes likely contribute to a proinflammatory and antitumor immune environment that maximizes ICI responsiveness. Most compellingly, fecal microbiota transplantation (FMT) from ICI responders to ICI nonresponders resensitized refractory patients to ICI treatment. This line of evidence provides the most convincing evidence for the causality and function of the microbiome in ICI responsiveness. This line of evidence shifts the focus from associative evidence to mechanistic and potentially actionable evidence (Jiang & Zhang, 2024; Procaccianti et al., 2023; Vongsavath et al., 2024; Yang et al., 2026). Collectively, this evidence shifts the conventional focus from the "tumor-centric" paradigm to a "tumor-host-microbiome ecosystem" that dictates treatment success or failure. The microbiome modulates drug metabolism, immune priming, tumor composition, and systemic inflammation, which intersect with classical genetic and immunologic determinants of resistance. This understanding has opened new avenues for therapeutic manipulation of the microbiome to circumvent resistance and improve treatment efficacy.

This chapter seeks to integrate contemporary evidence from mechanistic studies that define the role of the microbiome in modulating chemotherapeutic and immunotherapeutic resistance. By synthesizing emerging evidence from molecular biology, immunology, and microbiology, this chapter aims to provide a framework for understanding the emerging evidence for the role of the microbiome in modulating treatment resistance and potentially defining new avenues for future treatment strategies.

7.2 Classical mechanisms of chemotherapy and immunotherapy resistance

Despite these advances in cancer therapy, resistance to cancer drugs remains the major contributor to treatment failure, recurrence, and progression of cancer. Although advances in molecularly targeted therapies and immune-based therapies have shown improved patient survival in many types of cancer, both primary and secondary resistance have hindered long-term therapeutic success. Traditionally, cancer resistance has been viewed as a tumor-intrinsic process resulting from genetic instability and selective pressures from cancer therapies. The conventional chemotherapy resistance mechanism is a complex process in cancer cells, where multiple layers of cellular adaptations lead to a reduction in drug efficacy and failure to kill cancer cells. One of the best-characterized chemotherapy resistance mechanisms is the overexpression of ATP-binding cassette efflux transporters, such as P-glycoprotein (MDR1), which actively pump anticancer drugs out of the cell, resulting in a reduction in drug concentration below therapeutic levels (Fig. 7.1). This multidrug resistance mechanism allows cancer cells to escape a wide spectrum of structurally diverse drugs used in chemotherapy. Cancer cells also upregulate a number of detoxification enzymes, such as glutathione S-transferases and cytochrome P450 enzymes, to neutralize anticancer drugs through chemical modification, thereby inactivating their ability to produce DNA-damaging effects.

Target modifications also contribute to a reduction in chemotherapy efficacy. Alterations in drug-binding proteins, such as β-tubulin, topoisomerase I, and topoisomerase II, impair drug binding and decrease the potency of drugs such as taxanes, anthracyclines, and camptothecins. Cancer cells also upregulate DNA repair enzymes, such as those involved in homologous recombination repair, nucleotide excision repair, and mismatch repair, to rapidly repair DNA damage

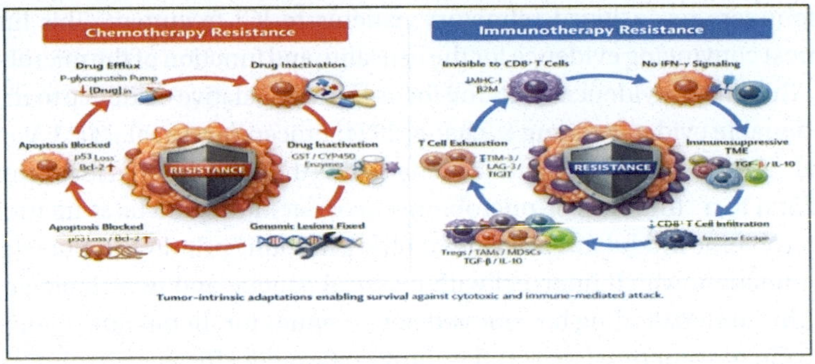

FIGURE 7.1 Traditional mechanisms of chemotherapy and immunotherapy resistance. Schematic representation of tumor resistance mechanisms. The left panel illustrates chemotherapy resistance driven by tumor-intrinsic adaptations including drug efflux via P-glycoprotein, enzymatic drug inactivation (GST/CYP450), target alterations, enhanced DNA repair, and apoptosis evasion (p53 loss, Bcl-2 upregulation). The right panel depicts immunotherapy resistance, highlighting impaired antigen presentation (↓MHC-I/β2M), defective IFN-γ signaling, T-cell exhaustion (TIM-3, LAG-3, TIGIT), immunosuppressive tumor microenvironment (Tregs, TAMs, MDSCs; TGF-β/IL-10), and reduced $CD8^+$ T-cell infiltration. The central tumor cell shielded by "RESISTANCE" denotes convergent mechanisms enabling survival against cytotoxic and immune-mediated attack. *IFN-γ*, Interferon-gamma; *IL-10*, interleukin-10; *MDSCs*, myeloid-derived suppressor cells; *MHC-I*, major histocompatibility complex class I; *LAG-3*, lymphocyte-activation gene 3; *TAMs*, tumor-associated macrophages; *TGF-β*, transforming growth factor-β; *TIGIT*, T-cell immunoreceptor with Ig and ITIM domains; *TIM-3*, T-cell immunoglobulin and mucin-domain containing 3; *Treg*, regulatory T cells.

induced by chemotherapy. The combination of these resistance mechanisms, together with apoptosis pathway deregulation, such as TP53 mutation and BCL2 overexpression, provides a potent mechanism to protect cancer cells from chemotherapy-induced cell death and to maintain cancer cell viability (Burgess et al., 2008; Mansoori et al., 2017; Shah et al., 2023).

In contrast, the mechanisms underlying immunotherapy resistance are complex tumor- and host-mediated phenomena, which are quite different from classical chemoresistance mechanisms. Since ICIs work by reinvigorating cytotoxic T-cell activity, the mechanisms underlying immunotherapy resistance are thought to involve the disruption of antigen presentation and immune recognition. Tumors develop immunotherapy resistance by downregulating the major histocompatibility complex class I (MHC-I) molecules and the β2-microglobulin gene, which render tumor cells less immunogenic to cytotoxic T cells. In addition, tumors develop immunotherapy resistance through defects in the interferon-γ signaling pathway, which is commonly the result of mutations in the JAK-STAT signaling pathway. Mechanisms of adaptive immunotherapy resistance include tumor-mediated mechanisms, which develop during immunotherapy. Tumors develop immunotherapy resistance by upregulating other immune checkpoint molecules, such as T-cell immunoglobulin and mucin-domain containing 3 (TIM-3), lymphocyte-activation gene 3 (LAG-3), and T-cell immunoreceptor with Ig and ITIM domains (TIGIT), which contribute to T-cell exhaustion even in the presence of PD-1 or CTLA-4 inhibitors. In addition, the tumor microenvironment is enriched with immunosuppressive cells, including Tregs, tumor-associated macrophages (TAMs), and myeloid-derived suppressor cells (MDSCs). Tregs, TAMs, and MDSCs contribute to immunotherapy resistance by secreting anti-inflammatory cytokines, including transforming growth factor-β (TGF-β) and interleukin-10

(IL-10), which inhibit T-cell activation and proliferation. In addition, these immunosuppressive cells inhibit dendritic cell activation and the proliferation of cytotoxic T cells, thereby rendering the tumor immunologically "cold" and resistant to immune-mediated destruction (Alsaafeen et al., 2025; Gongora et al., 2011).

While these classical resistance mechanisms are clearly important contributors to therapeutic failure, they cannot fully account for the striking interpatient heterogeneity commonly encountered in clinical oncology. Patients with similar tumor genetic profiles, PD-L1 expression signatures, tumor mutational burdens, and immune infiltrate compositions can have dramatically divergent responses to the same treatment regimen. This observation underscores the importance of extrinsic factors in drug resistance, beyond tumor genetics and intrinsic immune checkpoint controls. Among these extrinsic factors, the human microbiome has been identified as one of the most important nontumor-intrinsic contributors to drug resistance. The microbiome plays a critical role in xenobiotic metabolism, systemic inflammation, antigen presentation, and immune priming. It can modulate pharmacodynamics, influence immune checkpoint responses, and reshape the tumor microenvironment in a manner that interacts with, but clearly goes beyond, genetic and immunologic determinants of drug response. As such, knowledge of these classical resistance mechanisms provides a critical foundation, but understanding the roles played by the microbiome in drug resistance is clearly necessary to achieve a more complete model of therapeutic resistance in modern oncology (Xiang et al., 2024).

7.3 Clinical evidence supporting microbiome-mediated therapy resistance

Over the past decade, clinical data have increasingly supported the notion that the gut microbiome not only correlates with cancer therapy outcomes but also directly impacts them. Observational studies, prospective studies, and meta-analyses have all shown a strong association, suggesting that the microbial composition and diversity are critical in determining the outcome of cancer therapy, whether it be ICIs or traditional chemotherapy. In all of the studies, the common link among patients who have shown resistance to therapy has been the presence of a disrupted microbial balance, termed dysbiosis. One of the strongest clinical data sets supporting the link between the gut microbiome and the outcome of immunotherapy has been the studies assessing the impact of previous antibiotic use (Wang et al., 2025a). Antibiotics, while saving countless lives in the face of infectious diseases, have a profound impact on the microbial diversity of the human gut. Several clinical cohorts have shown that patients who have received antibiotics in the 30 to 60 days preceding the start of immune checkpoint inhibitor therapy have a decreased outcome.

These studies have been conducted in a range of cancer types, including melanoma, NSCLC, renal cell carcinoma, and urothelial carcinoma. Several meta-analyses have been performed, and all have shown a decreased PFS and OS in patients exposed to antibiotics compared to those who have not. Mechanistically, the loss of microbial diversity, or dysbiosis, has been shown to lead to a reduction in the levels of beneficial microbes, such as

Bifidobacterium, which are critical in the activation of dendritic cells and the subsequent priming of CD8+ T cells. Several prospective studies have shown that patients who have retained microbial diversity have a stronger interferon gamma signature, a greater density of tumor-infiltrating lymphocytes, and a greater response rate to PD-1/PDL-1 blockade. In contrast, patients who have received antibiotics have diminished immune activation and functionality.

On the other hand, certain microbial species have been reliably linked to favorable immunotherapy outcomes. Patients harboring enriched populations of *A. muciniphila, Ruminococcus,* and *B. longum* have shown improved objective response rates and improved survival in response to ICIs. The microbial species are believed to facilitate mucosal integrity, mature dendritic cells, and augment CD8+ T cell infiltration in tumors. An extensive 2025 narrative review, encompassing a critical analysis of 95 clinical studies conducted between 2015 and 2025, found that high microbial diversity and enriched populations of beneficial microbial species correlated with improved antitumor immunity in over 70% of cohorts, including patients with renal cell carcinoma and NSCLC. Importantly, these microbial species correlated with improved CD8+ T cell infiltration and downregulation of T cell exhaustion markers, thereby providing a functional validation of their immunomodulatory effects (Ciernikova et al., 2024; Yang et al., 2025; Yao et al., 2025).

More recently, intervention studies have provided compelling evidence to support a causal relationship between the microbiome and immunotherapy responsiveness. FMT from ICI responders to nonresponders has shown considerable promise in restoring responsiveness in refractory cohorts. FMT in phase I/II melanoma trials using PD-1 inhibitors resulted in a dramatic improvement in objective response rates from virtually 0% in refractory cohorts to ~65% in cohorts receiving FMT. Shotgun metagenomic sequencing revealed durable engraftment of donor-derived microbial communities, thereby correlating microbial transplantation with improved immune activation and clinical outcomes. Similar findings have been reported in refractory NSCLC cohorts, thereby providing conclusive evidence that the microbiome directly influences immunotherapy responsiveness rather than merely being a marker of underlying immune status.

The microbiome's influence is not restricted to immunotherapy. Clinical evidence also exists to support its involvement in chemotherapy resistance, particularly in colorectal cancer. Dysbiosis, in this case, characterized by overrepresentation of *Fusobacterium nucleatum,* has been correlated with resistance to 5-FU, a mainstay in chemotherapy in colorectal cancer. This microbe is able to metabolize chemotherapeutic drugs and initiate prosurvival signals in cancer cells, thereby diminishing their availability and efficacy. Clinical studies in advanced-stage colorectal cancer have also shown that lower microbial diversity is correlated with a higher rate of tumor recurrence postadjuvant chemotherapy. This demonstrates that microbial composition is not only important in immunotherapy but also in chemotherapy pharmacodynamics (Kostic et al., 2013a, 2013b; Nejman et al., 2020; Repass et al., 2016; Seely et al., 2022; Thomas, 2017; Zhang et al., 2025b).

Collectively, clinical evidence today far exceeds correlation. It demonstrates that the microbiome is a modifiable therapeutic determinant. From antibiotic treatment failure to microbiota-induced restoration of immunotherapy responsiveness, clinical evidence is rapidly accumulating to support the integration of microbial analysis in cancer treatment protocols. As this evidence evolves, the microbiome is emerging as a predictive biomarker and a therapeutic target in cancer treatment resistance.

7.3.1 The human microbiome in cancer

The human microbiome is a complex ecosystem consisting of a variety of microorganisms like bacteria, archaea, fungi, and viruses living symbiotically in association with the human body. The combined genetic material of these microbes, also referred to as the metagenome, far outweighs the coding capacity of the human genome, thereby offering a vast repertoire of metabolic and immunological functions. Though the highest microbial load is found in the gastrointestinal tract, which is dominated by phyla like Firmicutes, Bacteroidetes, Proteobacteria, and Actinobacteria, microbial populations are also found in other body sites.

Traditionally, several body sites were considered sterile under normal physiological conditions. However, recent advances in metagenomics, next-generation sequencing technologies, and culture-independent detection methods have revealed microbial populations at sites previously thought sterile. Recent studies have demonstrated the presence of microbial populations at sites like lung alveoli, pancreatic tissue, breast tissue, and even in the tumor microenvironment of extragastrointestinal tumors (Alanazi et al., 2024; Ericsson et al., 2015; Sun et al., 2025). This has revolutionized the way we think about the relationship between the host and the tumor microenvironment.

The process of cancer development and the treatment strategies that accompany it have significant effects on the balance of microbes. Cancer development itself results in changes to the host immune system and metabolic processes. These changes have significant effects on the balance of microbes. Cancer treatment strategies, which involve chemotherapy, radiation therapy, dietary changes, hospitalization, and antibiotics, also have effects on the balance of microbes. These changes to the balance of microbes result in dysbiosis, which is characterized by reduced microbial diversity and the presence of both reduced numbers of beneficial microbes and increased numbers of pathogenic microbes. This imbalance in microbes plays a significant role in the development of cancer and drug resistance.

The imbalance in microbes results in reduced effective antigen presentation due to reduced numbers of beneficial microbes that play a significant role in the regulation of major histocompatibility complex (MHC) class I molecules and CD8+ T-cell priming. Simultaneously, the presence of pathogen-associated molecular patterns from the predominant types of microbes results in the promotion of immunosuppressive pathways. These pathways involve the action of both regulatory T cells and myeloid-derived suppressor cells. Metagenome analysis of the types of microbes found in tumors revealed that the types of microbes found in tumors have distinct compositional and functional properties when compared to the types found in healthy tissue. These types of microbes found in tumors have significant effects on oncogenic pathways, drug metabolism, DNA repair mechanisms, and immune evasion pathways. This results in the generation of drug resistance mechanisms in addition to those found in the host DNA (Bai et al., 2025; Lin et al., 2025; Parajuli et al., 2025).

One of the strongest pieces of evidence demonstrating the functional involvement of the microbiome in cancer progression comes from animal model studies in a germ-free environment. Gopalakrishnan et al. (2018) conducted a landmark study in this direction, in which APCmin/+ mouse models were used to study colorectal cancer development in a germ-free environment. The study found that in mice lacking a microbiome, there was accelerated tumor growth with decreased $CD8^+$ T cell infiltration and interferon-gamma (IFN-γ) production in the tumor microenvironment. Importantly, FMT in these mice resulted in immune activation and reduced tumor burden, demonstrating the key role played by the microbiome in cancer immunity.

Overall, these studies demonstrate that the human microbiome is not a passive player in cancer but a key participant in cancer progression, and understanding the ecological roles played by microbes in cancer and in response to cancer therapies is a key step in understanding cancer biology and therapeutic resistance.

7.3.2 Microbiome and chemotherapy resistance

One of the most important and intriguing connections between the microbiome and anticancer pharmacotherapies was established when scientists found that microbes can directly metabolize chemotherapy drugs. Unlike other classical mechanisms of chemotherapy resistance, in which the genetics of the tumor cells are implicated, the study found that microbes can chemically alter chemotherapy agents before they can act on the tumor cells to induce their cytotoxic effects. Some bacterial species have enzymes that can metabolize, inactivate, and/or transform chemotherapeutic agents, thereby reducing their clinical efficacy.

One of the most important examples of the role of the microbiome in chemotherapy resistance was established in pancreatic ductal adenocarcinoma (PDAC). The study revealed that *Gammaproteobacteria* present in the PDAC tumor microenvironment have an enzyme that can metabolize the main chemotherapy agent used to treat PDAC, gemcitabine, to its inactive form, 2′,2′-difluorodeoxyuridine, through the action of the long isoform of the enzyme cytidine deaminase (CDD). This renders the chemotherapy agent ineffective, creating primary chemotherapy resistance that does not depend on the genetics of the tumor cells. More importantly, the study revealed that when the bacteria are depleted in the tumor microenvironment using specific antibiotics, the chemotherapy sensitivity of the tumor cells was restored, causing the tumor to regress (Böhm et al., 2025; Gou et al., 2021; Xu et al., 2025a, 2025c; Zhou et al., 2024).

Aside from localized intratumoral metabolism, the role of the gut microbiota in the systemic metabolism of chemotherapeutic agents has a significant impact on cancer treatment outcomes. For instance, most antineoplastic agents are metabolized in the liver and then excreted into the intestinal lumen in the form of inactive conjugates, primarily in the form of glucuronide conjugates. These conjugates, however, are then acted upon by β-glucuronidases, which are enzymes found in the gut microbiota, resulting in the formation of active drugs in the intestinal lumen, thereby causing tissue damage and diarrhea, as exemplified by the antineoplastic agent irinotecan, which is used in the treatment of colorectal cancer. Although this mechanism primarily causes toxicity, it also exemplifies the role of the gut microbiota in the systemic metabolism of drugs.

On the other hand, some gut microbiota can catabolize active drugs, effectively decreasing the systemic availability of drugs, thereby promoting subtherapeutic plasma concentrations of drugs, a condition that can create a pharmacological environment that favors tumor survival and resistance. The role of the gut microbiota in the systemic metabolism of drugs exemplifies the presence of a new organ of metabolism, which works in parallel with other organs of metabolism, including the liver and the kidneys (Jia et al., 2026; Li et al., 2026; Noh et al., 2017; Tian et al., 2026).

Furthermore, chemotherapy itself introduces another layer of complexity to this relationship by inducing significant changes in microbial composition. Chemotherapeutic agents, through their cytotoxic effects, often reduce the populations of beneficial commensals but simultaneously allow the overgrowth of proinflammatory pathogens and opportunistic microbes. This chemotherapy-induced dysbiosis results in compromised intestinal barrier function, systemic inflammation, and disruption of immune homeostasis. In turn, the proinflammatory environment may downregulate the antitumor immune response, thereby reducing the overall efficacy of the chemotherapy. In this manner, a vicious cycle may be initiated, where chemotherapy alters the microbial community, dysbiosis reduces the anticancer immune response and the overall efficacy of the drugs, and, in turn, resistance to the drugs is either developed or increased.

The role of the gut microbiome in the response to chemotherapy was beautifully demonstrated by the study conducted by Iida et al. (2013). In their study, the researchers demonstrated the importance of the gut microbiome in the response to chemotherapy using mouse sarcoma and MC38 mouse colon carcinoma models. In their study, the researchers found that antibiotic-induced dysbiosis reduced the efficacy of the chemotherapeutic agents oxaliplatin and cyclophosphamide. Germ-free mice were found to be nearly resistant to the chemotherapeutic drugs, which was attributed to the inability to produce reactive oxygen species (ROS) by myeloid cells infiltrating the tumor. Interestingly, the researchers found that the introduction of *Bacteroides* or *Bifidobacterium* to the germ-free mice restored the immune response to the chemotherapeutic drugs (Iida et al., 2013). Overall, these studies demonstrate the importance of the gut microbiome in the response to chemotherapy and the development of resistance to chemotherapeutic drugs. They demonstrate that the development of resistance to chemotherapy is not solely a tumor cell-intrinsic process but is also heavily influenced by the gut microbiome.

7.3.3 Microbiome and immunotherapy resistance

The recognition that the gut microbiome can affect the outcome of ICI therapy has been one of the most important breakthroughs in the field of oncology in recent years. ICI agents, including PD-1, PD-L1, and cytotoxic T-lymphocyte-associated protein 4 (CTLA-4) inhibitors, act by reawakening exhausted CD8+ cytotoxic T cells in the tumor microenvironment. The success of ICI agents does not depend only on the tumor's mutational burden and PD-L1 expression but also on the host's immune microenvironment. In recent years, it has become increasingly clear that the microbiome plays a key role in regulating the host's immune microenvironment, including systemic immune tone, dendritic cell maturation, antigen presentation, and T-cell priming.

Population-based clinical studies conducted on melanoma, NSCLC, and renal cell carcinoma (RCC) have consistently shown that gut microbial signature differences can distinguish between responders and nonresponders to ICI therapy. Patients with favorable responses to PD-1 and CTLA-4 inhibitors have been shown to have higher loads of specific beneficial microbes, including *A. muciniphila, Bifidobacterium* species, and *Faecalibacterium prausnitzii,* which are associated with increased CD8+ T-cell densities in the tumor microenvironment, improved interferon-γ signaling, and clinical outcomes, including higher objective response rates and improved PFS. These microbes have been shown to promote a more inflamed and immunologically active tumor microenvironment, thereby enhancing the efficacy of ICI therapy (Routy et al., 2018; Xu et al., 2025b; Yang & Shi, 2025).

In contrast, the perturbation of the gut microbiome, most often caused by antibiotics, has been consistently correlated with decreased immunotherapy response. Clinical studies have shown that the administration of antibiotics before or during ICI treatment is associated with decreased response rates and overall survival (OS). This reduction of commensal bacteria leads to decreased maturation and antigen presentation ability of dendritic cells, thereby impairing the activation of tumor-specific CD8+ T cells. Concurrently, the altered gut microbiome has also been shown to enhance the growth of immunosuppressive cells like regulatory T cells (Tregs) and MDSCs. These cells secrete cytokines that create an immunosuppressive microenvironment conducive to tumor growth. This leads to a shift from an immune-reactive state to an immune-tolerant state, thereby negating the very purpose of ICI treatment. Thus, the gut microbiome plays an important role in the development of immunotherapy resistance. Perhaps the most compelling evidence of the role of the gut microbiome in the development of immunotherapy resistance is provided by the clinical trials involving FMT. Studies have shown that the transfer of the gut microbiome of ICI responders to nonresponders has reversed the treatment-resistant state (Routy et al., 2025; Yu et al., 2021). This shows that the development of immunotherapy resistance is not an irreversible process but rather a dynamic state.

Preclinical studies have also helped to clarify the underlying mechanisms that account for the above findings. In one study by Sivan et al. (2015), germ-free mice with B16.SIY melanoma tumors showed suboptimal response to anti-PD-1 treatment in the absence of Bifidobacterium species. The absence of *Bifidobacterium* was related to suboptimal dendritic cell response and CD8+ T-cell activation. Notably, oral treatment with Bifidobacterium restored antitumor response and improved tumor control (Sivan et al., 2015).

In another study by Matson et al. (2018), 10 different species of microbes were found to be differentially represented in responders versus nonresponders to anti-PD-1 treatment in patients with melanoma, NSCLC, and RCC. Among them, *A. muciniphila* and *Ruminococcus* species were strongly associated with response to treatment, while *B. longum* was particularly related to improved survival in responders to treatment (Jin et al., 2019; Liao et al., 2025).

Overall, the above findings indicate that the role of the microbiome in the response to immune checkpoint inhibitor treatment is that of an "immunologic co-regulator," where the balance of different microbial species determines whether the tumor microenvironment is "cold" and nonresponsive is "hot" and responsive to treatment. Significantly, the above findings have opened up the possibility of manipulating the tumor microenvironment to overcome resistance to treatment and convert an otherwise untreatable condition into a treatable one.

7.3.4 Intratumoral microbiome: A local driver of therapy resistance

For decades, it was accepted that tumors are sterile environments devoid of microbial influence except in the case of infection-associated cancers. This perception was changed by advances in high-throughput DNA sequencing, metagenomics, spatial transcriptomics, and culture-independent microbial detection assays. These technologies have conclusively proven that many types of solid tumors contain distinct populations of bacteria in their microenvironment. These bacteria are not merely contaminants but are now known to be biologically active entities that play a crucial role in influencing the behavior of the tumor and the effectiveness of treatment interventions.

The microbial communities found in the tumor microenvironment are distinct from those found in the surrounding healthy tissue. The presence of these microbes adds a new dimension to the biology of the tumor, which operates independently of the genetic background of the tumor. These microbes are known to be derived from distant mucosal sites such as the gut and are found to be translocated to the tumor via hematogenous routes, the lymphatic system, and/or direct anatomical invasion. This phenomenon is seen in various types of cancers such as pancreatic, colorectal, lung, and oral cancers. Once translocated to the tumor environment, the microbes have to acclimatize to the hypoxic and nutrient-variable environment of the tumor. This environment is already known to be characterized by immune evasion and metabolic rewiring.

The bacteria found in the tumor environment have specialized enzymes that play a crucial role in influencing the effectiveness of treatment interventions. These bacteria have the capability to biotransform chemotherapeutic drugs, scavenge reactive oxygen species, and modulate DNA repair pathways. This enables them to influence the mechanisms by which chemotherapy and immunotherapy cause cytotoxic effects on the tumor cells. This influence is distinct from the effects seen by the systemic host microbiome, which influences the host immune system and metabolic pathways. The effects of the intratumoral microbes are localized and have the capability to create "microdomains of resistance" within the tumor tissue itself (Bautista et al., 2025; Liao et al., 2025; Zhang et al., 2025a).

The first study to provide evidence of the role of intratumoral bacteria in chemotherapy resistance was conducted by Geller et al. (2017). In PDAC, *Gammaproteobacteria* were found in tumor tissues expressing a long form of CDD, an enzyme that inactivates one of the primary chemotherapeutic agents used to target PDAC: gemcitabine. The inactivation of gemcitabine by CDD in tumor tissues was mediated by the production of 2′,2′-difluorodeoxyuridine, a metabolite of gemcitabine that lacks chemotherapeutic activity (Geller et al., 2017). The presence of *Gammaproteobacteria* in tumor tissues essentially renders tumor cells chemoresistant without any mutation in the tumor cells themselves. Moreover, depletion of *Gammaproteobacteria* from tumor tissues in murine models using specific antibiotics restored chemosensitivity to gemcitabine and led to regression of tumors. The study provided a new paradigm in drug resistance by identifying that microbial enzymes in tumor tissues could be responsible for primary chemoresistance.

In addition to their role in chemotherapy resistance, tumor-resident microbes have also been implicated in the modulation of tumor immunity in various cancers. For example, in colorectal and breast cancers, *Fusobacterium nucleatum* was found to invade tumor tissues and induce oncogenic signaling cascades that promote tumor progression and metastasis. Specifically, *F. nucleatum* activates the nuclear factor of kappa light chain enhancer (NF-κB) and β-catenin signaling cascades in tumor cells, leading to enhanced tumor proliferation and immune evasion. *F. nucleatum* was also found to induce PD-L1 expression in tumor cells, leading to reduced activity of cytotoxic T cells and reduced efficacy of anti-PD1-based immunotherapies in tumors. Moreover, *F. nucleatum* was found to reduce the presence of CD8+ T cells in tumor tissues, leading to an immunologically cold tumor microenvironment (Gao et al., 2021; Parhi et al., 2020; Yu et al., 2017).

Notably, these immunosuppressive activities have been demonstrated to be reversible. Depletion of *F. nucleatum* was achieved in experimental models through the administration of antibiotics or bacteriophage therapy. This improved the infiltrative ability of T cells and the response to immune checkpoint therapy. This series of discoveries has demonstrated the dynamic nature of the tumor-microbiome interface. It has also emphasized the potential for the tumor microbiome to offer a solution to the problem of therapy resistance. This is particularly the case when the genomics of the tumor cannot offer an explanation for the observed phenomena. It is now possible to perceive tumors as dynamic ecological systems rather than merely malignant cell communities. The presence of the tumor microbiome has introduced a localized and metabolically active component. This component has the potential to shape the response of the tumor to therapy (Fig. 7.2).

7.4 Molecular mechanisms linking the microbiome to cancer therapy resistance

The role of the microbiome in the therapeutic outcome of anticancer therapy can be described as follows: the microbiome plays a role in the outcome of anticancer therapy through a highly interconnected network of metabolic, immunologic, and molecular pathways that function in concert at the systemic, enteric, and tumor microenvironments at the same time. Rather than a single mechanism, the microbiome affects the outcome of therapy in a complex manner that involves layered interactions with host metabolism, immunologic priming, and tumor biology, and these mechanisms ultimately dictate the success or failure of chemotherapy and immunotherapy in the long term (Gazzaniga & Kasper, 2025; Zalila-Kolsi et al., 2025).

7.4.1 Microbial metabolites as immune and drug modulators

One of the major ways in which the microbiome modulates the response to treatment is through the production of bioactive metabolites. The commensal bacteria in the human gut have been

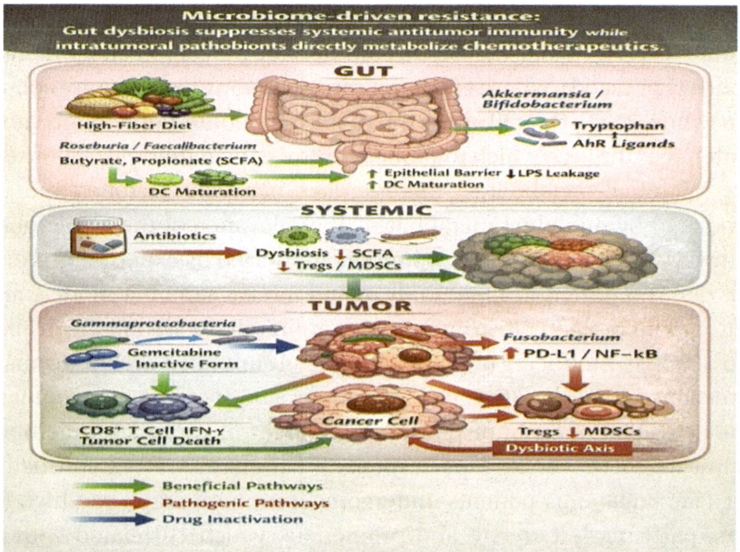

FIGURE 7.2 Microbiome-driven resistance to cancer therapy. This three-compartment model illustrates how gut microbiota influence systemic immunity and tumor response to therapy. In the gut, beneficial bacteria promote SCFA and AhR ligand production, enhancing epithelial integrity, dendritic cell maturation, and antitumor immune priming. In the systemic compartment, immune cells traffic to the tumor, while antibiotic-induced dysbiosis reduces SCFAs and promotes immunosuppressive Tregs and MDSCs. In the tumor, intratumoral bacteria directly mediate resistance by inactivating chemotherapeutic drugs and inducing immune evasion pathways. Green arrows indicate beneficial pathways, red arrows pathogenic mechanisms, and blue arrows drug inactivation. *Ahr*, aryl hydrocarbon receptor; *MDSCs*, myeloid-derived suppressor cells; *SCFA*, short-chain fatty acid; *Treg*, regulatory T cells.

shown to produce a wide variety of metabolites that have a significant effect on the host immune response and tumor progression.

One of the most studied metabolites in the context of cancer is the short-chain fatty acids (SCFAs), particularly butyrate and propionate, which are produced by the fermentation of fiber by the gut bacteria. The SCFAs have been shown to increase the strength of the intestinal epithelial lining, reduce systemic endotoxemia, and modulate the immune response through the balance between Tregs and effector T lymphocytes. The butyrate produced by the gut bacteria acts as a histone deacetylase inhibitor, leading to changes in the expression of various genes that promote the maturation of dendritic cells and the activation of cytotoxic CD8+ T cells. When there is a loss of biodiversity in the gut and the bacteria that produce SCFAs are reduced in number—a common feature in dysbiosis—the beneficial effects of the SCFAs are reduced. The reduced availability of SCFAs impairs antigen presentation by dendritic cells and CD8+ T-cell cytotoxicity, thereby reducing the efficacy of ICIs (Krishnamurthy et al., 2023).

Another key axis in this process is related to the metabolism of tryptophan, which is a critical amino acid in cancer therapy response. Tryptophan metabolism by microbes in the gut produces indole compounds, which in turn activate the aryl hydrocarbon receptor (AhR), a transcription factor required to preserve immune homeostasis in the mucosa and T cell fitness. The AhR pathway is required to preserve T cell persistence in tumors. However, disruption of this pathway by dysbiosis could lead to T cell exhaustion. Another key player in cancer therapy response is microbial secondary bile acids, whose effects on cancer therapy response are context-dependent (Zhu & Van den Eynde, 2024). Overall, these microbial metabolite-dependent pathways establish a "metabolic interface" through which microbes control cancer therapy response. This interface is mediated by microbial metabolites. This interface between microbes and cancer therapy response is mediated by microbial metabolites. The relevance of these microbial metabolite-dependent pathways to cancer therapy response is supported by experimental evidence.

Smith et al. (2013) reported in their study, using mouse sarcoma models maintained in a germ-free environment or in an environment with antibiotics added to the drinking water, that the elimination of SCFAs-producing microbes completely inhibited cyclophosphamide-induced Th1 immune responses and dendritic cell activation. However, butyrate supplementation restored immune activation and tumor rejection. The relevance of these microbial metabolite-dependent pathways to cancer therapy response in humans was established in a study in which 85 metastatic melanoma patients undergoing immunotherapy had high levels of SCFAs in their plasma, particularly butyrate and propionate, which correlated with favorable PFS. The high levels of these microbial metabolites correlated with high levels of *Ruminococcaceae* and CD8+/Treg in tumors. Overall, these microbial metabolite-dependent pathways establish a "metabolic interface" through which microbes control cancer therapy response (Smith et al., 2013).

7.4.2 Microbiome-driven immune remodeling

Apart from metabolite production, the microbiome also plays an influential role in the development of innate and adaptive immunity. The presence of beneficial commensal microorganisms stimulates the maturation of dendritic cells, increases antigen presentation efficiency, and stimulates tumor-specific CD8+ T-cell priming, which are essential in the treatment of tumors with ICI agents. On the contrary, an imbalance in the microbiome favors an immune response that is skewed toward immunosuppression, leading to increased Treg cells, reduced T-cell effector cytotoxicity, and increased MDSCs in the tumor microenvironment (Zeng et al., 2025a).

Microbial-associated molecular patterns (MAMPs), such as lipopolysaccharides (LPS) and peptidoglycan fragments, are sensed by innate immune cells through their interaction with Toll-like receptors (TLRs). The modulation of TLR signals is essential in the activation of dendritic cells and in the generation of antitumor immune responses. However, aberrant TLR signals have been implicated in chronic inflammation and immune exhaustion in tumors. The signals from the microbiome have also been shown to affect the production of cytokines, the expression of checkpoint ligands (e.g., PD-L1), and the efficiency of chemotherapy-induced immunogenic cell death, thereby affecting the outcome of immunotherapy and chemotherapy in tumors (Lu et al., 2025; Perl et al., 2025).

Clinical studies reinforce these mechanistic insights. A microbial consortium comprising *A. muciniphila, B. longum,* and *Ruminococcus* species has been identified as predictive of anti-PD-1 responsiveness in melanoma, NSCLC, and RCC populations. Importantly, fecal transplantation from responders into germ-free mice transferred PD-1 sensitivity and enhanced $CD8^+$ T-cell tumoricidal activity, demonstrating causality rather than mere association (Matson et al., 2018).

On the other hand, the impact of antibiotics on the microbiome offers strong clinical evidence for immune disruption. Cohort analyses have demonstrated that the administration of antibiotics before therapy reduces response rates, PFS, and OS in ICI-treated patients. Mechanistically, antibiotics have been shown to delete supportive cells of the dendritic cell compartment, reduce T cell priming, and increase the proportion of immunosuppressive cells, including Tregs and MDSCs. This leads to the development of "immunologically cold" tumors that are no longer susceptible to immune attack. Therefore, the microbiome is the master regulator of antitumor immunity. It determines whether ICI therapy is therapeutically reinvigorating or whether it is failing due to immune insufficiency (Pinato et al., 2019).

7.4.3 Tumor-resident microbiota and drug resistance

Besides a global suppression of immune functions, the microbiota that reside in the tumor have a direct effect on the phenotypic characterization of cancer cells. The intratumoral microbiome not localized to gastrointestinal sources regulates DNA damage responses, redox homeostasis, apoptotic thresholds, and intracellular signaling cascades. Some of the pathogenic species stimulate the pro-survival pathways, including NF-KB and STAT3, in tumor cells, which promotes proliferation, resistance to cytotoxic stress, and immune escape.

It is these microorganisms that thrive in the harsh conditions of the tumor microenvironment through the use of enzymatic pathways that reduce chemotherapy-induced oxidative stress and repair of DNA strand breaks. Intratumoral bacteria may also increase the apoptotic threshold of cancer cells by dampening the build-up of ROS and enhancing DNA-repair signaling, reducing the effectiveness of both chemotherapy and radiation therapy.

Moreover, the bacteria located in tumors might metabolize chemotherapeutic drugs locally, thus reducing their effective concentrations in tumor tissues. This local drug biotransformation can act in concert with tumor cell-intrinsic resistance processes to provide a dual-pronged model of resistance, one arm of which is microbial enzymatic inactivation of drugs, and another arm is microbe-mediated amplification of tumor survival pathways. The intratumoral microbiome will play a key role in the pathogenesis of therapeutic failure within this paradigm and will be independent of, and in some cases synergistic with, genetic mutations that confer intrinsic resistance (Jani et al., 2025; Xie et al., 2025; Zhou et al., 2025).

Taken together, these molecular mechanisms reveal that the microbiome influences cancer therapy through a multifaceted and dynamic network of interactions. From metabolite-mediated immune priming to tumor-localized drug inactivation, microbial communities shape therapeutic efficacy at every level of the tumor–host ecosystem. Appreciating this complexity is essential for developing microbiome-informed strategies that can overcome resistance and enhance precision oncology.

7.5 The tumor–microbiome–immune axis

The success or failure of cancer treatment is not determined solely by cancer genetics or drugs; rather, it is a result of a complex and dynamic interaction between cancer, immunity, and microbes. Although precision oncology has traditionally focused on genetic mutations, oncogenes, and molecular therapeutic targets, evidence is emerging to suggest that the microbiome is as important as cancer genetics in determining patient response to chemotherapy or immunotherapy. This understanding has led to the concept of a tripartite tumor–microbiome–immune axis in cancer treatment.

At a systemic level, gut microbiota play a key role in regulating immune homeostasis and metabolism. The production of bioactive metabolites such as SCFAs, indole derivatives from tryptophan metabolism, and secondary bile acids by commensal microbes can promote dendritic cell maturation, antigen presentation, and a balance between effector CD8+ T cells and regulatory T cells. This process is critical in generating a potent immune response against cancer, particularly in response to ICIs. The production of bioactive metabolites by a healthy, diverse microbiome can trigger a proinflammatory cascade, thereby optimizing T cell priming and creating a "hot" tumor microenvironment. On the other hand, a disrupted microbiome or dysbiosis can disrupt this immunologic balance. The disappearance or reduction of beneficial microbes and the expansion of proinflammatory or pathogenic microbes can lead to a higher number of Tregs, MDSCs, and upregulation of immune checkpoint molecules such as PD-L1 and CTLA-4 in the tumor microenvironment. This can lead to a failure in cancer treatment and a shift in the tumor-immune interface from a "cell kill" to a "cell tolerance" mechanism (Chung et al., 2024; Gunjur et al., 2024; Jamal et al., 2025).

Concomitantly, the tumor microbiome has localized oncogenic and pharmacological effects. In the tumor microenvironment, microbes may metabolize chemotherapeutic agents, thereby decreasing the concentration of drugs available to the tumor cells. In addition, the tumor microbiome activates prosurvival signaling pathways such as NF-κB and STAT3, thus promoting the proliferation of tumor cells and their survival against apoptosis. Moreover, the tumor microbiome may modulate the tumor cells' DNA repair mechanisms and their redox status, thus making the tumor cells more resistant to the cytotoxic effects of chemotherapy. Overall, the tumor microbiome and the immune system create a two-tiered tumor resistance mechanism, consisting of immunosuppression and localized chemotherapeutic resistance.

Collectively, the interplay between the tumor cells, the tumor microbiome, and the immune system creates a tumor microenvironment that is conducive to tumor development and therapeutic resistance. This novel tumor microenvironment is a dynamic tumor resistance platform superimposed over the inherent genetic tumor resistance mechanisms. This novel tumor microenvironment explains the therapeutic failure of immunotherapy in the presence of antibiotics, the therapeutic success of FMT in restoring chemotherapeutic sensitivity, and the therapeutic promise of tumor microbiome modulation. Overall, precision medicine may now transcend the traditional tumor-centric approach to a more holistic approach by including the tumor microbiome as a dynamic component in the development of novel cancer therapies (Bukowski et al., 2020; Ge et al., 2025; Kim et al., 2021).

7.6 Therapeutic modulation of the microbiome to overcome resistance

The recognition of the microbiome as a key player in cancer therapy resistance has created a brand-new therapeutic frontier. The microbiome is no longer regarded as a bystander or collateral damage in cancer treatment but rather as a therapeutic entity whose response can be modified to achieve a desired therapeutic outcome. This is a paradigm shift in cancer treatment and research, and it fits perfectly within the framework of precision medicine.

The advent of modern metagenomic sequencing technologies has enabled a detailed understanding of a patient's fecal microbiome. This includes understanding microbial diversity, identifying specific microbial components, and characterizing microbial metabolism. This information can then be correlated with genomic data from cancer patients to create a predictive algorithm to determine patient stratification based on their response to chemotherapy or immunotherapy. This will allow for early intervention in cancer treatment resistance, thereby preventing treatment failure.

This systems biology approach to cancer treatment also provides a framework to modulate the microbiome to achieve a therapeutic response. This includes FMT, probiotic therapy, fiber therapy, and microbial therapeutics to recode the tumor, microbiome, and immune response to cancer treatment. This will allow cancer treatment resistance to be averted and a therapeutic response to be achieved. The microbiome-directed therapies are no longer in the realm of imagination but have entered the realm of clinical validation (Petrelli et al., 2025; Spencer et al., 2021).

7.6.1 Probiotics, prebiotics, and diet

Of the various microbiome-targeted approaches, dietary modulation is one of the most accessible and physiologically logical interventions. The diet has a direct influence on the composition of the microbiome and the production of microbial metabolites. A high-fiber diet or the use of prebiotics and specific probiotics have shown their potential to increase the diversity of the gut microbiome and augment the antitumor immune potential.

Dietary fibers provide an important substrate that is fermented by commensal microbes like *Roseburia, Faecalibacterium*, and *Eubacterium* to produce SCFAs, especially butyrate and propionate. These metabolites are crucial in maintaining the integrity of the intestinal barrier, limiting endotoxin translocation, and regulating immune homeostasis. SCFAs have been shown to be essential in improving dendritic cell maturation, antigen presentation, and $CD8^+$ T-cell priming in the tumor microenvironment. In the tumor microenvironment, SCFAs have been shown to be important in limiting the accumulation of regulatory T cells, supporting the bioenergetics of effector T cells, and augmenting interferon gamma-mediated cytotoxic T-cell activity. A high-fiber diet thus converts immunologically "cold" tumors to inflamed tumors that are susceptible to immune checkpoint inhibitor therapy (Bautista et al., 2025; Bredon et al., 2024; Nguyen et al., 2024).

Preclinical models offer significant mechanistic evidence for these effects. For instance, in murine models of melanoma and colorectal cancer, high-fiber diets or inulin and pectin supplementation increased CD8+ T-cell infiltration into tumors and augmented the interferon-γ-mediated signaling cascade, significantly potentiating the effects of anti-PD-1 therapy. Conversely, fiber-deficient diets decreased SCFAs, increased tumor-infiltrating Tregs and MDSCs, and led to resistance against PD-1 inhibitor therapies. These adverse immune phenotypes, however, were absent in germ-free mice but could be replicated and corrected by fecal transplant and SCFA supplementation.

Preclinical models of specific probiotics suggest promising therapeutic effects in cancer treatment. For instance, colonization with *B. longum* and *A. muciniphila* has been shown in murine models of cancer to replicate the favorable responder phenotypes, significantly potentiating anti-PD-1 therapy by activating dendritic cells and priming T cells. These probiotics appear to activate a coordinated program of immune activation, which significantly potentiates PD-1 inhibitor therapies. In addition, fiber-replete diets supplemented with inulin and pectin increase tumor control and decrease Tregs, indicating a synergistic effect of diet and probiotics (Duan et al., 2025; Gamrath et al., 2025; Sardar et al., 2025; Ye et al., 2025; Zeng et al., 2025b).

Clinical validation of this evidence is also emerging. Observational and prospective studies in melanoma and NSCLC patient cohorts have indicated that improved objective response rates and PFS are associated with dietary fiber intake during immune checkpoint inhibitor therapy, irrespective of tumor mutational burden and PD-L1 expression. Metagenomic analysis in these cohorts also indicated enrichment of SCFAs and upregulation of interferon genes and antigen processing machinery. This evidence also points to the fact that indiscriminate probiotic consumption should be avoided since this may reduce microbial diversity and impair immunotherapy efficacy. Therefore, specific microbial modulation appears to be important.

Additional evidence for the therapeutic use of microbiome modulation was also obtained from phase I/II clinical trials in NSCLC and colorectal cancer. Probiotics containing *Lactobacillus rhamnosus* have also improved PFS when used in combination with ICIs. This may be due to the expansion of microbial networks containing SCFAs. Observational studies in 512 melanoma and NSCLC patients have indicated that prebiotic fiber consumption significantly improved response rates. However, this evidence was confounded by poor compliance with prebiotics (Fuller-Shavel et al., 2025; Malczewski et al., 2021; Somodi et al., 2025).

7.6.2 Fecal microbiota transplantation

FMT stands out as the most holistic approach to microbiome reconstitution. Unlike other approaches, such as dietary and probiotic interventions, that target specific microbial species, FMT offers the entire microbial ecosystem, allowing for rapid reconfiguration of the microbial community. This approach has emerged at the forefront in the treatment of immunotherapy resistance.

FMT, in transferring the microbial community from immunotherapy responders to non-responders, provides a complex immunomodulatory microbial community consisting of *A. muciniphila*, SCFA-producing *Clostridiales*, and beneficial bacteriophages, in addition to metabolically coordinated microbial networks. Unlike probiotics, which have difficulty in establishing long-lasting engraftment in chemotherapy and immunotherapy patients, FMT provides long-lasting microbial integration, including $CD8^+$ T-cell priming, myeloid reprogramming, and antitumor immune surveillance (Chen et al., 2019; Huang et al., 2022; Khoruts & Weingarden, 2014; Wu et al., 2025).

Mechanistically, FMT re-establishes immune pathways suppressed in ICI-refractory patients. Reconstitution with favorable microbes enhances intestinal barrier function, SCFA and indole production, dendritic cell activation, and tumor antigen presentation. This reduces Treg and MDSCs in the tumor microenvironment, relieving immune exhaustion. Germ-free or antibiotic-conditioned immunocompromised mouse melanoma (B16.SIY) and lung carcinoma (MC38) tumor models received FMT from ICI responders, which re-sensitized the tumors to PD-1 inhibition, enhancing intratumoral CD8+ T-cell density and tumor regression. In contrast, FMT from nonresponders did not provide these benefits (Bibbò et al., 2022; Ramesh et al., 2026; Wu et al., 2019).

Clinical trials have translated these findings into patient care. Landmark studies by Davar et al. (2021) and Baruch et al. (2021) demonstrated that melanoma patients refractory to prior PD-1 therapy achieved meaningful objective response rates following FMT from responder-derived donors combined with ICI rechallenge. These patients exhibited enhanced $CD8^+$ T-cell infiltration, increased interferon-γ expression, and microbial profiles resembling those of donors enriched in SCFA-producing taxa such as *F. prausnitzii* and *A. muciniphila*. Importantly, response rates were substantially higher than those of historical non-FMT controls (Baruch et al., 2021; Davar et al., 2021).

Although safety concerns, donor standardization, and regulatory complexities remain challenges, these studies establish FMT as a viable strategy for remodeling the tumor–microbiome–immune axis. The ability to overcome refractory immunotherapy resistance through microbial ecosystem transplantation signals the beginning of microbiome-directed precision immuno-oncology.

7.6.3 Microbiome-targeted drugs and engineered bacteria

Apart from the aforementioned ecological modulation of the microbiome by means of diet or FMT, new approaches are being developed to precisely engineer or manipulate the microbial community. Microbiome-based therapeutics are a more refined approach compared to the use of broad-spectrum antibiotics, which act indiscriminately on both good and bad microbes in the community.

Precision antibiotics and bacteriophage-based treatments are being developed to selectively eliminate pathogenic bacteria involved in drug metabolism and immunosuppression, while sparing immune-commensal microbes. These treatments target microbes involved in the inactivation of chemotherapeutic drugs and the induction of Treg populations, to restore the efficacy of drugs without affecting the microbial architecture as a whole (Allemailem, 2021; Harimoto & Danino, 2019; Wang et al., 2025b).

More promising are the recent advances in the field of engineered bacterial therapeutics. Recent advances in the field of synthetic biology have enabled the genetic engineering of microbes to produce immunomodulatory effects directly in the tumor microenvironment. Engineered microbes have the potential to produce aryl hydrocarbon receptor agonists, produce SCFAs locally, secrete cytokines, and degrade immunosuppressive metabolites. These living biotherapeutic agents allow precise spatiotemporal regulation of the immune microenvironment, which can be used to reprogram the tumor microenvironment.

Clinical trials conducted in melanoma and NSCLC patients have revealed the safety and preliminary efficacy of microbial therapies engineered to work in conjunction with checkpoint inhibitors. By shifting the immune balance from tolerogenic to effector-dominant immune states, these microbial therapies may be effective in overcoming the limitations of resistance mechanisms beyond the control of escalating drugs. In comparison to traditional probiotics, microbial therapeutics offer the advantage of targeted functionality, colonization, and immune modulation.

Overall, these precision microbiome therapies mark the dawn of a new era in the history of cancer therapy. Instead of targeting the tumor cells, it is likely that the focus of cancer therapy will be to modulate the microbiome to enhance the immune response and the sensitivity to drugs. By targeting the tumor–microbiome–immune axis at the levels of diet, ecology, drugs, and microbes, the therapeutic modulation of the microbiome is one of the most promising means to overcome the resistance mechanisms in the era of precision medicine (Allemailem, 2021; Farmer et al., 2025; Gurbatri et al., 2022).

7.7 Integration into precision oncology

The integration of microbiome science into precision oncology is arguably the most promising development in the evolution of cancer therapy in recent years. Precision medicine in oncology has traditionally relied on the identification of tumor-specific genomic alterations, including mutations and targets, to inform therapeutic decisions. Although the tumor-centric approach to precision medicine has revolutionized the field of oncology, it does not account for interpatient variability in response to therapy. The metagenomic and metabolomic analysis of the microbiome provides a more dynamic and functional approach to precision oncology, allowing for the assessment of real-time biological processes that can provide information on the competency of the host's immune system, its metabolic status, and its adaptability to therapy.

Somatic mutations, unlike the microbiome, are largely invariant once established and cannot be easily changed. Therefore, the adaptability of the microbiome to its microenvironment and its consequent potential to serve as a biomarker and/or therapeutic target render it an attractive entity in precision oncology. Advances in high-throughput sequencing have made it possible to obtain a detailed profile of the microbiome, including its functional metabolic pathways and the concentration of immunomodulatory metabolites, including SCFAs, indole derivatives, and secondary bile acids, and to correlate them with clinical endpoints, including response rate, PFS, and recurrence probability. More and more, such analyses have shown that the microbiome not only correlates with, but may also predict, the outcome of therapy (Conti et al., 2023; Ting et al., 2022).

Large clinical trials have now provided further support for the predictive potential of the microbiome. Indeed, across various tumor types, including melanoma, NSCLC, renal cell carcinoma, and gastrointestinal cancers, certain microbial profiles have been correlated with the likelihood of response to ICI therapy. These have included increased alpha diversity, the presence of certain microbes like **A. muciniphila**, **F. prausnitzii**, *Ruminococcaceae*, and increased SCFAs in the stool and plasma of the host. Such profiles have been associated with improved ORR, PFS, and OS in the setting of ICI therapy. Such an association of the microbiome with the likelihood of response to therapy has also provided the potential for the development of new stratification tools based on the host's microbiome profile. This is especially true when compared to genomic and immunological markers like TMB and PD-L1 expression (Derosa et al., 2022; Yousefi et al., 2024; Zhu et al., 2024). This is because the host's microbiome profile is likely to have an impact on the host's response to therapy. Indeed, the host's response to therapy is likely to be determined by the host's microbiome profile. This is especially true when compared to other host stratification tools like TMB and PD-L1 expression. This is because the host's response to therapy is likely to be determined by the host's microbiome profile. Indeed, the host's response to therapy is likely to be determined by the host's microbiome profile. This is especially true when compared to other host stratification tools like TMB and PD-L1 expression. This is because the host's response to therapy is likely to be determined by the host's microbiome profile. Indeed, the host's response to therapy is likely to be determined by the host's microbiome profile.

The microbiome, therefore, plays a dual role of prognostic sentinel and interventional nexus, and its results can be used to inform regimen selection, supportive care, and dosing strategies to limit unwanted ecological impact. Nutritional optimization and avoidance of unnecessary antibiotic use can be strategically implemented in the treatment regimen to maintain beneficial microbial networks.

These advances, therefore, collectively reposition the study of the microbiome as an essential component in the precision oncology paradigm, shifting the focus from the sole study of the tumor genome to the holistic stewardship of the tumor, host, and microbiome. The study of the microbiome can, therefore, be used to develop more holistic and dynamic approaches to personalizing cancer therapy, recognizing the microbiome's potential to serve as a prognostic and interventional tool in the process and to ultimately determine the success of the therapy itself (Dakal et al., 2025; Dey & Choubey, 2024).

7.8 Limitations

Despite increasing evidence indicating the significant role played by the microbiome in the modulation of resistance to cancer therapy, there are significant limitations to drawing definitive conclusions regarding causality and clinical applicability. Much of the current published data is based upon observational studies utilizing metagenomics approaches. Although this research indicates a strong association between the microbiome and therapy results, it does not allow for the assessment of causality versus consequence. For example, changes in the microbiome may be both a cause and a consequence of disease progression and treatment effects. Confounding variables such as disease stage, previous treatments, nutritional status, antibiotics, and host genetic background are often not controlled for in these studies.

Even though interventional studies have also been performed and have indicated promise for the use of FMT to modulate ICI resistance, there are significant limitations to drawing conclusions from this research. For example, FMT studies have indicated that approximately one-third of ICI nonresponders may be rendered responsive to therapy by the administration of the fecal microbiota from responders. Although this research provides a rare glimpse into causality, the studies performed to date have significant limitations. For example, although there is a variety of donor fecal microbiotas, there are significant limitations to the reproducibility of this research due to the lack of standardization for donor selection and response criteria. Survival endpoints have also not been fully characterized for this research (Barbosa et al., 2023; Tegegne & Savidge, 2025).

Another major challenge is the considerable heterogeneity of the human microbiome. For instance, the microbial composition varies among different geographic locations, ethnic groups, types of diets, environmental exposures, antibiotic use, co-existing diseases, and the genetic background of the individuals. For example, the microbial signatures of immunotherapy response in melanoma patients of Western descent are unlikely to be applicable to Asian patients suffering from NSCLC, or to patients suffering from different types of cancer. This heterogeneity of the human microbiome is a major limitation of the existing studies and indicates the need to conduct population-specific validation studies (Mallott et al., 2023).

Methodological limitations of the existing studies also include the sampling methods. For example, the existing studies have largely used fecal metagenomics as a surrogate marker of the human microbiome. Although fecal metagenomics has provided considerable insight into the human microbiome, it is unlikely to be a reliable indicator of the tumor microenvironment. For example, the microbial population in the tumor microenvironment, which directly interacts with cancer cells, tumor-infiltrating immune cells, and chemotherapeutic drugs, is anatomically and functionally different from the microbial population in the gut.

In addition, safety issues add another level of complexity to the translation of therapy. While FMT has been shown to be safe in the nononcologic setting, there are still safety issues related to the transmission of pathogens and the risk of opportunistic infections and ecological disturbances in the compromised host. Similarly, the indiscriminate administration of probiotics can have the unintended consequence of inhibiting the growth of native flora or delaying the return of the normal microbiome in the setting of antibiotic-induced dysbiosis. Indeed, new data suggest that some of these commercial preparations of probiotics can actually decrease diversity rather than increase it and thereby potentially negate the desired effects of therapy (Saha et al., 2021; Wang et al., 2016).

Lastly, the mechanistic basis of the therapy is still somewhat mysterious. While the association of certain microbes, for example, *A. muciniphila* or *F. prausnitzii*, with therapy is highly suggestive of the potential for therapy to impact the course of the disease, the molecular basis of the relationship of individual bacterial enzyme activity and the host signaling pathways to drug resistance is still an evolving area of research. Advanced integrative tools will likely be necessary to unravel the complex interactions of the host and the microbes to allow for precision-targeted therapy of the microbiome.

In conclusion, while the microbiome is an exciting new frontier in the treatment of oncology patients, there are still many hurdles to overcome before the full potential of the microbiome can be harnessed.

7.9 Future directions

The integration of microbiome science into precision oncology has tremendous potential, but its successful application in clinical practice will require simultaneous scientific, technological, and regulatory advances. As evidence mounts to support a relationship between microbial communities and therapeutic resistance or responsiveness, it is essential to go beyond associative evidence to predictive, mechanistic, and interventionist approaches.

The first step in this process is to integrate high-resolution microbiome analysis into prospective oncology clinical trials. Advanced metagenomics, metabolomics, transcriptomics, and high-resolution microbial taxonomic analysis should be incorporated into clinical research protocols. This will allow, in addition to microbial species identification, the determination of functional microbial metabolic pathways, enzymatic capabilities, and immune-modulatory metabolites. It is also important to note that longitudinal sampling, or sampling prior to, during, and after treatment, is a key element in this process. This will allow clinicians to identify dynamic microbial perturbations that precede therapeutic resistance, providing a window in which to intervene. Rather than merely detecting therapeutic resistance in a clinical patient, clinicians will eventually be able to predict it through microbial signatures and implement therapeutic prevention strategies such as dietary recalibration, microbial therapeutic intervention, or selective antibiotic therapy (Kumar et al., 2026; Zhang et al., 2019).

Another frontier to be addressed is to extend microbiome research beyond the gut to study the intratumoral microbiome. The microbes in tumors have a direct interaction with cancer cells, components of the tumor microenvironment, immune components, and pharmacological agents. The microbial communities in tumors have a direct effect on DNA repair, oxidative stress, drug metabolism, and immune checkpoint functions. Spatial microbiomics will be required to study the microbes in tumors and their symbiotic relationship with cancer and immune components. This could lead to a better understanding of cancer and could result in the discovery of new targets to interfere with microbe-induced drug resistance (Li et al., 2022). Another frontier in cancer treatment is to innovate cancer therapies. The current microbiome-based therapies, such as conventional probiotics and FMT, are still in their infancy and lack precision and reproducibility. The future could be in designing engineered microbial communities and synthetic biology-based approaches. Engineered microbes could be used to secrete immunostimulatory cytokines, produce aryl hydrocarbon receptor agonists, metabolize immunosuppressive compounds, and degrade tumor-protective compounds in the tumor microenvironment. Gene editing technologies such as CRISPR could be used to delete genes from microbes in tumors to prevent resistance to cancer drugs without affecting beneficial microbes. Another form of precision medicine could be achieved through bacteriophage therapy, in which bacteriophages could be used to target particular types of microbes in tumors, such as microbes involved in drug metabolism or immunosuppression. This could lead to a spatiotemporal control over microbes in tumors and could result in a cancer microbiome–immune axis that could be manipulated to achieve therapeutic effects (Nazir et al., 2024).

However, equally important to the development of microbiome science itself will be the integration of such data with genomic and immunophenotypic data using artificial intelligence and machine learning techniques. Cancer biology produces vast amounts of multidimensional data, and the addition of microbiome data will add yet another complex dimension to the analysis. AI techniques may be used to develop multiomics analyses that can process microbial diversity, metabolite concentration, tumor mutational burden, immunophenotypic infiltration, and treatment history in real-time and in concert with each other. Such techniques may be used to predict treatment response, identify patients at highest risk of developing resistance, and provide antibiotic and other microbiome-directed therapy in real-time. Such a convergence of microbiome science and computational oncology may lead to the development of a new approach to treatment stratification, away from the traditional approach of genome-based treatment and toward a more holistic approach to treatment based on the ecosystem itself (D'Urso & Broccolo, 2024; Hsu et al., 2026; McCoubrey et al., 2021).

Modulating the microbiome may become the key to the long-term extension of immunotherapy response, prevention of chemoresistance, and reprogramming the course of survival in cancer patients. Rather than seeing the development of resistance to immunotherapies and chemotherapy as an inevitable outcome, the clinician of the future may be able to intervene at the level of the microbial ecosystem to extend the period of antitumor immune response and reprogram the course of survival in cancer patients. Such a paradigm shift in the way in which we approach cancer treatment, away from the tumor itself and toward the ecosystem, has the potential to redefine the very way in which we approach the treatment of cancer in the future, not just in the genome, but in the microbiome itself.

7.10 Conclusions

The current cumulative scientific evidence now unequivocally confirms the human microbiome to be a key factor in influencing therapeutic responsiveness and resistance in modern oncology. No longer viewed as a mere bystander in the field of cancer biology, the human microbiome now appears to be an active and dynamic player in influencing treatment outcomes. Both GI tract and tumor-associated microbes play a pivotal role in the direct regulation of drug pharmacodynamics, immune homeostasis, and tumor architecture. Through the metabolic bioconversion of chemotherapeutic drugs, the generation of immunomodulatory metabolites, and the bidirectional regulation of innate and adaptive immune pathways, the human microbiome plays a profound role in influencing treatment success or failure.

Significantly, this chapter also focuses on the fact that dysbiosis in the human microbiome, caused by various factors such as chemotherapy, radiotherapy, hospitalization, dietary changes, and previous use of antibiotics, plays a significant role in compromising treatment efficacy. Loss of key microbial populations results in poor dendritic cell maturation, reduced priming of CD8+ T cells, and the creation of immunosuppressive niches rich in regulatory T cells and myeloid-derived suppressor cells. Conversely, the maintenance of eubiosis in the human microbiome results in improved immunosurveillance, maximized immune checkpoint inhibitor therapy efficacy, and re-established susceptibility to chemotherapeutic drugs. This association of improved treatment outcomes with microbial diversity and enrichment of specific microbial populations underscores the close association of microbial ecology with cancer treatment.

The convergence of these mechanistic, translational, and clinical data places the microbiome not merely as an associative biomarker but rather as a target for therapy itself. Preclinical models have established causal associations between microbial species and therapeutic responses, and early clinical trials of FMT have established the proof of principle that resistance to therapy can be at least partially overcome through microbial reconstitution. Dietary therapy, probiotics, responder-derived microbial consortia, and microbial engineering represent innovative therapeutic strategies that are progressing from preclinical to clinical application. These examples collectively support the notion that the tumor–microbiome–immune axis can be dynamically reprogrammed, and that the process of resistance, once considered an irreversible outcome, can be at least partially reversed.

However, to bring these and other promising strategies to routine clinical application, standardization, long-term safety assessment, and integration with existing oncologic practices will be important considerations in the future of precision oncology. The future of precision oncology may well depend on the simultaneous assessment of the tumor genome, the immune system, and the microbiome itself, and the potential benefits that such an approach may have in terms of improving the process of prognostication, therapy selection, and supportive care, including antibiotic therapy and nutritional support, among other things. The paradigm shift in the field of oncology is clear: effective cancer therapy can no longer be considered in the absence of the context in which the tumor itself exists.

Microbiome-based approaches promise a new dawn in the field of oncology, which extends beyond the traditional tumor-centric model and incorporates a holistic model of cancer therapy. In the process, precision medicine approaches are likely to achieve long-lasting and effective anti-tumor effects, minimize the emergence of resistance, and promote patient survival. As the field of cancer research advances, the microbiome has the potential to emerge as a crucial component of cancer therapy in the near future.

References

Adlakha, Y. K., & Chhabra, R. (2025). The human microbiome: Redefining cancer pathogenesis and therapy. *Cancer Cell International, 25*(1). https://doi.org/10.1186/s12935-025-03787-x.

Alanazi, A., Younas, S., Ejaz, H., Bi, B., Mazhari, Z., Abosalif, K., Abdalla, A. E., Alruwaili, M., Atif, M., & Junaid, K. (2024). Exploration of the human microbiome's role in health and disease through the lens of genetics. *Journal of Pure and Applied Microbiology, 18*(3), 1413–1423. https://doi.org/10.22207/jpam.18.3.61.

Allemailem, K. S. (2021). Innovative approaches of engineering tumor-targeting bacteria with different therapeutic payloads to fight cancer: A smart strategy of disease management. *International Journal of Nanomedicine, 16*, 8159–8184. https://doi.org/10.2147/IJN.S338272.

Alsaafeen, B. H., Ali, B. R., & Elkord, E. (2025). Resistance mechanisms to immune checkpoint inhibitors: Updated insights. *Emirates Molecular Cancer, 24*(1). https://doi.org/10.1186/s12943-024-02212-7.

Bai, B., Ma, J., Xu, W., Chen, X., Chen, X., Lv, C., Su, W., Li, Y., Sun, H., Zhang, B., Xiang, D., Li, Z., Wu, Y., Sun, J., & Yin, M. (2025). Gut microbiota and colorectal cancer: Mechanistic insights, diagnostic advances, and microbiome-based therapeutic strategies. *Frontiers in Microbiology, 16*. https://doi.org/10.3389/fmicb.2025.1699893.

Barbosa, E. C., Bucar, E. E. C., Jubé, G. R., Silveira, L. B., Silva, N. C. D., Faria, P. C. C., Ramos, P. L. C., Moraes, V. R. Y., & Barros, J. O. B. (2023). Fecal microbiota transplantation and its repercussions in patients with melanoma refractory to anti-PD-1 therapy: Scope review. *Revista do Colegio Brasileiro de Cirurgioes, 50*. https://doi.org/10.1590/0100-6991e-20233490-en.

Baruch, E. N., Youngster, I., Ben-Betzalel, G., Ortenberg, R., Lahat, A., Katz, L., Adler, K., Dick-Necula, D., Raskin, S., Bloch, N., Rotin, D., Anafi, L., Avivi, C., Melnichenko, J., Steinberg-Silman, Y., Mamtani, R., Harati, H., Asher, N., Shapira-Frommer, R., … Boursi, B. (2021). Fecal microbiota transplant promotes response in immunotherapy-refractory melanoma patients. *Science, 371*(6529), 602–609. https://doi.org/10.1126/science.abb5920.

Bautista, J., Fuentes-Yépez, M. P., Adatty-Molina, J., & López-Cortés, A. (2025). Microbial signatures in metastatic cancer. *Frontiers in Medicine, 12*. https://doi.org/10.3389/fmed.2025.1654792.

Bibbò, S., Ianiro, G., Giambò, F., Settanni, C. R., Cammarota, G., & Gasbarrini, A. (2022). Role of gut microbiome on immunotherapy efficacy in melanoma. *Human Vaccines and Immunotherapeutics, 18*(3). https://doi.org/10.1080/21645515.2021.1926759.

Birnboim-Perach, R., & Benhar, I. (2024). Using combination therapy to overcome diverse challenges of immune checkpoint inhibitors treatment. *International Journal of Biological Sciences, 20*(10), 3911–3922. https://doi.org/10.7150/ijbs.93697.

Böhm, D., Russ, E., Guchelaar, H. J., Ziemons, J., Penders, J., Smidt, M. L., van Best, N., & Deenen, M. J. (2025). The role of the gut microbiota in chemotherapy response, efficacy and toxicity: A systematic review. *npj Precision Oncology, 9*(1). https://doi.org/10.1038/s41698-025-01034-0.

Bredon, M., Danne, C., Pham, H. P., Ruffié, P., Bessede, A., Rolhion, N., Creusot, L., Brot, L., Alonso, I., Langella, P., Derosa, L., Cortot, A. B., Routy, B., Zitvogel, L., Segata, N., & Sokol, H. (2024). *Faecalibaterium prausnitzii* strain EXL01 boosts efficacy of immune checkpoint inhibitors. *OncoImmunology, 13*(1). https://doi.org/10.1080/2162402X.2024.2374954.

Bukowski, K., Kciuk, M., & Kontek, R. (2020). Mechanisms of multidrug resistance in cancer chemotherapy. *International Journal of Molecular Sciences, 21*(9), 3233. https://doi.org/10.3390/ijms21093233.

Burgess, D. J., Doles, J., Zender, L., Xue, W., Ma, B., McCombie, W. R., Hannon, G. J., Lowe, S. W., & Hemann, M. T. (2008). Topoisomerase levels determine chemotherapy response in vitro and in vivo. *Proceedings of the National Academy of Sciences, 105*(26), 9053–9058. https://doi.org/10.1073/pnas.0803513105.

Chacon, J., Faizuddin, F., McKee, J. C., Sheikh, A., Vasquez, V. M., Gadad, S. S., Mayer, G., Siby, S., McCabe, M., & Dhandayuthapani, S. (2025). Unlocking the microbial symphony: The interplay of human microbiota in cancer immunotherapy response. *Cancers, 17*(5), 813. https://doi.org/10.3390/cancers17050813.

Chen, D., Wu, J., Jin, D., Wang, B., & Cao, H. (2019). Fecal microbiota transplantation in cancer management: Current status and perspectives. *International Journal of Cancer, 145*(8), 2021–2031. https://doi.org/10.1002/ijc.32003.

Chung, I. Y., Kim, J., & Koh, A. (2024). The microbiome matters: Its impact on cancer development and therapeutic responses. *Journal of Microbiology, 62*(3), 137–152. https://doi.org/10.1007/s12275-024-00110-7.

Ciernikova, S., Sevcikova, A., & Mego, M. (2024). Targeting the gut and tumor microbiome in cancer treatment resistance. *American Journal of Physiology-Cell Physiology, 327*(6), C1433. https://doi.org/10.1152/ajpcell.00201.2024.

Conti, G., D'Amico, F., Fabbrini, M., Brigidi, P., Barone, M., & Turroni, S. (2023). Pharmacomicrobiomics in anticancer therapies: Why the gut microbiota should be pointed out. *Genes, 14*(1), 55. https://doi.org/10.3390/genes14010055.

Dakal, T. C., Xu, C., & Kumar, A. (2025). Advanced computational tools, artificial intelligence and machine-learning approaches in gut microbiota and biomarker identification. *Frontiers in Medical Technology, 6*. https://doi.org/10.3389/fmedt.2024.1434799.

Damodaran, C., Cho, J. Y., & Güngör, C. (2025). Therapeutic resistance and combination therapy for cancer: Recent developments and future directions. *Scientific Reports, 15*(1). https://doi.org/10.1038/s41598-025-12725-w.

Davar, D., Dzutsev, A. K., McCulloch, J. A., Rodrigues, R. R., Chauvin, J. M., Morrison, R. M., Deblasio, R. N., Menna, C., Ding, Q., Pagliano, O., Zidi, B., Zhang, S., Badger, J. H., Vetizou, M., Cole, A. M., Fernandes, M. R., Prescott, S., Costa, R. G. F., Balaji, A. K., ... Zarour, H. M. (2021). Fecal microbiota transplant overcomes resistance to anti-PD-1 therapy in melanoma patients. *Science, 371*(6529), 595–602. https://doi.org/10.1126/science.abf3363.

Derosa, L., Routy, B., Thomas, A. M., Iebba, V., Zalcman, G., Friard, S., Mazieres, J., Audigier-Valette, C., Moro-Sibilot, D., Goldwasser, F., Silva, C. A. C., Terrisse, S., Bonvalet, M., Scherpereel, A., Pegliasco, H., Richard, C., Ghiringhelli, F., Elkrief, A., Desilets, A., Blanc-Durand, F., ... Besse, B. (2022). Intestinal *Akkermansia muciniphila* predicts clinical response to PD-1 blockade in patients with advanced non-small-cell lung cancer. *Nature Medicine, 28*(2), 315–324. https://doi.org/10.1038/s41591-021-01655-5.

Dey, P., & Choubey, S. (2024). An urgent need for longitudinal microbiome profiling coupled with machine learning interventions. *Frontiers in Microbiology, 15*. https://doi.org/10.3389/fmicb.2024.1487841.

Duan, H., Xu, B., Luo, P., Chen, T., & Zou, J. (2025). Microbial metabolites and their influence on the tumor microenvironment. *Frontiers in Immunology, 16*. https://doi.org/10.3389/fimmu.2025.1675677.

D'Urso, F., & Broccolo, F. (2024). Applications of artificial intelligence in microbiome analysis and probiotic interventions—An overview and perspective based on the current state of the art. *Applied Sciences, 14*(19), 8627. https://doi.org/10.3390/app14198627.

Eiman, L., Moazzam, K., Anjum, S., Kausar, H., Sharif, E. A. M., & Ibrahim, W. N. (2025). Gut dysbiosis in cancer immunotherapy: Microbiota-mediated resistance and emerging treatments. *Frontiers in Immunology, 16*. https://doi.org/10.3389/fimmu.2025.1575452.

Elkrief, A., Pidgeon, R., Vareki, S. M., Messaoudene, M., Castagner, B., & Routy, B. (2025). The gut microbiome as a target in cancer immunotherapy: Opportunities and challenges for drug development. *Nature Reviews Drug Discovery, 24*(9), 685–704. https://doi.org/10.1038/s41573-025-01211-7.

Ericsson, A. C., Akter, S., Hanson, M. M., Busi, S. B., Parker, T. W., Schehr, R. J., Hankins, M. A., Ahner, C. E., Davis, J. W., Franklin, C. L., Amos-Landgraf, J. M., & Bryda, E. C. (2015). Differential susceptibility to colorectal cancer due to naturally occurring gut microbiota. *Oncotarget, 6*(32), 33689–33704. https://doi.org/10.18632/oncotarget.5604.

Farmer, S., Francis, O., & Goyal, N. (2025). Exploiting Salmonella typhimurium as a novel cancer therapeutic agent: From tumor colonization to metabolic engineering. *World Journal of Microbiology and Biotechnology, 41*(12). https://doi.org/10.1007/s11274-025-04716-w.

Fuller-Shavel, N., Davies, E. J., & Hasson, S. P. (2025). Nutritional strategies in supporting immune checkpoint inhibitor, PI3K inhibitor, and tyrosine kinase inhibitor cancer therapies. *Frontiers in Nutrition, 12*. https://doi.org/10.3389/fnut.2025.1670598.

Gamrath, L., Pedersen, T. B., Møller, M. V., Volmer, L. M., Holst-Christensen, L., Vestermark, L. W., & Donskov, F. (2025). Role of the microbiome and diet for response to cancer checkpoint immunotherapy: A narrative review of clinical trials. *Current Oncology Reports, 27*(1), 45–58. https://doi.org/10.1007/s11912-024-01622-6.

Gao, Y., Bi, D., Xie, R., Li, M., Guo, J., Liu, H. u, Guo, X., Fang, J., Ding, T., Zhu, H., Cao, Y., Xing, M., Zheng, J., Xu, Q., Xu, Q., Wei, Q., & Qin, H. (2021). *Fusobacterium nucleatum* enhances the efficacy of PD-L1 blockade in colorectal cancer. *Signal Transduction and Targeted Therapy, 6*(1). https://doi.org/10.1038/s41392-021-00795-x.

Gazzaniga, F. S., & Kasper, D. L. (2025). The gut microbiome and cancer response to immune checkpoint inhibitors. *Journal of Clinical Investigation, 135*(3). https://doi.org/10.1172/JCI184321.

Ge, M., Chen, X. Y., Huang, P., Fleishman, J. S., Yang, D. H., Wu, Z. X., Ke, Z. F., & Chen, Z. S. (2025). Understanding and overcoming multidrug resistance in cancer. *Nature Reviews Clinical Oncology, 22*(10), 760–780. https://doi.org/10.1038/s41571-025-01059-1.

Geller, L. T., Barzily-Rokni, M., Danino, T., Jonas, O. H., Shental, N., Nejman, D., Gavert, N., Zwang, Y., Cooper, Z. A., Shee, K., Thaiss, C. A., Reuben, A., Livny, J., Avraham, R., Frederick, D. T., Ligorio, M., Chatman, K., Johnston, S. E., Mosher, C. M., ... Straussman, R. (2017). Potential role of intratumor bacteria in mediating tumor resistance to the chemotherapeutic drug gemcitabine. *Science, 357*(6356), 1156–1160. https://doi.org/10.1126/science.aah5043.

Gongora, C., Vezzio-Vie, N., Tuduri, S., Denis, V., Causse, A., Auzanneau, C., Collod-Beroud, G., Coquelle, A., Pasero, P., Pourquier, P., Martineau, P., & Del Rio, M. (2011). New topoisomerase I mutations are associated with resistance to camptothecin. *Molecular Cancer, 10*. https://doi.org/10.1186/1476-4598-10-64.

Gopalakrishnan, V., Spencer, C. N., Nezi, L., Reuben, A., Andrews, M. C., Karpinets, T. V., Prieto, P. A., Vicente, D., Hoffman, K., Wei, S. C., Cogdill, A. P., Zhao, L., Hudgens, C. W., Hutchinson, D. S., Manzo, T., Petaccia De Macedo, M., Cotechini, T., Kumar, T., Chen, W. S., ... Wargo, J. A. (2018). Gut microbiome modulates response to anti-PD-1 immunotherapy in melanoma patients. *Science, 359*(6371), 97–103. https://doi.org/10.1126/science.aan4236.

Gou, W., Fu, Y., Yue, L., Chen, G. D., Cai, X., Shuai, M., Xu, F., Yi, X., Chen, H., Zhu, Y., Xiao, M. L., Jiang, Z., Miao, Z., Xiao, C., Shen, B., Wu, X., Zhao, H., Ling, W., Wang, J., Chen, Y. M., Guo, T., & Zheng, J. S. (2021). Gut microbiota, inflammation, and molecular signatures of host response to infection. *Journal of Genetics and Genomics, 48*(9), 792–802. https://doi.org/10.1016/j.jgg.2021.04.002.

Gunjur, A., Shao, Y., Rozday, T., Klein, O., Mu, A., Haak, B. W., Markman, B., Kee, D., Carlino, M. S., Underhill, C., Frentzas, S., Michael, M., Gao, B., Palmer, J., Cebon, J., Behren, A., Adams, D. J., & Lawley, T. D. (2024). A gut microbial signature for combination immune checkpoint blockade across cancer types. *Nature Medicine, 30*(3), 797–809. https://doi.org/10.1038/s41591-024-02823-z.

Gurbatri, C. R., Arpaia, N., & Danino, T. (2022). Engineering bacteria as interactive cancer therapies. *Science, 378*(6622), 858–864. https://doi.org/10.1126/science.add9667.

Harimoto, T., & Danino, T. (2019). Engineering bacteria for cancer therapy. *Emerging Topics in Life Sciences, 3*(5), 623–629. https://doi.org/10.1042/ETLS20190096.

Holohan, C., Van Schaeybroeck, S., Longley, D. B., & Johnston, P. G. (2013). Cancer drug resistance: An evolving paradigm. *Nature Reviews Cancer, 13*(10), 714–726. https://doi.org/10.1038/nrc3599.

Hsu, C. Y., Askar, S., Alshkarchy, S. S., Nayak, P. P., Attabi, K. A. L., Khan, M. A., Mayan, J. A., Sharma, M. K., Islomov, S., & Soleimani Samarkhazan, H. (2026). AI-driven multi-omics integration in precision oncology: Bridging the data deluge to clinical decisions. *Clinical and Experimental Medicine, 26*(1). https://doi.org/10.1007/s10238-025-01965-9.

Huang, J., Zheng, X., Kang, W., Hao, H., Mao, Y., Zhang, H., Chen, Y., Tan, Y., He, Y., Zhao, W., & Yin, Y. (2022). Metagenomic and metabolomic analyses reveal synergistic effects of fecal microbiota transplantation and anti-PD-1 therapy on treating colorectal cancer. *Frontiers in Immunology, 13*. https://doi.org/10.3389/fimmu.2022.874922.

Iida, N., Dzutsev, A., Stewart, C. A., Smith, L., Bouladoux, N., Weingarten, R. A., Molina, D. A., Salcedo, R., Back, T., Cramer, S., Dai, R. M., Kiu, H., Cardone, M., Naik, S., Patri, A. K., Wang, E., Marincola, F. M., Frank, K. M., Belkaid, Y., ... Goldszmid, R. S. (2013). Commensal bacteria control cancer response to therapy by modulating the tumor microenvironment. *Science, 342*(6161), 967–970. https://doi.org/10.1126/science.1240527.

Jamal, A., Kamal, M. A., Alqurashi, Y. E., Al-Malki, E. S., Naiyer, M. M., Hussain, S. A., & Hattiwale, H. M. (2025). The microbiome-cancer axis as a hidden contributor to early-onset tumorigenesis. *Medical Oncology, 42*(10). https://doi.org/10.1007/s12032-025-02988-8.

Jani, C. T., Edwards, K., Bhanushali, C., Zheng, X., Salazar, A. S., Lopes, G., & Watson, D. C. (2025). Leveraging beneficial microbiome-immune interactions via probiotic use in cancer immunotherapy. *Frontiers in Immunology, 16*. https://doi.org/10.3389/fimmu.2025.1713382.

Jia, J., Gao, W., Wang, C., Liu, L., Li, Y., Sun, Z., Yang, C., Chen, Y., Yu, H., & Cheng, Y. (2026). Intratumoral microbiota remodeling of the tumor microenvironment impact solid tumor immunotherapy. *Cell Death and Disease, 17*(1). https://doi.org/10.1038/s41419-025-08211-w.

Jiang, H., & Zhang, Q. (2024). Gut microbiota influences the efficiency of immune checkpoint inhibitors by modulating the immune system (Review). *Oncology Letters, 27*(2). https://doi.org/10.3892/ol.2024.14221.

Jin, Y., Dong, H., Xia, L., Yang, Y., Zhu, Y., Shen, Y., ... Lu, S. (2019). The diversity of gut microbiome is associated with favorable responses to anti-programmed death 1 immunotherapy in Chinese patients with NSCLC. *Journal of Thoracic Oncology, 14*(8), 1378–1389. https://doi.org/10.1016/j.jtho.2019.04.007.

Khoruts, A., & Weingarden, A. R. (2014). Emergence of fecal microbiota transplantation as an approach to repair disrupted microbial gut ecology. *Immunology Letters, 162*(2), 77–81. https://doi.org/10.1016/j.imlet.2014.07.016.

Kim, E., Ahn, H., & Park, H. (2021). A review on the role of gut microbiota in immune checkpoint blockade therapy for cancer. *Mammalian Genome, 32*(4), 223–231. https://doi.org/10.1007/s00335-021-09867-3.

Kostic, A. D., Chun, E., Robertson, L., Glickman, J. N., Gallini, C. A., Michaud, M., Clancy, T. E., Chung, D. C., Lochhead, P., Hold, G. L., El-Omar, E. M., Brenner, D., Fuchs, C. S., Meyerson, M., & Garrett, W. S. (2013). *Fusobacterium nucleatum* potentiates intestinal tumorigenesis and modulates the tumor-immune microenvironment. *Cell Host and Microbe, 14*(2), 207–215. https://doi.org/10.1016/j.chom.2013.07.007.

Krishnamurthy, H. K., Pereira, M., Bosco, J., George, J., Jayaraman, V., Krishna, K., Wang, T., Bei, K., & Rajasekaran, J. J. (2023). Gut commensals and their metabolites in health and disease. *Frontiers in Microbiology, 14*. https://doi.org/10.3389/fmicb.2023.1244293.

Kumar, A., Xu, C., & Dakal, T. C. (2026). Microbiome based precision medicine through integrated multiomics and machine learning. *Microbiological Research, 303*, 128384. https://doi.org/10.1016/j.micres.2025.128384.

Lei, W., Zhou, K., Lei, Y., Li, Q., & Zhu, H. (2025). Gut microbiota shapes cancer immunotherapy responses. *npj Biofilms and Microbiomes, 11*(1). https://doi.org/10.1038/s41522-025-00786-8.

Li, M. Y., Wu, X. Q., & Lee, T. K. W. (2026). Harnessing the microbiome: Unveiling the influence of the gut microbiota on hepatobiliary cancer therapeutic strategies. *Clinical and Molecular Hepatology, 32*(1), 91–126. https://doi.org/10.3350/cmh.2025.0476.

Li, S., Li, Q., & Lu, W. (2022). Intratumoral microbiome and gastrointestinal cancers. *Frontiers in Oncology, 12*. https://doi.org/10.3389/fonc.2022.1047015.

Liao, K., Wen, J., Liu, Z., Zhang, B., Zhang, X., Fu, Y., Zhang, W., Hu, H., Ai, K., Zhu, W., Xia, M., Lai, Y., Qian, Y., Xu, Y., Sun, F., Zhang, L., Zhong, Q., Huang, B., & Wang, X. (2025). The role of intratumoral microbiome in the occurrence, proliferation, metastasis of colorectal cancer and its underlying therapeutic strategies. *Ageing Research Reviews, 111*. https://doi.org/10.1016/j.arr.2025.102820.

Lin, A., Xiong, M., Jiang, A., Huang, L., Wong, H. Z. H., Feng, S., Zhang, C., Li, Y., Chen, L., Chi, H., Zhang, P., Ye, B., Zhang, H., Zhang, N., Zhu, L., Mou, W., Shen, J., Li, K., Xu, W., ... Luo, P. (2025). The microbiome in cancer. *iMeta, 4*(5). https://doi.org/10.1002/imt2.70070.

Lu, Y., Yuan, H., Liang, S., Li, D., Jiang, P., Wang, X., Zhang, K., & Liu, D. (2025). Microbial metabolite-driven immune reprogramming in tumor immunotherapy: Mechanisms and therapeutic perspectives. *Frontiers in Immunology, 16*. https://doi.org/10.3389/fimmu.2025.1603658.

Malczewski, A. B., Ketheesan, N., Coward, J. I. G., & Navarro, S. (2021). Enhancing checkpoint inhibitor therapy in solid tissue cancers: The role of diet, the microbiome & microbiome-derived metabolites. *Frontiers in Immunology, 12*. https://doi.org/10.3389/fimmu.2021.624434.

Mallott, E. K., Sitarik, A. R., Leve, L. D., Cioffi, C., Camargo, C. A., Hasegawa, K., & Bordenstein, S. R. (2023). Human microbiome variation associated with race and ethnicity emerges as early as 3 months of age. *PLoS Biology, 21*(8). https://doi.org/10.1371/journal.pbio.3002230.

Mansoori, B., Mohammadi, A., Davudian, S., Shirjang, S., & Baradaran, B. (2017). The different mechanisms of cancer drug resistance: A brief review. *Advanced Pharmaceutical Bulletin, 7*(3), 339–348. https://doi.org/10.15171/apb.2017.041.

Matson, V., Fessler, J., Bao, R., Chongsuwat, T., Zha, Y., Alegre, M. L., Luke, J. J., & Gajewski, T. F. (2018). The commensal microbiome is associated with anti-PD-1 efficacy in metastatic melanoma patients. *Science, 359*(6371), 104–108. https://doi.org/10.1126/science.aao3290.

McCoubrey, L. E., Elbadawi, M., Orlu, M., Gaisford, S., & Basit, A. W. (2021). Harnessing machine learning for development of microbiome therapeutics. *Gut Microbes, 13*(1), 1–20. https://doi.org/10.1080/19490976.2021.1872323.

Mcmillin, D. W., Negri, J. M., & Mitsiades, C. S. (2013). The role of tumour-stromal interactions in modifying drug response: Challenges and opportunities. *Nature Reviews Drug Discovery, 12*(3), 217–228. https://doi.org/10.1038/nrd3870.

Nazir, A., Hussain, F. H. N., & Raza, A. (2024). Advancing microbiota therapeutics: The role of synthetic biology in engineering microbial communities for precision medicine. *Emirates Frontiers in Bioengineering and Biotechnology, 12*. https://doi.org/10.3389/fbioe.2024.1511149.

Nejman, D., Livyatan, I., Fuks, G., Gavert, N., Zwang, Y., Geller, L. T., Rotter-Maskowitz, A., Weiser, R., Mallel, G., Gigi, E., Meltser, A., Douglas, G. M., Kamer, I., Gopalakrishnan, V., Dadosh, T., Levin-Zaidman, S., Avnet, S., Atlan, T., Cooper, Z. A., … Straussman, R. (2020). The human tumor microbiome is composed of tumor type-specific intracellular bacteria. *Science, 368*(6494), 973–980. https://doi.org/10.1126/science.aay9189.

Nguyen, N. T. A., Jiang, Y., & McQuade, J. L. (2024). Eating away cancer: The potential of diet and the microbiome for shaping immunotherapy outcome. *Frontiers in Immunology, 15*. https://doi.org/10.3389/fimmu.2024.1409414.

Noh, K., Kang, Y. R., Nepal, M. R., Shakya, R., Kang, M. J., Kang, W., Lee, S., Jeong, H. G., & Jeong, T. C. (2017). Impact of gut microbiota on drug metabolism: An update for safe and effective use of drugs. *Archives of Pharmacal Research, 40*(12), 1345–1355. https://doi.org/10.1007/s12272-017-0986-y.

Parajuli, B., Midya, V., Kiddle, R., Jager, N. D., Eggers, S., Spakowicz, D., Hoyd, R., Salhia, B., Chan, C. H. F., Churchman, M. L., Rounbehler, R. J., Yao, S., Rutkowski, M. R., Tarhini, A. A., Mudaranthakam, D. P., Masood, A., Bocklage, T. J., Lentz, R. W., Hatoum, H., … Bosch, D. E. (2025). Primary tumor microbiomes predict distant metastasis of colorectal cancer. *npj Precision Oncology, 9*(1). https://doi.org/10.1038/s41698-025-01188-x.

Parhi, L., Alon-Maimon, T., Sol, A., Nejman, D., Shhadeh, A., Fainsod-Levi, T., Yajuk, O., Isaacson, B., Abed, J., Maalouf, N., Nissan, A., Sandbank, J., Yehuda-Shnaidman, E., Ponath, F., Vogel, J. ö, Mandelboim, O., Granot, Z., Straussman, R., & Bachrach, G. (2020). Breast cancer colonization by *Fusobacterium nucleatum* accelerates tumor growth and metastatic progression. *Nature Communications, 11*(1). https://doi.org/10.1038/s41467-020-16967-2.

Perl, M., Fante, M. A., Herfeld, K., Scherer, J. N., Poeck, H., & Orberg, E. T. (2025). Microbiota-derived metabolites: Key modulators of cancer immunotherapies. *Med, 6*(8), 100773. https://doi.org/10.1016/j.medj.2025.100773.

Petrelli, F., Ghidini, A., Dottorini, L., Ghidini, M., Zaniboni, A., & Tomasello, G. (2025). Clinical evidence for microbiome-based strategies in cancer immunotherapy: A state-of-the-art review. *Medicina, 61*(9), 1595. https://doi.org/10.3390/medicina61091595.

Pinato, D. J., Howlett, S., Ottaviani, D., Urus, H., Patel, A., Mineo, T., Brock, C., Power, D., Hatcher, O., Falconer, A., Ingle, M., Brown, A., Gujral, D., Partridge, S., Sarwar, N., Gonzalez, M., Bendle, M., Lewanski, C., Newsom-Davis, T., … Bower, M. (2019). Association of prior antibiotic treatment with survival and response to immune checkpoint inhibitor therapy in patients with cancer. *JAMA Oncology, 5*(12), 1774–1778. https://doi.org/10.1001/jamaoncol.2019.2785.

Procaccianti, G., Roggiani, S., Conti, G., Brigidi, P., Turroni, S., & D'amico, F. (2023). *Bifidobacterium* in anticancer immunochemotherapy: Friend or foe? *Microbiome Research Reports, 2*(3). https://doi.org/10.20517/mrr.2023.23.

Ramesh, A., Subbarayan, R., Shrestha, R., & Adtani, P. N. (2026). Exploring fecal microbiota transplantation: Potential benefits, associated risks, and challenges in cancer treatment. *Cancer Reports, 9*(1). https://doi.org/10.1002/cnr2.70455.

Repass, J., Maherali, N., & Owen, K. (2016). Reproducibility project: Cancer biology. Registered report: *Fusobacterium nucleatum* infection is prevalent in human colorectal carcinoma. *Elife, 5*, 299–306.

Routy, B., Le Chatelier, E., Derosa, L., Duong, C. P. M., Alou, M. T., Daillère, R., ... Zitvogel, L. (2018). Gut microbiome influences efficacy of PD-1–based immunotherapy against epithelial tumors. *Science, 359*(6371), 91–97. https://doi.org/10.1126/science.aan3706.

Routy, B., Rafie, E., & Elkrief, A. (2025). Antibiotic-related dysbiosis in cancer immunotherapy: From preclinical insights to practice-changing evidence. *Nature Cancer, 6*(12), 1909–1912. https://doi.org/10.1038/s43018-025-01055-5.

Saha, S., Mara, K., Pardi, D. S., & Khanna, S. (2021). Long-term safety of fecal microbiota transplantation for recurrent *Clostridioides difficile* infection. *Gastroenterology, 160*(6), 1961. https://doi.org/10.1053/j.gastro.2021.01.010.

Sardar, P., Beresford-Jones, B. S., Xia, W., Shabana, O., Suyama, S., Ramos, R. J. F., Soderholm, A. T., Tourlomousis, P., Kuo, P., Evans, A. C., Imianowski, C. J., Conti, A. G., Wesolowski, A. J., Baker, N. M., McCord, E. A. L., Okkenhaug, K., Whiteside, S. K., Roychoudhuri, R., Bryant, C. E., ... Pedicord, V. A. (2025). Gut microbiota-derived hexa-acylated lipopolysaccharides enhance cancer immunotherapy responses. *Nature Microbiology, 10*(3), 795–807. https://doi.org/10.1038/s41564-025-01930-y.

Seely, K. D., Morgan, A. D., Hagenstein, L. D., Florey, G. M., & Small, J. M. (2022). Bacterial involvement in progression and metastasis of colorectal neoplasia. *Cancers, 14*(4). https://doi.org/10.3390/cancers14041019.

Sevcikova, A., Izoldova, N., Stevurkova, V., Kasperova, B., Chovanec, M., Ciernikova, S., & Mego, M. (2022). The impact of the microbiome on resistance to cancer treatment with chemotherapeutic agents and immunotherapy. *International Journal of Molecular Sciences, 23*(1), 488. https://doi.org/10.3390/ijms23010488.

Shah, D., & Ajazuddin, S. B. (2023). Role of natural P-gp inhibitor in the effective delivery for chemotherapeutic agents. *Journal of Cancer Research and Clinical Oncology, 149*(1), 367–391. https://doi.org/10.1007/s00432-022-04387-2.

Sivan, A., Corrales, L., Hubert, N., Williams, J. B., Aquino-Michaels, K., Earley, Z. M., Benyamin, F. W., Lei, Y. M., Jabri, B., Alegre, M. L., Chang, E. B., & Gajewski, T. F. (2015). Commensal *Bifidobacterium* promotes antitumor immunity and facilitates anti-PD-L1 efficacy. *Science, 350*(6264), 1084–1089. https://doi.org/10.1126/science.aac4255.

Smith, P. M., Howitt, M. R., Panikov, N., Michaud, M., Gallini, C. A., Bohlooly-Y, M., Glickman, J. N., & Garrett, W. S. (2013). The microbial metabolites, short-chain fatty acids, regulate colonic T reg cell homeostasis. *Science, 341*(6145), 569–573. https://doi.org/10.1126/science.1241165.

Somodi, C., Dora, D., Horváth, M., Szegvari, G., & Lohinai, Z. (2025). Gut microbiome changes and cancer immunotherapy outcomes associated with dietary interventions: A systematic review of preclinical and clinical evidence. *Journal of Translational Medicine, 23*(1). https://doi.org/10.1186/s12967-025-06586-0.

Spencer, C. N., McQuade, J. L., Gopalakrishnan, V., McCulloch, J. A., Vetizou, M., Cogdill, A. P., Wadud Khan, M. A., Zhang, X., White, M. G., Peterson, C. B., Wong, M. C., Morad, G., Rodgers, T., Badger, J. H., Helmink, B. A., Andrews, M. C., Rodrigues, R. R., Morgun, A., Kim, Y. S., ... Wargo, J. A. (2021). Dietary fiber and probiotics influence the gut microbiome and melanoma immunotherapy response. *Science, 374*(6575), 1632–1640. https://doi.org/10.1126/science.aaz7015.

Sun, J., Song, S., Liu, J., Chen, F., Li, X., & Wu, G. (2025). Gut microbiota as a new target for anticancer therapy: From mechanism to means of regulation. *npj Biofilms and Microbiomes, 11*(1). https://doi.org/10.1038/s41522-025-00678-x.

Tegegne, H. A., & Savidge, T. C. (2025). Gut microbiome metagenomics in clinical practice: Bridging the gap between research and precision medicine. *Gut Microbes, 17*(1). https://doi.org/10.1080/19490976.2025.2569739.

Thomas, H. (2017). Intra-tumour bacteria promote gemcitabine resistance in pancreatic adenocarcinoma. *Nature Reviews Gastroenterology & Hepatology, 14*(11), 632. https://doi.org/10.1038/nrgastro.2017.142.

Tian, M., Soleimani Samarkhazan, H., Shahabedin Alemohammad, S., Fakhraei Manesh, M., Tavakoli, F., Shams, A., & Zeynalabadi, A. (2026). Microbiome dysbiosis and chemotherapy resistance in acute myeloid leukemia (AML). *npj Biofilms and Microbiomes, 12*(1). https://doi.org/10.1038/s41522-025-00891-8.

Ting, N. L.-N., Lau, H. C.-H., & Yu, J. (2022). Cancer pharmacomicrobiomics: Targeting microbiota to optimise cancer therapy outcomes. *Gut, 71*(7), 1412–1425. https://doi.org/10.1136/gutjnl-2021-326264.

Vongsavath, T., Rahmani, R., Min Tun, K., & Manne, V. (2024). The use of fecal microbiota transplant in overcoming and modulating resistance to Anti-PD-1 therapy in patients with skin cancer. *Cancers, 16*(3), 499. https://doi.org/10.3390/cancers16030499.

Wang, H., Xie, J., Li, N. a, Liu, Q., Song, W., Chen, W., Peng, C., & Tang, H. (2025a). Unraveling immunotherapy resistance in solid tumors: Decoding mechanisms and charting future therapeutic landscapes. *Oncology Research, 33*(12), 3789–3800. https://doi.org/10.32604/or.2025.067592.

Wang, M., Liu, M., Wang, D., Yang, D., Zeng, Y., Lan, Y., & Wang, Q. (2025b). Engineered bacteria for cancer therapy: Advancements, challenges, and future directions. *Chinese Medical Journal, 138*(24), 3224–3250. https://doi.org/10.1097/cm9.0000000000003807.

Wang, S., Xu, M., Wang, W., Cao, X., Piao, M., Khan, S., Yan, F., Cao, H., Wang, B., & Grivennikov, S. (2016). Systematic Review: Adverse events of fecal microbiota transplantation. *PLOS ONE, 11*(8), e0161174. https://doi.org/10.1371/journal.pone.0161174.

Wu, X., Zhang, T., Chen, X., Ji, G., & Zhang, F. (2019). Microbiota transplantation: Targeting cancer treatment. *Cancer Letters, 452*, 144–151. https://doi.org/10.1016/j.canlet.2019.03.010.

Wu, Y., Chen, X. i, Wu, Q., & Wang, Q. (2025). Research progress on fecal microbiota transplantation in tumor prevention and treatment. *Open Life Sciences, 20*(1). https://doi.org/10.1515/biol-2022-0954.

Xiang, Y., Liu, X., Wang, Y., Zheng, D., Meng, Q., Jiang, L., Yang, S., Zhang, S., Zhang, X., Liu, Y., & Wang, B. (2024). Mechanisms of resistance to targeted therapy and immunotherapy in non-small cell lung cancer: Promising strategies to overcoming challenges. *Frontiers in Immunology, 15*. https://doi.org/10.3389/fimmu.2024.1366260.

Xie, Z., Wu, Z., Liu, Y., Gu, Y. u, Niu, J., & Lv, K. (2025). Intratumoral microbiota: Implications for cancer progression and treatment. *Frontiers in Microbiology, 16*. https://doi.org/10.3389/fmicb.2025.1551515.

Xu, G., Jiang, Y., Sun, C., Brandt, B. W., Nazmi, K., Morelli, L., Lencioni, G., Giovannetti, E., & Deng, D. (2025a). Role of oral bacteria in mediating gemcitabine resistance in pancreatic cancer. *Biomolecules, 15*(7), 1018. https://doi.org/10.3390/biom15071018.

Xu, J., Song, J., Fu, Z., Zhou, H., Zhang, Y., & Shi, C. (2025b). Unraveling gut microbiome interferences in cancer immunotherapy: A meta-analysis of diverse drug effects. *BMC Cancer, 25*(1). https://doi.org/10.1186/s12885-025-15094-9.

Xu, L., Hu, B., He, J., Fu, X., & Liu, N. (2025c). Intratumor microbiome-derived butyrate promotes chemo-resistance in colorectal cancer. *Frontiers in Pharmacology, 15*. https://doi.org/10.3389/fphar.2024.1510851.

Yang, D., Chen, L., Rong, L., & Lang (2025). Tumor-associated microbiota: Multi-cancer landscape, mechanistic insights and clinical translation. *Oncology Letters, 30*(5), 527.

Yang, Y., & Shi, X. (2025). Big lessons from the little *Akkermansia muciniphila* in hepatocellular carcinoma. *Frontiers in Immunology, 16*. https://doi.org/10.3389/fimmu.2025.1524563.

Yang, Z., Liang, L., Li, X., Peng, X., Qian, X., Huang, Z., Wang, X., Hu, Q., & Fu, X. (2026). *Akkermansia muciniphila* enhances the antitumour efficacy of αPD-1 therapy in gastric cancer by remodelling the tumour immune microenvironment. *Toxicology and Applied Pharmacology, 507,* 117711. https://doi.org/10.1016/j.taap.2026.117711.

Yao, R., Sun, L., Gao, R., Mei, Y., Xue, G., & Yu, D. (2025). PTTM: Dissecting the profile of tumor tissue microbiome to reveal microbiota features and associations with host transcriptome. *Briefings in Bioinformatics, 26*(1). https://doi.org/10.1093/bib/bbaf057.

Ye, M., Ju, H., Ren, G., & Hu, J. (2025). The role of microbiome in immunotherapy: Insights and perspectives. *Seminars in Cancer Biology, 117,* 131–151. https://doi.org/10.1016/j.semcancer.2025.11.001.

Yousefi, Y., Baines, K. J., & Vareki, S. M. (2024). Microbiome bacterial influencers of host immunity and response to immunotherapy. *Cell Reports Medicine, 5*(4). https://doi.org/10.1016/j.xcrm.2024.101487.

Yu, T. C., Guo, F., Yu, Y., Sun, T., Ma, D., Han, J., Qian, Y., Kryczek, I., Sun, D., Nagarsheth, N., Chen, Y., Chen, H., Hong, J., Zou, W., & Fang, J. Y. (2017). *Fusobacterium nucleatum* promotes chemoresistance to colorectal cancer by modulating autophagy. *Cell, 170*(3), 548. https://doi.org/10.1016/j.cell.2017.07.008.

Yu, Y., Zheng, P., Gao, L., Li, H., Tao, P., Wang, D., Ding, F., Shi, Q., & Chen, H. (2021). Effects of antibiotic use on outcomes in cancer patients treated using immune checkpoint inhibitors: A systematic review and meta-analysis. *Journal of Immunotherapy, 44*(2), 76–85. https://doi.org/10.1097/CJI.0000000000000346.

Zalila-Kolsi, I., Dhieb, D., Osman, H. A., & Mekideche, H. (2025). The gut microbiota and colorectal cancer: Understanding the link and exploring therapeutic interventions. *Biology, 14*(3), 251. https://doi.org/10.3390/biology14030251.

Zeng, J., He, Z., Wang, G., Ma, Y., & Zhang, F. (2025a). Interaction between microbiota and immunity: Molecular mechanisms, biological functions, diseases, and new therapeutic opportunities. *MedComm, 6*(7). https://doi.org/10.1002/mco2.70265.

Zeng, L. i, Qian, Y., Cui, X., Zhao, J., Ning, Z., Cha, J., Wang, K., Ge, C., Jia, J., Dou, T., Chen, H., Liu, L., Bao, Z., & Jian, Z. (2025b). Immunomodulatory role of gut microbial metabolites: Mechanistic insights and therapeutic frontiers. *Frontiers in Microbiology, 16.* https://doi.org/10.3389/fmicb.2025.1675065.

Zhang, S., Huang, J., Jiang, Z., Tong, H., Ma, X., & Liu, Y. (2025a). Tumor microbiome: Roles in tumor initiation, progression, and therapy. *Molecular Biomedicine, 6*(1). https://doi.org/10.1186/s43556-025-00248-9.

Zhang, W., Xiang, Y., Ren, H. e, Liu, Y., Wang, Q. i, Ran, M., Zhou, W., Tian, L., Zheng, X., Qiao, C., Liu, Y., & Yan, M. (2025b). The tumor microbiome in cancer progression: Mechanisms and therapeutic potential. *Molecular Cancer, 24*(1). https://doi.org/10.1186/s12943-025-02403-w.

Zhang, X., Li, L., Butcher, J., Stintzi, A., & Figeys, D. (2019). Advancing functional and translational microbiome research using meta-omics approaches. *Microbiome, 7*(1). https://doi.org/10.1186/s40168-019-0767-6.

Zhou, L., Li, B., Ren, J., Wang, S., & Wang, J. (2025). Microbiome-mediated regulation of chemoradiotherapy response. *Frontiers in Oncology, 15.* https://doi.org/10.3389/fonc.2025.1659467.

Zhou, Y., Tao, L., Qiu, J., Xu, J., Yang, X., Zhang, Y. U, Tian, X., Guan, X., Cen, X., & Zhao, Y. (2024). Tumor biomarkers for diagnosis, prognosis and targeted therapy. *Signal Transduction and Targeted Therapy, 9*(1). https://doi.org/10.1038/s41392-024-01823-2.

Zhu, J., & Van den Eynde, B. J. (2024). AHR and tryptophan metabolism: A collaborative dynamics of immune regulation. *Genes and Immunity, 25*(2), 170–171. https://doi.org/10.1038/s41435-023-00235-6.

Zhu, Z., Huang, J., Zhang, Y., Hou, W., Chen, F., Mo, Y. Y., & Zhang, Z. (2024). Landscape of tumoral ecosystem for enhanced anti-PD-1 immunotherapy by gut *Akkermansia muciniphila. Cell Reports, 43*(6). https://doi.org/10.1016/j.celrep.2024.114306.

8

Cancer pharmacomicrobiomics: Targeting microbiota to optimize cancer therapy outcomes

Salome Satya Vani Punuri[a], Wandeep Dagar[b], Shirisha Vodnala[a], Bhupinder Bhyan[c] and Sarita Jangra[b]

[a]DEPARTMENT OF PHARMACY PRACTICE, SRI VENKATESHWARA COLLEGE OF PHARMACY, HYDERABAD, TELANGANA, INDIA [b]CHITKARA COLLEGE OF PHARMACY, CHITKARA UNIVERSITY, RAJPURA, PUNJAB, INDIA [c]SCHOOL OF PHARMACEUTICAL SCIENCES, RIMT UNIVERSITY, MANDI GOBINDGARH, PUNJAB, INDIA

8.1 Introduction

Personalized therapy, commonly referred to as precision medicine, represents an evolving clinical framework that incorporates individual cellular, molecular, and genetic characteristics to guide therapeutic selection, dosing, and timing in cancer management (Ngoc et al., 2024). Among all the therapeutic areas, cancer treatment has experienced rapid advancements in precision medicine because of the heterogeneity of tumors, interindividual differences in drug response, and toxicity with cancer treatment (Tsimberidou et al., 2020). Despite these advances, tumor genomics and host genetics are the main focuses of current personalized cancer treatment, which ignores the impact of human microbiota (Huang et al., 2023)

Human microbiota is a constantly changing dynamic community of about 40 trillion microorganisms encompassing diverse bacterial, fungal, and viral species that collectively contribute to host physiological and immunological functions (Sender et al., 2016). These microbes primarily reside on the body's epithelial surfaces, such as the gastrointestinal tract, skin, and various mucosal linings (Sepich-Poore et al., 2021). An imbalance in their natural makeup will disrupt their healthy equilibrium and is referred to as dysbiosis (Fan & Pedersen, 2021). This altered state can cause neurological, gastrointestinal, and metabolic disorders (Zhuang et al., 2019). In addition, accumulating evidence demonstrates that certain gut microbes also contribute to the development of cancer, especially gastrointestinal tract malignancies (Tilg et al., 2018). For

The Microbiome and Cancer Treatment: Overcoming Resistance and Enhancing Efficacy.
DOI: https://doi.org/10.1016/B978-0-443-33206-7.00011-X

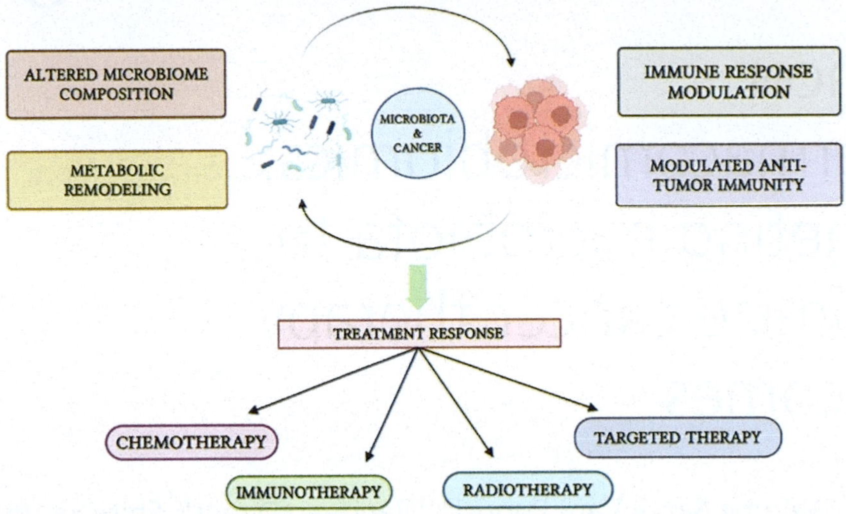

FIGURE 8.1 The dynamic relationship between the microbiota and cancer influences therapeutic responses by shaping tumor biology, modulating immune surveillance, regulating inflammation, and altering drug metabolism—thereby impacting the efficacy, resistance, and toxicity profiles of chemotherapy, radiotherapy, targeted therapy, and immunotherapy.

example, the adhesin FadA produced by *Fusobacterium nucleatum* promotes colorectal cancer development by interacting with epithelial E-cadherin, thereby activating downstream Wnt/β-catenin signaling pathways that enhance oncogenic transcriptional programs (Rubinstein et al., 2013). Additionally, some microbes impede immune surveillance or promote inflammation, thereby indirectly contributing to cancer development (Wilson et al., 2019).

8.1.1 Emergence of pharmacomicrobiomics in precision oncology

Pharmacomicrobiomics is a rapidly evolving field that explores how microbiomes influence drug response through modifications in pharmacokinetics, pharmacodynamics, and therapeutic outcomes (Roden et al., 2019). Integration of patient-specific microbiome profiles into therapeutic decision-making enables the design of individualized treatment strategies and enhances the optimization of drug efficacy and response.

In cancer treatment, microbiota significantly influences responses to chemotherapy, affecting both treatment efficacy and toxicity through immune and metabolic mechanisms (Alexander et al., 2017). Recognition of these influences gives promising opportunities to mitigate treatment-related toxicity and enhance efficacy by deliberately targeting the microbiota (Alexander et al., 2017). Growing evidence from experimental and clinical studies suggests that the gut microbiota affects host responses across multiple anticancer modalities, including cytotoxic chemotherapy, radiation therapy, molecularly targeted agents, and immunotherapeutic approaches (Fig. 8.1)(Alexander et al., 2017; Shiao et al., 2021; Wong et al., 2021).

8.1.2 The conceptual framework and historical development of pharmacomicrobiomics

Over the past 20 years, developments in genetics, molecular biology, and computational sciences have significantly changed the concept of precision medicine. The primary focus of early precision medicine efforts was pharmacogenomics, which emphasizes how inherited variation in drug-metabolizing enzymes, transporters, and molecular targets affects therapeutic response and toxicity. Pharmacogenomics has made drug selection better in some circumstances, but its ability to predict is still limited in cancer treatment, where therapy response reflects complex, dynamic interactions beyond host genetics alone (Relling & Evans, 2015; Weinshilboum & Wang, 2017). A key limitation of pharmacogenomic models is their inability to account for ecological and environmental factors that influence drug disposition. Among these, the human microbiota has shown itself to be an important but unknown factor affecting treatment responses (Kuntz & Gilbert, 2017). Later, it was discovered that commensal bacteria have metabolic capacities similar to those of the liver, which led to the emergence of pharmacomicrobiomics (Maier et al., 2018).

Early metabolomics research revealed that metabolites originating from the microbiota can alter the bioavailability of the drug and influence host signaling pathways, thereby contributing to interindividual variation in drug response (Weinshilboum & Wang, 2017). Further research has shown that, independent of human enzymatic systems, microbial enzymes metabolize a variety of drugs, including anticancer agents (Kuntz & Gilbert, 2017; Sepich-Poore et al., 2021). The microbial genome has a large metabolic reservoir that can undergo quick functional changes in response to diet, treatment, and illness, in contrast to the stable human genome (Maier et al., 2018). This dynamic host-microbe interaction is especially important in cancer. Microbial ecosystems interact with tumor heterogeneity, immunological variability, and treatment-induced changes to influence therapeutic outcomes (Relling & Evans, 2015). The microbiota also influences immune monitoring, systemic inflammation, and the composition of the tumor microenvironment (TME) (Tilg et al., 2018). Therefore, it is feasible to consider the role of pharmacomicrobiomics in cancer treatment as an integrated network linking microbiome, host system, and tumor genome (Ting et al., 2022). The microbiome interacts with both axes by influencing immune differentiation, cytokine signaling, metabolic programming, and drug metabolism; tumor genetics determines intrinsic drug sensitivity; and host immunity controls response to immunomodulatory therapy (Sharon et al., 2016). Crucially, microbial influences are not limited to the gut. Although tumors were assumed to be sterile environments, emerging studies have shown unique microbial populations within tumor tissues, broadening the scope of pharmacomicrobiomics from systemic to spatially specific tumor contexts (Dohlman et al., 2022). Thus, the transition from pharmacogenomics to pharmacomicrobiomics shows a trend toward integrated precision oncology frameworks.

8.2 Microbiota and chemotherapy response

Alexander et al. (2017) demonstrated that gut microbiota influence chemotherapy efficacy and toxicity through a complex network of chemical signaling pathways, exerting both direct and indirect effects at systemic and intratumoral levels. To conceptualize these interactions, the authors introduced the TIMER mechanistic framework, which encompasses microbial translocation, immunomodulation, drug metabolism, and enzymatic degradation, as well as alterations in microbial diversity and ecological balance that collectively shape chemotherapeutic outcomes (Alexander et al., 2017). Conceptually, these microbiome–tumor interactions align with broader ecological models such as the bacterial driver–passenger hypothesis proposed by Tjalsma et al. (2012), which describes dynamic microbial succession during colorectal cancer development.

8.2.1 Direct microbiota–drug interactions

8.2.1.1 Microbial enzymatic modification of chemotherapeutic agents

Gut bacteria have millions of protein-coding genes, enabling them to directly metabolize chemotherapeutic agents through enzyme-mediated reactions (Spanogiannopoulos et al., 2016). Drugs are directly converted into active, inactive, or potentially toxic metabolites by microbial enzymes. These conversions can result in drug activation, inactivation, or conversion into toxic metabolites, thereby influencing the pharmacokinetics and therapeutic outcomes (Spanogiannopoulos et al., 2016). Host carboxylesterases transform the topoisomerase I inhibitor irinotecan (CPT-11), which is frequently used as a first-line treatment for metastatic colorectal cancer, into its active metabolite SN-38. After being glucuronidated in the liver to produce SN-38 glucuronide (SN-38G), this metabolite is subsequently removed by the bile (Bailly, 2019; Nagar & Blanchard, 2006). Microbial β-glucuronidase activity in the gut can convert SN-38G back into the active toxic metabolite SN-38, causing injury to the intestinal tissues and resulting in dose-limiting gastrointestinal toxicity, most notably severe diarrhea (Stringer et al., 2008). The main sources of intestinal β-glucuronidase activity are bacterial groups belonging to *Clostridium* clusters XIVa and IV, including genera such as *Clostridium, Eubacterium*, and *Ruminococcus* (McIntosh et al., 2012). Importantly, irinotecan treatment itself has been shown to promote the expansion of these taxa, thereby exacerbating treatment-associated toxicity (Lin et al., 2012). Targeted inhibition of microbial β-glucuronidases using small-molecule compounds, including pyrazolo[4,3-c]quinoline derivatives (e.g., TCH-3562) and uronic isofagomine analogs, has demonstrated therapeutic potential by mitigating irinotecan-induced intestinal toxicity without compromising antitumor efficacy (Bhatt et al., 2020; Wallace et al., 2010).

8.2.2 Indirect microbiota-mediated mechanisms

8.2.2.1 Microbial metabolic support of chemotherapeutic efficacy

The activation and efficacy of some chemotherapeutic agents may depend on bacterial metabolism. Studies conducted using *Caenorhabditis elegans* models revealed that the activation of 5-fluorouracil (5-FU) into its cytotoxic RNA-damaging metabolites requires bacterial genes involved in ribonucleotide metabolism and vitamin B6 and B9 biosynthesis. The dependence of chemotherapy on microbial cometabolism is implied by the fact that disruption of these bacterial metabolic pathways reduces 5-FU efficacy. Notably, concomitant drugs like metformin can reduce the anticancer effects of 5-FU by inhibiting bacterial one-carbon metabolism (García-González et al., 2017). These results demonstrate the clinical significance of drug–microbiome interactions, especially in cancer patients with other comorbid conditions.

8.2.2.2 Immunomodulatory effects of gut microbiota on chemotherapy response

Beyond metabolism, the gut microbiota also influences chemotherapy-induced anticancer immunity. Certain chemotherapeutic agents exert immunostimulatory effects that require microbial participation (Galluzzi et al., 2020). Cyclophosphamide (CTX), a widely used alkylating chemotherapeutic agent, exerts part of its antitumor activity through immune modulation, notably by reducing immunosuppressive regulatory T-cell populations and favoring Th1-polarized responses (Galluzzi et al., 2020). CTX-induced disruption of intestinal barrier integrity further enables selective commensal bacteria, including *Enterococcus hirae* and *Lactobacillus johnsonii*, to translocate to secondary lymphoid tissues, where they promote the expansion of pathogenic Th17 cells and memory Th1 subsets required for optimal therapeutic efficacy (Viaud et al., 2013). In contrast, *Barnesiella intestinihominis* remains localized within the colon yet enhances systemic antitumor immunity by stimulating polyfunctional $CD8^+$ cytotoxic T-cell responses and Th1 immunity, thereby supporting intratumoral recruitment of interferon-γ-producing $\gamma\delta$ T cells (Daillère et al., 2016). These microbiota-driven immunostimulatory effects are mediated through nucleotide-binding oligomerization domain-containing protein 2 (NOD2)-dependent signaling pathways, highlighting the potential for host–microbiome-targeted strategies to augment CTX responsiveness (Cheng et al., 2020).

8.2.2.3 Microbiota-dependent reactive oxygen species and metabolite signaling

Platinum-based anticancer drugs such as oxaliplatin and cisplatin rely on microbiota-dependent immune priming for their cytotoxic effects (Iida et al., 2013; Lokody, 2014). Through myeloid differentiation primary response 88 (MYD88)-dependent signaling in myeloid cells, certain Gram-positive gut bacteria can increase immune activity within tumors by encouraging the production of reactive oxygen species (ROS) (Iida et al., 2013). Additionally, immunogenic gut commensals enhance CD8 T cell memory formation and B cell responses by stimulating dendritic cell–T follicular helper cell interactions (Roberti et al., 2020). Microbial metabolites also influence chemotherapy responses. Short-chain fatty acids (SCFAs), particularly butyrate, improve oxaliplatin-induced anticancer immunity through histone deacetylase inhibition and upregulation of inhibitor of DNA binding 2 (ID2), thereby promoting interleukin-12-dependent cytotoxic T-cell activity (Bachem et al., 2019; He et al., 2021).

8.2.3 Intratumoral microbiota–drug interactions

8.2.3.1 Enzymatic inactivation of chemotherapy within tumors

Beyond the gut, microbes residing within tumor tissue can directly modulate chemotherapeutic efficacy (Geller et al., 2017; Liu et al., 2021). In pancreatic ductal adenocarcinoma (PDAC), intratumoral bacteria, mainly Gammaproteobacteria, express the long isoform of cytidine deaminase

(CDD-L), which metabolizes gemcitabine into an inactive compound. This microbial inactivation contributes to intrinsic and acquired chemoresistance (Geller et al., 2017). *Mycoplasma hyorhinis* confers gemcitabine resistance despite lacking CDD-L, indicating the involvement of microbial processes other than CDD isoforms (Geller et al., 2017). Preclinical research supported the functional significance of intratumoral microbiota by showing that coadministration of antibiotics such as ciprofloxacin can reverse gemcitabine resistance (Geller et al., 2017).

8.2.4 Chemoresistance and chemosensitization mediated by microbiota

There is growing evidence that microbial communities also play a role in intrinsic and acquired resistance to treatment, even though gut and tumor-associated microbes can increase the effectiveness of chemotherapy (Spanogiannopoulos et al., 2016). The integrated mechanisms that give rise to microbiota-driven resistance include enzymatic drug inactivation, activation of tumor-protective signaling pathways, metabolic changes in cancer cells, and modifications of the TME toward immune evasion and stem cell preservation (Spanogiannopoulos et al., 2016).

8.2.4.1 Microbiota-driven activation of pro-survival signaling pathways

Pathogen-associated molecular patterns (PAMPs) and microbial metabolites can trigger oncogenic signaling cascades that prevent chemotherapy-induced apoptosis. In tumor and stromal cells, lipopolysaccharides and peptidoglycans from Gram-positive and Gram-negative bacteria trigger Toll-like receptor (TLR) signaling, which activates nuclear factor-κB (NF-κB) and upregulates antiapoptotic genes like survivin and BCL-2 (Rakoff-Nahoum & Medzhitov, 2009). *Fusobacterium nucleatum* increases oxaliplatin and 5-fluorouracil resistance in colorectal cancer by initiating autophagy pathways via TLR4–MYD88 signaling, enabling tumor cells to endure chemotherapeutic stress (Yu et al., 2017). The association between high intratumoral abundance and lower disease-free survival and recurrence highlights the therapeutic significance of *F. nucleatum* (Mima et al., 2016).

8.2.4.2 Modulation of cancer stem cell phenotypes

According to recent studies, bacteria can affect the growth and survival of cancer stem cells (CSCs), a type of tumor that can regenerate itself and is resistant to conventional chemotherapy (Batlle & Clevers, 2017). Chemicals derived from the microbiota can influence stemness-associated phenotypes by changing signaling pathways like Wnt/β-catenin and Notch, which are involved in CSC maintenance. Since dysbiotic microbiota manipulation increases chemosensitivity and decreases stemness traits in experimental models, targeting microbiota-driven CSC habitats may be a practical strategy to overcome chemoresistance (Batlle & Clevers, 2017).

8.2.4.3 Microbiota-mediated metabolic reprogramming of tumors

Chemotherapy response is further affected by the metabolic interactions between microbiota and malignancies. Tumor glycolysis, oxidative phosphorylation, and nucleotide biosynthesis are all impacted by microbial metabolites, which change the body's vulnerability to antimetabolites and agents that damage DNA (Vander Heiden et al., 2009). For instance, tumor reliance on folate pathways is impacted by microbial modification of one-carbon metabolism, which influences antifolate medication responsiveness (Newman & Maddocks, 2017). Furthermore, the context affects how SCFAs affect chemotherapy. Butyrate can enhance immune-mediated tumor clearance in some circumstances, but excessive butyrate can boost resistance by inducing epigenetic modifications that promote cell cycle arrest and DNA repair (Donohoe et al., 2012). These contradictory effects emphasize the significance of microbial balance rather than enrichment of individual metabolites.

8.2.5 Methods for characterizing the microbiome of cancer

The study of microbiomes in oncology has been greatly accelerated by rapid advances in computational biology, metabolomics, and high-throughput genome sequencing (Kuntz & Gilbert, 2017). Accurate characterization of microbial composition and activity is essential for understanding microbiota–therapy relationships and incorporating pharmacomicrobiomics into clinical practice. Since each analytical method has distinct benefits and drawbacks, its complementary application has proven crucial to current cancer microbiome research (Integrative HMP Research Network Consortium, 2019; Knight et al., 2017).

8.2.5.1 Sequencing of the 16S rRNA gene

Sequencing the 16S ribosomal RNA (rRNA) gene has become a common first step in analyzing bacterial communities. This method amplifies and sequences both variable and conserved regions of the bacterial 16S rRNA gene. It allows for taxonomic classification at the genus level or, in some cases, at the species level (Knight et al., 2017). This technique has been widely used in clinical oncology studies to connect gut microbiota composition with the results of chemotherapy and immunotherapy because it has established analytical processes and is relatively less expensive. However, there are inherent limits to 16S rRNA sequencing. It does not detect components such as fungi and viruses. It also has low taxonomic resolution and cannot reliably distinguish closely related species (Kuntz & Gilbert, 2017). Additionally, it offers limited insight into the functional abilities of microbes, which is often more relevant to immune response and drug metabolism. As a result, higher-resolution methods are increasingly being used alongside 16S-based research.

8.2.5.2 Metagenomic sequencing by shotgun

Shotgun metagenomic sequencing solves many problems associated with 16S profiling by sequencing all microbial DNA from a sample. This method allows for a complete examination of microbial gene composition and metabolic potential. It also provides species- and strain-level detail (Integrative HMP Research Network Consortium, 2019). Metagenomics has uncovered functional pathways linked to immune modulation, drug metabolism, and the adaptation of microbes associated with tumors in cancer research. Metagenomic analysis has enabled the identification of microbial enzymes that alter chemotherapy drugs and the discovery of microbial signatures specific to different tumor types (Maier et al., 2018). However, practical challenges still exist, including higher costs, greater computing requirements, and vulnerability to host DNA contamination, especially in tumor tissue samples.

8.2.5.3 Functional activity profiling and metatranscriptomics

Metatranscriptomics reveals genes that are actively expressed in specific situations, while metagenomics identifies microbial genes. By sequencing microbial RNA, metatranscriptomic analyses capture the dynamic responses of microbes to environmental changes and cancer treatments (Franzosa et al., 2018). This approach is valuable for understanding how immunotherapy or chemotherapy impacts microbial activity instead of just community structure. However, metatranscriptomics faces technical challenges due to RNA instability, lower microbial RNA levels compared to host RNA, and complex data interpretation (Franzosa et al., 2018). Consequently, its application in large-scale clinical cancer research is still limited, though it is expected to increase as methods improve.

8.2.5.4 Metabolomics and metabolites produced by microorganisms

Metabolomics improves sequencing-based methods by directly measuring microbial and host metabolites in biological samples. Among the important metabolites produced by the microbiota that support immune regulation and affect responses to cancer treatment are substances like SCFAs, indoles, polyamines, and bile acids (Koh et al., 2016). Recent studies have linked specific metabolic signatures to the effectiveness of immunotherapy and treatment-related side effects using both targeted and untargeted metabolomic analyses. Metabolomics creates a direct connection between microbial composition and biological effects since metabolites are the active byproducts of host-microbiome interactions (Nicholson et al., 2012). Nevertheless, differentiating between host-derived and microbial metabolites and considering dietary factors remains a significant challenge.

8.2.5.5 Tumor-localized microorganisms and spatial microbiomics

Recent findings show that microbes can be found in tumor tissues, often living inside immune and cancer cells. Spatial microbiomics techniques like fluorescence in situ hybridization (FISH), imaging mass spectrometry, and spatial transcriptomics enable the identification and localization of microorganisms within the tumor microenvironment. These methods have uncovered tumor-type-specific distributions of microbes and their relationships with immune infiltration and treatment resistance (Nejman et al., 2020; Poore et al., 2020). Spatial context is crucial because stool-based methods cannot fully capture drug metabolism within tumors and localized immune regulation.

8.2.5.6 Integration of single-cell and multiomics

New single-cell technologies enable profiling of microbial presence, host gene expression, and immune traits at the cellular level. By integrating metagenomics, transcriptomics, metabolomics, and host genomics within multiomics frameworks, researchers can achieve a system-level understanding of interactions between the microbiota, host, and tumors (Sepich-Poore et al., 2021). Machine-learning algorithms that identify complex patterns predicting therapy responses are increasingly supporting these integrated methods. While multiomics integration is primarily limited to research settings, it represents an important step toward using microbiome insights in precision oncology (Sepich-Poore et al., 2021). These technologies collaborate to form the foundation of cancer pharmacomicrobiomics. To capture the compositional, functional, and geographic complexity of the cancer microbiome and transform microbiome findings into effective therapies, complementary techniques must be carefully selected and integrated.

8.3 Microbiota and immunotherapy response

Cancer cells exert a variety of immunosuppressive strategies to reduce antitumor immunity, most notably by activating immune checkpoint signaling pathways that limit T-cell activity (Pardoll, 2012). Immune checkpoint inhibitors (ICIs), specifically monoclonal antibodies that target cytotoxic T-lymphocyte-associated antigen-4 (CTLA-4) and programmed cell death protein-1 (PD-1) or its ligand PD-L1, have significantly advanced cancer treatment by restoring antitumor immune responses (Ribas & Wolchok, 2018). The Food and Drug Administration (FDA) has approved several ICIs, which are now widely indicated in many cancers (Vaddepally et al., 2020). Despite the advancements, only a subset of patients, around 10%–30%, have shown the efficacy of ICI therapy and are often limited by heterogeneity, with resistance and side effects (Sharma et al., 2017). Research shows that gut microbiota composition significantly affects systemic and intratumoral immune responses. This composition influences the effectiveness and toxicity of immune checkpoint blockade (Zitvogel et al., 2018a).

8.3.1 Microbiota modulation of cytotoxic T-lymphocyte-associated antigen-4 blockade responses

Ipilimumab, a monoclonal antibody that targets CTLA-4, is commonly used to treat metastatic melanoma (Hodi et al., 2010). Recent studies suggest that the success of ipilimumab treatment is influenced by gut microbiota composition, especially the role of Bacteroides species. Preclinical studies revealed that germ-free or antibiotic-treated mice exhibit impaired responses to CTLA-4 blockade, underscoring the necessity of microbial signals for therapeutic activity (Vétizou et al., 2015). Reconstitution with *Bacteroides fragilis* restores responsiveness to CTLA-4 inhibition and is accompanied by reduced tumor burden (Pitt et al., 2016). By promoting IL-12-mediated Th1 responses in tumor-associated lymphoid sites and supporting dendritic cell maturation within the tumor microenvironment, certain commensal bacteria, most notably *B. fragilis*, contribute to antitumor priming (Pitt et al., 2016). These immune effects re-establish sensitivity to CTLA-4 blockade while simultaneously mitigating treatment-induced colitis (Dubin et al., 2016). Clinical studies further support these findings, showing enrichment of *B. fragilis* and other beneficial taxa, including *Bifidobacterium* species, in patients responding favorably to ipilimumab (Frankel et al., 2017).

8.3.2 Microbiota influence on programmed death-1/programmed death ligand-1 immunotherapy

Similar microbiota dependencies have been identified for PD-1 and PD-L1 blockade (Routy et al., 2018). Both animal and human studies demonstrated that favorable clinical responses are associated with distinct microbial signatures rather than single bacterial species. Enrichment of taxa such as *Akkermansia muciniphila, Faecalibacterium, Bifidobacterium, Enterococcus hirae,* and certain *Clostridiales* correlates with improved outcomes across melanoma, nonsmall-cell lung cancer, and renal cell carcinoma (Gopalakrishnan et al., 2018). Functionally, these microbes enhance dendritic cell activation, promote $CD8^+$ T-cell priming, and increase intratumoral T-cell infiltration, thereby strengthening antitumor immunity (Matson et al., 2018). On the other hand, dysbiosis marked by an overrepresentation of potentially harmful taxa, like *Bacteroidales*, has been linked to resistance to PD-1/PD-L1 therapy. Notably, poorer immunotherapy outcomes are consistently correlated with antibiotic-induced dysbiosis, supporting the microbiota's causative role (Derosa et al., 2018). Crucially, variations in tumor type, host genetics, immunological environment, and analytical techniques are reflected in interstudy heterogeneity in microbial markers. These findings highlight the importance of ecosystem-level balance by demonstrating that immunotherapy response is determined by the structure and function of microbial communities rather than isolated species (Zitvogel et al., 2018).

8.3.3 Immune-related adverse events and microbiota

ICIs promote anticancer immunity by releasing inhibitory immune signals. However, this immune activation can extend beyond tumors and lead to immune-related adverse events (irAEs), which can damage organs like the skin, liver, lungs, gut, and endocrine tissues. These toxicities significantly limit immunotherapy. They do not arise from direct drug toxicity but from issues with immune tolerance (Postow et al., 2018; Sharma & Allison, 2015). Research shows that the gut microbiome plays an important role in maintaining immune balance, affecting both the severity and likelihood of experiencing irAEs (Zitvogel et al., 2018).

8.3.3.1 Microbiota control of immune tolerance and inflammatory balance

Commensal microbiota help maintain immune tolerance by managing regulatory T cells (Tregs), keeping the epithelial barrier intact, and altering proinflammatory cytokine signaling (Vétizou et al., 2015; Zitvogel et al., 2018). Dysbiosis increases the chance of immune overactivation after ICI treatment by disrupting these regulatory processes. Cohort studies show that patients with severe irAEs have different microbiome profiles compared to those who are tolerant. They often have lower microbial diversity and weaker functional capacity (Chaput et al., 2017; Dubin et al., 2016). Importantly, the therapeutic benefit does not always align with microbial effects on toxicity. It can be challenging to distinguish effectiveness from harm during immune checkpoint inhibition. Some microbiota enhance sensitivity to inflammatory damage while also boosting effector T-cell activation and anticancer immunity (Zitvogel et al., 2018).

8.3.3.2 Immune-mediated colitis and microbiota

The most common and significant irAE related to CTLA-4 and PD-1/PD-L1 inhibitors is immune-mediated colitis. Research indicates that the risk of colitis is linked to dysbiosis, which features reduced microbial richness and a decline in immunoregulatory taxa (Chaput et al., 2017; Vétizou et al., 2015). An increased abundance of *Bacteroides* species has been linked to a lower risk of colitis in patients receiving ipilimumab. This may happen through increased Treg induction and immune suppression mediated by interleukin-10 (Chaput et al., 2017; Frankel et al., 2017). Conversely, a surplus of proinflammatory microbial communities can lead to severe gastrointestinal toxicity, mucosal immune infiltration, and damage to the epithelial barrier (Dubin et al., 2016). Evidence from germ-free and antibiotic-treated animal models further supports the important role of the microbiota in regulating intestinal immune toxicity during checkpoint inhibitor therapy (Vétizou et al., 2015).

8.3.3.3 Immune-related hepatitis and the microbiota-liver axis

Another less common but serious irAE is immune-mediated hepatitis, especially in patients receiving combination ICIs. Since microbial metabolites and pathogen-associated molecular patterns reach the liver through the portal circulation, the gut-liver axis plays a crucial role in maintaining liver immune tolerance (Tripathi et al., 2018). Changes in bile acid metabolism and signaling molecules from microbes, influenced by dysbiosis, affect the activation of Kupffer cells, hepatic natural killer T-cell responses, and the production of inflammatory cytokines. These factors can determine susceptibility to ICI-induced hepatitis (Ma et al., 2018; Tripathi et al., 2018). Clinical findings suggest that an intact microbial diversity and metabolic balance are linked to a lower frequency of severe liver toxicity (Ma et al., 2018).

8.3.3.4 Pulmonary immune toxicity and microbiota

Although rare, immune-related pneumonitis can be a deadly side effect of ICIs. Recent evidence demonstrates that the gut microbiota composition influences lung immune balance through cytokine regulation and systemic immune priming (Wang et al., 2018). Patients may be more prone to lung inflammation during checkpoint suppression if dysbiosis promotes irregular T-cell activation and proinflammatory signaling. Clinical links between antibiotic use and a higher risk of pneumonitis support the idea of microbiota-mediated immune modulation, but further research is needed for a deeper understanding (Derosa et al., 2018).

8.3.3.5 The severity of immune-related adverse events, dysbiosis, and antibiotics

Exposure to antibiotics is a significant modifiable risk factor for the development of irAEs. Broad-spectrum antibiotics can harm immune regulatory networks that usually manage excessive inflammation by seriously disrupting microbial diversity and functional resilience (Derosa et al., 2018). Clinical studies indicate that patients who receive antibiotics before or during immunotherapy experience a higher rate of severe irAEs, such as hepatitis and colitis, often linked to reduced treatment effectiveness (Derosa et al., 2018; Routy et al., 2018). These results signify the importance of strategies that maintain microbiota and careful management of antibiotic use in patients undergoing immune checkpoint treatment.

8.3.3.6 Predictive and therapeutic implications

Microbiome-based predictors of irAEs have emerged as useful tools for evaluating toxicity risk. Metabolites derived from microbiota, active metabolic pathways, and baseline microbial diversity have shown potential as biomarkers for predicting susceptibility to irAEs

(Gopalakrishnan et al., 2018; Zitvogel et al., 2018). In cases of resistant immune-mediated colitis, therapeutic strategies like dietary changes and fecal microbiota transplantation (FMT) have shown promise; however, careful evaluation is needed to avoid compromising anticancer immunity (Wang et al., 2018). Overall, these findings support integrating microbiome profiling into immunotherapy safety measures and establish the microbiota as a crucial factor in immune-related toxicity management.

8.3.4 Microbiome-based biomarkers for response toward cancer treatment

Significant differences in how individuals respond to cancer therapy remain unclear, even with progress in immune profiling and tumor genetics. Growing evidence suggests that gut microbiota can provide useful biomarkers to predict toxicity and success in various cancer treatments (Gopalakrishnan et al., 2018; Zitvogel et al., 2018). Research indicates that having a more diverse gut microbiome, which supports a strong immune system, is associated with better outcomes. This is especially true for patients using ICIs (Dubin et al., 2016; Routy et al., 2018). In addition to diversity, distinctive microbial community structures distinguish responders from nonresponders, highlighting ecosystem-level organization as a determinant of responses rather than individual taxa. However, due to differences in geography, diet, and research methods, specific taxonomic markers may not consistently predict outcomes across different groups. Despite this, certain bacterial types like *A. muciniphila, Faecalibacterium,* and *Bifidobacterium* species have often been linked to favorable outcomes in immunotherapy (Gopalakrishnan et al., 2018; Routy et al., 2018). Thus, functional aspects of the microbiome are being recognized as more reliable and broadly applicable indicators.

Metagenomic and metabolomic studies reveal that microbial pathways involved in producing SCFAs, transforming bile acids, and metabolizing amino acids are closely linked to treatment response (Zitvogel et al., 2018). Microbial activity influences treatment effects through compounds like butyrate and inosine, which directly affect immune cell differentiation, activation of dendritic cells, and the function of cytotoxic T-cells. The discovery of bacteria residing in tumors adds another layer to potential biomarkers. Microorganisms present in tumors might influence local drug metabolism, immune cell infiltration, and resistance to treatment, while stool-based profiles can reflect systemic immune changes (Nejman et al., 2020). Therefore, combining systemic and localized microbiome data helps build a more comprehensive approach to predicting treatment responses. Despite their promise, microbiome-based biomarkers have limitations. These include variability between individuals, the impact of diet and antibiotics, and changes over time (Falony et al., 2016). For these biomarkers to be clinically useful, they must be validated and integrated with those from the host and tumor. Nonetheless, creating biomarkers that consider the microbiome is a vital step toward personalized cancer treatment.

8.4 Microbiota and radiotherapy response

The effectiveness and toxicity of radiotherapy, a crucial cancer treatment, vary significantly between patients because of variations in immune activation. The microbiota, a crucial regulator of host immunity, has a major impact on therapeutic results because radiation triggers both innate and adaptive immune responses (Shiao et al., 2021). In animal studies of melanoma and breast cancer, using antibiotics to reduce gut bacteria made radiotherapy less effective. In contrast, removing commensal fungi improved anticancer responses (Yang et al., 2021). The fungal sensor Dectin-1, which was also linked to survival in breast cancer patients, had to be expressed intratumorally for these effects to occur (Shiao et al., 2021; Yang et al., 2021).

Radiation responses are further modulated by microbial metabolites. Increased butyrate-producing gut bacterial abundance was inversely correlated with radiation efficacy in models of melanoma and colorectal cancer (Dong et al., 2021). By blocking TBK1 and IRF3 phosphorylation, butyrate inhibited the Stimulator of interferon genes (STING)-dependent type I interferon signaling in dendritic cells, thereby reducing radiation-induced cytotoxic T-cell responses without directly protecting tumor cells. Hepatocellular cancer has been linked to similar microbiota–STING interactions (Li et al., 2022). Beyond the gut, changes in the oral microbiota encouraged the translocation of *Fusobacterium nucleatum* to colorectal cancers, which decreased the effectiveness of radiotherapy; these effects were restored by antibiotic intervention (Venkidesh et al., 2023). Because gut or vaginal dysbiosis contributes to gastrointestinal and gynecologic side effects, which can be alleviated through microbiota regulation, microbiota also affects radiation-induced toxicity (Tsementzi et al., 2021).

8.4.1 Environmental, dietary, and lifestyle factors affecting the cancer microbiota

Various host-related and environmental factors affect the dynamic makeup and capabilities of the human microbiota. These include microbial diversity, metabolic output, and immune interactions, all of which are significantly influenced by diet, lifestyle choices, and environmental exposures (Integrative HMP Research Network Consortium, 2019; Knight et al., 2017). Understanding how these external factors shape microbial communities is vital for improving cancer treatment outcomes and advancing precision oncology, especially since the microbiota influences responses to chemotherapy, immunotherapy, and radiotherapy (Helmink et al., 2019).

8.4.1.1 Microbial diversity and dietary patterns

Diet is a key factor in determining gut microbiota composition. Long-term eating habits influence metabolite production, the structure of microbial communities, and microbial diversity. This, in turn, shapes immune responses essential for cancer treatment (David et al., 2014). Greater microbial diversity and an abundance of taxa that produce SCFA, such as *Faecalibacterium, Roseburia,* and *Eubacterium,* are linked to plant-based, fiber-rich diets like the Mediterranean diet. These microorganisms help maintain immune balance and support the intestinal barrier, enhancing anticancer immunity. Western-style diets that are high in fats and processed carbohydrates but low in fiber tend to encourage potentially harmful microbes, lower microbial diversity, and lead to dysbiosis (Turnbaugh et al., 2006). These dietary patterns are linked to weaker responses to ICIs and a higher risk of treatment-related side effects. Clinical studies show that cancer patients with higher baseline microbial diversity and fiber intake experience better progression-free survival after anti-PD-1 treatment (Spencer et al., 2021).

8.4.1.2 Microbial metabolites and dietary fiber

Fermenting dietary fiber by gut microbes produces SCFAs like acetate, propionate, and butyrate. These metabolites have various effects on tumor biology, immune function, and epigenetic regulation. For example, butyrate aids in the development of memory T-cells, enhances cytotoxic T-cell activity, and alters regulatory T-cell behavior by inhibiting histone deacetylase (He et al., 2021; Koh et al., 2016). However, the effects of SCFAs can vary depending on the circumstances. In some cases, excessive butyrate production might reduce dendritic cell activation and weaken type I interferon signaling. This can lower the effectiveness of immunotherapy or radiation, even though moderate levels may benefit immune-mediated tumor control (Li et al., 2022). These findings stress the importance of balanced microbial communities over random metabolite enrichment.

8.4.1.3 Metabolism of amino acids, fatty acids, and polyphenols

Certain dietary components, in addition to fiber, affect how the microbiome responds to cancer treatments. Gut bacteria also convert polyphenols from foods such as fruits, vegetables, tea, and coffee into bioactive compounds that have anti-inflammatory and anticancer effects (Selma et al., 2009). These metabolites enhance T-cell responses, improve antigen presentation, and help manage oxidative stress. Conditions like obesity and metabolic syndrome are associated with chronic low-grade inflammation, altered bile acid metabolism, and microbial imbalance (Costantini et al., 2017). Additionally, host and microbial enzymes break down amino acids such as arginine and tryptophan, producing metabolites that influence immune checkpoint signaling and T-cell growth (Routy et al., 2018). Changes in microbial amino acid metabolism have been linked to resistance to immunotherapy, underscoring the role of dietary changes.

8.4.1.4 Microbiota dysregulation, metabolic syndrome, and obesity

Obesity and metabolic syndrome are associated with chronic low-grade inflammation, altered bile acid metabolism, and gut dysbiosis (Tilg & Moschen, 2014). People with obesity often have more harmful microbial taxa and lower microbial diversity, which can weaken anticancer immune responses and reduce treatment effectiveness. Clinical evidence has connected obesity-related dysbiosis to increased immune-related side effects and poorer ICI responses (McQuade et al., 2018). The microbiota can also affect bile acid composition, which influences immune cell differentiation and tumor growth, via the Farnesoid X receptor (FXR) and TGR5 signaling pathways (Fiorucci & Distrutti, 2015). Together, these findings highlight the strong link between microbiota composition and metabolic health, both of which can affect cancer treatment results.

8.4.1.5 Microbiota-influencing lifestyle factors

Lifestyle choices such as exercise, smoking, drinking, and sleep habits also affect the microbiota. Regular exercise boosts immune function and lowers inflammation by increasing SCFA-producing bacteria and microbial diversity (Allen et al., 2018). Conversely, smoking and heavy drinking can lead to dysbiosis, disrupt the gut barrier, and cause systemic inflammation, negatively impacting cancer prognosis and treatment response (Biedermann & Rogler, 2015). Disrupting circadian rhythms, which often happens to cancer patients due to stress and treatment schedules, can also interfere with microbial activity and immune regulation (Leone et al., 2015). Recent studies suggest that timing treatments to align with circadian cycles and microbiota activity may enhance treatment effectiveness.

8.4.1.6 Environmental exposures and concomitant medications

Environmental factors, including exposure to antibiotics, proton pump inhibitors, and commonly prescribed medications like metformin, significantly influence microbiota composition (Imhann et al., 2016). Antibiotic-induced dysbiosis has been repeatedly linked to lower survival rates and reduced immunotherapy effectiveness (Huang et al., 2019). On the other hand, while its effects depend on the context, metformin can modify immune responses against tumors and impact microbial metabolism (García-González et al., 2017). Collectively, these findings highlight the importance of considering diet, lifestyle, and environmental exposures in microbiome-informed precision oncology. Tailoring interventions based on these factors may improve treatment effectiveness, reduce side effects, and enhance long-term outcomes.

8.5 Microbiota and molecularly targeted therapy

By specifically blocking oncogenic signaling pathways necessary for tumor growth, survival, and angiogenesis, molecularly targeted therapies constitute a fundamental component of contemporary oncology. Agents that target key signaling pathways, such as mitogen-activated protein kinase (MAPK), vascular endothelial growth factor (VEGF), and epidermal growth factor receptor (EGFR) pathways, have shown notable clinical benefits across various cancer types. Significant interindividual variation in treatment efficacy, toxicity, and resistance persists as a significant clinical challenge despite these advancements (Sawyers, 2004). Increasing evidence shows that the gut microbiota influences therapeutic outcomes beyond tumor-intrinsic genetic changes by influencing drug absorption, metabolism, immune signaling, and resistance pathways (Kuntz & Gilbert, 2017; Zmora et al., 2018).

8.5.1 Interactions between microbiota and epidermal growth factor receptor-targeted treatments

EGFR tyrosine kinase inhibitors (TKIs), like gefitinib and erlotinib, are commonly used to treat nonsmall-cell lung cancer and other epithelial cancers with activating EGFR mutations. Although patient selection mainly depends on tumor genomic profiling, growing research indicates that microbial composition may also impact treatment response and toxicity (Lynch et al., 2004). Preclinical studies demonstrate that gut microbiota may affect the pharmacokinetics of EGFR-TKIs by changing enterohepatic circulation, intestinal permeability, and epithelial transport (Maier et al., 2018). Increased gastrointestinal toxicity, which may require dose adjustments or treatment breaks, has been associated with dysbiosis, characterized by lower microbial diversity and an increase in proinflammatory bacteria. In addition, the microbiota may indirectly influence how the liver clears drugs by affecting bile acid metabolism, which can change overall drug levels in the body (Ridlon et al., 2006). EGFR inhibition also alters immune signaling in the TME. The microbiota may shape the immune response by affecting baseline immune activity and cytokine production. Together, these findings indicate that interactions between the host and microbiome significantly contribute to the success of EGFR-targeted therapy, along with tumor genetics (Ridlon et al., 2006).

8.5.2 Modulation of microbiota in antiangiogenic treatments

Bevacizumab and VEGF receptor inhibitors are antiangiogenic drugs that target the VEGF pathway to suppress tumor blood vessel growth and restore abnormal blood vessel structure. New research indicates that gut microbial composition may affect angiogenic signaling and how well patients respond to VEGF-targeted therapies (Folkman, 1995). Microbial metabolites, including SCFAs and secondary bile acids, play a role in regulating endothelial cell function and inflammatory pathways related to blood vessel formation (Koh et al., 2016). A dysbiotic microbiota may create an environment that promotes blood vessel growth and suppresses the immune response, which can be driven by increased overall inflammation and the expansion of myeloid-derived suppressor cells, thereby reducing the effectiveness of VEGF inhibition (Gabrilovich, 2017). Conversely, antiangiogenic treatments can disrupt gut balance, causing injury to the intestinal lining and altering the microbiota. This two-way interaction highlights the complexity of drug and microbiota interactions and underscores the importance of monitoring microbial changes during treatment (Imhann et al., 2016).

8.5.3 Microbiota influence on BRAF and MEK inhibitor responses

BRAF and MEK inhibitors are crucial for treating BRAF-mutant melanoma and other cancers that activate the MAPK pathway. These treatments primarily target signaling pathways within tumors, but their success increasingly appears to depend on immune responses influenced by the microbiota (Flaherty et al., 2012). A favorable gut microbiota composition has been associated with enhanced immune cell infiltration and better tumor responses in patients using MAPK pathway inhibitors (Routy et al., 2018). On the other hand, dysbiosis can trigger early resistance by creating an immunosuppressive tumor environment and activating alternative signaling pathways. Microbes might modify cytokine networks and antigen presentation, affecting both the strength and duration of the body's response to BRAF and MEK inhibition (Long et al., 2014).

8.5.4 Microbiota-driven resistance signaling pathways

The microbiota impacts drug metabolism and the immune system but also directly affects resistance signaling in tumor cells. Microbial components activate pattern recognition receptors, including Toll-like receptors. This activation triggers signaling pathways like NF-κB, STAT3, and MAPK, which help tumor cells endure treatment and resist drugs

(Rakoff-Nahoum & Medzhitov, 2009). Chronic inflammation caused by the microbiota can drive changes in cells that promote cancer. These changes include epithelial–mesenchymal transition and the development of cancer stem cell traits, hindering the effectiveness of targeted therapies (Batlle & Clevers, 2017). These resistance mechanisms resemble those seen in chemotherapy and immunotherapy, indicating that microbiota-driven signaling plays a significant role in therapeutic resistance across various cancer treatments.

8.5.5 Clinical implications

The effect of microbiota on patient responses to targeted therapy highlights the limitations of focusing solely on tumor characteristics in precision medicine. Incorporating microbiome profiling into clinical practice could improve patient classification, identify those at risk for side effects, and guide effective treatment combinations. Additionally, modifying the microbiota through dietary changes or targeting specific microbes might boost the effectiveness of targeted therapies, especially when approached in a personalized and controlled manner (Zmora et al., 2018).

8.6 Microbiota-targeted strategies to optimize cancer therapeutic outcomes

The recognition of the microbiota as a determinant of anticancer therapy response has transformed it from a confounding variable into a therapeutic target, highlighting its potential to be deliberately modulated to enhance treatment efficacy, overcome therapeutic resistance, and reduce treatment-related toxicity (Kouidhi et al., 2023). Strategies that target the microbiome can be tailored to match the specific microbiome profile of each patient (Kouidhi et al., 2023; Ngoc et al., 2024). The following are a few strategies for modifying the microbiota to optimize cancer therapeutic outcomes (Fig. 8.2).

8.6.1 Antibiotics

Antibiotics are widely used in patients with cancer to prevent and treat infections, but they can disrupt gut microbiota and can affect the clinical outcomes of immunotherapy (Kim et al., 2019). According to mounting clinical and preclinical evidence, reduced therapeutic responses to ICIs are linked to microbial disruption caused by antibiotics (Huang et al., 2019). In murine models of lung cancer or melanoma, antibiotics like vancomycin and ampicillin can disrupt the cells that help fight cancer, facilitating tumor metastasis (Cheng et al., 2014). Additionally, clinical research indicates that patients with lung and renal cancers who were exposed to antibiotics prior to receiving ICI treatment have a lower overall survival (OS) and progression-free survival (PFS) rate (Derosa et al., 2018). However, some evidence suggests the potential benefit when antibiotics are administered near ICI initiation (Fessas et al., 2021).

Meta-analyses indicate that avoiding the use of antibiotics within 42–60 days before immunotherapy improves OS, consistent with the microbiota recovery timelines

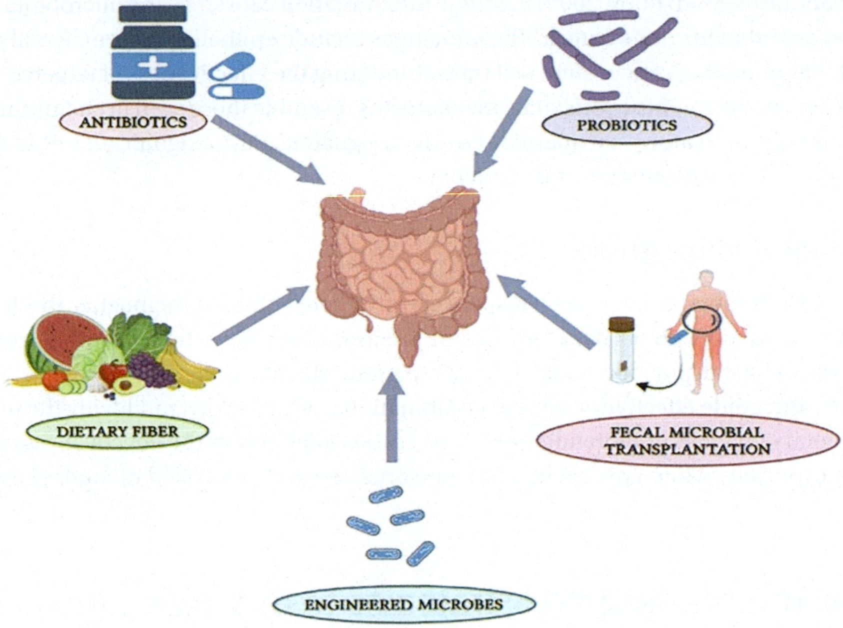

FIGURE 8.2 Harnessing microbiota-based interventions to optimize cancer therapy outcomes by modulating gut microbial composition, enhancing host immune responses, reducing treatment-associated toxicities, and improving the efficacy of chemotherapy, radiotherapy, and immunotherapy through precision-targeted microbial therapeutics.

(Wilson et al., 2020). Broad-spectrum antibiotics exert more profound effects on microbiota when compared with narrow-spectrum agents (Ahmed et al., 2018). Antibiotics may prevent microbial activity that promotes tumors, such as *Clostridium* species that produce androgens, and decrease the effectiveness of androgen restriction therapy for prostate cancer (Pernigoni et al., 2021). In microbiota-rich malignancies like pancreatic cancer, where antibiotics lessen microbial-driven immunosuppression and improve ICI efficacy, localized antibiotic treatments have shown beneficial effects (Pushalkar et al., 2018). In general, the use of antibiotics should be customized according to microbiome profile, immunological status, and tumor type (Wilson et al., 2020).

8.6.2 Probiotics

Probiotics are live microbial preparations that show beneficial physiological effects on the host upon administration in adequate amounts (Hill et al., 2014). According to the preclinical studies, it was demonstrated that *Bifidobacterium bifidum* K57 promotes $CD4^+$, $CD8^+$ T-cell activation and cytokine release, functioning in conjunction with anti-PD-1 therapy (Lee et al., 2021), whereas *B. pseudolongum* generates inosine that promotes T-cell adenosine A2A signaling (Martins et al., 2019). *Akkermansia* is a probiotic that promotes immunotherapy, according to next-generation sequencing (NGS)-based studies. TLR2 signaling is activated, Tfh cells are increased, and immunosuppressive Treg populations are decreased by the outer membrane protein Amuc (Ansaldo et al., 2019). Clinically, probiotics stimulate butyrate-producing bacteria primarily from the *Firmicutes* phylum, like *Roseburia, Eubacterium, Clostridium, Ruminococcus,* etc., linked to antitumor immunity, decreased postoperative infections, and reduced damage caused by radiation and chemotherapy (Jiang et al., 2019). Probiotic-based cancer treatment is still constrained by the lack of standardization, strain variability, and trial paucity despite encouraging outcomes (Spencer et al., 2021). Evidence also suggests that high dietary fiber consumption without probiotic supplementation may maximize the effectiveness of immunotherapy (Spencer et al., 2021).

8.6.3 Fecal microbiota transplantation

FMT originated from traditional Chinese medicine. It has gained renewed interest because it can restore microbial diversity and affect host metabolism and immunity. This method involves transferring stool from a healthy or treatment-responsive donor into a patient's gastrointestinal tract to restore or change the gut microbial community (Zitvogel et al., 2018). It was first studied in metabolic disorders, where microbiota from lean donors improved insulin sensitivity in obese recipients. This effect links to an increase in butyrate-producing bacteria (Grigorescu & Dumitrascu, 2016). These findings provided a rationale for extending FMT to cancer therapy. Preclinical studies show that FMT from patients who respond well to anticancer treatments improves effectiveness in mouse models (Routy et al., 2018). Clinical trials evaluating FMT in cancer immunotherapy are largely confined to early phases (Table 8.1)(US National Library of Medicine. ClinicalTrials.gov Identifier, 2025, US National Library of Medicine. ClinicalTrials.gov Identifier, 2024, US National Library of Medicine. ClinicalTrials.gov Identifier, 2021, US National Library of Medicine. ClinicalTrials.gov Identifier, 2025, US National Library of Medicine. ClinicalTrials.gov Identifier, 2024 Recipients of FMT from responders display more $CD8^+$ cytotoxic T cells and innate immune effector cells, along with fewer immunosuppressive myeloid and regulatory T-cell populations. In contrast, FMT from nonresponders slows antitumor immunity and speeds up tumor growth (Baruch et al., 2021; Routy et al., 2018). These findings imply that a healthy gut microbiome can enhance immune responses in the tumor and systemically throughout the body, particularly increasing the efficacy of ICIs (Baruch et al., 2021). Although FMT is widely used, it is only approved for recurrent *Clostridium difficile* infections. Its application in cancer therapy is restricted to clinical trials (Wang et al., 2018). Emerging evidence indicates that FMT could improve the effectiveness of immunotherapy in colorectal cancer and melanoma, while also reducing treatment-related side effects, such as chemotherapy-induced gastrointestinal issues (Davar et al., 2021). Despite its potential, challenges like choosing donors, standardizing protocols, finding the right dose, and safety concerns, including the risk of infection and immune-related side effects, make routine clinical use difficult. Still, FMT is a promising microbiome-based strategy in precision oncology (Zitvogel et al., 2018). Several clinical trials are currently investigating FMT as an adjuvant strategy to enhance the efficacy and overcome resistance to ICIs in cancer therapy (Table 8.1).

Table 8.1 Clinical trials evaluating FMT with immunotherapy.

Clinical trial phase (Trial id)	Subjects (n)	Type of cancer	Immuno therapy regimen	FMT donor type	FMT route	Outcome
I(NCT03772899) (US National Library of Medicine. ClinicalTrials.gov Identifier, 2025)	20	Melanoma	αPD-1 mAb	ICI responder	Oral capsules	Safety
II(NCT03341143) (US National Library of Medicine. ClinicalTrials.gov Identifier, 2024)	18	Melanoma	αPD-1 mAb	ICI responder	Colonoscopy ± capsules	Objective response rate
I(NCT05008861) (US National Library of Medicine. ClinicalTrials.gov Identifier, 2021)	20	NSCLC	αPD-1 mAb and chemotherapy	NR*	Capsules	Adverse events, objective response rate
I(NCT04163289) (US National Library of Medicine. ClinicalTrials.gov Identifier, 2025)	20	Renal cancer	αPD-1 mAb or αCTLA-4 mAb	Healthy Donor	Oral capsules	Immune-related colitis
I(NCT04130763) (US National Library of Medicine. ClinicalTrials.gov Identifier, 2024)	10	Gastro intestinal cancer	αPD-1 mAb	NR*	Colonoscopy	Objective response rate, abnormal vital signs, adverse events

*NR denotes not reported in the trial registry.

αCTLA-4, anticytotoxic T-lymphocyte-associated antigen-4; *αPD-1*, antiprogrammed death-1; *FMT*, fecal microbiota transplantation; *ICI*, immune checkpoint inhibitors; *NSCLC*, nonsmall-cell lung cancer.

8.6.4 Emerging engineered microbiome approaches

The engineering of microbes that precisely colonize tumors and modify the TME has improved anticancer immunity through recent developments in synthetic biology (Zitvogel et al., 2018). Immunostimulatory molecules or therapeutic compounds can be delivered locally by engineered strains of *Salmonella, Escherichia coli,* and *Bifidobacterium* (Chowdhury et al., 2019). For instance, modified *E. coli* Nissle 1917 increases CD4 and CD8+ cytotoxic T lymphocyte infiltration and improves anti-PD-L1 therapeutic responsiveness by converting tumor-derived ammonia into L-arginine, a crucial metabolite for T-cell survival (Canale et al., 2021). In preclinical models, other modified bacteria are made to lyse inside tumors and produce immune modulators such as anti-CD47 nanobodies, which improve tumor phagocytosis, stimulate tumor-infiltrating T-cells, inhibit metastasis, and extend survival. In addition to engineered microbial strains, several microbiome-based strategies are being studied to improve immunotherapy outcomes. Genetically modified commensal bacteria, like *Staphylococcus epidermidis,* altered to express tumor antigens, can stimulate tumor-specific T-cell responses that may inhibit both primary and metastatic cancers (Chen et al., 2018). Tumor suppression can be aided by the delivery of immunomodulatory chemicals and antigens by bacterial extracellular vesicles and outer membrane vesicles generated from *Bifidobacterium* and *Lactobacillus* (Luo et al., 2024). Other strategies include microbial metabolites like valproic acid that function as histone deacetylase inhibitors and work in conjunction with ICIs (Yang et al., 2023); microbiota-derived peptides like EO2401 that mimic tumor-associated antigens and activate memory T cells, showing clinical benefit in glioblastoma patients (Talpin et al., 2024); and phage therapy to reshape the microbiota and TME (Hsu et al., 2019). Collectively, these strategies highlight the growing potential of synthetic consortia, microbial products, and engineered microbes as accurate and durable cancer immunotherapy modalities (Zitvogel et al., 2018).

8.6.5 Advanced techniques for modulating the microbiome in precision oncology

Probiotics, FMT, and modified bacteria are types of live microbial therapies that can affect anticancer immunity. However, safety issues, differences between strains, and complex regulations limit their practical use (Baruch et al., 2021; Martins et al., 2019; Zitvogel et al., 2018). Consequently, nonliving or indirect microbiome-modulation techniques that change host-microbiome interactions and microbial activity without introducing live organisms have gained more attention (Kuntz & Gilbert, 2017; Ting et al., 2022). These methods include bacteriophages, prebiotics, postbiotics, dietary changes, and fecal virome transplantation (FVT). They offer safer, scalable, and more practical ways to integrate microbiome science into precision oncology (Hsu et al., 2019; Knight et al., 2017; Koh et al., 2016).

8.6.5.1 Dietary modulation as a foundational microbiome intervention

Diet significantly influences gut microbiome composition and metabolic activity. In cancer patients, diet quickly and consistently impacts microbial diversity, metabolite production, epithelial barrier integrity, and immune function (David et al., 2014; Knight et al., 2017). Dietary fiber intake, in particular, is important for boosting antitumor immunity (Spencer et al., 2021; Zitvogel et al., 2018). High-fiber diets increase SCFA-producing bacteria in the *Ruminococcaceae* and *Lachnospiraceae* families. The bacteria are associated with better responses to ICIs and greater intratumoral $CD8^+$ T-cell infiltration (Bachem et al., 2019; Koh et al., 2016; Spencer et al., 2021). On a mechanistic level, when microbes ferment dietary fiber, they produce SCFAs like butyrate, propionate, and acetate. These substances regulate immune responses through various pathways (Koh et al., 2016; Nicholson et al., 2012). SCFAs inhibit histone deacetylases, promote dendritic cell maturation, enhance antigen presentation, and influence T-cell differentiation and memory formation (Bachem et al., 2019; He et al., 2021). Importantly, these effects are context-dependent; excessive SCFA exposure may induce T-cell quiescence or impair effector function under certain metabolic conditions, highlighting the necessity of balanced microbial ecosystems rather than indiscriminate metabolite enrichment (Donohoe et al., 2012; Vander Heiden et al., 2009). Overall, these findings suggest that dietary changes could play a crucial role in a patient-centered approach to microbiome-informed precision oncology (Zitvogel et al., 2018; Zmora et al., 2018).

8.6.5.2 Selective ecosystem reconfiguration and prebiotics

Prebiotics provide a targeted way to change the microbiome by promoting the proliferation and metabolic activity of beneficial microbes (Knight et al., 2017; Kuntz & Gilbert, 2017). Unlike probiotics, which introduce new strains that may or may not establish themselves successfully, prebiotics work with existing microbial communities that are already adapted to the host (Kuntz & Gilbert, 2017; Zmora et al., 2018). Common prebiotics include inulin, fructo-oligosaccharides, resistant starches, and substances rich in polyphenols, all of which affect microbial structure and function differently (Koh et al., 2016; Selma et al., 2009). Research shows that giving prebiotics can increase SCFA production, enhance antitumor immune responses, including improved sensitivity to ICIs, and restore microbial diversity after chemotherapy or antibiotic treatment (Alexander et al., 2017; Bachem et al., 2019; Zitvogel et al., 2018). However, responses to prebiotics can vary widely from person to person, influenced by dietary habits, metabolic states, and baseline microbiome composition (Falony et al., 2016; Knight et al., 2017). These findings underline the importance of characterizing the microbiome when applying prebiotic strategies in precision cancer treatment (Kuntz & Gilbert, 2017; Zmora et al., 2018).

8.6.5.3 Microbial metabolites and postbiotics as immunomodulators

Postbiotics, a rapidly growing type of therapy derived from the microbiome, consist of nonviable microbial metabolites with biological effects (Koh et al., 2016; Yang et al., 2023). These include microbial nucleosides, indoles, polyamines, bile acid derivatives, and SCFAs that directly influence metabolic and immune pathways (Koh et al., 2016; Nicholson et al., 2012). For example, inosine has a significant role in improving immunotherapy responses, enhancing T-cell effector function through signaling at the adenosine A2A receptor, especially in tumor environments with metabolic restrictions (He et al., 2021; Yang et al., 2023). Secondary bile acids modify immune tolerance by influencing liver natural killer T cells and myeloid cell activation through interactions along the gut-liver axis (Ma et al., 2018; Tripathi et al., 2018). Importantly, the effects of postbiotics depend on the host's metabolic conditions, tumor type, and immune state. Therefore, therapies based on postbiotics must be carefully dosed to avoid unwanted immune suppression (Donohoe et al., 2012; Vander Heiden et al., 2009).

8.6.5.4 Virome-targeted modulation and bacteriophages

The gut virome, especially bacteriophages, has also become a major factor in human immunity and microbial ecology (Dohlman et al., 2022; Hsu et al., 2019). Bacteriophages influence bacterial populations through predation, gene transfer, and metabolic changes, indirectly affecting immune responses (Hsu et al., 2019; Knight et al., 2017). Phage-mediated microbiome modifications offer a precise method for targeting harmful or immunosuppressive bacterial types while preserving beneficial communities (Hsu et al., 2019; Zmora et al., 2018). Research indicates that phage therapy can alter metabolite profiles, reorganize microbial networks, and influence inflammatory signaling crucial for cancer growth and treatment responses (Cheng et al., 2020; Hsu et al., 2019). While its application in oncology is still developing, phage-based methods show promise as precision tools for microbiome editing with fewer side effects than broad-spectrum antibiotics (Derosa et al., 2018; Hsu et al., 2019).

8.6.5.5 Fecal virome transplantation and nonbacterial components

FVT is an emerging method that targets only the viral components of the gut environment (Dohlman et al., 2022; Hsu et al., 2019). FVT aims to restore microbial balance by delivering virus-like particles that do not contain live bacteria, reducing the risk of infections (Hsu et al., 2019). Preclinical studies suggest that FVT can replicate some benefits of FMT, like restoring microbial diversity and immune balance, through bacteriophage-mediated control of bacterial populations (Hsu et al., 2019; Knight et al., 2017). Despite the limited data in oncology, FVT highlights the broader importance of nonbacterial microbiome components in regulating immune function and treatment responses (Dohlman et al., 2022; Hsu et al., 2019). As methods improve for characterizing and manipulating the virome, FVT may offer an additional or alternative approach for modifying the microbiome in cancer patients (Franzosa et al., 2018; Knight et al., 2017).

8.7 Challenges, limitations, and future directions toward integrative precision oncology

The integration of microbiome-informed methods into routine cancer care is still limited by conceptual, technical, and clinical barriers, despite major advancements in understanding microbiome-host-tumor interactions (Helmink et al., 2019; Zitvogel et al., 2018). The diversity, changeability, and differences in microbiome across individuals complicate standardization and clinical decision-making. Preclinical and early clinical studies show that microbial ecosystems influence treatment effectiveness and side effects (Gopalakrishnan et al., 2018; Knight et al., 2017). To incorporate microbiome science into future precision oncology, several challenges must be addressed (Kuntz & Gilbert, 2017).

8.7.1 Interindividual variability and biological complexity

Interindividual variability and biological complexity. The vast range of microbial communities among individuals stands as one of the biggest challenges for microbiome-based cancer treatments (Falony et al., 2016; Knight et al., 2017). Even in clinically similar populations, significant differences in microbiome composition and function can arise from host genetics, nutrition, geography, age, other health conditions, prior antibiotic use, and prior cancer treatments (Falony et al., 2016). Consequently, microbial profiles associated with treatment responses in one group often fail to repeat in other studies, limiting their usefulness as general biomarkers (Frankel et al., 2017; Knight et al., 2017). Microbial functions are also highly dynamic (Nicholson et al., 2012). Microbial gene expression and metabolic outputs change rapidly in response to factors such as diet, treatment, inflammation, and disease progression, unlike the more stable human genome (Maier et al., 2018; Nicholson et al., 2012). This variability emphasizes the need for longitudinal sampling methods and raises concerns about the usefulness of microbiome data collected at a single time point for guiding long-term treatment decisions (Franzosa et al., 2018; Integrative HMP Research Network Consortium, 2019).

8.7.2 Causality versus correlation

A continuing challenge in this field is telling apart causal microbial effects from mere associations (Knight et al., 2017; Zitvogel et al., 2018). Many clinical studies identify correlations between microbial taxa or metabolites and treatment outcomes, but definitive causal inference remains difficult because of confounding variables like diet, medication exposure, and severity of the disease (Knight et al., 2017; Kuntz & Gilbert, 2017) The intricacy of the human immune system and microbiome cannot be fully replicated by germ-free and antibiotic-treated animal models, despite the fact that they have yielded insightful information (Knight et al., 2017; Viaud et al., 2013). Interventional studies, including dietary changes, antibiotic use, and microbiome transfer techniques, can provide stronger evidence of causality, but they tend to be limited in scale and scope (Derosa et al., 2018; Spencer et al., 2021). Strong validation of causality will require well-designed, randomized trials that stratify based on microbiome data and focus on functional outcomes rather than just taxonomic relationships (Franzosa et al., 2018; Integrative HMP Research Network Consortium, 2019).

8.7.3 Analytical and methodological constraints

Another major hurdle is the technical variation among microbiome studies (Integrative HMP Research Network Consortium, 2019; Knight et al., 2017). Inconsistent results and limited study comparability arise from variations in sample collection, sequencing technologies, storage, bioinformatic workflows, and statistical analyses (Franzosa et al., 2018; Knight et al., 2017). Furthermore, commonly used 16S rRNA sequencing does not capture nonbacterial components like fungi, viruses, and phages, which are increasingly recognized as important regulators of the immune response (Dohlman et al., 2022; Franzosa et al., 2018). Although methods like metatranscriptomics, metabolomics, and shotgun metagenomics offer deeper functional insights, their high costs, complexity, and susceptibility to contamination from host DNA, especially in tumor samples, limit their clinical use (Franzosa et al., 2018; Nejman et al., 2020). There is a critical need for the development of clinically viable tests and the standardization of analytical processes (Integrative HMP Research Network Consortium, 2019; Kuntz & Gilbert, 2017).

8.7.4 Safety, ethics, and regulatory considerations

Interventions targeting the microbiome raise specific ethical and safety concerns (Helmink et al., 2019). Treatments like probiotics, FMT, and modified bacteria come with risks of infection, gene transfer, and unintended immune activation, particularly in cancer patients with weakened immune systems (Martins et al., 2019; Wang et al., 2018). Even nonliving therapies, such as postbiotics and dietary changes, may have context-dependent adverse effects if not applied carefully (Donohoe et al., 2012; Spencer et al., 2021). Regulatory frameworks for microbiome-based treatments are still underdeveloped (Kuntz & Gilbert, 2017; Zmora et al., 2018). Inconsistent classifications hinder large-scale clinical applications and complicate regulatory procedures for pharmaceuticals, biologics, live treatments, and dietary supplements (Hill et al., 2014; Kuntz & Gilbert, 2017). To bring microbiome-informed therapies beyond experimental stages, consistent manufacturing practices, clear regulatory guidance, and long-term safety monitoring are essential (Helmink et al., 2019; Hill et al., 2014).

8.7.5 Precision oncology and the microbiome

The future of microbiome-informed oncology lies in integrated systems-level frameworks that consider the microbiome alongside tumor genetics, host immunology, metabolism, and environmental factors rather than relying on isolated therapies (Ngoc et al., 2024; Tsimberidou et al., 2020). The characteristics of the microbiome should be considered as factors that modify treatment environments, affecting drug metabolism, immune activity, and the risk of side effects, rather than as standalone therapies (Cheng et al., 2020; Ting et al., 2022). A key step toward this goal is integrating multiple omics types. Combining metagenomics, transcriptomics, metabolomics, tumor genomes, and immune profiling allows for the identification of functional microbial pathways that influence treatment response and resistance (Franzosa et al., 2018; Integrative HMP Research Network Consortium, 2019). Although clinical validation is still limited, machine learning methods applied to these integrated datasets have shown promise in identifying prognostic signatures that outperform single-modality biomarkers (Wong et al., 2021; Knight et al., 2017).

8.8 Conclusion

Therapeutic resistance and treatment-related toxicity remain as major challenges in cancer treatment. Mounting evidence underscores the significant role of the microbiota in influencing carcinogenesis, antitumor immune responses, and the effectiveness of anticancer therapies. Although strategies aimed at modulating the gut microbiota are associated with limitations and safety concerns, these approaches have demonstrated promising potential to improve and optimize therapeutic outcomes. Despite these results, major challenges remain. Advancing pharmacomicrobiomics through integrated longitudinal human studies that combine metagenomics with other multiomics approaches, functional analyses, and well-designed clinical trials is essential to identify key microbial drivers of treatment outcomes and to translate the current insights into safe and effective personalized cancer therapies.

References

Ahmed, J., Kumar, A., Parikh, K., Anwar, A., Knoll, B. M., Puccio, C., Chun, H., Fanucchi, M., & Lim, S. H. (2018). Use of broad-spectrum antibiotics impacts outcome in patients treated with immune checkpoint inhibitors. *OncoImmunology, 7*(11). https://doi.org/10.1080/2162402x.2018.1507670.

Alexander, J. L., Wilson, I. D., Teare, J., Marchesi, J. R., Nicholson, J. K., & Kinross, J. M. (2017). Gut microbiota modulation of chemotherapy efficacy and toxicity. *Nature Reviews Gastroenterology and Hepatology, 14*(6), 356–365. https://doi.org/10.1038/nrgastro.2017.20.

Allen, J. M., Mailing, L. J., Niemiro, G. M., Moore, R., Cook, M. D., White, B. A., Holscher, H. D., & Woods, J. A. (2018). Exercise alters gut microbiota composition and function in lean and obese humans. *Medicine and Science in Sports and Exercise, 50*(4), 747–757. https://doi.org/10.1249/MSS.0000000000001495.

Ansaldo, E., Slayden, L. C., Ching, K. L., Koch, M. A., Wolf, N. K., Plichta, D. R., Brown, E. M., Graham, D. B., Xavier, R. J., Moon, J. J., & Barton, G. M. (2019). *Akkermansia muciniphila* induces intestinal adaptive immune responses during homeostasis. *Science, 364*(6446), 1179–1184. https://doi.org/10.1126/science.aaw7479.

Bachem, A., Makhlouf, C., Binger, K. J., de Souza, D. P., Tull, D., Hochheiser, K., Whitney, P. G., Fernandez-Ruiz, D., Dähling, S., Kastenmüller, W., Jönsson, J., Gressier, E., Lew, A. M., Perdomo, C., Kupz, A., Figgett, W., Mackay, F., Oleshansky, M., Russ, B. E., … Bedoui, S. (2019). Microbiota-derived short-chain fatty acids promote the memory potential of antigen-activated CD8+ T cells. *Immunity, 51*(2), 285. https://doi.org/10.1016/j.immuni.2019.06.002.

Bailly, C. (2019). Irinotecan: 25 years of cancer treatment. *Pharmacological Research, 148*, 104398. https://doi.org/10.1016/j.phrs.2019.104398.

Baruch, E. N., Youngster, I., Ben-Betzalel, G., Ortenberg, R., Lahat, A., Katz, L., Adler, K., Dick-Necula, D., Raskin, S., Bloch, N., Rotin, D., Anafi, L., Avivi, C., Melnichenko, J., Steinberg-Silman, Y., Mamtani, R., Harati, H., Asher, N., Shapira-Frommer, R., … Boursi, B. (2021). Fecal microbiota transplant promotes response in immunotherapy-refractory melanoma patients. *Science, 371*(6529), 602–609. https://doi.org/10.1126/science.abb5920.

Batlle, E., & Clevers, H. (2017). Cancer stem cells revisited. *Nature Medicine, 23*(10), 1124–1134. https://doi.org/10.1038/nm.4409.

Bhatt, A. P., Pellock, S. J., Biernat, K. A., Walton, W. G., Wallace, B. D., Creekmore, B. C., Letertre, M. M., Swann, J. R., Wilson, I. D., Roques, J. R., Darr, D. B., Bailey, S. T., Montgomery, S. A., Roach, J. M., Azcarate-Peril, M. A., Sartor, R. B., Gharaibeh, R. Z., Bultman, S. J., & Redinbo, M. R. (2020). Targeted inhibition of gut bacterial β-glucuronidase activity enhances anticancer drug efficacy. *Proceedings of the National Academy of Sciences, 117*(13), 7374–7381. https://doi.org/10.1073/pnas.1918095117.

Biedermann, L., & Rogler, G. (2015). The intestinal microbiota: Its role in health and disease. *European Journal of Pediatrics, 174*(2), 151–167. https://doi.org/10.1007/s00431-014-2476-2.

Canale, F. P., Basso, C., Antonini, G., Perotti, M., Li, N., Sokolovska, A., Neumann, J., James, M. J., Geiger, S., Jin, W., Theurillat, J. P., West, K. A., Leventhal, D. S., Lora, J. M., Sallusto, F., & Geiger, R. (2021). Metabolic modulation of tumours with engineered bacteria for immunotherapy. *Nature, 598*(7882), 662–666. https://doi.org/10.1038/s41586-021-04003-2.

Chaput, N., Lepage, P., Coutzac, C., Soularue, E., Le Roux, K., Monot, C., Boselli, L., Routier, E., Cassard, L., Collins, M., Vaysse, T., Marthey, L., Eggermont, A., Asvatourian, V., Lanoy, E., Mateus, C., Robert, C., & Carbonnel, F. (2017). Baseline gut microbiota predicts clinical response and colitis in metastatic melanoma patients treated with ipilimumab. *Annals of Oncology, 28*(6), 1368–1379. https://doi.org/10.1093/annonc/mdx108.

Chen, Y. E., Fischbach, M. A., & Belkaid, Y. (2018). Skin microbiota–host interactions. *Nature, 553*(7689), 427–436. https://doi.org/10.1038/nature25177.

Cheng, M., Qian, L., Shen, G., Bian, G., Xu, T., Xu, W., Shen, G., & Hu, S. (2014). Microbiota modulate tumoral immune surveillance in lung through a γδT17 immune cell-dependent mechanism. *Cancer Research, 74*(15), 4030–4041. https://doi.org/10.1158/0008-5472.can-13-2462.

Cheng, W. Y., Wu, C. Y., & Yu, J. (2020). The role of gut microbiota in cancer treatment: Friend or foe? *Gut, 69*(10), 1867–1876. https://doi.org/10.1136/gutjnl-2020-321153.

Chowdhury, S., Castro, S., Coker, C., Hinchliffe, T. E., Arpaia, N., & Danino, T. (2019). Programmable bacteria induce durable tumor regression and systemic antitumor immunity. *Nature Medicine, 25*(7), 1057–1063. https://doi.org/10.1038/s41591-019-0498-z.

Costantini, L., Molinari, R., Farinon, B., & Merendino, N. (2017). Impact of omega-3 fatty acids on the gut microbiota. *International Journal of Molecular Sciences, 18*(12), 2645. https://doi.org/10.3390/ijms18122645.

Daillère, R., Vétizou, M., Waldschmitt, N., Yamazaki, T., Isnard, C., Poirier-Colame, V., Duong, C. P. M., Flament, C., Lepage, P., Roberti, M. P., Routy, B., Jacquelot, N., Apetoh, L., Becharef, S., Rusakiewicz, S., Langella, P., Sokol, H., Kroemer, G., Enot, D., … Zitvogel, L. (2016). *Enterococcus hirae* and *Barnesiella intestinihominis* facilitate cyclophosphamide-induced therapeutic immunomodulatory effects. *Immunity, 45*(4), 931–943. https://doi.org/10.1016/j.immuni.2016.09.009.

Davar, D., Dzutsev, A. K., McCulloch, J. A., Rodrigues, R. R., Chauvin, J. M., Morrison, R. M., Deblasio, R. N., Menna, C., Ding, Q., Pagliano, O., Zidi, B., Zhang, S., Badger, J. H., Vetizou, M., Cole, A. M., Fernandes, M. R., Prescott, S., Costa, R. G. F., Balaji, A. K., … Zarour, H. M. (2021). Fecal microbiota transplant overcomes resistance to anti-PD-1 therapy in melanoma patients. *Science, 371*(6529), 595–602. https://doi.org/10.1126/science.abf3363.

David, L. A., Maurice, C. F., Carmody, R. N., Gootenberg, D. B., Button, J. E., Wolfe, B. E., Ling, A. V., Devlin, A. S., Varma, Y., Fischbach, M. A., Biddinger, S. B., Dutton, R. J., & Turnbaugh, P. J. (2014). Diet rapidly and reproducibly alters the human gut microbiome. *Nature, 505*(7484), 559–563. https://doi.org/10.1038/nature12820.

Derosa, L., Hellmann, M. D., Spaziano, M., Halpenny, D., Fidelle, M., Rizvi, H., Long, N., Plodkowski, A. J., Arbour, K. C., Chaft, J. E., Rouche, J. A., Zitvogel, L., Zalcman, G., Albiges, L., Escudier, B., & Routy, B. (2018). Negative association of antibiotics on clinical activity of immune checkpoint inhibitors in patients with advanced renal cell and non-small-cell lung cancer. *Annals of Oncology, 29*(6), 1437–1444. https://doi.org/10.1093/annonc/mdy103.

Dohlman, A. B., Klug, J., Mesko, M., Gao, I. H., Lipkin, S. M., Shen, X., & Iliev, I. D. (2022). A pan-cancer mycobiome analysis reveals fungal involvement in gastrointestinal and lung tumors. *Cell, 185*(20), 3807. https://doi.org/10.1016/j.cell.2022.09.015.

Dong, J., Li, Y., Xiao, H., Zhang, S., Wang, B., Wang, H., Li, Y., Fan, S., & Cui, M. (2021). Oral microbiota affects the efficacy and prognosis of radiotherapy for colorectal cancer in mouse models. *Cell Reports, 37*(4), 109886. https://doi.org/10.1016/j.celrep.2021.109886.

Donohoe, D. R., Collins, L. B., Wali, A., Bigler, R., Sun, W., & Bultman, S. J. (2012). The Warburg effect dictates the mechanism of butyrate-mediated histone acetylation and cell proliferation. *Molecular Cell, 48*(4), 612–626. https://doi.org/10.1016/j.molcel.2012.08.033.

Dubin, K., Callahan, M. K., Ren, B., Khanin, R., Viale, A., Ling, L., No, D., Gobourne, A., Littmann, E., Huttenhower, C., Pamer, E. G., & Wolchok, J. D. (2016). Intestinal microbiome analyses identify melanoma patients at risk for checkpoint-blockade-induced colitis. *Nature Communications, 7*(1). https://doi.org/10.1038/ncomms10391.

Falony, G., Joossens, M., Vieira-Silva, S., Wang, J., Darzi, Y., Faust, K., Kurilshikov, A., Bonder, M. J., Valles-Colomer, M., Vandeputte, D., Tito, R. Y., Chaffron, S., Rymenans, L., Verspecht, C., Sutter, L., Lima-Mendez, G., D'hoe, K., Jonckheere, K., Homola, D., … Raes, J. (2016). Population-level analysis of gut microbiome variation. *Science, 352*(6285), 560–564. https://doi.org/10.1126/science.aad3503.

Fan, Y., & Pedersen, O. (2021). Gut microbiota in human metabolic health and disease. *Nature Reviews Microbiology, 19*(1), 55–71. https://doi.org/10.1038/s41579-020-0433-9.

Fessas, P., Naeem, M., Pinter, M., Marron, T. U., Szafron, D., Balcar, L., Saeed, A., Jun, T., Dharmapuri, S., Gampa, A., Wang, Y., Khan, U., Muzaffar, M., Navaid, M., Lee, P.-C., Bulumulle, A., Yu, B. o, Paul, S., Nimkar, N., … Pinato, D. J. (2021). Early antibiotic exposure is not detrimental to therapeutic effect from immunotherapy in hepatocellular carcinoma. *Liver Cancer, 10*(6), 583–592. https://doi.org/10.1159/000519108.

Fiorucci, S., & Distrutti, E. (2015). Bile acid-activated receptors, intestinal microbiota, and the treatment of metabolic disorders. *Trends in Molecular Medicine, 21*(11), 702–714. https://doi.org/10.1016/j.molmed.2015.09.001.

Flaherty, K. T., Infante, J. R., Daud, A., Gonzalez, R., Kefford, R. F., Sosman, J., Hamid, O., Schuchter, L., Cebon, J., Ibrahim, N., Kudchadkar, R., Burris, H. A., Falchook, G., Algazi, A., Lewis, K., Long, G. V., Puzanov, I., Lebowitz, P., Singh, A., … Weber, J. (2012). Combined BRAF and MEK inhibition in melanoma with BRAF V600 mutations. *New England Journal of Medicine, 367*(18), 1694–1703. https://doi.org/10.1056/NEJMoa1210093.

Folkman, J. (1995). Angiogenesis in cancer, vascular, rheumatoid and other disease. *Nature Medicine, 1*(1), 27–30. https://doi.org/10.1038/nm0195-27.

Frankel, A. E., Coughlin, L. A., Kim, J., Froehlich, T. W., Xie, Y., Frenkel, E. P., & Koh, A. Y. (2017). Metagenomic shotgun sequencing and unbiased metabolomic profiling identify specific human gut microbiota associated with immune checkpoint therapy efficacy in metastatic melanoma. *Cancer Immunology Research, 5*(10), 848–860. https://doi.org/10.1158/2326-6066.CIR-17-0140.

Franzosa, E. A., McIver, L. J., Rahnavard, G., Thompson, L. R., Schirmer, M., Weingart, G., Lipson, K. S., Knight, R., Caporaso, J. G., Segata, N., & Huttenhower, C. (2018). Species-level functional profiling of metagenomes and metatranscriptomes. *Nature Methods, 15*(11), 962–968. https://doi.org/10.1038/s41592-018-0176-y.

Gabrilovich, D. I. (2017). Myeloid-derived suppressor cells. *Cancer Immunology Research, 5*(1), 3–8. https://doi.org/10.1158/2326-6066.CIR-16-0297.

Galluzzi, L., Humeau, J., Buqué, A., Zitvogel, L., & Kroemer, G. (2020). Immunostimulation with chemotherapy in the era of immune checkpoint inhibitors. *Nature Reviews Clinical Oncology, 17*(12), 725–741. https://doi.org/10.1038/s41571-020-0413-z.

García-González, A. P., Ritter, A. D., Shrestha, S., Anderson, E. C., Yilmaz, L. S., & Walhout, A. J. M. (2017). Bacterial metabolism affects the Caenorhabditis elegans response to cancer chemotherapeutics. *Cell, 169*, 431–445.e12. https://doi.org/10.1016/j.cell.2017.03.043.

Geller, L. T., Barzily-Rokni, M., Danino, T., Jonas, O. H., Shental, N., Nejman, D., Gavert, N., Zwang, Y., Cooper, Z. A., Shee, K., Thaiss, C. A., Reuben, A., Livny, J., Avraham, R., Frederick, D. T., Ligorio, M., Chatman, K., Johnston, S. E., Mosher, C. M., … Straussman, R. (2017). Potential role of intratumor bacteria in mediating tumor resistance to the chemotherapeutic drug gemcitabine. *Science, 357*(6356), 1156–1160. https://doi.org/10.1126/science.aah5043.

Gopalakrishnan, V., Spencer, C. N., Nezi, L., Reuben, A., Andrews, M. C., Karpinets, T. V., Prieto, P. A., Vicente, D., Hoffman, K., Wei, S. C., Cogdill, A. P., Zhao, L., Hudgens, C. W., Hutchinson, D. S., Manzo, T., Petaccia De Macedo, M., Cotechini, T., Kumar, T., Chen, W. S., … Wargo, J. A. (2018). Gut microbiome modulates response to anti-PD-1 immunotherapy in melanoma patients. *Science, 359*(6371), 97–103. https://doi.org/10.1126/science.aan4236.

Grigorescu, I., & Dumitrascu, D. L. (2016). Implication of gut microbiota in diabetes mellitus and obesity. *Acta Endocrinologica, 12*(2), 206–214. https://doi.org/10.4183/aeb.2016.206.

He, Y., Fu, L., Li, Y., Wang, W., Gong, M., Zhang, J., Dong, X., Huang, J., Wang, Q., Mackay, C. R., Fu, Y.-X., Chen, Y., & Guo, X. (2021). Gut microbial metabolites facilitate anticancer therapy efficacy by modulating cytotoxic CD8+ T cell immunity. *Cell Metabolism, 33*(5), 988. https://doi.org/10.1016/j.cmet.2021.03.002.

Helmink, B. A., Khan, M. A. W., Hermann, A., Gopalakrishnan, V., & Wargo, J. A. (2019). The microbiome, cancer, and cancer therapy. *Nature Medicine, 25*(3), 377–388. https://doi.org/10.1038/s41591-019-0377-7.

Hill, C., Guarner, F., Reid, G., Gibson, G. R., Merenstein, D. J., Pot, B., Morelli, L., Canani, R. B., Flint, H. J., Salminen, S., Calder, P. C., & Sanders, M. E. (2014). Expert consensus document: The international scientific association for probiotics and prebiotics consensus statement on the scope and appropriate use of the term probiotic. *Nature Reviews Gastroenterology and Hepatology, 11*(8), 506–514. https://doi.org/10.1038/nrgastro.2014.66.

Hodi, F. S., O'Day, S. J., McDermott, D. F., Weber, R. W., Sosman, J. A., Haanen, J. B., Gonzalez, R., Robert, C., Schadendorf, D., Hassel, J. C., Akerley, W., Van Den Eertwegh, A. J. M., Lutzky, J., Lorigan, P., Vaubel, J. M., Linette, G. P., Hogg, D., Ottensmeier, C. H., Lebbé, C., … Urba, W. J. (2010). Improved survival with ipilimumab in patients with metastatic melanoma. *New England Journal of Medicine, 363*(8), 711–723. https://doi.org/10.1056/NEJMoa1003466.

Hsu, B. B., Gibson, T. E., Yeliseyev, V., Liu, Q., Bry, L., Yeliseyev, V., Silver, P. A., & Gerber, G. K. (2019). Bacteriophages dynamically modulate gut microbiota and host immunity. *Cell Host Microbe, 25*, 803–814.e5. https://doi.org/10.1016/j.chom.2019.05.004.

Huang, X., Zhu, M., Chen, R., Ni, J., Zhao, W., Li, S., Lu, X., Jiao, H., & Cao, X. (2023). Innovative drugs promote precision cancer therapy. *Clinical Cancer Bulletin, 2*(1). https://doi.org/10.1007/s44272-023-00002-8.

Huang, X. Z., Gao, P., Song, Y. X., Xu, Y., Sun, J. X., Chen, X. W., Zhao, J. H., & Wang, Z. N. (2019). Antibiotic use and the efficacy of immune checkpoint inhibitors in cancer patients: A pooled analysis of 2740 cancer patients. *OncoImmunology, 8*(12). https://doi.org/10.1080/2162402X.2019.1665973.

Iida, N., Dzutsev, A., Stewart, C. A., Smith, L., Bouladoux, N., Weingarten, R. A., Molina, D. A., Salcedo, R., Back, T., Cramer, S., Dai, R. M., Kiu, H., Cardone, M., Naik, S., Patri, A. K., Wang, E., Marincola, F. M., Frank, K. M., Belkaid, Y., … Goldszmid, R. S. (2013). Commensal bacteria control cancer response to therapy by modulating the tumor microenvironment. *Science, 342*(6161), 967–970. https://doi.org/10.1126/science.1240527.

Imhann, F., Bonder, M. J., Vila, A. V., Fu, J., Mujagic, Z., Vork, L., Tigchelaar, E. F., Jankipersadsing, S. A., Cenit, M. C., Harmsen, H. J. M., Dijkstra, G., Franke, L., Xavier, R. J., Jonkers, D., Wijmenga, C., Weersma, R. K., & Zhernakova, A. (2016). Proton pump inhibitors affect the gut microbiome. *Gut, 65*(5), 740–748. https://doi.org/10.1136/gutjnl-2015-310376.

Integrative HMP Research Network Consortium. (2019). The integrative human microbiome project. *Nature, 569*(7758), 641–648. 10.1038/s41586-019-1238-8.

Jiang, C., Wang, H., Xia, C., Dong, Q., Chen, E. n, Qiu, Y., Su, Y., Xie, H., Zeng, L., Kuang, J., Ao, F., Gong, X., Li, J., & Chen, T. (2019). A randomized, double-blind, placebo-controlled trial of probiotics to reduce the severity of oral mucositis induced by chemoradiotherapy for patients with nasopharyngeal carcinoma. *Cancer, 125*(7), 1081–1090. https://doi.org/10.1002/cncr.31907.

Kim, H., Lee, J. E., Hong, S. H., Lee, M. A., Kang, J. H., & Kim, I.-H. (2019). The effect of antibiotics on the clinical outcomes of patients with solid cancers undergoing immune checkpoint inhibitor treatment: A retrospective study. *BMC Cancer, 19*(1). https://doi.org/10.1186/s12885-019-6267-z.

Knight, R., Callewaert, C., Marotz, C., Hyde, E. R., Debelius, J. W., McDonald, D., et al. (2017). The microbiome and human biology. *Science, 356*(6340), eaan5047. https://doi.org/10.1126/science.aam5106.

Koh, A., De Vadder, F., Kovatcheva-Datchary, P., & Bäckhed, F. (2016). From dietary fiber to host physiology: Short-chain fatty acids as key bacterial metabolites. *Cell, 165*(6), 1332–1345. https://doi.org/10.1016/j.cell.2016.05.041.

Kouidhi, S., Zidi, O., Belkhiria, Z., Rais, H., Ayadi, A., Ayed, F. B., Mosbah, A., Cherif, A., & El Gaaied, A. B. A. (2023). Gut microbiota, an emergent target to shape the efficiency of cancer therapy. *Exploration of Targeted Anti-tumor Therapy, 4*(2), 240–265. https://doi.org/10.37349/etat.2023.00132.

Kuntz, T. M., & Gilbert, J. A. (2017). Introducing the microbiome into precision medicine. *Trends in Pharmacological Sciences, 38*(1), 81–91. https://doi.org/10.1016/j.tips.2016.10.001.

Ngoc, K. L, Pham, T. T. H., Nguyen, T. K., & Huong, P. T. (2024). Pharmacomicrobiomics in precision cancer therapy: Bench to bedside. *Frontiers in Immunology, 15*. https://doi.org/10.3389/fimmu.2024.1428420.

Lee, S.-H., Cho, S.-Y., Yoon, Y., Park, C., Sohn, J., Jeong, J.-J. u, Jeon, B. u-N., Jang, M., An, C., Lee, S., Kim, Y. Y., Kim, G., Kim, S., Kim, Y., Lee, G. B., Lee, E. J. u, Kim, S. G., Kim, H. S., Kim, Y., … Park, H. (2021). *Bifidobacterium bifidum* strains synergize with immune checkpoint inhibitors to reduce tumour burden in mice. *Nature Microbiology, 6*(3), 277–288. https://doi.org/10.1038/s41564-020-00831-6.

Leone, V., Gibbons, S. M., Martinez, K., Hutchison, A. L., Huang, E. Y., Cham, C. M., Pierre, J. F., Heneghan, A. F., Nadimpalli, A., Hubert, N., Zale, E., Wang, Y., Huang, Y., Theriault, B., Dinner, A. R., Musch, M. W., Kudsk, K. A., Prendergast, B. J., Gilbert, J. A., & Chang, E. B. (2015). Effects of diurnal variation of gut microbes and high-fat feeding on host circadian clock function and metabolism. *Cell Host & Microbe, 17*(5), 681–689. https://doi.org/10.1016/j.chom.2015.03.006.

Li, Z., Zhang, Y., Hong, W., Wang, B., Chen, Y., Yang, P., Zhou, J., Fan, J., Zeng, Z., & Du, S. (2022). Gut microbiota modulate radiotherapy-associated antitumor immune responses against hepatocellular carcinoma Via STING signaling. *Gut Microbes, 14*(1). https://doi.org/10.1080/19490976.2022.2119055.

Lin, X. B., Dieleman, L. A., Ketabi, A., Bibova, I., Sawyer, M. B., Xue, H., Field, C. J., Baracos, V. E., & Gänzle, M. G. (2012). Irinotecan (CPT-11) chemotherapy alters intestinal microbiota in tumour bearing rats. *PLoS ONE, 7*(7). https://doi.org/10.1371/journal.pone.0039764Canada.

Liu, W., Zhang, X., Xu, H., Li, S., Lau, H. C.-H., Chen, Q., Zhang, B., Zhao, L., Chen, H., Sung, J. J.-Y., & Yu, J. (2021). Microbial community heterogeneity within colorectal neoplasia and its correlation with colorectal carcinogenesis. *Gastroenterology, 160*(7), 2395–2408. https://doi.org/10.1053/j.gastro.2021.02.020.

Lokody, I. (2014). Bacterial balance affects cancer treatment. *Nature Reviews Cancer, 14*(1), 11. https://doi.org/10.1038/nrc3658.

Long, G. V., Fung, C., Menzies, A. M., Pupo, G. M., Carlino, M. S., Hyman, J., Shahheydari, H., Tembe, V., Thompson, J. F., Saw, R. P., Howle, J., Hayward, N. K., Johansson, P., Scolyer, R. A., Kefford, R. F., & Rizos, H. (2014). Increased MAPK reactivation in early resistance to dabrafenib/trametinib combination therapy of BRAF-mutant metastatic melanoma. *Nature Communications, 5*. https://doi.org/10.1038/ncomms6694.

Luo, Z, Cheng, X, Feng, B, Fan, D, Liu, X, Xie, R, … Zeng, W (2024 Sep). Engineering versatile bacteria-derived outer membrane vesicles: an adaptable platform for advancing cancer immunotherapy. *Advanced Science, 11*(33), 2400049. doi:10.1002/advs.202400049.

Lynch, T. J., Bell, D. W., Sordella, R., Gurubhagavatula, S., Okimoto, R. A., Brannigan, B. W., Harris, P. L., Haserlat, S. M., Supko, J. G., Haluska, F. G., Louis, D. N., Christiani, D. C., Settleman, J., & Haber, D. A. (2004). Activating mutations in the epidermal growth factor receptor underlying responsiveness of non-small-cell lung cancer to gefitinib. *New England Journal of Medicine, 350*(21), 2129–2139. https://doi.org/10.1056/NEJMoa040938.

Ma, C., Han, M., Heinrich, B., Fu, Q., Zhang, Q., Sandhu, M., Agdashian, D., Terabe, M., Berzofsky, J. A., Fako, V., Ritz, T., Longerich, T., Theriot, C. M., McCulloch, J. A., Roy, S., Yuan, W., Thovarai, V., Sen, S. K., Ruchirawat, M., … Greten, T. F. (2018). Gut microbiome–mediated bile acid metabolism regulates liver cancer via NKT cells. *Science, 360*(6391). https://doi.org/10.1126/science.aan5931.

Maier, L., Pruteanu, M., Kuhn, M., Zeller, G., Telzerow, A., Anderson, E. E., Brochado, A. R., Fernandez, K. C., Dose, H., Mori, H., Patil, K. R., Bork, P., & Typas, A. (2018). Extensive impact of non-antibiotic drugs on human gut bacteria. *Nature, 555*(7698), 623–628. https://doi.org/10.1038/nature25979.

Martins, F., Sofiya, L., Sykiotis, G. P., Lamine, F., Maillard, M., Fraga, M., Shabafrouz, K., Ribi, C., Cairoli, A., Guex-Crosier, Y., Kuntzer, T., Michielin, O., Peters, S., Coukos, G., Spertini, F., Thompson, J. A., & Obeid, M. (2019). Adverse effects of immune-checkpoint inhibitors: Epidemiology, management and surveillance. *Nature Reviews Clinical Oncology, 16*(9), 563–580. https://doi.org/10.1038/s41571-019-0218-0.

Matson, V., Fessler, J., Bao, R., Chongsuwat, T., Zha, Y., Alegre, M. L., Luke, J. J., & Gajewski, T. F. (2018). The commensal microbiome is associated with anti-PD-1 efficacy in metastatic melanoma patients. *Science, 359*(6371), 104–108. https://doi.org/10.1126/science.aao3290.

McIntosh, F. M., Maison, N., Holtrop, G., Young, P., Stevens, V. J., Ince, J., Johnstone, A. M., Lobley, G. E., Flint, H. J., & Louis, P. (2012). Phylogenetic distribution of genes encoding β-glucuronidase activity in human colonic bacteria and the impact of diet on faecal glycosidase activities. *Environmental Microbiology, 14*(8), 1876–1887. https://doi.org/10.1111/j.1462-2920.2012.02711.x.

Mima, K., Nishihara, R., Qian, Z. R., Cao, Y., Sukawa, Y., Nowak, J. A., Yang, J., Dou, R., Masugi, Y., Song, M., Kostic, A. D., Giannakis, M., Bullman, S., Milner, D. A., Baba, H., Giovannucci, E. L., Garraway, L. A., Freeman, G. J., Dranoff, G., … Ogino, S. (2016). *Fusobacterium nucleatum* in colorectal carcinoma tissue and patient prognosis. *Gut, 65*(12), 1973–1980. https://doi.org/10.1136/gutjnl-2015-310101.

Nagar, S., & Blanchard, R. (2006). Pharmacogenetics of uridine diphosphoglucuronosyltransferase (UGT) 1A family members and its role in patient response to irinotecan. *Drug Metabolism Reviews, 38*(3), 393–409. https://doi.org/10.1080/03602530600739835.

Nejman, D., Livyatan, I., Fuks, G., Gavert, N., Zwang, Y., Geller, L. T., Rotter-Maskowitz, A., Weiser, R., Mallel, G., Gigi, E., Meltser, A., Douglas, G. M., Kamer, I., Gopalakrishnan, V., Dadosh, T., Levin-Zaidman, S., Avnet, S., Atlan, T., Cooper, Z. A., … Straussman, R. (2020). The human tumor microbiome is composed of tumor type-specific intracellular bacteria. *Science, 368*(6494), 973–980. https://doi.org/10.1126/science.aay9189.

Newman, A. C., & Maddocks, O. D. K. (2017). One-carbon metabolism in cancer. *British Journal of Cancer, 116*(12), 1499–1504. https://doi.org/10.1038/bjc.2017.118.

Nicholson, J. K., Holmes, E., Kinross, J., Burcelin, R., Gibson, G., Jia, W., & Pettersson, S. (2012). Host-gut microbiota metabolic interactions. *Science, 336*(6086), 1262–1267. https://doi.org/10.1126/science.1223813.

Pardoll, D. M. (2012). The blockade of immune checkpoints in cancer immunotherapy. *Nature Reviews Cancer, 12*(4), 252–264. https://doi.org/10.1038/nrc3239.

Pernigoni, N., Zagato, E., Calcinotto, A., Troiani, M., Mestre, R. P., Calì, B., Attanasio, G., Troisi, J., Minini, M., Mosole, S., Revandkar, A., Pasquini, E., Elia, A. R., Bossi, D., Rinaldi, A., Rescigno, P., Flohr, P., Hunt, J., Neeb, A., … Alimonti, A. (2021). Commensal bacteria promote endocrine resistance in prostate cancer through androgen biosynthesis. *Science, 374*(6564), 216–224. https://doi.org/10.1126/science.abf8403.

Pitt, J. M., Vétizou, M., Daillère, R., Roberti, M. P., Yamazaki, T., Routy, B., Lepage, P., Boneca, I. G., Chamaillard, M., Kroemer, G., & Zitvogel, L. (2016). Resistance mechanisms to immune-checkpoint blockade in cancer: Tumor-intrinsic and -extrinsic factors. *Immunity, 44*(6), 1255–1269. https://doi.org/10.1016/j.immuni.2016.06.001.

Poore, G. D., Kopylova, E., Zhu, Q., Carpenter, C., Fraraccio, S., Wandro, S., Kosciolek, T., Janssen, S., Metcalf, J., Song, S. J., Kanbar, J., Miller-Montgomery, S., Heaton, R., Mckay, R., Patel, S. P., Swafford, A. D., & Knight, R. (2020). Microbiome analyses of blood and tissues suggest cancer diagnostic approach. *Nature, 579*(7800), 567–574. https://doi.org/10.1038/s41586-020-2095-1.

Postow, M. A., Sidlow, R., & Hellmann, M. D. (2018). Immune-related adverse events associated with immune checkpoint blockade. *New England Journal of Medicine, 378*(2), 158–168. https://doi.org/10.1056/NEJMra1703481.

Pushalkar, S., Hundeyin, M., Daley, D., Zambirinis, C. P., Kurz, E., Mishra, A., Mohan, N., Aykut, B., Usyk, M., Torres, L. E., Werba, G., Zhang, K., Guo, Y., Li, Q., Akkad, N., Lall, S., Wadowski, B., Gutierrez, J., Rossi, J. A. K., … Miller, G. (2018). The pancreatic cancer microbiome promotes oncogenesis by induction of innate and adaptive immune suppression. *Cancer Discovery, 8*(4), 403–416. https://doi.org/10.1158/2159-8290.cd-17-1134.

Rakoff-Nahoum, S., & Medzhitov, R. (2009). Toll-like receptors and cancer. *Nature Reviews Cancer, 9*(1), 57–63. https://doi.org/10.1038/nrc2541.

Relling, M. V., & Evans, W. E. (2015). Pharmacogenomics in the clinic. *Nature, 526*(7573), 343–350. https://doi.org/10.1038/nature15817.

Ribas, A., & Wolchok, J. D. (2018). Cancer immunotherapy using checkpoint blockade. *Science, 359*(6382), 1350–1355. https://doi.org/10.1126/science.aar4060.

Ridlon, J. M., Kang, D. J., & Hylemon, P. B. (2006). Bile salt biotransformations by human intestinal bacteria. *Journal of Lipid Research, 47*(2), 241–259. https://doi.org/10.1194/jlr.R500013-JLR200.

Roberti, M. P., Yonekura, S., Duong, C. P. M., Picard, M., Ferrere, G., Tidjani Alou, M., Rauber, C., Iebba, V., Lehmann, C. H. K., Amon, L., Dudziak, D., Derosa, L., Routy, B., Flament, C., Richard, C., Daillère, R., Fluckiger, A., Van Seuningen, I., Chamaillard, M., … Zitvogel, L. (2020). Chemotherapy-induced ileal crypt apoptosis and the ileal microbiome shape immunosurveillance and prognosis of proximal colon cancer. *Nature Medicine, 26*(6), 919–931. https://doi.org/10.1038/s41591-020-0882-8.

Roden, D. M., McLeod, H. L., Relling, M. V., Williams, M. S., Mensah, G. A., Peterson, J. F., & Van Driest, S. L. (2019). Pharmacogenomics. *The Lancet., 394*(10197), 521–532. https://doi.org/10.1016/S0140-6736(19)31276-0.

Routy, B., Le Chatelier, E., Derosa, L., Duong, C. P. M., Alou, M. T., Daillère, R., Fluckiger, A., Messaoudene, M., Rauber, C., Roberti, M. P., Fidelle, M., Flament, C., Poirier-Colame, V., Opolon, P., Klein, C., Iribarren, K., Mondragón, L., Jacquelot, N., Qu, B., … Zitvogel, L. (2018). Gut microbiome influences efficacy of PD-1-based immunotherapy against epithelial tumors. *Science, 359*(6371), 91–97. https://doi.org/10.1126/science.aan3706.

Rubinstein, M. R., Wang, X., Liu, W., Hao, Y., Cai, G., & Han, Y. W. (2013). *Fusobacterium nucleatum* promotes colorectal carcinogenesis by modulating E-Cadherin/β-catenin signaling via its FadA adhesin. *Cell Host & Microbe., 14*(2), 195–206. https://doi.org/10.1016/j.chom.2013.07.012.

Sawyers, C. (2004). Targeted cancer therapy. *Nature, 432*(7015), 294–297. https://doi.org/10.1038/nature03095.

Selma, M. V., Espín, J. C., & Tomás-Barberán, F. A. (2009). Interaction between phenolics and gut microbiota: Role in human health. *Journal of Agricultural and Food Chemistry, 57*(15), 6485–6501. https://doi.org/10.1021/jf902107d.

Sender, R., Fuchs, S., & Milo, R. (2016). Revised estimates for the number of human and bacteria cells in the body. *PLOS Biology, 14*(8), e1002533. https://doi.org/10.1371/journal.pbio.1002533.

Sepich-Poore, G. D., Zitvogel, L., Straussman, R., Hasty, J., Wargo, J. A., & Knight, R. (2021). The microbiome and human cancer. *Science, 371*(6536). https://doi.org/10.1126/science.abc4552.

Sharma, P., Hu-Lieskovan, S., Wargo, J. A., & Ribas, A. (2017). Primary, adaptive, and acquired resistance to cancer immunotherapy. *Cell, 168*(4), 707–723. https://doi.org/10.1016/j.cell.2017.01.017.

Sharma, P., & Allison, J. P. (2015). The future of immune checkpoint therapy. *Science, 348*(6230), 56–61. https://doi.org/10.1126/science.aaa8172.

Sharon, G., Sampson, T. R., Geschwind, D. H., & Mazmanian, S. K. (2016). The central nervous system and the gut microbiome. *Cell, 167*(4), 915–932. https://doi.org/10.1016/j.cell.2016.10.027.

Shiao, S. L., Kershaw, K. M., Limon, J. J., You, S., Yoon, J., Ko, E. Y., Guarnerio, J., Potdar, A. A., McGovern, D. P. B., Bose, S., Dar, T. B., Noe, P., Lee, J., Kubota, Y., Maymi, V. I., Davis, M. J., Henson, R. M., Choi, R. Y., … Underhill, D. M. (2021). Commensal bacteria and fungi differentially regulate tumor responses to radiation therapy. *Cancer Cell, 39*(9), 1202. https://doi.org/10.1016/j.ccell.2021.07.002.

Spanogiannopoulos, P., Bess, E. N., Carmody, R. N., & Turnbaugh, P. J. (2016). The microbial pharmacists within us: A metagenomic view of xenobiotic metabolism. *Nature Reviews Microbiology, 14*(5), 273–287. https://doi.org/10.1038/nrmicro.2016.17.

Spencer, C. N., McQuade, J. L., Gopalakrishnan, V., McCulloch, J. A., Vetizou, M., Cogdill, A. P., Wadud Khan, M. A., Zhang, X., White, M. G., Peterson, C. B., Wong, M. C., Morad, G., Rodgers, T., Badger, J. H., Helmink, B. A., Andrews, M. C., Rodrigues, R. R., Morgun, A., Kim, Y. S., … Wargo, J. A. (2021). Dietary fiber and probiotics influence the gut microbiome and melanoma immunotherapy response. *Science, 374*(6575), 1632–1640. https://doi.org/10.1126/science.aaz7015.

Stringer, A. M., Gibson, R. J., Logan, R. M., Bowen, J. M., Yeoh, A. S. J., & Keefe, D. M. K. (2008). Fecal microflora and β-glucuronidase expression are altered in an irinotecan-induced diarrhea model in rats. *Cancer Biology and Therapy, 7*(12), 1919–1925. https://doi.org/10.4161/cbt.7.12.6940.

Talpin, A, Maia, A, Carpier, JM, Kulakowski, G, Gaal, C, Strozzi, F, … Mersceman, T (2024 Jun). A Mimicry-Based Strategy Between Human and Commensal Antigens for the Development of a New Family of Immune Therapies for Cancer. *bioRxiv, 1*, 2024. doi:10.1101/2024.05.27.596102.

Tilg, H., Adolph, T. E., Gerner, R. R., & Moschen, A. R. (2018). The intestinal microbiota in colorectal cancer. *Cancer Cell, 33*(6), 954–964. https://doi.org/10.1016/j.ccell.2018.03.004.

Tilg, H., & Moschen, A. R. (2014). Microbiota and diabetes: An evolving relationship. *Gut, 63*(9), 1513–1521. https://doi.org/10.1136/gutjnl-2014-306928.

Ting, N. L. N., Lau, H. C. H., & Yu, J. (2022). Cancer pharmacomicrobiomics: Targeting microbiota to optimise cancer therapy outcomes. *Gut, 71*(7), 1412–1425. https://doi.org/10.1136/gutjnl-2021-326264.

Tjalsma, H., Boleij, A., Marchesi, J. R., & Dutilh, B. E. (2012). A bacterial driver-passenger model for colorectal cancer: Beyond the usual suspects. *Nature Reviews Microbiology, 10*(8), 575–582. https://doi.org/10.1038/nrmicro2819.

Tripathi, A., Debelius, J., Brenner, D. A., Karin, M., Loomba, R., Schnabl, B., & Knight, R. (2018). The gut-liver axis and the intersection with the microbiome. *Nature Reviews Gastroenterology and Hepatology, 15*(7), 397–411. https://doi.org/10.1038/s41575-018-0011-z.

Tsementzi, D., Meador, R., Eng, T., Patel, P., Shelton, J., Arluck, J., Scott, I., Dolan, M., Khanna, N., Konstantinidis, K. T., & Bruner, D. W. (2021). Changes in the vaginal microbiome and associated toxicities following radiation therapy for gynecologic cancers. *Frontiers in Cellular and Infection Microbiology, 11*. https://doi.org/10.3389/fcimb.2021.680038.

Tsimberidou, A. M., Fountzilas, E., Nikanjam, M., & Kurzrock, R. (2020). Review of precision cancer medicine: Evolution of the treatment paradigm. *Cancer Treatment Reviews, 86*, 102019. https://doi.org/10.1016/j.ctrv.2020.102019.

Turnbaugh, P. J., Ley, R. E., Mahowald, M. A., Magrini, V., Mardis, E. R., & Gordon, J. I. (2006). An obesity-associated gut microbiome with increased capacity for energy harvest. *Nature, 444*(7122), 1027–1031. https://doi.org/10.1038/nature05414.

McQuade, J. L., Daniel, C. R., Hess, K. R., Mak, C., Wang, D. Y., Rai, R. R., … Lane, S. (2018). Association of body-mass index and outcomes in patients with metastatic melanoma treated with targeted therapy, immunotherapy, or chemotherapy: a retrospective, multicohort analysis. *The Lancet Oncology, 19*(3), 310–322.

US National Library of Medicine. ClinicalTrials.gov Identifier. (2024). https://clinicaltrials.gov/ct2/show/NCT03341143.

US National Library of Medicine. ClinicalTrials.gov Identifier. (2025). https://clinicaltrials.gov/ct2/show/NCT03772899

US National Library of Medicine. ClinicalTrials.gov Identifier, (2024). https://clinicaltrials.gov/ct2/show/NCT04130763

US National Library of Medicine. ClinicalTrials.gov Identifier. (2025). https://clinicaltrials.gov/study/NCT04163289

US National Library of Medicine. ClinicalTrials.gov Identifier. (2021). https://clinicaltrials.gov/ct2/show/NCT05008861

Vaddepally, R. K., Kharel, P., Pandey, R., Garje, R., & Chandra, A. B. (2020). Review of indications of FDA-approved immune checkpoint inhibitors per NCCN guidelines. *Cancers (Basel), 12*(3), 738. https://doi.org/10.3390/cancers12030738.

Vander Heiden, M. G., Cantley, L. C., & Thompson, C. B. (2009). Understanding the Warburg effect: The metabolic requirements of cell proliferation. *Science, 324*(5930), 1029–1033. https://doi.org/10.1126/science.1160809.

Venkidesh, B. S., Shankar, S. R., Narasimhamurthy, R. K., Rao, S. B. S., & Mumbrekar, K. D. (2023). Radioprotective potential of probiotics against gastrointestinal and neuronal toxicity: A preclinical study. *Clinical and Translational Oncology, 25*(11), 3165–3173. https://doi.org/10.1007/s12094-023-03184-8.

Vétizou, M., Pitt, J. M., Daillère, R., Lepage, P., Waldschmitt, N., Flament, C., Rusakiewicz, S., Routy, B., Roberti, M. P., Duong, C. P. M., Poirier-Colame, V., Roux, A., Becharef, S., Formenti, S., Golden, E., Cording, S., Eberl, G., Schlitzer, A., Ginhoux, F., … Zitvogel, L. (2015). Anticancer immunotherapy by CTLA-4 blockade relies on the gut microbiota. *Science., 350*(6264), 1079–1084. https://doi.org/10.1126/science.aad1329.

Viaud, S., Saccheri, F., Mignot, G., Yamazaki, T., Daillère, R., Hannani, D., Enot, D. P., Pfirschke, C., Engblom, C., Pittet, M. J., Schlitzer, A., Ginhoux, F., Apetoh, L., Chachaty, E., Woerther, P.-L., Eberl, G., Bérard, M., Ecobichon, C., Clermont, D., … Zitvogel, L. (2013). The intestinal microbiota modulates the anticancer immune effects of cyclophosphamide. *Science, 342*(6161), 971–976. https://doi.org/10.1126/science.1240537.

Wallace, B. D., Wang, H., Lane, K. T., Scott, J. E., Orans, J., Koo, J. S., Venkatesh, M., Jobin, C., Yeh, L. A., Mani, S., & Redinbo, M. R. (2010). Alleviating cancer drug toxicity by inhibiting a bacterial enzyme. *Science, 330*(6005), 831–835. https://doi.org/10.1126/science.1191175.

Wang, Y., Wiesnoski, D. H., Helmink, B. A., Gopalakrishnan, V., Choi, K., DuPont, H. L., Jiang, Z.-D., Abu-Sbeih, H., Sanchez, C. A., Chang, C.-C., Parra, E. R., Francisco-Cruz, A., Raju, G. S., Stroehlein, J. R., Campbell, M. T., Gao, J., Subudhi, S. K., Maru, D. M., Blando, J. M., … Jenq, R. R. (2018). Fecal microbiota transplantation for refractory immune checkpoint inhibitor-associated colitis. *Nature Medicine, 24*(12), 1804–1808. https://doi.org/10.1038/s41591-018-0238-9.

Wang, Y, Wiesnoski, DH, Helmink, BA, Gopalakrishnan, V, Choi, K, DuPont, HL, … Parra, ER (2018 Dec). Fecal microbiota transplantation for refractory immune checkpoint inhibitor-associated colitis. *Nature medicine, 24*(12), 1804–1808.

Weinshilboum, R. M., & Wang, L. (2017). Pharmacogenomics: Precision medicine and drug response. *Mayo Clinic Proceedings, 92*(11), 1711–1722. https://doi.org/10.1016/j.mayocp.2017.09.001.

Wilson, B. E., Routy, B., Nagrial, A., & Chin, V. T. (2020). The effect of antibiotics on clinical outcomes in immune-checkpoint blockade: A systematic review and meta-analysis of observational studies. *Cancer Immunology, Immunotherapy, 69*(3), 343–354. https://doi.org/10.1007/s00262-019-02453-2.

Wilson, M. R., Jiang, Y., Villalta, P. W., Stornetta, A., Boudreau, P. D., Carrá, A., Brennan, C. A., Chun, E., Ngo, L., Samson, L. D., Engelward, B. P., Garrett, W. S., Balbo, S., & Balskus, E. P. (2019). The human gut bacterial genotoxin colibactin alkylates DNA. *Science, 363*(6428). https://doi.org/10.1126/science.aar7785.

Wong, C. W., Yost, S. E., Lee, J. S., Gillece, J. D., Folkerts, M., Reining, L., Highlander, S. K., Eftekhari, Z., Mortimer, J., & Yuan, Y. (2021). Analysis of Gut microbiome using explainable machine learning predicts risk of diarrhea associated with tyrosine kinase inhibitor neratinib: A pilot study. *Frontiers in Oncology, 11*. https://doi.org/10.3389/fonc.2021.604584.

Yang, K., Hou, Y., Zhang, Y., Liang, H., Sharma, A., Zheng, W., Wang, L., Torres, R., Tatebe, K., Chmura, S. J., Pitroda, S. P., Gilbert, J. A., Fu, Y.-X., & Weichselbaum, R. R. (2021). Suppression of local type I interferon by gut microbiota–derived butyrate impairs antitumor effects of ionizing radiation. *Journal of Experimental Medicine, 218*(3). https://doi.org/10.1084/jem.20201915.

Yang, Q, Wang, B, Zheng, Q, Li, H, Meng, X, Zhou, F, & Zhang, L (2023 May). A review of gut microbiota-derived metabolites in tumor progression and cancer therapy. *Advanced Science, 10*(15), 2207366.

Yu, T. C., Guo, F., Yu, Y., Sun, T., Ma, D., Han, J., Qian, Y., Kryczek, I., Sun, D., Nagarsheth, N., Chen, Y., Chen, H., Hong, J., Zou, W., & Fang, J.-Y. (2017). *Fusobacterium nucleatum* promotes chemoresistance to colorectal cancer by modulating autophagy. *Cell, 170*(3), 548. https://doi.org/10.1016/j.cell.2017.07.008.

Zhuang, L., Chen, H., Zhang, S., Zhuang, J., Li, Q., & Feng, Z. (2019). Intestinal microbiota in early life and its implications on childhood health. *Genomics, Proteomics & Bioinformatics, 17*(1), 13–25. https://doi.org/10.1016/j.gpb.2018.10.002.

Zitvogel, L., Ma, Y., Raoult, D., Kroemer, G., & Gajewski, T. F. (2018a). The microbiome in cancer immunotherapy: Diagnostic tools and therapeutic strategies. *Science, 359*(6382), 1366–1370. https://doi.org/10.1126/science.aar6918.

Zitvogel, L., Ma, Y., Raoult, D., Kroemer, G., & Gajewski, T. F. (2018b). The microbiome in cancer immunotherapy. *Nature Review Immunology, 18*(2), 85–100. https://doi.org/10.1126/science.aar6918.

Zmora, N., Zeevi, D., Korem, T., Segal, E., & Elinav, E. (2018). Taking it personally: Personalized utilization of the human microbiome in health and disease. *Cell, 174*(6), 1388–1405. https://doi.org/10.1016/j.cell.2018.08.001.

9

Gut microbiome in modulating immune checkpoint inhibitors

Jyotchna Devi Bade[a], Abdul Rahaman[b], Kanaka Durga Devi Nelluri[c], Sunjana Nelluri[a] and Bhavana Alaparthi[c]

[a]DEPARTMENT OF BIOCHEMISTRY, GREAT EASTERN MEDICAL SCHOOL AND HOSPITAL, SRIKAKULAM, ANDHRA PRADESH, INDIA [b]DEPARTMENT OF PHARMACEUTICAL SCIENCES, VIGNAN'S FOUNDATION FOR SCIENCE, TECHNOLOGY AND RESEARCH, GUNTUR, ANDHRA PRADESH, INDIA [c]DEPARTMENT OF PHARMACEUTICAL SCIENCES, KVSR SIDDHARTHA COLLEGE OF PHARMACEUTICAL SCIENCES, VIJAYAWADA, ANDHRA PRADESH, INDIA

9.1 Introduction

The gut microbiome, a large community of microbes living in the gastrointestinal tract, is an important modulator of the immune response to cancer treatment, especially with the use of immune checkpoint inhibitors (ICIs). This dynamic interaction influences therapeutic response and patient outcome, and the gut microbiome is thus a central area of interest in cancer immunotherapy. Several research studies have found that gut microbiota diversity and composition could be considerably different in responding versus nonresponding individuals to ICIs, indicating that certain microbial communities can promote or suppress therapeutic activity (Gazzaniga & Kasper, 2025; Lin et al., 2024; Zhang et al., 2023). Evidence suggests alpha diversity, or microbial species diversity within the gut, is linked with enhanced response to immunotherapy, especially in melanoma patients undergoing programmed death 1 (PD-1) blockade (Kang et al., 2024; Li et al., 2022b). The gut microbiome is also reported to produce metabolites like short-chain fatty acids (SCFAs), which can augment immune function and be responsible for the efficacy of ICIs by modulating T cell activation and inducing antitumor responses (Cani, 2018; Pesheva, 2024). In addition, the development of tools like the Integrated Microbiome Prediction Index holds the promise to predict nonresponse to immunotherapy and thereby detect patients who will most likely benefit from treatments targeting the microbiota (Kang et al., 2024; Pesheva, 2024; Zhang et al., 2024). Although the therapeutic benefit of the gut microbiome for augmenting the effectiveness of ICI is enticing, it carries limitations, for example, dysbiosis that may result in immune-related adverse events (irAEs) and complicate treatment (Chang et al., 2024; Verheijden et al., 2025). The bidirectional interaction between the immune system and gut

The Microbiome and Cancer Treatment: Overcoming Resistance and Enhancing Efficacy.
DOI: https://doi.org/10.1016/B978-0-443-33206-7.00012-1

Table 9.1 Immune checkpoint inhibitors and their mechanisms of action.

Checkpoint target	Drug name	Mechanism of action
PD-1 (Programmed death-1)	Nivolumab, Pembrolizumab	Block PD-1 receptor on activated T cells, B cells, and NK cells, preventing interaction with PD-L1, restoring T-cell activation and function.
PD-L1 (Programmed death-ligand 1)	Atezolizumab, Durvalumab, Avelumab	Block PD-L1 on tumor cells and antigen-presenting cells (APCs), preventing binding to PD-1, allowing immune cells to effectively recognize and attack tumors.
CTLA-4 (Cytotoxic T-lymphocyte-associated protein 4)	Ipilimumab, Tremelimumab	Block CTLA-4, preventing suppression of T-cell activation by APCs, leading to enhanced and prolonged antitumor immune response.

NK, natural killer.

microbiome, regulated by psychological stress and heredity, highlights the complexity of these relationships and the urgency for continued investigations into how the microbiome needs to be optimally maintained so that cancer therapy can be advanced (Pesheva, 2024; Verheijden et al., 2025). With immunotherapy evolving the paradigm of cancer treatment, the crossroads of gut microbiome science holds the potential to optimize therapeutic intervention, enhance patient selection, and reduce complications from therapy. This complex interplay can be utilized in the form of more tailored and effective cancer therapy and thereby maximize the overall efficacy of ICIs in clinical application (Griffin & Hang, 2022; Jiang & Zhang, 2024; Yi et al., 2018).

9.2 Immune checkpoint inhibitors and their mechanism of action

9.2.1 Immune checkpoint inhibitors

ICIs represent a groundbreaking discovery in cancer immunotherapy that holds an incredibly powerful way of activating and enhancing the immune system to detect and eliminate cancer cells. Immune checkpoints, in natural circumstances, represent systems of suppression that avoid overreaction of the immune system by avoiding autoimmunity. Cancer in most instances subverts such checkpoints to elude immune observation, and cancer cells can expand unrestrained. ICIs have the function of inhibiting such inhibitory mechanisms and hence reactivating immune cells, particularly cytotoxic T lymphocytes, to produce a better and more persistent antitumor immune response, as shown in Table 9.1. The most clinically proven ICIs target three immune checkpoint proteins: PD-1, programmed death ligand 1 (PD-L1), and cytotoxic T-lymphocyte-associated protein 4 (CTLA-4). PD-1 is an inhibitory checkpoint receptor present on activated T cells, B cells, and natural killer (NK) cells. When PD-1 is bound to PD-L1, which is otherwise overexpressed on the surface of tumor cells and antigen-presenting cells (APCs), it prevents T-cell function and activation, allowing immune escape. PD-1 inhibitors nivolumab and pembrolizumab block this binding, effectively restoring the tumor-targeting function of T cells. Similarly, PD-L1 inhibitors like atezolizumab, durvalumab, and avelumab block PD-L1 from binding to PD-1 to allow the immune system to target and kill the tumor cells more effectively (Ciernikova et al., 2024; Gut, 2018; Hu et al., 2024; Routy et al., 2017).

9.2.2 Mechanisms of action

9.2.2.1 Programmed death 1 and programmed death ligand 1 inhibition

PD-1 is an immune-inhibitory receptor that is found on the majority of immune cells, such as T cells, B cells, NK cells, dendritic cells (DCs), tumor-infiltrating lymphocytes (TILs), and myeloid cells. PD-1 is very important in keeping the immune system in check and stopping autoimmunity by limiting excessive immune response. But several cancers hijack this process to avoid immune attack. Its ligand, PD-L1, is found on the surface of APCs, tumor cells, endothelial cells, and stromal cells. Under the physiological situation, PD-L1/PD-1 interaction acts as a check on T-cell activation to modulate T-cell-mediated immune-mediated tissue inflammation and damage. In the tumor microenvironment (TME), however, PD-L1 is expressed on cancer cells either constitutively or in a signal-inducible manner following inflammatory signals like interferon-gamma (IFN-γ) to dampen antitumor immune responses. When PD-L1 is occupied by PD-1 on T cells, it initiates suppressive signals that repress T-cell receptor (TCR) signaling, cytokine production, and T-cell exhaustion. This makes the immune response futile, allowing the avoidance of immune surveillance by the cancer cells and the sustainment of growth. Apart from directly inhibiting T-cell activation, PD-1 and PD-L1 interaction also affect other immune cells like B cells and NK cells, reducing the immune system's ability to mount an antitumor response (Gut, 2018; Hu et al., 2024).

In an attempt to counteract this immune evasion process, ICIs of PD-1 or PD-L1 have been created. PD-1 inhibitors such as nivolumab and pembrolizumab block PD-1 directly, thereby preventing it from interacting with PD-L1 and restoring T-cell function. PD-L1 inhibitors such as atezolizumab, durvalumab, and avelumab block PD-L1 itself, thereby preventing PD-1 from interacting with it and allowing immune cells to bind and destroy tumors. These therapies have been excellent in clinical efficacy in the management of a wide range of cancers like melanoma, nonsmall cell lung cancer (NSCLC), renal cell carcinoma (RCC), bladder cancer, and Hodgkin lymphoma.

However, PD-1/PD-L1 inhibitor response in patients is heterogeneous, and there are resistance mechanisms. Tumor-intrinsic resistance processes such as low tumor mutational burden (TMB), loss of antigen presentation (for example, loss of major histocompatibility complex, MHC), and overexpression of alternative immune checkpoint molecules such as TIM-3 and LAG-3 may overcome the PD-1 blockade. TME is also implicated, in which immune-suppressive cells such as regulatory T cells (Tregs) and myeloid-derived suppressor cells (MDSCs) and cytokines such as TGF-β and IL-10 would be implicated in downregulating the immune cell activation. To circumvent these limitations, combination regimens have been developed that combine PD-1/PD-L1 inhibitors with CTLA-4 inhibitors (such as ipilimumab), chemotherapy, radiation, cancer vaccines, and microbiome-targeted therapies to maximize immune activation and response rates. With further investigation, it will be crucial in realizing the maximum therapeutic potential of immune checkpoint blockade to learn how to optimize PD-1/PD-L1 inhibition using biomarker-based patient selection, new combination strategies, and immune microenvironment modulation (Table 9.1) (Ciernikova et al., 2024; Routy et al., 2017).

9.2.2.2 Cytotoxic T-lymphocyte-associated protein 4 inhibition and its role in cancer immunotherapy

Cytotoxic T-lymphocyte-associated protein 4, or CTLA-4, is a critical immune checkpoint receptor expressed predominantly on activated T cells and Tregs. It functions as an immune response-negative regulator by competing with CD28, a costimulatory molecule necessary for T-cell activation. Such competition is crucial for immune homeostasis to prevent hyperimmune responses and maintain self-tolerance. However, tumors usurp this pathway to evade immune recognition, and CTLA-4 is therefore a critical target for ICIs. In normal situations, APCs express the costimulatory ligands CD80 (B7-1) and CD86 (B7-2), which can bind T-cell CD28 or CTLA-4. CD28 binding to CD80/CD86 transduces a positive costimulation that leads to T-cell activation, proliferation, and cytokine production—a process necessary to generate a successful immune response to infection and tumor. However, CTLA-4 engages with CD80 and CD86 with much greater affinity than CD28 does, so it is capable of displacing CD28 from these molecules. This results in the prevention of T cell activation and a suppression of the overall immune response.

In addition, CTLA-4 is constitutively overexpressed on Tregs, immune-suppressive cells that assist with immune tolerance through suppression of exuberant inflammation and autoimmunity. Through active suppression of effector T cell activity and sequestration of CD80/CD86, Tregs assist with the development of an immunosuppressive TME that allows cancer cells to evade immune detection. ICIs such as CTLA-4 target agents ipilimumab and tremelimumab work by inhibiting the interaction between CTLA-4 and CD80/CD86. This action, in turn, inhibits the competitive inhibition activity against CD28, hence enhancing T-cell activation and promoting the immune response against the tumor cells. By inhibiting CTLA-4, such ICIs enhance the growth of tumor-specific T cells and inhibit the immunosuppressive action of Tregs, resulting in a more effective antitumor immune response.

9.2.3 Clinical applications of immune checkpoint inhibitors

ICIs have revolutionized cancer treatment by providing long-term and durable responses in most cancers such as melanoma, NSCLC, RCC, urothelial carcinoma, and Hodgkin's lymphoma, as mentioned in Fig. 9.1. Unlike the conventional chemotherapy and targeted therapy drugs, which are mostly active by either killing the cancer cells directly or blocking oncogenic pathways, ICIs work by restoring the body's immune system to recognize and eliminate tumors. Perhaps the most striking clinical advantage of ICIs is their ability to provoke long-term remission, even after stopping treatment. This durability is especially noted in tumors such as melanoma, where individuals with complete or partial response can be progression-free for years, at times without the need for additional therapy. Clinical trials have demonstrated that a subpopulation of patients

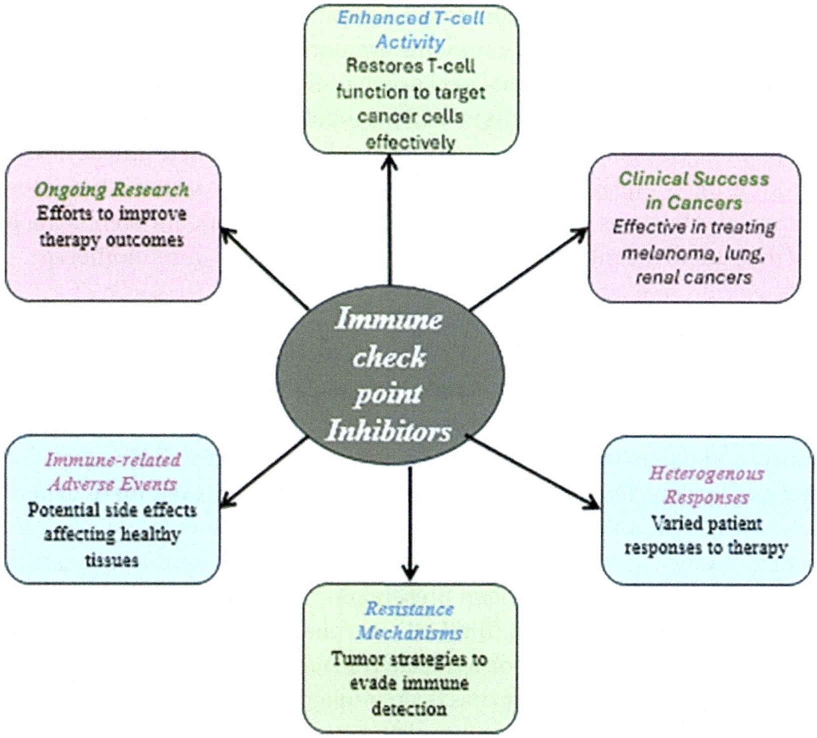

FIGURE 9.1 Mechanism of action and clinical implications of immune checkpoint inhibitors (ICIs) in cancer therapy. Immune checkpoint inhibitors (ICIs) block inhibitory receptors such as PD-1/PD-L1 and CTLA-4 on T cells, thereby restoring antitumor immune responses and enhancing cytotoxic T-cell–mediated cancer cell destruction. Clinically, ICIs have transformed cancer therapy by improving survival across multiple malignancies, though they are associated with immune-related adverse events due to systemic immune activation. *CTLA-4*, cytotoxic T-lymphocyte-associated protein 4; *PD-1*, programmed death 1; *PD-L1*, programmed death ligand 1.

who received treatment with ICIs, including PD-1 inhibitors (nivolumab and pembrolizumab) and CTLA-4 inhibitors (ipilimumab), have long-term survival, much better than standard treatments. While ICIs are effective, they are highly heterogeneous and are determined by numerous factors. The TME determines sensitivity to ICIs. Those tumors with an immunologically "hot" TME, i.e., having high proportions of TILs, proinflammatory cytokines, and PD-L1 expression, will be responsive to ICIs. On the other hand, immunosuppressive "cold" TME tumors, which lack immune infiltration and are high in Tregs and MDSCs, are refractory to ICIs (Hakozaki et al., 2020).

The gut microbiome is also another determinant that has been explored to determine ICI efficacy. Gut microbiota composition and diversity have been shown to play a central role in predicting the success of immunotherapy, according to studies. Some bacterial populations, including *Akkermansia muciniphila* and *Faecalibacterium prausnitzii*, were found to promote increased antitumor immunity, while dysbiosis (microbiota intestinal imbalance) might result in resistance to ICIs. Other therapies, including fecal microbiota transplantation (FMT), probiotics, and diet-based interventions, are also being investigated as possible ways of manipulating the microbiome to enhance the effectiveness of ICI. Despite the revolutionary efficacy of ICIs, not every patient responds to such therapy, and some eventually develop primary or secondary resistance. Combination regimens with dual checkpoint inhibition (e.g., PD-1 + CTLA-4 inhibitors), combination with chemotherapy, radiation, and personalized immunotherapy strategies are being pursued vigorously to circumvent resistance and enhance treatment efficacy. With continued research decoding the complex associations between the immune system, the biology of cancer, and environmental influences such as the microbiome, the therapeutic significance of ICIs will grow, paving the path to the future of more selective and effective immunotherapy.

9.2.4 Clinical efficacy and resistance

Though ICIs have signaled unparalleled accomplishment within oncology, to date, their remedial usefulness still remains minimalistic because fewer than half of patients have evidenced an initial response, and plenty of other patients have become resistant during the allotted period. ICI resistance can be depicted as primary (inherent) or secondary (acquired), where the cancer does not show a response, and individuals initially prosper yet ultimately deteriorate. Resistance can be due to a number of mechanisms, some of which include tumor-intrinsic mechanisms such as decreased TMB, impaired antigen presentation, and overexpression of other immune checkpoints such as LAG-3 and TIM-3. The TME also plays a critical role in supporting immune cells such as Tregs, MDSCs, and tumor-associated macrophages (TAMs), which inhibit T-cell activation. Secondly, the gut microbiota has been implicated in mediating ICI efficacy, in which particular microbial communities evoke a greater response and dysbiosis results in resistance. To avoid such complications, researchers are exploring combination therapy such as double checkpoint blockade (PD-1 + CTLA-4 inhibitors), ICIs and chemotherapy along with radiotherapy, and targeting immunosuppressive cells or molecules within the TME. In addition, microbiome-directed therapies, including FMT and probiotics, are being investigated to enhance treatment outcomes. As resistance remains the most important issue, its mechanisms and how to develop personalized therapeutic approaches will be crucial to optimizing the duration and effectiveness of ICIs in cancer therapy.

9.2.5 Adverse effects and patient stratification

Usage of ICIs has also been associated with a number of irAEs, which must be carefully monitored and managed during therapy. Identification of patient subsets who will respond to ICI therapy is an area of much ongoing research, particularly in terms of personalizing immunotherapy and decreasing the occurrence of serious adverse effects.

9.2.5.1 Overview of immune-related adverse events caused by immune checkpoint inhibitors

ICIs have revolutionized the treatment of cancer by enhancing the immune system to recognize and eliminate cancer. This enhanced immune activity, however, can also lead to irAEs, in which the immune system mistakenly targets nontumor tissues. These toxicities are of different extents and affect more than one organ system, the most common of which include dermatological (pruritus, rash), gastrointestinal (colitis, hepatitis, diarrhea), endocrine (thyroiditis, adrenal insufficiency, hypophysitis), and pulmonary (pneumonitis) toxicities. Severe toxicities in certain instances involve cardiovascular (myocarditis, pericarditis), neurological (encephalitis, neuropathy), renal, and hematologic toxicities, which are uncommon but can be life-threatening. The development of irAEs is unforeseen, happening within weeks to months of treatment onset, and even after therapy is stopped in some instances.

IrAEs must be handled by an interdisciplinary team with an emphasis on early diagnosis and timely treatment. Mild irAEs can normally be managed by symptomatic therapy, and moderate to severe irAEs typically require corticosteroids to manage the inappropriate activation of the immune system. In case of corticosteroid failure, alternative immunosuppressive medications like tumor necrosis factor (TNF) inhibitors or mycophenolate mofetil are employed. Despite these measures, some irAEs are recalcitrant or lead to autoimmune diseases of prolonged duration needing long-term medical therapy.

One of the most crucial parts of achieving optimization of ICI therapy is choosing patients who can benefit from treatment with minimal risk of irAEs. Prediction of response and toxicity can be made using baseline gut microbiota, genetic background, underlying autoimmune conditions, and systemic inflammatory markers, as reported in recent literature. For instance, those patients with higher heterogeneity of the gut microbiota have experienced better responses to ICIs, whereas microbial reconfigurations have been linked to risk for irAEs. Circulating T-cell subsets, cytokines, and autoantibodies are also being investigated to further stratify the patient population. By integrating predictive biomarkers, microbiome-directed therapies, and customized treatment approaches, clinicians can maximize patient safety and therapeutic outcomes. Additional research in maximizing patient selection and minimizing irAEs will be critical to maximizing the clinical benefit of ICIs. Immunotherapy's destiny will depend on delicately tuning antitumor immunity with immune tolerance and ultimately enhancing patient outcomes without additional treatment-related toxicities (Kang et al., 2024; Wang & Geng, 2023).

9.3 Gut microbiome

Gut microbiota is the flora of microbes living within the human intestine and coevolving in association with the host for the establishment of a sophisticated ecosystem. The microbes are engaged in food digestion, nutrient absorption, and body homeostasis through interaction with the immune system. Recent research showed that the composition of gut microbiota could serve as a potential biomarker for the indication of whether cancer patients are likely to respond to immunotherapy with ICIs. Some gut microbes, such as those of the genus *Bifidobacterium*, have been found to be accountable for improved immune responses to immunotherapy. Metabolic products produced by gut microbiota, including SCFAs, have been reported to alter the TME and control immune cell function. The metabolites can enhance immune cells' cytotoxicity against tumor cells, thereby improving the efficacy of immunotherapy. However, ICI administration can disrupt the balance between inflammation and tolerance, leading to immune system imbalance. This disruption can lead to enhanced proinflammatory processes and reduced anti-inflammatory responses in the gut, with enhanced T cell recruitment and proinflammatory cell differentiation, and suppressed anti-inflammatory cell differentiation. Diet exerts powerful influences on gut microbiota composition, and high-fiber and plant food diets, including the Mediterranean Diet, have beneficial influences on microbial diversity. Grasping the dialogue between gut microbiota, diet, and immune response is central to enhancing immunotherapy modalities and deriving enhanced clinical advantage in cancer patients.

9.3.1 Composition and diversity

Composition and diversity of the gut microbiome are at the heart of immune response determination and the impact of cancer immunotherapy. Gut microbiome diversity refers to microbial species richness and evenness in the gut, with greater diversity correlating with greater immune regulation and increased immunity to ICIs. Antitumor immunity is improved through a healthy diversity of the gut microbiome, boosting T-cell activation as well as the suppression of irAEs. Decreased diversity, or dysbiosis, has, in contrast, been associated with chronic inflammation and weaker immunotherapy. Not only is diversity key, but also the specific types of gut microbes are crucial, as certain bacterial genera have been found to be helpful or detrimental regarding immunotherapy. Supportive microbes, i.e., *A. muciniphila, F. prausnitzii,* and *Bifidobacterium* spp., maintain gut barrier integrity, immune tolerance, and the generation of SCFAs, all of which enhance therapy responses. On the other hand, an overabundance of putative pathobionts like *Clostridium* spp. and *Escherichia coli* may play roles in immune suppression and inflammation, resulting in a deteriorating effect on the response to therapy. Since microbiome diversity and composition play a vital role in immunotherapy, strategies such as probiotics, diet interventions, and FMT are being investigated in order to maximize the gut microbiota and enhance the outcomes of cancer therapy. A study has revealed that the gut microbiome and mycobiome composition can differ significantly between individuals, especially between responders to immunotherapy (DCB group) and nonresponders (NDB group). Following immunotherapy, stability in microbial composition was observed at the phylum level in both groups, whereas species-level fluctuations were more pronounced, suggesting that certain microbial communities may be associated with therapeutic responses.

9.3.2 Interaction with the immune system

The gut microbiota plays a vital role in immune modulation, and its interaction with the immune system can influence cancer patients' response to ICIs. The gut microbiota interacts with the immune system through several mechanisms, including regulation of immune cell activation, synthesis of immunomodulatory metabolites, and control of systemic inflammation. Health-promoting bacteria, like *F. prausnitzii* and *Prevotella copri*, also play a role in antitumor immunity through the augmentation of regulatory and effector T-cell activity, with a resultant balance in the immune microenvironment supporting ICI responsiveness. These bacteria are known to produce SCFAs, including butyrate, which are effective in preserving the integrity of gut barriers, decreasing inflammation, and facilitating antigen presentation by DCs. Furthermore, the gut microbiome also affects cytokine levels, as indicated by reduced serum IL-18 levels in responders to ICI therapy. IL-18 has been linked with chronic inflammation and immune suppression, and implies that a balanced microbiota could contribute to modulating proinflammatory signaling. The fact that both the benefiters' and healthy individuals' microbiota composition are comparable also highlights that a well-preserved microbial community plays a key role in sustaining immune homeostasis. Thus, modulation of the gut microbiota by dietary interventions, probiotics, or FMT has the potential to enhance the outcomes of cancer immunotherapy by augmenting the host's endogenous immune response against cancer. Investigation of how nonmolecular factors influence treatment response is a key area of investigation that may lead to new therapeutic approaches.

9.3.3 Gut microbiota's metabolic activities

The gut microbiota participates in sophisticated metabolic reactions that are crucial for human health. It produces numerous metabolites, such as SCFAs and secondary bile acids, which are significant for energy and nutrition. SCFAs, which are generated via the fermentation of dietary fibers by gut microbes, have also been found to possess anti-inflammatory effects and could play a protective role in cancer and ICI therapy (Griffin & Hang, 2022; Kang et al., 2024). Bile acids, however, play roles in nutrient metabolism and absorption, with some of these acids being altered by bacteria in the gut to produce secondary bile acids, which in turn affect immune reactions (Routy et al., 2017; Verheijden et al., 2025).

9.4 Gut microbiome interaction with immune checkpoint inhibitors

The gut microbiome is important for the modulation of ICI efficacy and toxicity. The bacteria coevolve with the host to create an intricate ecosystem affecting numerous physiological activities, such as immune response and inflammation control. The composition of the gut microbiome could be a candidate biomarker predicting outcomes in cancer patients after ICI therapy, especially immune checkpoint blockade targeting the PD-1/PD-L1 and CTLA-4 pathways, as shown in Fig. 9.2.

9.4.1 Gut microbiota and programmed death 1/programmed death ligand 1 inhibition

Gut microbiota has a vital function to provide in regulating immune response, particularly the effectiveness of PD-1/PD-L1 ICIs as cancer therapy agents. Research has also proved that some bacterial communities, including *Bifidobacterium, A. muciniphila,* and *Faecalibacterium,* are positively associated with improved ICI responses. These microorganisms influence the immune system by modulating the TME, antigen presentation, and T cell activation, thus improving the body's ability to recognize and destroy cancer cells. One of the mechanisms through which these

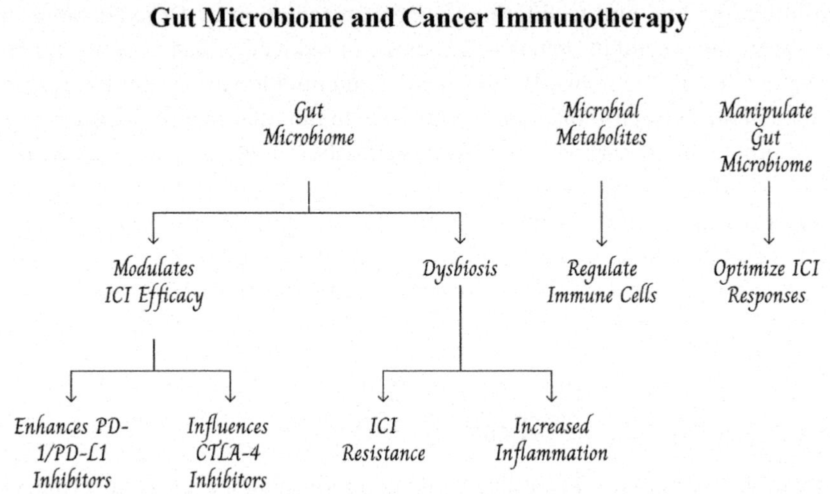

FIGURE 9.2 The role of gut microbiome in modulating immune checkpoint inhibitor efficacy and toxicity. The gut microbiome influences immune checkpoint inhibitor (ICI) efficacy by shaping systemic and tumor-specific immune responses, where certain commensal bacteria enhance antigen presentation, T-cell activation, and response to PD-1/PD-L1 and CTLA-4 blockade. Conversely, dysbiosis can reduce therapeutic benefit and increase immune-related adverse events, highlighting the potential of microbiome modulation strategies—such as probiotics, prebiotics, diet, and fecal microbiota transplantation—to optimize ICI outcomes. *CTLA-4*, cytotoxic T-lymphocyte-associated protein 4; *PD-1*, programmed death 1; *PD-L1*, programmed death ligand 1.

bacteria enhance the efficacy of ICI is through the production of SCFAs such as butyrate, propionate, and acetate that not only improve the intestinal barrier but also promote T cell differentiation, inhibit inflammation, and improve antigen presentation by DCs. *Bifidobacterium* has also been identified to increase DCs' transcription, leading to increased secretion of proinflammatory cytokines such as IL-12 and TNF-α, which are pivotal for the activation of CD8+ cytotoxic T lymphocytes—the prevailing immune cells responsible for tumor removal. In addition, gut microbiota can also regulate tumor cell surface expression of PD-L1 indirectly to modulate immune escape. Supplementation of commensal gut bacteria has been found in mouse models of early-stage cancer to increase tumor infiltration by T cells, promote IFN-γ production, and prolong survival when used together with PD-1 blockade. Dysbiosis—imbalance in gut microbiota—has, on the contrary, been associated with ICI resistance, augmented inflammation, as well as greater susceptibility to irAEs. Interestingly, those patients who received broad-spectrum antibiotics that wipe out gut microbial diversity have poor responses to ICIs and poor survival rates. These findings speak to the therapeutic potential of microbiome-based therapy, including probiotics, prebiotics, diet modification, and fecal microbiota transplants (FMTs) as powerful agents to optimize cancer immunotherapy. In the future, integration of real-time microbiome analysis into practice may allow personalized immunotherapy strategies and allow clinicians to predict patient response and accordingly adjust treatments for more effective therapies (Ciernikova et al., 2024; Lee et al., 2022; Zheng et al., 2020).

9.4.2 Cytotoxic T-lymphocyte-associated protein 4 blockade and microbiota dynamics

CTLA-4 blockade has increasingly come to be a treatment whose efficacy is regulated by the dynamics of gut microbiota, which have an integral role in modulating immune responses. Experiments have established that the presence and density of gut microbiota had a colossal impact on CTLA-4 inhibitor efficacy, as discovered through experiments by Marie Vetizou et al. SPF mice fared dramatically better with CTLA-4 blockade compared to germ-free or antibiotic-treated mice in their research, proving that the healthy microbiome needs to be present to maximize therapeutic effect. The research also found *Bacteroides thetaiotaomicron* and *B. uniformis* to be the prevailing microbial species behind increased responses. The bacteria are credited with promoting DC maturation and antigen presentation, thereby strengthening T-cell activation and the antitumor immune response.

Furthermore, significant changes in the composition of gut microbial communities have been observed following CTLA-4 blockade therapy, suggesting that the therapy itself reorganizes the microbiome in a way highly likely to influence immunity. A particularly intriguing observation was that *B. fragilis*, an immunomodulatory bacterium, did not change during treatment. This stability suggests that *B. fragilis* is potentially implicated in maintaining immune homeostasis and mitigating excessive irAEs associated with CTLA-4 blockade. The pathways through which *B. fragilis* has been found to modulate immune responses are through the production of immunostimulatory compounds such as PSA that enhance the activities of T-helper 1 cells and additionally contribute to the generation of an antitumor microenvironment (Sitthideatphaiboon et al., 2024; The microbiome in cancer Nature, 2024).

Besides such microbiome components, other possible therapeutic modalities involving the microbiome to maximize CTLA-4 blockade efficacy also exist. Preclinical models show that FMT from ICI-refractory patients can trigger a response in resistant individuals through the replenishment of healthy microbe levels. Moreover, probiotic treatments and nutritional changes that expand the presence of healthy bacteria might offer a noninvasive method to enhance patient outcomes. While the complex interplay between gut microbiota and immune checkpoint therapy remains to be uncovered, potential studies in the future may concentrate on individualized microbiome-directed treatment that boosts the efficacy of CTLA-4 inhibitors with the least amount of toxicity, providing the gateway toward more specific and personalized cancer immunotherapy.

9.4.3 Impact on immune cells

The gut microbiota plays a key role in regulating innate and adaptive immunity, immune homeostasis, inflammation, and the efficacy of immunotherapy. One of the major barriers to control by gut microbiota over the immune system is the secretion of microbial metabolites like SCFAs, tryptophan metabolites, and polyamines, and these have been found to regulate immune cell function and preserve intestinal barrier function. These metabolites have been shown to repress hyper-inflammation, promote immune tolerance, and enhance the capacity of the body to elicit a potent antitumor immune response.

On the adaptive immune front, gut microbiota are involved in Tregs that ensure the prevention of autoimmune response and immune homeostasis. Tregs, under normal conditions, inhibit over-activation of the immune response, limiting inflammation and preventing tissue injury. Under immunotherapy, modulation of Treg activity—perhaps through the agency of certain microbial strains—can increase antitumor immunity by alleviating immune suppression of the TME. Moreover, gut microbiota have the potential to control other types of T-cell activations and differentiations, such as Th1, Th17, and cytotoxic CD8+ T cells, each playing a vital role in orchestrating host immune responses against cancer (Gut microbiome may influence immunotherapy response | News releases American Association for Cancer Research (AACR), 2019).

Aside from adaptive immunity, the gut microbiota also controls innate immune cells such as DCs, macrophages, and NK cells. Microbial stimuli directly regulate antigen-presenting DCs and affect their ability to prime T cells and evoke optimal immune responses. In the same way, macrophage polarization to proinflammatory (M1) or anti-inflammatory (M2) phenotypes can be controlled by microbial-derived signals, whereby the immune system promotes or inhibits tumor growth. NK cells, being the first line of defense against cancer, have also been found to be controlled by gut microbiota, whereby specific bacterial species augment their cytotoxicity and tumor-lytic activity. New evidence indicates that by modulating gut microbiota in a directed manner—via probiotics, prebiotics, FMT, or diet—ICI activity may be enhanced while minimizing immune-related toxicities. Enhanced understanding of these microbial-immune interactions has the potential to be applied to precision immunotherapy approaches, optimizing the therapeutic benefit by leveraging the gut microbiome to enhance anticancer immunity while preserving immune tolerance.

9.4.4 Microbial metabolites as immunomodulatory mediators

Microbial metabolites like (SCFAs: butyrate, acetate, propionate), tryptophan-derived AhR ligands, secondary bile acids, inosine, and polyamines are powerful immunomodulatory agents that, upon interaction with host receptors, can lead to immune response changes via metabolic reprogramming and epigenetic modifications. SCFAs originating from the fermentation of dietary fiber signal via G- protein coupled receptors and also through the inhibition of histone deacetylases alter gene expression in APCs as well as lymphocytes; this usually results in DCs becoming more tolerant, showing less expression of costimulatory molecules, producing less IL, 12, and at the same time promoting Foxp3 expression and the proliferation of Tregs. Microbial indoles and other AhR agonists, which are metabolites of tryptophan, likewise modulate the functioning and thus the phenotype of DCs, enhance the epithelial barrier function, and stimulate IL-22 and IL-10, associated pathways that limit excessive Th1 inflammatory responses. Secondary bile acids that are a product of microbial conversion of host bile salts can bind to nuclear and G-protein-coupled bile-acid receptors (e.g., FXR, TGR5) and thereby modulate innate immune responses as well as support immune regulatory microenvironments in mucosal tissues. Polyamines regulate several major cellular pathways, including growth, autophagy, and differentiation. These pathways may serve as a basis for T-cell memory formation, while at the same time making a connection to immunoregulatory, IL-10-biased situations. On the other hand, inosine-an evolutionarily conserved purine nucleoside whose levels are regulated by the microbiota-has been shown to potentiate antitumor immunity through modulation of adenosine/purinergic signaling and support the metabolic fitness of tumor, reactive CD8+ T cells, thus enhancing responses to PD1-blockade in preclinical and translational studies. In summary, these metabolites modulate a few critical biochemical factors, such as receptor signaling, epigenetic remodeling, and metabolic reprogramming, which in turn allow APC function, the cytokine milieu, and T-cell fate decisions to be rebalanced.

These mechanistic effects lead to predictable consequences for CD8+ T cells, DC maturation, the Treg-Th1 axis, and cytokine landscapes, although the results are very different depending on the context. By driving tolerogenic DC programs (less IL-12, fewer costimulatory signals), SCFAs, AhR ligands, secondary bile acids, and polyamines generally inhibit robust Th1 priming and aggressive CD8+ effector differentiation; instead, they promote Treg induction and increased IL-10 production to maintain mucosal homeostasis and to prevent immunopathology. In many steady-state and barrier contexts, this is advantageous, as it limits tissue damage while maintaining immune tolerance. However, metabolite action is not always suppressive: acetate is able to enhance antiviral CD8+ responses in certain tissues, and inosine has been demonstrated to remodel TMEs toward increased IL-12/IFN-γ signaling and better CD8+ mediated tumor elimination when combined with checkpoint blockade. Therefore, the overall cytokine profile-whether dominated by IL-10 and correspondingly decreased IL-12/IFN (tolerance) or by increased IL-12 and IFN (activation) is a function of the metabolite nature, concentration, tissue milieu, and the immune signals present at the same time. From a translational perspective, these data rationalize therapeutic approaches that either elevate the levels of regulatory metabolites in order to ameliorate inflammatory diseases or increase proeffector metabolites (or inhibit suppressive ones) to potentiate the effectiveness of vaccines and cancer immunotherapy, while always being mindful of the contextual duality of microbial small molecules (Calvo-Barreiro et al., 2023; Donia & Fischbach, 2015; Liu et al., 2025).

9.4.5 Tumor microenvironment remodeling by gut microbiota

The gut microbiome regulates the TME through complex and diverse interactions of both the adaptive and innate immune systems, vascular remodeling, interferon pathways, as well as epigenetic and metabolic changes of myeloid cells. The composition of microbiota and microbial metabolites impacts the presence, types, and activity of TILs: a good microbial signature or the movement of commensals inside the tumor can lead to more CD8+ T-cell infiltration and increased effector activity, while dysbiosis or signals that attract suppressive myeloid cells are linked to fewer TILs and reduced function. MDSCs and TAMs represent the main targets of microbiome-driven remodeling; microbial signals and tumor-secreted factors that interact with the microbiota can lead to higher MDSC/TAM recruitment and their immunosuppressive differentiation (e.g., through chemokine axes discussed in obesity-related models), thus facilitating TIL apoptosis and immunotherapy resistance. One of the central mechanisms through which the TME is rendered immunosuppressive involves metabolic reprogramming, especially changed fatty-acid uptake and storage in lipid droplets within MDSCs and TAMs, which connects

Table 9.2 Factors affecting gut microbiome influence on immune checkpoint inhibitors.

Factor	Details
Composition of the gut microbiome	The presence of beneficial bacteria (*Akkermansia muciniphila, Bacteroides, Faecalibacterium*) is linked to improved immune checkpoint inhibitors (ICIs) response, while dysbiosis can lead to resistance or toxicity.
Dietary influences	A fiber-rich diet supports beneficial microbiota, while high-fat or processed foods may promote dysbiosis, impacting ICI efficacy.
Role of probiotics	Probiotics and fecal microbiota transplantation (FMT) may enhance gut microbiome diversity and improve response to ICIs.
Immune-related adverse effects (irAEs)	An imbalanced gut microbiome can trigger excessive inflammation, increasing the risk of autoimmune-like toxicities associated with ICIs.

microbial metabolites and host lipid handling to epigenetic and functional changes in myeloid cells. Similarly, angiogenesis is indirectly modulated by microbes via inflammatory and stromal signaling pathways, which in turn change vascular normalization and hence the trafficking of immune cells and drug delivery to tumors. Basically, microbes in tumors or microbial-derived signals can amplify innate sensing pathways like STING, thereby elevating type I interferon responses that strengthen antigen presentation and antitumor immunity, subsequently resulting in better responses to therapies such as CD47 or checkpoint blockade in preclinical models. Cumulatively, these associations reveal a microbiome-epigenetic/metabolic axis that dictates the resulting equilibrium of immune activation and suppression in the TME and hence identifies therapeutic possibilities for reprogramming MDSCs/TAMs, reviving TIL function, normalizing vasculature, and utilizing interferon signaling for immunotherapy sensitization of tumors (Hamze Sinno et al., 2024; Raychaudhuri et al., 2015; Shi et al., 2020; Siddiqui & Glauben, 2022).

9.5 Factors of gut microbiome effect on immune checkpoint inhibitors

The gut microbiota are significant regulators of the efficacy of ICIs because they control their efficacy as well as their toxicity. This is attributed to several reasons, as they are mentioned in Table 9.2.

9.5.1 Composition of the gut microbiome

The gut microbiome is a diverse community of trillions of microbes such as bacteria, viruses, fungi, and archaea that play a role in the formation of the immune system and ICI response. There is recent evidence that the diversity and composition of gut microbiota have a strong correlation with the success of ICI therapy, wherein certain bacterial species promote or suppress the treatment effect. They have identified probiotic bacterial genera that are advantageous, such as

A. muciniphila, Bifidobacterium, Faecalibacterium, and *Ruminococcaceae*, and are associated with positive responses to ICIs. Such microbes contribute to antitumor immunity by modifying the activation of immune cells, antigen presentation, and establishment of a proinflammatory environment for successful cancer therapy. For example, *A. muciniphila* was shown to increase DC and cytotoxic T cell recruitment and activation to increase the immune response of the body against cancer. Similarly, *Faecalibacterium* species are known to secrete SCFAs, such as butyrate, with anti-inflammatory properties as well as preserving intestinal barrier function to suppress inappropriate immune suppression.

Conversely, a disruption of the intestinal microbiome, or dysbiosis, can negatively impact ICI efficacy. Certain immunosuppressive or pathogenic bacteria, such as *E. coli, Prevotella*, and *Bacteroides*, have been linked with poor responses to immunotherapy. They may perpetuate chronic inflammation, suppress effector T-cell activity, or increase Treg cells and produce an immunosuppressive TME where cancer cells become resistant to immune attack. Furthermore, patients with low microbial diversity or patients who have previously received broad-spectrum antibiotics before or in the course of ICI treatment have worse outcomes, further implicating a balanced microbiome. With these discoveries in mind, there are attempts being made to modulate the gut microbiota to maximize ICI therapy. Those efforts include FMT, probiotic supplementation, prebiotic nutritional therapy, and microbial-derived metabolite therapy to increase ICI activity. Elucidation of the precise role of the gut microbiome in cancer immunotherapy could lead to more personalized treatment approaches, enabling us to find out which patients are most likely to benefit from ICIs and to design microbiome-targeted interventions to increase the response to therapy.

9.5.2 Dietary effects on gut microbiome and immune checkpoint inhibitor response

Diet is also a critical factor in determining the gut microbiome, which then impacts immune function and the activity of ICIs. Fiber has been highlighted among dietary constituents as a prime regulator of gut microbial composition and beneficial immune effects. A diet high in fiber, fruits, vegetables, whole grains, and legumes has been linked with increased microbial diversity and bacterial species enrichments that enhance antitumor immunity. Observational studies in melanoma and cancer patients have revealed that patients having high-fiber diets respond positively to ICI therapy compared with patients having low-fiber diets. The action is thought to be mediated by the action of fiber-fermenting bacteria like *F. prausnitzii, Bifidobacterium*, and *A. muciniphila* that release SCFAs such as butyrate, propionate, and acetate. SCFAs are important metabolites that control immune function through the facilitation of the activation of DCs, increased cytotoxic T-cell response, and inhibition of systemic inflammation.

Preclinical experiments in mouse models also corroborate these results, showing that consumption of dietary fiber is associated with retarded tumor growth. Mice on a high-fiber diet showed increased antitumor immunity, as reflected by enhanced CD8+ T cell infiltration into tumors and improved ICI efficacy. Interestingly, such effects were not seen in germ-free mice, highlighting the central role of gut microbiota in mediating dietary fiber's immunostimulatory effect. Besides fiber, other dietary constituents such as polyphenols (berries, green tea, dark chocolate) and omega-3 fatty acids (fish and flaxseeds) have been investigated for their ability to impact the gut microbiota and to improve ICI efficacy. In contrast, diets typical of the Western diet pattern with high fat and low fiber intake have been associated with gut dysbiosis, systemic inflammation, and low response rates to ICIs.

Such findings stress the potential role of nutrition interventions as a strategy to boost cancer immunotherapy. Personalized nutrition therapy, such as counseling for higher fiber intake or prebiotic and probiotic supplements, can modulate the composition of the gut microbiota and clinical response in ICI-treated individuals. Additional clinical trials are nevertheless necessary to determine optimal dietary recommendations and their mechanistic correlations with cancer therapy immune responses (Davar et al., 2021; Gamrath et al., 2025; Roviello et al., 2021).

9.5.3 Role of probiotics

Probiotics—living microorganisms with health benefits that are delivered upon consumption in suitable quantities—have been in the spotlight as putative modulators of the gut microbiome for the improvement of ICI therapy. Probiotics may enhance the immune system of the host and respond better to immunotherapy by promoting a healthy composition of gut microbiota. Following amassing evidence suggesting that gut microbiota diversity is involved in defining the effectiveness of ICIs, researchers have been studying the role of probiotics to enhance immune functions and antitumor activity. Multiple preclinical and clinical studies demonstrate the therapeutic potential of treatment with probiotics, namely *Bifidobacterium, Lactobacillus,* and *A. muciniphila* strains, in terms of cancer therapy. These gut-dwelling bacteria maintain homeostasis, augment the biosynthesis of SCFAs, and modulate inflammation, factors accountable for potent immune surveillance of cancer. Certain probiotic strains have been reported to increase CD8+ T cell infiltration into the TME, enhance DC antigen presentation, and inhibit immunosuppressive Tregs, thereby triggering a more potent antitumor immune response.

In addition to conventional probiotic supplementation, FMT has been a very promising therapeutic strategy to manipulate the gut microbiome and enhance ICI efficacy. Clinical evidence in melanoma patients has revealed that fecal microbiota transfer from ICI-responsive individuals into nonresponders could increase treatment response. FMT was found to reinstate gut microbial diversity and amplify systemic immune activity, which might reverse ICI resistance in some patients. While these promising findings, the use of probiotics in cancer immunotherapy is a complex area of study. While there are studies to indicate benefits, others find that unregulated use of probiotics can have negative consequences, including an increase in certain types of bacteria that may suppress immunity. Further, the efficacy of probiotic supplementation appears to depend on the probiotic strains being used, the patient's microbiome composition, and the nature of the cancer being treated (Humphries & Daud, 2018).

9.5.4 Immune-related adverse effects

Gut microbiome is not only important for regulating the potency of ICIs but also for the development and severity of immune-related adverse effects (irAEs). The irAEs occur as a result of excessive activation of the immune system, producing inflammation and autoimmunity in multiple organs, such as the gastrointestinal tract, liver, lungs, and endocrine glands. Recent data suggest that some microbial signatures are a protective factor or risk factor for irAEs. For example, there have been reports of studies linking increased abundance of some commensal bacteria such as *F. prausnitzii* and *Bacteroides* with reduced risk of severe irAEs, depending on how they may modulate immune homeostasis and act in an anti-inflammatory manner. Conversely, *Enterococcus faecium* and *E. coli* detection have been linked with increased risk of adverse effects because these bacteria have the potential to trigger proinflammatory processes that exacerbate immune dysregulation.

Moreover, alterations in gut microbial diversity, or dysbiosis, have been identified in those with severe irAEs, particularly colitis, one of the most common toxicities associated with ICIs. Reducing microbial diversity, including the loss of regulatory and anti-inflammatory bacteria, may lead to immune hyperactivation and tissue injury. The identification of these patterns in microorganisms represents a promising starting point for forecasting and preventing toxicities induced by ICI. Therapeutic methods like FMT, selective probiotic supplementation, and nutrition-based therapy to restore microbalance have been tested as plausible methods for minimizing irAEs with no compromise in the therapeutic efficacy of ICIs. As the science evolves, a tailored strategy for immunotherapy that takes into account the composition of the gut microbiome may result in improved patient stratification, enabling clinicians to recognize those at increased risk for irAEs and adopt preemptive microbiome-modulating therapies. This may ultimately enhance patient outcomes by improving the tolerability of ICIs without compromising their powerful anticancer activity (Lynn et al., 2021).

9.6 Tracking gut microbiome profiles

Supervising gut microbiome profiles is important for comprehending the intricate relationships between gut microbiota and immune systems, especially in light of ICIs. Improvements in sequencing and analytical techniques have substantially increased the capacity to profile gut microbiome composition. Two of the most common methods are 16S ribosomal RNA gene sequencing (16S rRNA-seq) and metagenomic sequencing, both providing different types of information on microbial communities. Though 16S rRNA-seq is generally known to detect up to the level of bacterial genus, metagenomic sequencing identifies bacteria at the species level, providing a better representation of microbial diversity as well as richness (Davar et al., 2021; Humphries & Daud, 2018). A further key technique used for dissecting gut microbiome data is the incorporation of machine learning methods. These approaches enable the combination of different data types, which can allow researchers to identify correlations between microbial profiles and clinical responses to ICIs. Machine learning, through the use of large datasets, can detect predictive patterns that can be used to guide individualized treatment approaches (Jiang & Zhang, 2024; Lynn et al., 2021). In addition, fecal samples are widely utilized as surrogates for gut microbiota because they are noninvasive to collect and contain a rich source of information about microbial communities (Roviello et al., 2021) . Such a variation in profiles of gut microbiota can notably affect patient therapeutic responses, and it is thus required to monitor the profiles continuously in the long run. Such continuous dynamic assessment gives researchers and doctors a better clue about the therapeutic modulation by the gut microbiota and directs an individualized form of treatment strategy (The fundamentals of open access and open research Springer Nature (n.d.) ;Zheng et al., 2020).

9.6.1 Multiomics approaches in microbiome research

At present, research on microbiomes utilizes an extensive multiomics toolset, which includes 16S rRNA amplicon sequencing, shotgun metagenomics, meta-transcriptomics, metabolomics, and proteomics, which are sometimes combined with tumor genomics. This combination can reveal, among other things, taxonomic composition, functional potential, active gene expression, small-molecule mediators, and protein effectors that contribute to tumor microbiome networks. While 16S rRNA sequencing still stands as a readily available, inexpensively viable method to profile bacterial community structure down to genus and occasionally species level. It thus allows for large-scale diversity and association studies. On the other hand, shotgun metagenomics not only gives strain-level resolution but also gene catalogs that enable functional inference and the detection of virulence or metabolic pathways. Further, metatranscriptomics records microbial and host-microbe crosstalk in situ, highlighting transcriptional pathways actively expressed in the TME or gut. Metabolomics is concerned with the identification of microbial metabolites (SCFAs, bile acids, purines, polyamines) that have a direct impact on immune and stromal cells, whereas proteomics is a method of identifying both secreted and cellular proteins from microbes and hosts that are responsible for carrying out biological functions. Combining microbial omics with tumor genomics (mutational burden, neoantigen load, transcriptomic immune signatures) not only reveals mechanisms, e.g., microbial routes associated with tumor immune infiltration or resistance mechanisms, but it also facilitates the testing of causal hypotheses in preclinical models and the generation of biomarkers for clinical translation (reviews and multiomics roadmaps). Due to the high dimensionality and compositional characteristics of microbiome data, AI and machine, learning techniques such as (regularized regression, random forests, gradient boosting, deep learning, and ensemble methods) are being more and more employed to create predictive models that embed omic layers, identify stable features, and classify samples; standardized computational workflows and thorough validation remain crucial for reproducibility and interpretability (methodological assessments and ML guidance). The signature predictive of patients' response to ICIs derived from the microbiome through these approaches in several cohorts has also been used in the design of stratified clinical trials and the identification of interventional strategies (microbiome modulation, metabolite supplementation) to sensitize tumors to immunotherapy (Aguiar-Pulido et al., 2016; Campagna et al., 2024; Deek et al., 2024; Wu et al., 2023).

9.6.2 Biomarker development and predictive signatures

Biomarker development in oncology is increasingly focusing on the utilization of microbial diversity indices along with the identification of specific microbial taxa to help in patient stratification, prediction of ICI responses, and anticipation of therapy-induced complications. Usually, ecological indices like Shannon diversity correlate well with favorable outcomes, e.g., higher alpha diversity tends to be linked with more vigorous antitumor immunity. Besides, selective signatures that are composed of beneficial microbial taxa such as *A. muciniphila*, different species of *Bifidobacterium*, and *F. prausnitzii* have been consistently found in studies to be characteristic of ICI responders and, thus, associated with enhanced CD8+ T, cell infiltration and interferon signaling; these microbial strains may also constitute parts of multifeature classifiers retrieved through machine learning (e.g., random forests, support vector machines, elastic net) that integrate taxonomic, functional (metagenomic pathways), metabolomic, and clinical variables to predict response with higher precision than single markers. A key aspect of developing powerful classifiers is to pay attention to potential confounders: a history of antibiotic treatment, either before or during the therapy, has the effect of lowering the microbiome diversity, disrupting beneficial signatures, and leading to worse outcomes of ICI therapy; hence, it is essential to take medication history into account and adjust for baseline disruptions when constructing predictive models. Baseline microbiome stratification determines a patient's microbiome cluster or enterotype and can direct personalized interventions (such as fecal microbiota transplant, probiotics, dietary modulation, metabolite supplementation) aimed at transforming treatment nonresponders into responders. However, for the model to be generalizable, it needs to be validated in large multicohort studies with standardized sampling/processing. Recent multiomics clinical studies and computational frameworks have stressed the importance of cross-cohort harmonization, feature stability assessment, and thorough external validation to help prevent overfitting and to yield clinically actionable microbiome biomarkers for immunotherapy decision-making (Li et al., 2022a).

9.7 Strategies for control of the gut microbiome to improve immune checkpoint inhibitor therapy

The gut microbiome is also being considered as a major immune system regulator, modulating the efficacy and toxicity of ICIs used in cancer treatment. Keeping this in view, scientists are designing different strategies for manipulating the microbiome to enhance the impact of ICI. They are dietary manipulation, probiotic supplementation, FMTs, and designed microbiomes. By modulating the gut microbiota, practitioners attempt to enhance antitumor immunity, decrease irAEs, and improve overall patient outcomes, as mentioned in Fig. 9.3.

9.7.1 Dietary interventions

9.7.1.1 Plant-based diets and high-fiber intake

Diet strongly shapes the makeup of the gut microbiome. Plant-based diets rich in fiber, like the Mediterranean Diet, have been associated with greater microbial diversity, and it has been demonstrated that greater microbial diversity is correlated with better responses to ICI treatment. These diets contain prebiotic fiber that stimulates growth of healthful gut bacteria, which, in turn, produce essential metabolites such as SCFAs, such as butyrate, acetate, and propionate.

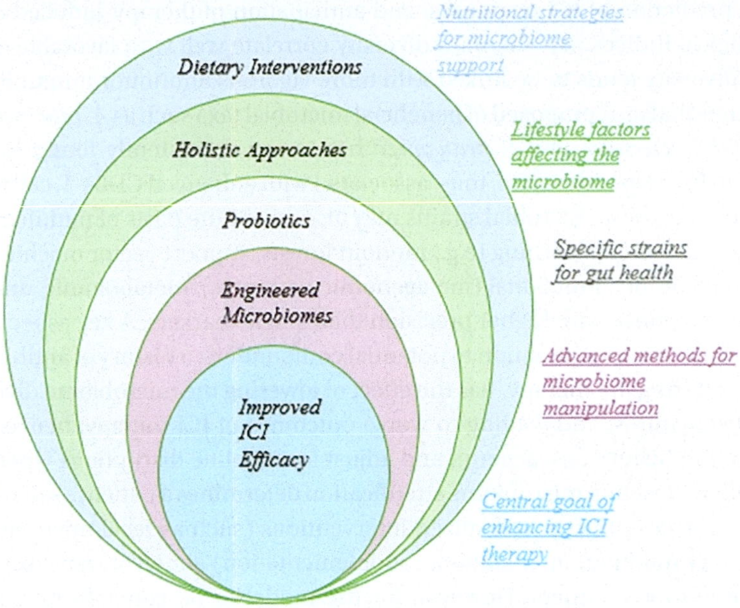

FIGURE 9.3 Strategies for modulating the gut microbiome to enhance immune checkpoint inhibitor therapy. Gut microbiome modulation strategies—such as high-fiber diets, targeted probiotics/prebiotics, fecal microbiota transplantation, and careful antibiotic stewardship—aim to restore beneficial microbial diversity that enhances T-cell activation and response to immune checkpoint inhibitors. Emerging approaches, including defined microbial consortia and engineered bacteria, offer precision tools to improve ICI efficacy while minimizing immune-related toxicity. *ICI*, immune checkpoint inhibitors.

These SCFAs:

- Regulate intestinal immune homeostasis.
- Increase differentiation of Tregs to enhance immune tolerance.
- Regulate DC stimulation to enhance antitumor immunity.
- Suppress systemic inflammation, which is crucial to offset immune activation upon ICI treatment.

Some observational studies have shown that cancer patients who take more than 30 g of fiber a day and eat more than 30 different plant species per week have better response rates to ICIs than those on low-fiber diets. Western and high-fat diets, with high consumption of processed food and red meat, however, have been linked with gut dysbiosis, higher proinflammatory bacterial loads, and lower ICI responses (Gazzaniga & Kasper, 2025; Pesheva, 2024).

9.7.1.2 Fermented foods and polyphenols

Fermented foods like yogurt, kimchi, and sauerkraut carry live probiotic bacteria, which can boost gut microbial diversity. Likewise, polyphenol-rich foods like berries, green tea, and dark chocolate have been reported to modulate the gut microbiota composition and function to favor beneficial bacterial species while suppressing inflammation.

9.7.1.3 Low-protein diets and amino acid restriction

Latest evidence indicates that heavy animal protein consumption (particularly processed and red meat) could cause the richness in proinflammatory bacteria of the gut to increase, thus secondary bile acids become present in high numbers and impair the immune system negatively. In contrast, high dietary intake of proteins from plants (legumes, seeds, nuts) has been linked to a better gut microbiome with protective functions against tumors and antitumor immune responses (Pesheva, 2024; Zheng et al., 2020).

9.7.2 Holistic approaches

9.7.2.1 The role of lifestyle factors

Holistic approaches highlight that the health of the gut microbiome not only depends on diet but also on the level of stress, the level of exercise, and sleeping patterns. Long-term stress and insomnia have been associated with gut dysbiosis and immune disorders, which may undermine the efficacy of ICI.

Exercise has been shown to improve microbiome diversity, antitumor immunity, and reduce inflammation.

Stress management interventions such as meditation and yoga may improve microbial composition by reducing cortisol-mediated dysbiosis.

Holistic treatments are not intended as an alternative to conventional cancer therapy but as a complement to ICI treatment, improving immune response through microbiome-nurturing lifestyle adjustments (Chang et al., 2024; Routy et al., 2017).

9.7.3 Probiotics

9.7.3.1 Lactobacillus *and* Bifidobacterium *strains*

Probiotic supplementation is another possible route for microbiome modulation. Some *Lactobacillus* and *Bifidobacterium* species have been demonstrated to enhance antitumor immunity by:

- Enhancing intestinal barrier function, inhibiting bacterial translocation, and reducing inflammation.
- Sensitizing cytotoxic T cell activation, which is crucial for tumor clearance.
- Modulating regulatory T cell (Treg) function, reversing excessive immune suppression (Davar et al., 2021; Roviello et al., 2021).

9.7.3.2 Key probiotic strains examined in immune checkpoint inhibitor treatment

L. paracasei: Increases microbial diversity and preserves immune homeostasis.

L. rhamnosus: Downregulates inflammation through Treg modulation and DC regulation.

Bifidobacterium breve: Potentiates DC maturation and strengthens anti-PD-1 response (Chang et al., 2024; Roviello et al., 2021).

9.7.3.3 Caution when applying probiotics

Although promising, recent studies have shown that unlimited use of probiotics can lower microbiome diversity, leading to reduced ICI responses in some patients. This means that the best approach is most probably tailored probiotic treatment—according to one's own microbiome pattern (Davar et al., 2021; Roviello et al., 2021).

9.7.4 Engineered microbiomes in treating cancer

The gut microbiome also plays a crucial role in the regulation of the immune system, and the latest studies have discovered the possibility of utilizing it to enhance the success of cancer therapy. Among the more encouraging approaches in this respect is the use of engineered microbiomes, including FMT and synthetic bacterial consortia. These treatments seek to alter the microbial flora among cancer patients, especially those receiving ICI therapy, in an attempt to enhance immune response and the effectiveness of the treatments.

9.7.4.1 Fecal microbiota transplantation

FMT is the transplantation of gut microbiota from ICI-responsive donors into nonresponders, essentially changing the recipient's microbial community. This method has worked well in clinical trials, especially for patients with melanoma. The research has shown enhanced responses to ICIs in patients receiving FMT, solidifying the gut microbiome's position in mediating immune checkpoint blockade efficacy. FMT has also been associated with elevated levels of beneficial bacterial species like *A. muciniphila*, which play a role in enhanced response to anti-PD-1 therapy. It is thus indicated that manipulation of gut microbiota may be a potential approach to increasing cancer immunotherapy success (Davar et al., 2021).

9.7.4.2 Synthetic microbial consortia

In addition to FMT, scientists are designing engineered microbiomes with synthetic bacterial consortia programmed to generate precise immunomodulatory metabolites. These are SCFAs such as butyrate and propionate, which sustain anti-inflammatory pathways, polysaccharides that stimulate DC and T cell activation, and bile acid metabolites that affect regulatory T cell differentiation. Through adjustment of the immune response, synthetic microbial consortia provide a regulated and accurate pathway to modulate ICI efficacy with the potential for minimized irAEs (Roviello et al., 2021).

9.7.5 Microbiome editing technologies

CRISPR-based bacterial engineering, phage therapy, selective microbial depletion, synthetic biology platforms, and bacterial drug-delivery systems are collectively a rapidly maturing toolkit for microbiome editing that holds great translational promise. CRISPR methods (delivered via conjugative plasmids, phage vectors or engineered carriers) allow, for example, precise in situ editing of commensals or pathogens to disrupt virulence factors, delete resistance genes, or reprogram metabolic outputs, which is durable, targetable modulation beyond broad antibiotics; bacteriophages-natural predators of bacteria can be engineered for narrow-spectrum killing, payload delivery (including CRISPR cargo), or modulation of community structure with high specificity and low collateral damage to beneficial taxa; selective microbial depletion strategies (narrow-spectrum antimicrobials, engineered probiotics that outcompete pathogens, or targeted bacteriocins) allow deleterious strains removal while community functions are preserved; synthetic biology platforms, which help design programmable microbial therapeutics that, for instance, can sense disease signals and hence respond by producing therapeutic molecules (cytokines, enzymes, immunomodulatory metabolites) or self-limiting circuits for safety control; and bacterial drug-delivery systems that are engineered strains or biomaterial-armed microbes localize to tumors or mucosal niches to release anticancer agents, immune stimulants, or checkpoint modulators with spatial precision, thus enhancing efficacy and reducing systemic toxicity. The translational potential is pretty great. Such methods have the capacity to change correlative microbiome-disease relationships into causal treatments (e.g., replenishing beneficial metabolites, undoing antibiotic resistance, changing TMEs), allow for personalized microbiome therapeutics (strain-level editing guided by multiomics), and combine with existing modalities like immunotherapy or antibiotics to overcome resistance or increase responses. However, there are still significant translational difficulties in delivery efficiency in complicated ecosystems, horizontal gene transfer and ecological impacts, off-target effects, regulatory pathways, manufacturing scale-up, and rigorous safety/ethical frameworks, but improvements in phage engineering, programmable CRISPR, transposase systems, and containment circuits are solving these issues and pushing some strategies to clinical evaluation. In general, microbiome editing technologies represent a flexible, mechanistic way to therapeutic modulation of host-microbe interactions with a very high degree of specificity and the potential for long-lasting effects in infectious disease, cancer, and chronic inflammatory conditions (Fooladi et al., 2023; Roberts et al., 2025).

9.8 Future directions

As studies of the gut microbiome in the modulation of ICIs are developing, a number of important future directions become apparent for further investigation.

9.8.1 Understanding mechanisms of interaction

One of the important areas for further research is to clarify the mechanisms through which the gut microbiota affects the activity of ICIs. It involves identifying the microbial species beneficial or detrimental to therapy and how they interact with the host immune system. One of these mechanisms under investigation includes the modulation of systemic immune reactions by gut microbiota. Certain bacterial genera such as *A. muciniphila* and *F. prausnitzii* have been implicated in enhanced responsiveness to ICIs by their ability to modulate immune cell activation and generate antitumor immunity. These pathogens produce metabolites such as SCFAs and polyamines, which regulate the activity of Tregs, cytotoxic T cells, and APCs and thus decide the immune landscape that is needed for successful immunotherapy.

Subsequent research should also investigate how microbial-derived molecules engage with major immune pathways, including the PD-1/PD-L1 and CTLA-4 axes, which are the main targets of ICIs. Elucidation of these complex molecular interactions may open the door to microbiome-directed therapeutic approaches, including probiotics, prebiotics, and microbiota transplantation, to maximize cancer immunotherapy responses.

9.8.2 Personalized microbiome-based therapies

Tailored microbiome-mediated therapies are an innovative strategy for maximizing the therapeutic efficacy of ICIs by tapping the immunomodulatory potential of the gut microbiome. Researchers can identify the patient's microbial signatures that predict better therapeutic benefits by examining their microbiome profiles and constructing individualized interventions based on them. These interventions may include the administration of probiotics or prebiotics to promote the development of beneficial bacteria, absorption modifications to provide sustenance to a healthy microbiota, or FMTs for the restoration of microbial diversity in dysbiosis patients. These intervention-driven techniques can enhance ICI responses and decrease immune-related adverse reactions, which can ultimately lead to more potent and tolerable cancer immunotherapy (Gunjur et al., 2024; Hwang et al., 2023).

9.8.3 Large-scale clinical trials

Large-scale clinical trials must be conducted to confirm the gut microbiome's role in predicting the efficacy of ICIs. While early studies have shown correlations between specific microbial patterns and outcomes, robust validation across different patient groups is required to ensure that the findings are generalizable to a large population. Standardized microbiome analysis techniques need to be incorporated in such trials to establish reproducible biomarkers that predict patient outcomes to ICIs. The study of variations in microbiome composition across different populations, cancers, and therapeutic regimens can also optimize the application of individualized immunotherapy. With the integration of microbiome information into routine clinical practice, subsequent trials will potentially result in microbiome-directed patient stratification to enable more personalized therapeutic approaches that optimize effectiveness while minimizing toxicity (Bakdash et al., 2025).

9.8.4 Examining other combinations for therapeutics

Exploring the gut microbiome's interaction with other therapies for cancer, including chemotherapy and targeted therapies, is an important area for future study. The microbiome has been found to play a role in drug metabolism, immune modulation, and inflammation, all of which can affect responses to treatment. For instance, some gut bacteria have the ability to make chemotherapeutic drugs more effective by modulating the host immune system or by directly metabolizing drugs into more bioactive substances. Conversely, microbial imbalances may lead to treatment resistance or increased toxicity. These complex interactions may be decoupled by the creation of combination therapies that leverage the microbiome to improve patient outcomes. Microbiome-targeting interventions, including probiotics, prebiotics, and FMTs, may render existing treatments more effective with reduced side effects. By integrating microbiome analysis into cancer treatment, physicians could potentially individualize the treatment so that it is as effective as possible and leads to improved survival and an acceptable quality of life for patients (Gunjur et al., 2024).

9.8.5 Longitudinal studies

Longitudinal studies are crucial for uncovering how gut microbiome dynamics shape the effectiveness and safety of ICI therapy over time. By monitoring microbiome changes continuously before, during, and after treatment, scientists can discover microbial signatures pointing to good or bad treatment outcomes, mechanisms of resistance, and irAEs. For instance, beneficial bacteria such as *A. muciniphila* correlate with enhanced ICI responses, and some microbial imbalances may be the cause of resistance. These experiments also make it possible to predict irAEs by observing microbial alterations that are correlated with side effects and potentially initiate early intervention. In addition, on-line microbiome analysis may lead to personalized treatment strategies, in which treatments are adjusted based on an individual's microbial makeup. Advances in sequencing technologies and AI-driven microbiome analysis further augment such efforts, ultimately optimizing ICI therapy, enhancing response rates, and reducing therapy-related complications (Bakdash et al., 2025; Zheng et al., 2020).

9.9 Conclusion

The gut microbiome has been recognized as one of the key factors determining the impact of ICI by affecting the activation of the antitumor immune response and the overall clinical outcomes. An increasing number of studies suggest that microbial diversity, an increase in beneficial bacterial species, and their metabolic products, especially SCFAs, promote T-cell activation and, therefore, potentiate antitumor immunity. This chapter shows that the microbiota is a very important factor in modulating the effects of ICIs in the TME. On the other hand, microbiome-associated dysbiosis might be one of the causes for irAEs as well as the reduced effectiveness of the therapy. The relationship between the genetics of the host, diet, lifestyle, and psychological stress also makes microbiome-immune system interactions more complicated, thus pointing to the requirement for combined and mechanistic studies. Microbiome-targeting strategies, such as probiotic supplementation, diet changes, and FMT, are potential adjunct therapies to optimize the effects of ICI, which can be used in combination with other treatments. On the other hand, newly developed predictive tools, such as comprehensive microbial-based indices, can help identify which patients might benefit most, thereby enabling a more personalized therapeutic approach. In turn, deeper insights into the microbiome-immune interactions at the molecular level could not only allow the accurate identification of patients who will most likely benefit from immunotherapy, but they can also reduce irAEs while improving the overall efficacy of the treatment. Ultimately, bringing microbiome research into oncology clinics will likely result in more patient-specific and long-lasting responses to ICIs.

Acknowledgment

The authors are very much thankful to the Management of Vignan's Foundation for Science, Technology and Research, Guntur; Great Eastern Medical School and Hospital (GEMS), Srikakulam; and KVSR Siddhartha College of Pharmaceutical Sciences, Vijayawada, for their support and constant encouragement.

References

Aguiar-Pulido, V., Huang, W., Suarez-Ulloa, V., Cickovski, T., Mathee, K., & Narasimhan, G. (2016). Metagenomics, metatranscriptomics, and metabolomics approaches for microbiome analysis: Supplementary issue: Bioinformatics methods and applications for big metagenomics data. *Evol Bioinform Online, 12*(Suppl 1), 5–16. http://dx.doi.org/10.4137/EBO.S36436.

Bakdash, G., Popple, A., Klisko, D., Hudson, R., Castan, L., Villemin, C., Schreiber, F., Berlato, C., Corrie, P., Sharpington, T., Lawley, T. D., & Robinson, M. J. (2025). Abstract B102: Clinical response to checkpoint inhibitors is associated with distinct gut bacteria that promote anti-tumor immunity through different mechanisms. *Cancer Immunology Research, 13*(2_Supplement), B102. https://doi.org/10.1158/2326-6074.io2025-b102.

Calvo-Barreiro, L., Zhang, L., Abdel-Rahman, S. A., Naik, S. P., & Gabr, M. (2023). Gut microbial-derived metabolites as immune modulators of T helper 17 and regulatory T cells. *International Journal of Molecular Sciences, 24*(2), 1806. http://dx.doi.org/10.3390/ijms24021806.

Campagna, A., Clasen, F., Portlock, T., Zampini, M., Ficara, F., Crisafulli, L., Brindisi, M., Martano, G., Saba, E., Ubezio, M., Russo, A., Todisco, G., Maggioni, G., Lanino, L., Buizza, A., Pinocchio, N., Ventura, D., Viviani, F., Torre, E., Antunes Dos Reis, R., & Shoaie, S. (2024). Clinical relevance of the integrative analysis of gut microbiome and metabolomics in myeloid neoplasms: Correlations with genomic profiles, treatment response/complications and clinical outcome. *Blood, 144*(Supplement 1), 104. http://dx.doi.org/10.1182/blood-2024-204635.

Cani, P. D. (2018). Human gut microbiome: Hopes, threats and promises. *Gut, 67*(9), 1716–1725. https://doi.org/10.1136/gutjnl-2018-316723.

Chang, J. W.-C., Hsieh, J.-J., Tsai, C.-Y., Chiu, H.-Y., Lin, Y.-F., Wu, C.-E., Shen, Y.-C., Hou, M.-M., Chang, C.-Y., Chen, J.-A., Chen, C.-L., Chiu, C.-T., Yeh, Y.-M., & Chiu, C.-H. (2024). Gut microbiota and clinical response to immune checkpoint inhibitor therapy in patients with advanced cancer. *Biomedical Journal, 47*(5), 100698. https://doi.org/10.1016/j.bj.2024.100698.

Ciernikova, S., Sevcikova, A., Novisedlakova, M., & Mego, M. (2024). Insights into the relationship between the gut microbiome and immune checkpoint inhibitors in solid tumors. *Cancers, 16*(24), 4271. https://doi.org/10.3390/cancers16244271.

Davar, D., Dzutsev, A. K., McCulloch, J. A., Rodrigues, R. R., Chauvin, J. M., Morrison, R. M., Deblasio, R. N., Menna, C., Ding, Q., Pagliano, O., Zidi, B., Zhang, S., Badger, J. H., Vetizou, M., Cole, A. M., Fernandes, M. R., Prescott, S., Costa, R. G. F., Balaji, A. K., … Zarour, H. M. (2021). Fecal microbiota transplant overcomes resistance to anti-PD-1 therapy in melanoma patients. *Science, 371*(6529), 595–602. https://doi.org/10.1126/science.abf3363.

Deek, R. A., Ma, S., Lewis, J., & Li, H. (2024). Statistical and computational methods for integrating microbiome, host genomics, and metabolomics data. *Elife, 13*. http://dx.doi.org/10.7554/eLife.88956.

Donia, M. S., & Fischbach, M. A. (2015). Human microbiota. Small molecules from the human microbiota. *Science, 349*(6246), 1254766. http://dx.doi.org/10.1126/science.1254766.

Fooladi, S., Rabiee, N., & Iravani, S. (2023). Genetically engineered bacteria: A new frontier in targeted drug delivery. *Journal of Materials Chemistry B Materials for Biology and Medicine, 11*(42), 10072–10087. http://dx.doi.org/10.1039/d3tb01805a.

Gamrath, L., Pedersen, T. B., Møller, M. V., Volmer, L. M., Holst-Christensen, L., Vestermark, L. W., & Donskov, F. (2025). Role of the microbiome and diet for response to cancer checkpoint immunotherapy: A narrative review of clinical trials. *Current Oncology Reports, 27*(1), 45–58. https://doi.org/10.1007/s11912-024-01622-6.

Gazzaniga, F. S., & Kasper, D. L. (2025). The gut microbiome and cancer response to immune checkpoint inhibitors. *Journal of Clinical Investigation, 135*(3). https://doi.org/10.1172/jci184321.

Griffin, M. E., & Hang, H. C. (2022). Microbial mechanisms to improve immune checkpoint blockade responsiveness. *Neoplasia, 31*, 100818. https://pmc.ncbi.nlm.nih.gov/articles/PMC9284443/.

Gunjur, A., Shao, Y., Rozday, T., Klein, O., Mu, A., Haak, B. W., Markman, B., Kee, D., Carlino, M. S., Underhill, C., Frentzas, S., Michael, M., Gao, B., Palmer, J., Cebon, J., Behren, A., Adams, D. J., & Lawley, T. D. (2024). A gut microbial signature for combination immune checkpoint blockade across cancer types. *Nature Medicine, 30*(3), 797–809. https://doi.org/10.1038/s41591-024-02823-z.

Gut bacteria affect immunotherapy response Cancer.gov. (2018). Retrieved from: https://www.cancer.gov/news-events/cancer-currents-blog/2018/gut-bacteria-checkpoint-inhibitors.(Accessed: 17 February 2026)

Gut microbiome may influence immunotherapy response | News releases American Association for Cancer Research (AACR). (2019) Retrieved from: https://www.aacr.org/about-the-aacr/newsroom/news-releases/dietary-factors-affecting-gut-microbiome-may-influence-response-to-immunotherapy-in-melanoma-patients/.

Hakozaki, T., Richard, C., Elkrief, A., Hosomi, Y., Benlaïfaoui, M., Mimpen, I., Terrisse, S., Derosa, L., Zitvogel, L., Routy, B., & Okuma, Y. (2020). The gut microbiome associates with immune checkpoint inhibition outcomes in patients with advanced non–small cell lung cancer. *Cancer Immunology Research, 8*(10), 1243–1250. https://doi.org/10.1158/2326-6066.cir-20-0196.

Hamze Sinno, S., Imperatore, J. A., Bai, S., Gomes-Jourdan, N., Mafarachisi, N., Coronnello, C., Zhang, L., Jašarević, E., Osmanbeyoglu, H. U., Buckanovich, R. J., & Cascio, S. (2024). Egfl6 promotes ovarian cancer progression by enhancing the immunosuppressive functions of tumor-associated myeloid cells. *Journal of Clinical Investigation, 134*(21). http://dx.doi.org/10.1172/JCI175147.

Hu, M., Lin, X., Sun, T., Shao, X., Huang, X., Du, W., Guo, M., Zhu, X., Zhou, Y., Tong, T., Guo, F., Han, T., Wu, X., Shi, Y., Xiao, X., Zhang, Y., Hong, J., & Chen, H. (2024). Gut microbiome for predicting immune checkpoint blockade-associated adverse events. *Genome Medicine, 16*(1). https://doi.org/10.1186/s13073-024-01285-9.

Humphries, A., & Daud, A. (2018). The gut microbiota and immune checkpoint inhibitors. *Human Vaccines & Immunotherapeutics, 14*(9), 2178–2182. https://doi.org/10.1080/21645515.2018.1442970.

Hwang, S. W., Kim, M. K., & Kweon, M. N. (2023). Gut microbiome on immune checkpoint inhibitor therapy and consequent immune-related colitis: A review. *Intestinal Research, 21*(4), 433–442. https://doi.org/10.5217/ir.2023.00019.

Jiang, H., & Zhang, Q. (2024). Gut microbiota influences the efficiency of immune checkpoint inhibitors by modulating the immune system (Review). *Oncology Letters, 27*(2). https://doi.org/10.3892/ol.2024.14221.

Kang, X., Lau, H. C. H., & Yu, J. (2024). Modulating gut microbiome in cancer immunotherapy: Harnessing microbes to enhance treatment efficacy. *Cell Reports Medicine, 5*(4), 101478. https://doi.org/10.1016/j.xcrm.2024.101478.

Lee, K. A., Thomas, A. M., Bolte, L. A., Björk, J. R., De Ruijter, L. K., Armanini, F., Asnicar, F., Blanco-Miguez, A., Board, R., Calbet-Llopart, N., Derosa, L., Dhomen, N., Brooks, K., Harland, M., Harries, M., Leeming, E. R.,

Lorigan, P., Manghi, P., Marais, R., … Segata, N. (2022). Cross-cohort gut microbiome associations with immune checkpoint inhibitor response in advanced melanoma. *Nature Medicine, 28*(3), 535–544. https://www.nature.com/articles/s41591-022-01695-5#citeas.

Li, P., Luo, H., Ji, B., & Nielsen, J. (2022a). Machine learning for data integration in human gut microbiome. *Microbial Cell Factories, 21*(1), 241. http://dx.doi.org/10.1186/s12934-022-01973-4.

Li, X., Zhang, S., Guo, G., Han, J., & Yu, J. (2022b). Gut microbiome in modulating immune checkpoint inhibitors. *EBioMedicine, 82*, 104163. https://doi.org/10.1016/j.ebiom.2022.104163.

Lin, Y., Xie, M., Lau, H. C. H., Zeng, R., Zhang, R., Wang, L., Li, Q., Wang, Y., Chen, D., Jiang, L., Damsky, W., & Yu, J. (2024). Effects of gut microbiota on immune checkpoint inhibitors in multi-cancer and as microbial biomarkers for predicting therapeutic response. *Cell Press, 6*(3). https://doi.org/10.1016/j.medj.2024.10.007.

Liu, H., Xiong, X., Zhu, W., Wang, S., Huang, W., Zhu, G., & Xu, H. (2025). Gut microbial metabolites in cancer immunomodulation. *Molecular cancer, 25*(1), 8. http://dx.doi.org/10.1186/s12943-025-02521-5.

Lynn, D. J., Benson, S. C., Lynn, M. A., & Pulendran, B. (2021). Modulation of immune responses to vaccination by the microbiota: Implications and potential mechanisms. *Nature Reviews Immunology, 22*(1), 33–46. https://www.nature.com/articles/s41577-021-00554-7#citeas.

Pesheva, B. E. (2024). To boost cancer immunotherapy's fighting power, look to the gut. *Harvard Medical School.* https://hms.harvard.edu/news/boost-cancer-immunotherapys-fighting-power-look-gut.

Raychaudhuri, B., Rayman, P., Huang, P., Grabowski, M., Hambardzumyan, D., Finke, J. H., & Vogelbaum, M. A. (2015). Myeloid derived suppressor cell infiltration of murine and human gliomas is associated with reduction of tumor infiltrating lymphocytes. *Journal of Neuro-Oncology [Internet], 122*(2), 293–301. http://dx.doi.org/10.1007/s11060-015-1720-6.

Roberts, A., Adler, B. A., Cress, B. F., Doudna, J. A., & Barrangou, R. (2025). Phage-based delivery of CRISPR-associated transposases for targeted bacterial editing. *Proceedings of the National Academy of Sciences USA., 122*(30), e2504853122. http://dx.doi.org/10.1073/pnas.2504853122.

Routy, B., Chatelier, E. L., Derosa, L., Duong, C. P. M., Alou, M. T., Daillère, R., Fluckiger, A., Messaoudene, M., Rauber, C., Roberti, M. P., Fidelle, M., Flament, C., Poirier-Colame, V., Opolon, P., Klein, C., Iribarren, K., Mondragón, L., Jacquelot, N., Qu, B., … Zitvogel, L. (2017). Gut microbiome influences efficacy of PD-1-based immunotherapy against epithelial tumors. *Science, 359*(6371), 91–97. https://doi.org/10.1126/science.aan3706.

Roviello, G., Iannone, L. F., Bersanelli, M., Mini, E., & Catalano, M. (2021). The gut microbiome and efficacy of cancer immunotherapy. *Pharmacology & Therapeutics, 231*, 107973. https://doi.org/10.1016/j.pharmthera.2021.107973.

Shi, Y., Zheng, W., Yang, K., Harris, K. G., Ni, K., Xue, L., Lin, W., Chang, E. B., Weichselbaum, R. R., & Fu, Y.-X. (2020). Intratumoral accumulation of gut microbiota facilitates CD47-based immunotherapy via STING signaling. *Journal of Experimental Medicine, 217*(5). http://dx.doi.org/10.1084/jem.20192282.

Siddiqui, S., & Glauben, R. (2022). Fatty acid metabolism in myeloid-derived suppressor cells and tumor-associated macrophages: Key factor in cancer immune evasion. *Cancers (Basel), 14*(1), 250. http://dx.doi.org/10.3390/cancers14010250.

Sitthideatphaiboon, P., Somlaw, N., Zungsontiporn, N., Ouwongprayoon, P., Sukswai, N., Korphaisarn, K., Poungvarin, N., Aporntewan, C., Hirankarn, N., Vinayanuwattikun, C., & Yu, J. (2024). Dietary pattern and the corresponding gut microbiome in response to immunotherapy in Thai patients with advanced non-small cell lung cancer (NSCLC). *Scientific Reports, 14*(1). https://www.nature.com/articles/s41598-024-79339-6#citeas.

The fundamentals of open access and open research Springer Nature (n.d.) Retrieved from: https://www.springernature.com/gp/open-research/about/the-fundamentals-of-open-access-and-open-research. (Accessed: 17 February 2026).

The microbiome in cancer Nature. 2024. Retrieved from: https://www.nature.com/collections/gahafacddj.

Verheijden, R. J., Van Eijs, M. J. M., Paganelli, F. L., Viveen, M. C., Rogers, M. R. C., Top, J., May, A. M., van de Wijgert, J. H. H. M., & Suijkerbuijk, K. P. M. (2025). Gut microbiome and immune checkpoint inhibitor toxicity. *European Journal of Cancer, 216*, 115221. https://doi.org/10.1016/j.ejca.2025.115221.

Wang, X., & Geng, S. (2023). Diet-gut microbial interactions influence cancer immunotherapy. *Frontiers in Oncology, 13*. https://doi.org/10.3389/fonc.2023.1138362.

Wu, J., Singleton, S. S., Bhuiyan, U., Krammer, L., & Mazumder, R. (2023). Multi-omics approaches to studying gastrointestinal microbiome in the context of precision medicine and machine learning. *Frontiers in Molecular Biosciences, 10*, 1337373. http://dx.doi.org/10.3389/fmolb.2023.1337373.

Yi, M., Yu, S., Qin, S., Liu, Q., Xu, H., Zhao, W., Chu, Q., & Wu, K. (2018). Gut microbiome modulates efficacy of immune checkpoint inhibitors. *Journal of Hematology & Oncology, 11*(1). https://doi.org/10.1186/s13045-018-0592-6.

Zhang, H., Hong, Y., Wu, T., Ben, E., Li, S., Hu, L., & Xie, T. (2024). Role of gut microbiota in regulating immune checkpoint inhibitor therapy for glioblastoma. *Frontiers in Immunology, 15*. https://doi.org/10.3389/fimmu.2024.1401967.

Zhang, M., Liu, J., & Xia, Q. (2023). Role of gut microbiome in cancer immunotherapy: From predictive biomarker to therapeutic target. *Experimental Hematology and Oncology, 12*(1). https://doi.org/10.1186/s40164-023-00442-x.

Zheng, D., Liwinski, T., & Elinav, E. (2020). Interaction between microbiota and immunity in health and disease. *Cell Research, 30*(6), 492–506. https://doi.org/10.1038/s41422-020-0332-7.

10

Microbiome-based diagnostics and biomarkers: The search for mechanistic connections

Neema Kumari[a], Shailaja Allani[b], Anna Knapinska[c] and Ajay Bommareddy[d]

[a]MALLA REDDY INSTITUTE OF MEDICAL SCIENCES, MALLA REDDY VISHWAVIDYAPEETH, HYDERABAD, TELANGANA, INDIA [b]CENTRE FOR MOLECULAR BIOLOGY AND BIOTECHNOLOGY, FLORIDA ATLANTIC UNIVERSITY, BOCA RATON, FL, UNITED STATES [c]DEPARTMENT OF CHEMISTRY & BIOCHEMISTRY, FLORIDA ATLANTIC UNIVERSITY, BOCA RATON, FL, UNITED STATES [d]DEPARTMENT OF BIOMEDICAL SCIENCE, CHARLES E SCHMIDT COLLEGE OF MEDICINE, FLORIDA ATLANTIC UNIVERSITY, BOCA RATON, FL, UNITED STATES

10.1 Introduction

Cancer is an uncontrolled proliferation of cells requiring space and excess nutrients in the human body and is the second most common cause of death worldwide (World Health Organization Cancer, 2025). It is a complex disease caused by several factors, such as calcium dysregulation (Bong & Monteith, 2018; Capiod et al., 2007; Kumari et al., 2024), chemoresistance (Kumari et al., 2021; Ramos et al., 2021; Zheng, 2017), tumor microenvironment (Anderson & Simon, 2020; Baghban et al., 2020; de Visser & Joyce, 2023), genetic and epigenetic alterations (Herceg & Hainaut, 2007; Takeshima & Ushijima, 2019; Teh & Fearon, 2019), weakened immunity (Finn, 2012; Lee et al., 2022), and environmental influences (Boffetta & Nyberg, 2003; Wilson et al. 2002). Apart from these factors, another major factor linked to cancer is microbiota dysregulation (Khan et al., 2022). The human microbiota is the community of microorganisms that live inside and outside the human body and includes numerous microbes, including bacteria, fungi, viruses, and protozoa (Xavier et al., 2020). These microbiota are found in almost every organ of the body, including the skin, nose, mouth, lungs, breast, gut, and urogenital tract (Ealla et al., 2024; Hou et al., 2022; Kandalai et al., 2023). Microbiota were linked to cancer in the 19th century by Rous (1911). Around 15%–20% of cancers are caused when the normal microbiota is disrupted, releasing toxins and carcinogenic metabolites and initiating chronic inflammatory

The Microbiome and Cancer Treatment: Overcoming Resistance and Enhancing Efficacy.
DOI: https://doi.org/10.1016/B978-0-443-33206-7.00004-2

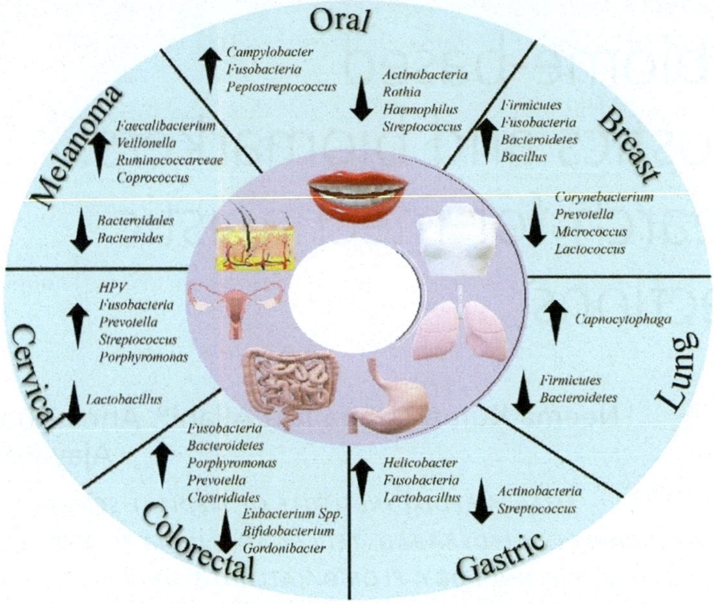

FIGURE 10.1 Overview of the microbes increased (↑) or decreased (↓) in different cancers. *Source: Adapted from Aitmanaitė, L., Širmonaitis, K., & Russo, G., (2023). Microbiomes, their function, and cancer: How metatranscriptomics can close the knowledge gap.* International Journal of Molecular Sciences, 24 *(18), 13786, https://doi.org/10.3390/ijms241813786. This article is an open-access article distributed under the terms and conditions of the Creative Commons Attribution (CC BY) license (https://creativecommons.org/licenses/by/4.0/).*

reactions (DiMaio et al., 2022; Khan et al., 2022; Verma, 2017; Xavier et al., 2020). They have been shown to affect cancer initiation, development, and response to therapies (Khan et al., 2022; Xavier et al., 2020). Microbes such as *Helicobacter pylori, Porphyromonas gingivalis, Chlamydia trachomatis, Mycobacterium tuberculosis, Escherichia coli,* and *Salmonella enterica* are linked to gastric, oral, cervical, lung, colorectal, and gallbladder cancer, respectively (Khan et al., 2022). Fig. 10.1 presents the list of microbes that increase or decrease in different cancers (Aitmanaitė et al., 2023).

The expression of specific parameters in the body is often explored to detect cancer and its abnormal presence. For example, biological molecules found in various body fluids, including urine, blood, and body tissues, are checked for their presence, absence, or abnormal expression. These biological molecules, also called biomarkers, have been used for cancer detection since the mid-20th century (Zhou et al., 2024). The genetic composition of microbiota has been investigated to serve as biomarkers and their interaction with the host. Therefore, microbiota, along with their collective genomes, are called microbiomes (Qasem & El-Sayed, 2025). The term "microbiome" is used hereafter in the chapter to maintain consistency.

Despite the available links of microbiome dysregulation to cancer, establishing a mechanistic connection is still challenging due to its complex and dynamic nature and its interactions with the host. Due to genetics, diet, lifestyle, and environment, the unique microbiome in each human makes it challenging to identify consistent microbial patterns associated with specific cancers. Moreover, the resilient nature of microbiomes complicates the identification of consistent biomarkers linked to cancer. Additionally, microbial dynamics and treatment interventions make it challenging to differentiate between cause and correlation, i.e., whether microbiome dysregulation is due to cancer or vice versa. Longitudinal studies can help determine whether microbial dysregulation causes cancer or vice versa. However, such studies require a significant amount of time and resources. Furthermore, the complex interplay between microbes and immune responses makes it challenging to understand the mechanistic links because of the modulation of immune responses by microbial metabolites (Verma, 2017).

Technical limitations also add to the challenges. To characterize the microbiome accurately, techniques such as metatranscriptomics, metaproteomics, metabotyping, and bioinformatics tools are required to handle vast and complex data sets efficiently. Sample collection also requires careful handling to avoid contamination, which can lead to misleading results. To identify a clear mechanistic connection, it is also necessary that all microbes be studied; however, most studies focus on bacteria (Verma, 2017).

10.2 Mechanistic link between microbiomes and cancer

Studies have shown that microbiomes influence cancer cells through metabolites, oxidative stress and inflammation, immune modulation, and pathway modulation (Qasem & El-Sayed, 2025). Understanding all these factors can help in understanding the various mechanisms by which microbiomes play a role in cancer. Additionally, it will also help determine the biomarkers that can serve in cancer diagnosis and treatment.

10.2.1 Metabolites

Metabolites are generated by bacteria from dietary sources or endogenous products such as bile acids and cholesterol. These metabolites could be end-products, intermediates, or derived from the conversion of the existing metabolites (Zhang et al., 2024). Additionally, these metabolites could be either carcinogenic or anticancer in nature.

Toxins that affect host DNA and chromosomes by inducing mutations in genes such as tumor suppressor genes or proto-oncogenes are known as genotoxins. This genetic damage can lead to cancer development (Qasem & El-Sayed, 2025; Zechner & Kienesberger, 2024). Metabolites can also have cytotoxic effects by damaging the cellular structure and function, causing cellular inflammation and stress, which, in the long term, leads to carcinogenesis. These metabolites are known as cytotoxins (Aktories & Barbieri, 2005). Pathways are crucial to regulate cellular activities systematically. Any dysregulation or deviation in the pathways can lead cells to proliferate uncontrollably, undergo apoptosis, or undergo abnormal growth. This can result in the development of cancer or other diseases. Microbiomes are known to target cellular pathways through their metabolites, which can result in cancer development. These metabolites can be detected in body samples such as serum, feces, and mucous. These samples are then analyzed using techniques such as gas chromatography, liquid chromatography, matrix-assisted laser desorption/ionization, capillary electrophoresis, and nuclear magnetic resonance (Liu et al., 2023). Below are some of the metabolites involved in carcinogenesis, briefly described:

Adenovirus-like protease regulator A (AvrA) is secreted by *Salmonella* spp. as a type 3 secretion system effector protein. AvrA causes colorectal cancer (CRC) by modulating ubiquitination and acetylation of target proteins, thereby modulating inflammation and proliferation (Lu et al., 2014,2016; Wibowo et al., 2023; Ye et al., 2007). AvrA inhibits ubiquitination and degradation of β-catenin. This leads to enhanced β-catenin signaling, inhibited apoptosis, and increased intestinal epithelial cell proliferation (Lu et al., 2014; Wibowo et al., 2023). β-catenin, being a negative regulator of nuclear factor kappa-light-chain-enhancer of activated B cells (NF-κB), inhibits it, thus suppressing proinflammatory responses. AvrA also inhibits NF-κB by inhibiting ubiquitination of inhibitor of NF-κB alpha (IκBα) (Ye et al., 2007). Additionally, AvrA activates the signal transducer and activator of transcription 3 (STAT3) pathway by upregulating interleukin-6 (IL-6). This, in turn, increases the levels of proliferating cell nuclear antigen, a marker of epithelial cell proliferation, thereby indicating the role of AvrA in inducing colonic inflammation and proliferation (Lu et al., 2016).

1. *Adenosine diphosphate (ADP)-heptose* is an intermediate generated during the heptose biosynthesis pathway. It serves as a pathogen-associated molecular pattern of Gram-negative bacteria (Duizer & de Zoete, 2023). ADP-heptose activates NF-κB signaling through the cytosolic alpha protein kinase one (ALPK1) receptor. Upon recognition of ADP-heptose, ALPK1 phosphorylates TIFA (tumor necrosis factor (TNF) receptor-associated factor (TRAF) interacting protein with forkhead associated domain) at threonine (position 9). This leads to the oligomerization of TIFA with adjacent TIFA through its forkhead-associated domain, thus forming TIFAsomes, large TIFA oligomers. These complexes then recruit TRAF6, which initiates downstream signaling cascades that lead to NF-κB activation (Duizer & de Zoete, 2023; García-Weber et al., 2023; Neuper et al., 2024). ADP-heptose also increases the release of inflammatory cytokines and chemokines such as IL-6, TNF, interferon-γ, etc., as shown in murine models (Zhou et al., 2018).
2. *Bacteroides fragilis toxin (BFT)* is a zinc-dependent metalloprotease toxin with a 20 kDa molecular weight. BFT activates STAT3, which helps in cell proliferation, inflammation, metastasis, and angiogenesis. BFT also alters signaling pathways and induces reactive oxygen species (ROS) production. ROS causes DNA damage and E-cadherin cleavage. E-cadherin is a tumor suppressor protein, and cleavage causes the accumulation of β-catenin in the cytoplasm, from where it is transported to the nucleus. In the nucleus, β-catenin binds to the transcription factor/lymphoid enhancer-binding factor. It also increases the transcription of the proto-oncogene coding for the cyclin D1 protein. Additionally, BFT causes tissue injury in the gut by damaging tight junctions and increasing permeability (Cheng et al., 2020a; Dadgar-Zankbar et al., 2023). BFT induces carcinogenesis by targeting cellular pathways and inducing mutations in the tumor suppressor protein p53. BFT also induces the expression of cyclooxygenase-2 (a prostaglandin-endoperoxide synthase 2) in epithelial cells during inflammation and thus serves as a biomarker for inflammation and colon cancer screening (Cheng et al., 2020a; Minghetti, 2004).

3. *Colibactin* is a peptide polyketide, a secondary metabolite released mainly by polyketide synthase-positive (pks$^+$) *E. coli* and other *Enterobacteriaceae* members. It contains two electrophilic cyclopropane warheads, which can bind to adenine and cause DNA crosslinking (Dougherty & Jobin, 2021; Dubinsky et al., 2020; Duizer & de Zoete, 2023). Adenine in DNA is alkylated by pks$^+$*E. coli*, leading to the formation of colibactin–DNA adducts, a covalent DNA modification (Duizer & de Zoete, 2023). Colibactin also alters Wnt proteins, protects β-catenin from degradation, induces the generation of ROS, and causes double-strand breaks in DNA by copper-mediated oxidative cleavage. DNA damage thus inhibits the cell cycle, resulting in cell death (Zhang & Sun, 2024). However, if the damage is not repaired and the cell does not undergo death, the mutations or alterations in DNA lead to cancer development. In a study on a colitis-susceptible IL10$^+$ mouse strain, the authors concluded that inflammation affects both the host and microbiota. Inflammation causes microbiota to adhere to the colonic mucosa by reducing the production of protective mucins and antimicrobial peptides. This adherence makes colibactin reach the epithelium of host cells and promote colon tumorigenesis (Arthur et al., 2012).
4. *Cytotoxin-associated gene A (CagA)* is an effector protein with a 125–145 kDa molecular weight. It is produced mainly by *H. pylori* (Ansari & Yamaoka, 2020), with 50%–70% of *H. pylori* strains having the gene for CagA (Zhong et al., 2021). CagA is transported inside the cells with the help of the bacterial type 4 secretory system and host phosphatidylserine. Once inside the cell, the EPIYA (glutamic acid–proline–isoleucine–tyrosine–alanine) motif at the C-terminal of CagA is phosphorylated and interacts with the Src homology 2 (SH2) domain of proteins such as pro-oncogene SH2 phosphatases, phosphoinositide 3-kinase (PI3K), CT10 regulator of kinase, and the adaptor protein "growth factor receptor-bound protein 2," and thereby dysregulates cell signaling pathways. Dysregulated cell signaling pathways disrupt cell adhesion, proliferation, elongation, and IL-8 expression (Ansari & Yamaoka, 2020; Lai et al., 2021; Sakatani et al., 2023). Additionally, in a study, CagA was shown to increase the expression of apoptosis-related protein (B-cell lymphoma 2: Bcl-2), proliferation-related protein (cyclin D1), invasion-related proteins (N-cadherin), and autophagy-related proteins (microtubule-associated protein 1 light chain 3 beta II/I (LC3B II/LC3B-I)) in colon cancer cells, thus supporting cancer growth (Zhong et al., 2021).
5. *Cytolethal distending toxin (CDT)* is the first well-characterized bacterial genotoxin and is produced by Gram-negative bacteria such as *Campylobacter jejuni, Salmonella spp., E. coli, H. hepaticus,* etc. (Akbar et al., 2022; Lai et al., 2021; Qasem & El-Sayed, 2025). CDT helps these bacteria in tissue colonization, where they target the host's immunity by arresting the cell cycle, thus causing epithelial cell death and altering macrophage functions due to the high sensitivity of lymphocytes to CDT cytotoxicity (Lai et al., 2021). CDT enters the cells with the action of its three subunits: CdtA, CdtB, and CdtC. The genes *cdtA, cdtB,* and *cdtC* coding these subunits are conserved within the same species but differ among species (Lai et al., 2021). CdtA and CdtC are binding subunits that interact with cell membrane lipid rafts and help CdtB enter the cell and reach the nucleus. CdtB is a catalytic subunit with deoxyribonuclease activity. CdtB induces double-strand breaks in DNA, thus initiating a DNA damage response through the ataxia-telangiectasia

mutated-dependent phosphorylation of the H2A histone family member X protein. The activated ataxia-telangiectasia mutated pathway leads to the inhibition of the cell cycle by targeting the G2/M transition and thus apoptosis (Bezine et al., 2016; Lai et al., 2021; Lin et al., 2017). When DNA damage is not repaired correctly, the risk of cancer increases. However, in a study, CDT is also shown to induce radiosensitivity in pancreatic cancer cells by inducing double-stranded DNA breaks and inhibiting autophagy (Lin et al., 2017).

6. *Indole metabolites* are generated by the gut microbiome by metabolizing tryptophan via the indole pathway. Generally, tryptophan is metabolized by two major pathways, the kynurenine and serotonin pathways. While the kynurenine pathway accounts for ~90%–95% of tryptophan metabolism, the serotonin pathway accounts for 1%–2% of tryptophan metabolism. Both these pathways generate products distinct from indole and its derivatives, which are primarily generated through microbial metabolism (Badawy, 2017; Tsuji et al., 2023). Microbiomes involved in this metabolism are *Bacteroides, Bifidobacterium, Clostridium, E. coli, Lactobacillus, Parabacteroides, Peptostreptococcus,* and *Proteus vulgaris* (Jia et al., 2024; Tennoune et al., 2022). The metabolism generates Indole-3-pyruvate, Indole-3-lactic acid (ILA), Indole acrylic acid (IA), Indole-3-propionic acid, Indole-3-acetaldehyde (IAAld), Indole acetic acid (IAA), Indole-3-aldehyde (IAld), Indole-3-carboxylic acid (ICA), Indole-3-acetamide (IAM), and indolimine either directly or by conversion of one metabolite to another (Jia et al., 2024). ILA, produced by *Lactobacillus gallinarum (L. gallinarum),* possesses anticancer activity in CRC by inhibiting cell proliferation and prompting apoptosis by binding to tumor cells' aryl hydrocarbon receptor (AHR) (Jia et al., 2024; Kandalai et al., 2023; Zhang et al., 2023). The ILA from *L. plantarum* L168 activates $CD8^+$ T cells and reduces the expression of the serum amyloid A3 (Saa3) gene (Jia et al., 2024; Zhang et al., 2023). The Saa3 gene encodes a high-density lipoprotein-associated acute-phase protein that plays a role in inflammatory reactions (Tannock et al., 2018). ILA by *L. reuteri* reduces T helper cells (Jia et al., 2024). Indolimine is produced through the condensation of IAld with a primary amine during tryptophan metabolism. Indolimine activates the AHR, leading to the upregulation of the *Cyp1a1* gene (Duizer & de Zoete, 2023; Patel et al., 2023). Cytochrome P450, family 1, subfamily A, member 1 (CYP1A1) metabolizes carcinogens like benzo(a)pyrene and generates reactive benzo[a]pyrene-7,8-dihydrodiol-9,10-epoxide, which is an endocrine disruptor and forms a DNA adduct, thus inducing carcinogenesis. Additionally, CYP1A1 increases the expression of IL-6, a proinflammatory cytokine (Ling et al., 2004; Patel et al., 2023).

7. *Polyamines,* released by both host cells and gut bacteria such as *Bacteroides spp.* and *Fusobacterium* spp., are small polycationic alkylamines in cells at tightly regulated intracellular levels. They include putrescine, cadaverine, spermidine, and spermine. In healthy cells, they are required for cellular activities such as gene regulation, protein synthesis, ion channel regulation, cell division, and differentiation. However, dysregulation in the metabolism of polyamines is often seen in cancers, leading to elevated intracellular levels of polyamines. This increased level of polyamines is maintained by enzymes for polyamine synthesis and oncogenes such as MYC, JUN, FOS, KRAS, and BRAF (Hanus et al., 2021; Holbert et al., 2022; Soda, 2011; Tofalo et al., 2019). Generally, ornithine decarboxylase

converts ornithine into putrescine. But oncogenes such as MYC regulate the enzyme to increase its activity in cancer to generate more polyamines (Hanus et al., 2021). Elevated levels of polyamines help cancer cells in metastasis, angiogenesis, colonizing secondary tumor sites, and escaping detection by the immune system (Soda, 2011). In CRC, biofilm formation has been associated with altered and increased polyamine metabolites, thus suggesting that the polyamines can increase tumor development (Hanus et al., 2021).

8. *Short-chain fatty acids (SCFAs)* are produced by microbes by fermenting carbohydrates in the stomach and small intestine. SCFA synthesis increases with certain food items such as sourdough bread, dairy products, and vinegar. Furthermore, a metagenomic study has identified multiple bacterial enzymes and genes that are involved in SCFA synthesis. The enzymes involved are propionyl-CoA transferase, CO dehydrogenase/acetyl-CoA synthase complex, and butyrate acetoacetate CoA transferase. The genes include *yciA, tesA, tesB*, and *menI* (Gou et al., 2024; Mirzaei et al., 2021; Zhang et al., 2021a, 2024). These SCFAs possess both procancer and anticancer effects (Mirzaei et al., 2021; Zhang et al., 2024). SCFAs demonstrate anticancer effects by targeting $CD8^{+}$T cell responses and improving adaptive immunity (Zhang et al., 2023). Acetate, butyrate, and propionate are the most common SCFAs, with a molar ratio of 60:20:20 (Gou et al., 2024; Hanus et al., 2021; Zhang et al., 2024). While acetate and propionate are produced by *Bacteroidetes*, butyrate is produced by *Firmicutes* (den Besten et al., 2013). Of these, butyrate remains primarily in the colon, and acetate and propionate are absorbed into the circulation. Host cell receptors such as GPR41/FFAR3, GPR43/FFAR2, and GPR109A/HCAR2 or transporters such as MCT1/SLC16A1 and SMCT1/SLC548 interact with these SCFAs (Hanus et al., 2021). Butyrate serves as an essential energy source for colonic epithelial cells and exhibits antitumor activity due to its histone deacetylase activity. However, butyrate can promote or inhibit colonocyte development depending on physiological conditions. Similarly, acetate and propionate can promote or inhibit tumors, but their activity is less evident than that of butyrate (Zhang et al., 2024).

9. *Secondary bile acids (SBA)* are the bile acids produced by bacteria in the intestine by the dehydroxylation of the primary bile acids, i.e., the bile acids produced by the liver. SBAs include deoxycholic acid and lithocholic acid, derived from primary bile acids such as cholic and chenodeoxycholic acids (Ajouz et al., 2014; Lenci et al., 2023; Liu et al., 2022; Wahlström et al., 2016). In a two-step manner, cholic acid and chenodeoxycholic acid are converted to deoxycholic acid and lithocholic acid, respectively, with the help of microbiome bile salt hydrolase and 7α-hydroxysteroid dehydrogenase (Yang & Qian, 2022). First, cholesterol is oxidized with the help of cytochromes P450 to form cholic and chenodeoxycholic acids, which are then conjugated to glycine. Once these acids are translocated into the small intestine, taurine is removed (deconjugated) by bacterial bile salt hydrolases, producing SBAs. Released taurine is then used by gut microbiota as a nutrient, thus potentially developing bile resistance and colonization in the gastrointestinal tract (Gou et al., 2024). Bacteria with bile salt hydrolase activity include *Firmicutes, Clostridium, Bacteroidetes, Lactobacillus, Methanobrevibacter smithii, Actinobacteria, Proteobacteria,* and others. Bacteria with 7α-hydroxysteroid dehydrogenase include

Clostridium, Eubacterium, Ruminococcus, Trichospiraceae, and *Desulfovibrionales* (Yang & Qian, 2022). SBAs induce CRC cell proliferation by the activation of epidermal growth factor receptors (EGFR), mitogen-activated protein kinase (MAPK), Wnt/β-catenin, and PI3K/Akt/IκB/NF-κB pathways, increased ROS and reactive nitrogen species, mutagenesis, and oxidative DNA damage (Ajouz et al., 2014; Liu et al., 2022).

10. *Tilimycin* is a tricyclic pyrrolobenzodiazepine synthesized in a nonribosomal peptide synthetase pathway. Tilimycin is generated by *til*-gene-carrying *Klebsiella spp.,* specifically *Klebsiella oxytoca,* which is usually present in 2%–9% of healthy humans. The normal presence of *K. oxytoca* exposes humans to low doses of tilimycin throughout their lives. Tilimycin forms a DNA adduct and induces single-strand and double-strand breaks in DNA, thus causing chromosomal instability and cell cycle arrest at the G1 or S phase (Alexander et al., 2020; Pöltl et al., 2023; Unterhauser et al., 2019). In a study on colonic stem cells, the authors indicated that tilimycin induces mutation in murine colorectal epithelial stem cells, resulting in stabilized monoclonal mutant crypts. Thus, exposure to tilimycin can cause somatic mutations in the colon and increase the risk of CRC in humans having the *til-* gene-carrying *Klebsiella* spp. (Pöltl et al., 2023).
11. *Vacuolating cytotoxin A (VacA)* is a multifunctional protein toxin secreted by *H. pylori.* It induces vacuolation, depolarization of membrane potential, disruption of mitochondrial functions, autophagy, inhibition of T-cell proliferation, and apoptosis (Palframan et al., 2012; Yuan et al., 2021). VacA creates anion-selective channels on the host cell membrane through which chloride ions enter the cell and cause osmotic swelling and vacuolation. Apoptosis is caused by the release of cytochrome c from mitochondria. It is worth noting that VacA counteracts the effects of CagA, another metabolite secreted by *H. pylori,* by interfering with EGFR and Erk1/2 pathways. In contrast, CagA inhibits apoptosis and vacuolation induced by VacA by inhibiting the activity of the Src kinase family. Additionally, CagA inhibits the transport of VacA to late endosomes by blocking its colocalization with lysosome-associated membrane protein 1, a glycoprotein found on the membranes of lysosomes and endosomes (Palframan et al., 2012).

Table 10.1 summarizes the list of cancer-inducing metabolites, the microbiomes producing them, the mechanism, and the associated cancer (s).

10.2.2 Oxidative stress, inflammation, and immune modulation

The microbiome influences ROS levels, promoting cell proliferation. An imbalance in ROS increases oxidative stress, thereby damaging critical biomolecules and cells (Qasem & El-Sayed, 2025; Reuter et al., 2010). The microbes involved in ROS regulation belong to four primary phyla: *Actinobacteria, Bacteroidetes, Firmicutes,* and *Proteobacteria. Bacteroidetes* and *Firmicutes* comprise 90% of the total gut bacteria (Qasem & El-Sayed, 2025). The microbes initiate an inflammatory response by generating formylated peptides, which bind to G-protein-coupled receptors of macrophages and neutrophils. The initiated inflammatory response then leads to the generation of superoxide radicals by nicotinamide adenine dinucleotide phosphate oxidase 1,

Table 10.1 Microbiota metabolites, mechanisms, and cancer associated with them.

Metabolite	Microbiome	Mechanism	Cancer	References
AvrA	*Salmonella spp.*	Inhibits NF-κB and activates β-catenin	Colorectal	Ye et al. (2007), Lu et al. (2014)
ADP-heptose	*Streptomyces fimbriatus, S. hygroscopicus, Escherichia coli, Helicobacter pylori*	Binds to alpha kinase 1 and activates NF-κB via Tumor Necrosis Factor Receptor-Associated Factor (TRAF) 2/6, TIFA. Also increases inflammatory cytokines and chemokines	Gastric	Duizer and de Zoete (2023), Neuper et al. (2024), Zhou et al. (2018)
BFT	Enterotoxigenic *Bacteroides fragilis*	Activates STAT3, induces ROS, cleaves E-cadherin, activates β-catenin, damages the tight junctions, mutates tumor protein p53, and induces cyclooxygenase-3 expression	Colorectal	Cheng et al. (2020a), Qasem and El-Sayed (2025), Dadgar-Zankbar et al. (2023), Minghetti (2004)
Colibactin	Polyketide synthase *(pks)*$^{+}$ *E. coli, Klebsiella pneumoniae, K. aerogenes, Citrobacter koseri*	Crosslinks DNA, alters Wnt proteins, protects β-catenin, and induces ROS	Colorectal	Kandalai et al. (2023), Qasem and El-Sayed (2025), Zechner and Kienesberger (2024), Dougherty and Jobin (2021), Zhang and Sun (2024)
CagA	*H. pylori*	Dysregulates cell signaling pathways such as NF-κB, PI3K/Akt, MAPK, Rat sarcoma- Extracellular signal-regulated kinase (RAS-ERK), Wnt/β-catenin	Gastric, intestinal, MALT lymphoma	Ansari and Yamaoka (2020), Lai et al. (2021), Sakatani et al. (2023), Ding et al. (2010), Neal et al. (2013), Song et al. (2015); Duan et al. (2025)

(continued on next page)

Table 10.1 Microbiota metabolites, mechanisms, and cancer associated with them—cont'd

Metabolite	Microbiome	Mechanism	Cancer	References
CDT	*S. enterica, Escherichia, Campylobacter spp., H. hepaticus, H. ducreyi, Aggregatibacter actinomycetemcomitans*	Induces double-strand breaks in DNA and activates ataxia-telangiectasia mutated pathways	Colorectal, Hepatocellular, Intestinal	Qasem and El-Sayed (2025), Lai et al. (2021), Akbar et al. (2022), Bezine et al. (2016), Ge et al. (2007), He et al. (2019)
Indole metabolites (e.g., ILA and indolimine)	*Bacteroides, Bifidobacterium, Clostridium, E. coli, Lactobacillus, Parabacteroides, Peptostreptococcus, P. vulgaris, Morganella morganii*	ILA: inhibits cell proliferation, induces apoptosis, reduces Saa3 expression, and reduces T helper cells Indolimine: activates AHR→ upregulates Cypla1 gene	Colorectal	Zechner and Kienesberger (2024), Duizer and de Zoete (2023), Tennoune et al. (2022), Patel et al. (2023), Ling et al. (2004)
Polyamines	*Bacteroides spp., Fusobacterium spp., E. coli, Enterococcus faecalis, Bifidobacterium spp.,*	Modulate DNA-protein and protein–protein interactions	Gastric, breast, prostate, colon, lung, skin	Tofalo et al. (2019), Thomas* and Thomas (2001), Nowotarski et al. (2013)
Short-chain fatty acids	*Bacteroidetes, Firmicutes*	$CD8^+$T cell response modulation, histone deacetylase activity	Colorectal, bladder, breast, gastric, liver, lung, pancreatic, prostate	Zhang et al. (2023, 2024), Mirzaei et al. (2021)
Secondary bile acids	*Clostridium, Firmicutes, Bacteriodetes, Lactobacillus, Methanobrevibacter, Actinobacter, Proteobacteria, Eubacterium, Ruminococcus, Trichospiraceae, Desulfovibrionales*	Activation of EGFR, MAPK, Wnt/β-catenin, and PI3K/Akt/i-b/NF-κB pathways induces ROS and reactive nitrogen species, mutagenesis, and oxidative DNA damage	Liver, colorectal	Ajouz et al. (2014), Liu et al. (2022), Yang and Qian (2022), Ridlon et al. (2014)

(continued on next page)

Tilimycin	*Klebsiella spp.*	Induces single-strand and double-strand DNA breaks	Colorectal	Zechner and Kienesberger (2024), Unterhauser et al. (2019), Alexander et al. (2020), Pöltl et al. (2023)
Vacuolating cytotoxin A	*H. pylori*	Vacuolation, depolarization of membrane potential, disruption of mitochondrial functions, autophagy, inhibition of T-cell proliferation, and apoptosis	Gastric	Palframan et al. (2012), Yuan et al. (2021), Duan et al. (2025)

ADP-heptose, adenosine diphosphate; *AHR*, aryl hydrocarbon receptor; *AvrA*, adenovirus-like protease regulator A; *BFT, Bacteroides fragilis toxin; CDT*, cytolethal distending toxin; *EGFR*, epidermal growth factor receptors; *ILA*, indole-3-lactic acid; *MAPK*, mitogen-activated protein kinase; NF-κB, nuclear factor kappa B; *PI3K*, phosphoinositide 3-kinase; *ROS*, reactive oxygen species; *STAT3*, signal transducer and activator of transcription 3.

thus forming ROS such as nitric oxide (NO). NO is formed by *Lactobacilli* and *Bifidobacteria* converting nitrate and nitrites into NO. Another pathway of NO formation is converting L-arginine to NO with the help of NO synthase by *Streptococcus* and *Bacilli* (Qasem & El-Sayed, 2025).

The persistent inflammatory reaction and oxidative stress over a prolonged period could damage healthy epithelial and stromal cells, leading to cancer formation at the site. ROS mediate cancer formation either directly or through the signaling pathways. The direct mode includes oxidation, nitration, and halogenation of nuclear DNA, RNA, and lipids. ROS induces breaks, point mutations, and aberrant cross-linking in DNA and mutations in tumor suppressor genes and proto-oncogenes at high concentrations. Low ROS levels can promote cellular proliferation and activate cell survival signaling pathways (Reuter et al., 2010).

The stress induced by oxidants is countered by the endogenous protective systems in the body, such as superoxide dismutase, glutathione peroxidase, catalase, peroxiredoxins, vitamins A, C, and E (Azzimonti et al., 2023). The microbiome influences the transcription factor nuclear factor erythroid 2–related factor 2 (Nrf2), which regulates the responses of antioxidant enzymes, including glutathione-S-transferase, nicotinamide adenine dinucleotide phosphate quinone reductase 1, and glutamate cysteine ligase (de la Vega et al., 2018). Redox homeostasis, the balance between pro-oxidants and antioxidants, can interfere with every step, from tumor progression to drug resistance (Xing et al., 2022). It was shown that the Nrf2 pathway functions as a protective pathway in the early stages of cancer by rescuing from ROS-induced damage. Still, in many cancers at later stages (Azzimonti et al., 2023), there was an upregulation of Nrf2 and superoxide dismutase, leading to metastasis and resistance to chemotherapeutic drugs (Chaisiriwong et al., 2016; Khamari et al., 2018; Kim et al., 2010; Matsuoka et al., 2022). Dysbiosis of the microbiome can create an environment conducive to pathogenic bacteria that can promote tumor development in the gut, liver, skin, lung, prostate, breast, and other organs (Azzimonti et al., 2023).

CRC, oxidative stress, and the microbiome: CRC is the second most diagnosed cancer in males and third in females, and several studies have demonstrated that intestinal dysbiosis strongly correlates with various stages of CRC (Cheng et al., 2020b). The alpha bug hypothesis has supported the manifestation of CRC (Sears & Pardoll, 2011), where bacterial species, including enterogenic *Bifidobacterium fragilis* producing the *B. fragilis* toxin, *Fusobacterium nucleatum*, and *Enterococcus faecalis,* outnumber the protective gut bacteria; and the driver–passenger model, where intestinal bacteria produce toxins that provide flora for opportunistic bacteria such as *Fusobacterium* spp. that induce carcinogenicity (Cheng et al., 2020b; Tjalsma et al., 2012). Studies in animal and cell culture models have demonstrated that *E. faecalis* induces superoxide and hydroxyl radical production, resulting in DNA strand breaks and point mutations (Wang & Huycke, 2007). This could create a mutagenic environment by accumulating stepwise mutations, elevating the risk for CRC. Patients with chronic inflammatory diseases such as inflammatory bowel disease, ulcerative colitis, and Crohn's disease are at a serious risk of CRC (Beaugerie & Itzkowitz, 2015). The intestinal microbiome creates a tumorigenic environment, promoting chronic inflammation that results in tumor initiation and progression (Cheng et al., 2020b). *Streptococcus bovis*, a pathogenic bacterium, is found at increased levels in CRC patients and drives tumor progression through inflammation (Gupta et al., 2010).

A recent pilot study on metatranscriptome analysis of 10 CRC and non-CRC fecal samples has revealed a dominant and complex role of oxidative stress genes, suggesting an altered microbial ROS/reactive nitrogen species scavenging environment and directly indicating that ROS are a primary reason for the accumulation of stepwise mutations in CRC development. The study identified a differential pattern of oxidative stress pathways encompassing a reduced expression of protective hydrogen peroxide-scavenging genes but upregulated NO-scavenging genes (Lamaudière et al., 2023).

Skin and other cancers, oxidative stress, and microbiome: Exposure to UV radiation or particulate aromatic hydrocarbons, inducing inflammation, ROS production, DNA damage, and mutations progressing into skin cancer, is a typical example of inflammation and oxidative damage leading to cancer (Azzimonti et al., 2023). Despite the lack of precise understanding of whether oxidative stress is a cause or effect of skin cancer or dysbiosis, the microbiome plays a significant role in modulating the cancer environment. The administration of certain probiotic bacteria, such as *L. casei* and *L. reuteri*, with their antioxidant properties, increased overall survival by reducing metastasis in melanoma mouse models (Luo et al., 2020; Matsuzaki et al., 1987); lower amounts of RoxP, an antioxidant secreted by *Cutibacterium acnes*, were evident in basal cell carcinoma tissues (Andersson et al., 2019). In contrast, microbial species such as *Malassezia furfur* yeast and *Staphylococcus aureus* have been implicated in the elevation of pro-oxidant species that secrete increased levels of toxins, upregulating the AHR pathways, leading to further progression of cancer (Magiatis et al., 2013; Voigt et al., 2022). Chronic inflammation triggered by the virulent factor peptide modulin phenol soluble-alpha of *S. aureus* was identified to be involved in different stages of squamous cell carcinoma. Altered production of lithocholic acid, a metabolite that regulates oxidative stress pathways and halts the proliferation of tumor cells, correlates with a poor prognosis of breast cancer (Kovács et al., 2019). Bile acids, bioactive gut metabolites, have been shown to induce apoptosis in prostate cancer development by disrupting mitochondrial membrane potential (Goldberg et al., 2013). Conversely, at higher concentrations, bile acids initiated the promotion of CRC (Ou et al., 2013).

Inflammation and the immune system: Cross-talk exists between oxidative stress and chronic inflammation; the host's immune system and the microbiome modulate tumorigenic processes. Inflammatory cells produce ROS, and ROS further exacerbates inflammatory pathways such as the nuclear factor kappa B (NF-κB) transcription factor that can activate more than 150 genes involving the release of inflammatory cytokines and thereby connecting the immune system (Jabłońska-Trypuć, 2023).

A dysregulated immune system contributes to cancer development by initiating inflammatory reactions (Gonzalez et al., 2018). The microbiome plays a critical role in modulating the inflammatory response of the tumor microenvironment. Inflammasomes, consisting of nucleotide-binding oligomerization domain-like receptors, detect signals that the host and the microbiota release, producing cytokines such as IL-18 (Elinav et al., 2011). The release of protective cytokines such as IL-18 maintains the integrity of the intestinal epithelial membrane, and animal models with a deficiency in IL-18 are sensitized to chemical-induced CRCs (Zaki et al., 2010). IL-18 protects the intestinal mucosa by activating the STAT3 pathway and stimulating the production of IL-22, which can modulate tissue repair (Jabłońska-Trypuć, 2023).

In contrast, in the classic example of bacteria-induced carcinogenesis, continued exposure to the pathogenic *H. pylori* releases toxic factors that regulate the NF-κB pathway and mitogen-activated pathways and lead to elevated levels of proinflammatory cytokines, including IL-1, IL-6, IL-8, and TNF-α (Sun et al., 2023). These proinflammatory cytokines alter the tumor microenvironment and promote an aggressive cancer phenotype, enabled by angiogenesis and metastasis (Jabłońska-Trypuć, 2023). Studies in CRC have suggested the creation of a proinflammatory environment by *F. nucleatum* through activating the NF-κB pathway and increased levels of IL-17 that further activate the STAT3 pathway and cell proliferation (Cheng et al., 2020b). Furthermore, *F. nucleatum* activates toll-like receptor 4 (TLR4) and produces 12,13-EpOME conducive to epithelial–mesenchymal transformation, advancing CRC metastasis (Kong et al., 2021).

Gut microbiome and brain tumor pathology: The bidirectional communication between the brain and gut microbiome is a biological process conveyed through various pathways and is identified as the gut-brain axis. Dysbiosis of gut microbiota and subsequent alterations in the gut-brain axis throughout life have been associated with various brain disorders and diseases (Ratsika et al., 2023). Recent studies have suggested the role of gut microbiota and its dysbiosis in influencing the development of glioblastoma through various processes, including therapeutic resistance, pathogenesis, immune modulation, and changes in metabolism (Hanif et al., 2017). Glioblastoma, an aggressive brain tumor of glial origin, is one of the deadliest tumors and is characterized by poor prognosis (Glioblastoma Multiforme, 2024). Exposure to high doses of ionizing radiation has been identified as a causative factor for glioblastoma occurrence and is primarily diagnosed in adults with a median age of 64 years (Mohamed et al., 2025). In addition to glioblastoma being a cold tumor evading immune responses, standard approaches of surgical resection, radiotherapy (RT), and chemotherapy with temozolomide pose a challenging situation for its treatment. For example, Fan et al. showed that the development of glioma in mice contributed to a decrease in the abundance of *Bacteroidetes* and an increase in the abundance of *Firmicutes*, including *Clostridia* species (Fan et al., 2022). After fecal microbiota transplantation, the abundance of *Bacteroidia* was supplemented in the microbiota of the mice, which slowed down glioma, suggesting that decreased abundance of *Bacteroidia* could be one of the reasons for the progressive growth of glioma (Fan et al., 2022). The authors also demonstrated that antibiotic treatment contributed to gut microbiome dysbiosis, downregulated the expression of FoxP3 in the mouse brain, and played a role in the development of glioma in mice. It was concluded that maintaining the balance of the gut microbiome in mice could upregulate FoxP3 expression in the brain and slow down the growth of glioma (Fan et al., 2022). In a different study, Rosito et al. also demonstrated that antibiotic-induced gut dysbiosis affects the glioma tumor microenvironment. The authors concluded that increased levels of glycine, which resulted in part due to antibiotic-induced dysbiosis and its effects on microglia, glioma, and endothelial cells, established a proangiogenic environment in the brain tumor area and led to tumor progression (Rosito et al., 2024). Emerging studies corroborate the direct effects of chemotherapeutic agents on microbiome composition and subsequent outcomes associated with their efficacy and toxicity (Keane et al., 2025). For example, temozolomide, a second-generation alkylating agent used in the treatment of glioblastoma, is shown to have attenuated efficacy contributed by the antibiotic-mediated depletion of microbiota. Furthermore, recruitment of immune cells was also altered by deletion of microbiota, and antibiotic treatment accelerated glioma development, reversed the antitumor effect of temozolomide, and aggravated immunosuppression (Hou et al., 2023). The authors concluded that gut bacteria could serve as a predictive biomarker and a therapeutic target for the clinical utility of temozolomide.

The gut microbiome and liver cancer: Hepatocellular carcinoma (HCC) is one of the most commonly diagnosed cancers that develops exclusively in patients with chronic liver disease, driven by multiple factors over several years. Studies have provided evidence toward the role of gut microbiome in promoting the development of liver diseases and HCC (Yu & Schwabe, 2017). Multiple mechanisms, including increased hepatic exposure to gut-derived microbiota-associated molecular patterns such as lipopolysaccharide (LPS) that promote hepatic inflammation, fibrosis, proliferation, and upregulation of antiapoptotic signals, along with the release of cancer-promoting and senescence-promoting metabolites such as deoxycholic acid from dysbiotic bacteria, have been known to promote liver diseases and HCC (Yu & Schwabe, 2017). A study conducted by Zhang et al. (2021b) showed that prolonged high dietary cholesterol intake induced spontaneous and progressive development of nonalcoholic fatty liver disease-associated liver cancer (NAFLD-HCC) in male mice by modulating the gut microbiota. The authors concluded that cholesterol-induced increase in taurocholic acid and decrease in 3-indole propionic acid through microbiota alterations contributed to lipid accumulation and cell proliferation in the liver, leading to NAFLD-HCC development. Furthermore, it was shown that anticholesterol inhibition completely abrogated dietary cholesterol-induced NAFLD-HCC development (Zhang et al., 2021b). In a different study, Wang et al. (2025) showed that HCC-associated gut dysbiosis mediated by *K. pneumoniae* through gut barrier dysfunction and translocation to the liver exacerbated HCC development through the penicillin-binding protein 1B–TLR4 axis in the HCC mouse model. The authors concluded that targeting *K. pneumoniae* could help in the prevention and treatment of HCC (Wang et al., 2025). Another recent study that constructed a human flora-associated intrahepatic metastatic HCC mouse model confirmed dysbiosis of microbiota as an important contributor to the development of intrahepatic metastasis of HCC. It was shown that the abundance of beneficial bacterial strains, including *Anaerotruncus colihominis* and *Dysosmobacter welbionis*, was significantly reduced, resulting in dysbiosis that eventually contributed to HCC intrahepatic metastasis by promoting neutrophil inflammatory activation, excessive neutrophil extracellular trap formation, and facilitation of tissue necrosis and tumor vascular growth. The authors also identified that healthy fecal microbiota transfer suppressed dysbiosis and the processes involved in intrahepatic metastasis of HCC (Deng et al., 2025). A study that investigated the role of probiotics in the prevention and treatment of HCC established that daily supplementation with *Akkermansia muciniphila* ameliorates liver steatosis and effectively attenuates tumor growth in an orthotopic metabolic dysfunction-associated fatty liver disease (MAFLD)–HCC mouse model. The authors showed that *A. muciniphila* repairs the intestinal lining, with a decrease in LPS and bile acid metabolites, and, in combination with programmed cell death protein 1 (PD-1) treatment, exerts a maximal growth-suppressive effect with increased infiltration and activation of T cells (Wu et al., 2025). It was concluded that *A. muciniphila* could serve as a noninvasive predictive biomarker of the PD-1 response in patients with HCC.

10.3 Microbiome biomarkers in cancer

Biomarkers are biological molecules that indicate normal and abnormal processes occurring in the body. Microbiomes and their metabolites can both serve as biomarkers in disease detection. Abnormal conditions in the body, i.e., diseases, often cause these biomarkers to be overexpressed or underexpressed in diseased tissues compared to normal tissues. Hence, they can be used for early cancer detection and for designing drugs and medical devices (Califf, 2018; Zwezerijnen-Jiwa et al., 2023).

Based on their applications, these biomarkers are categorized into diagnostic, monitoring, pharmacodynamic/response, predictive, and prognostic (Califf, 2018). These biomarkers can be obtained from body fluids and waste, including oral mucosa, blood, urine, and feces (Zwezerijnen-Jiwa et al., 2023).

10.3.1 Role of microbiome as diagnostic biomarker

Diagnostic biomarkers are used to detect cancer at an early stage. These biomarkers help in noninvasive cancer diagnosis even before the onset of symptoms. Microbiomes or metabolites, such as SCFAs or polyamines, of specific gut microbiomes, such as *F. nucleatum, E. coli,* and *B. fragilis,* can be detected in fecal samples. Additionally, several products of bacterial metabolism, such as SBAs, have been implicated in cancers such as CRC. Currently, the diagnosis of CRC is based on invasive colonoscopy or sigmoidoscopy for biopsy of suspicious lesions. Noninvasive diagnostic screening stool tests, including guaiac-based fecal occult blood test, fecal immunochemical test, and multitargeted stool DNA test (Cologuard), are utilized frequently for early diagnosis. Despite the beneficial utility of these available diagnostic tests, certain limitations associated with these approaches warrant the development of other noninvasive approaches with high specificity and selectivity that help with early diagnosis, prognosis, and treatment outcomes. The diversity of fecal microbiomes in different stages of CRC lends itself as a basis for exploring biomarkers that could provide valuable information for the early detection of CRC.

Detection of metabolites has been reported in the body fluids as a noninvasive and cost-effective approach for early diagnosis and prognosis of CRC. A comprehensive review by Raza et al. (2022) summarizes information on liquid biopsy markers, including oral microbiota-related bacterial networks, gut-microbiome-associated serum metabolites, along with circulating tumor DNAs, microRNAs, and long noncoding RNAs, and their role in CRC diagnosis, prognosis, and treatment outcome. For example, analysis of matched saliva and stool samples from CRC patients and healthy individuals showed that four bacterial strains, *S. koreensis, S. anginosis, Solobacterium moorei,* and *Peptostreptococcus stomatis,* were detected at high levels in the oral cavity of CRC patients (Uchino et al., 2021).

A recent study reported a novel integrated model based on changes in gut microbiome-associated serum metabolites that can distinguish patients with CRC and adenoma from healthy subjects more efficiently than the clinical marker carcinoembryonic antigen (CEA) (Chen et al., 2022). In the study, the authors performed an integrated analysis of serum metabolomics and metagenome sequencing of paired fecal samples. They identified a set of serum metabolites in patients with CRC and adenoma that exhibited a close association with the gut microbiome. The authors concluded that by focusing on gut microbiome-associated serum metabolites, their model could acquire a tumor detection panel more specific to colon cancer and achieve a sensitivity of 83.5% and specificity of 84.9% in the independent validation cohort, which is higher than other serum panels.

In a retrospective analysis of patients hospitalized for bacteremia, it was reported that patients who developed bacteremia from *B. fragilis, S. gallolyticus, and F. nucleatum* were diagnosed more frequently with CRC than uninfected individuals. The authors also identified new species, including *Clostridium perfringens* and *Gemella morbillorum,* that were enriched in the CRC microbiota and could play a role in CRC development (Kwong et al., 2018).

In a meta-analysis that included a total of 1056 samples with published 16S rRNA data from multiple studies, the authors evaluated gut microbiome changes as CRC progresses (from control stage to adenoma to cancer) to identify biomarkers specific to adenoma for early diagnosis and treatment of CRC (Wu et al., 2021). The authors performed a pooled functional analysis based on phylogenetic investigation of communities by reconstructing unabsorbed states that revealed an altered microbiome by increased ADP-heptose biosynthesis in adenoma and elevated menaquinol-10 biosynthesis in CRC.

Antimicrobial antibodies have also been investigated as reliable markers for CRC diagnosis. *F. nucleatum* infection can elicit a strong humoral immune response. The antibodies (IgA and IgG) against this infection were significantly higher in the sera from CRC patients than in those of healthy subjects and those with benign colon disease (Wang et al., 2016). The authors also demonstrated that serum levels of IgA combined with CEA and carbohydrate antigen 19-9 (CA19-9) have a superior sensitivity compared with CEA or CA19-9 alone in detecting early-stage CRC, and that *F. nucleatum*-IgA antibodies could be a potential and valid diagnostic marker for early CRC (Wang et al., 2016).

10.3.2 Role of microbiome as prognostic and predictive biomarker

The gut microbiome, as a predictive and/or prognostic biomarker, can predict the clinical outcome of patients, their response to treatment approaches, and possible side effects associated with treatment. Various microbial genes, microbiota-related serological markers, and metabolites, including SCFAs, SBAs, LPS, indole, branched-chain amino acids, etc., found in samples of biological fluids, tumor tissue, feces, and oral cavity samples could serve to predict the outcome of therapeutic interventions.

Pomyen et al. (2021) reported that p-cresol sulfate could be responsible for gut dysbiosis and HCC pathogenesis. P-cresol is primarily produced by *C. difficile* and is metabolized in the liver through a conjugation process (sulfonation) to produce a less toxic form, p-cresol sulfate. It was identified that p-cresol sulfate can activate EGFR and contribute to the survival of HCC cells in the late stage of the disease by interacting with E-cadherin and β-catenin (Kim et al., 2019; Pomyen et al., 2021; Sun et al., 2015).

A recent prospective clinical study that included patients with unresectable HCC receiving immunotherapy investigated microbiome metabolites, including formononetin, alpha-D-glucose, galactaric acid, 13-L-hydroperoxylinoleic acid, and arachidonic acid associated with *Ruminococcus, Klebsiella, Bifidobacterium,* and *Lactobacillus* species (Wu et al., 2022). The authors studied potential biomarkers for predicting the response status of anti-PD-1-based immunotherapy. They concluded that *Ruminococcus* species was enriched in responders and positively correlated with serum galactaric acid, while *Klebsiella* was positively associated with 3-methylindole and lenticin. Similarly, *Coprococcus* was negatively correlated with formononetin, 13-L-hydroxyperoxy linoleic acid, and 12-hydroxy dodecanoic acid, and *Hemophilus,* traditionally identified as a pathogenic bacterium, was positively associated with sebacic acid. Gok Yavuz et al. (2023) extensively reviewed the importance of gut microbiome through modulation of the immune system as a diagnostic and predictive marker in HCC.

Studies found that fecal microbiome biomarkers have the potential to predict the presence of mutations in CRC-related genes that could provide helpful information in identifying individuals at high risk of developing CRC and also in the rational selection of therapeutic regimens. For example, a study by Liang et al. (2020) examined the association of highly pathogenic adenomatous polyposis coli mutation with the gut microbiome and found that three bacterial species, *B. pseudocatenulatum, Faecalibacterium prausnitzii,* and *F. mortiferum,* were potentially related to adenomatous polyposis coli gene mutations in patients with intestinal adenomatous polyps.

A recent study found a distinctive microbiota profile that could distinguish BRAF-mutated cases among CRCs and could serve as a reliable noninvasive clinical biomarker for patient-tailored diagnostic and therapeutic applications (Trivieri et al., 2020). The authors analyzed gut microbial profiles in mice and patients' BRAF wild-type samples and found lower diversity and richness compared with healthy controls.

10.4 Microbiome-based diagnostic tool

Microbiota, along with their metabolites and cellular contents such as DNA, RNA, and extracellular vesicles, expressed in body fluids such as blood, cerebrospinal fluid, gastric juice, intestinal fluid, saliva, and urine (Connal et al., 2023; Luo et al., 2024), could be promising diagnostic tools. A liquid biopsy is a procedure that involves testing these fluids for the presence of microbiota, their metabolites, or cellular components for cancer screening. Thus, liquid biopsy provides a noninvasive solution for cancer detection. Also, since body fluid collection is a convenient process, it can be repeated at different stages of cancer, thus helping in early and advanced cancer detection and monitoring (Luo et al., 2024).

Early cancer-derived genetic biomarkers are not always found in blood or are present at very low concentrations; therefore, detecting early cancer through liquid biopsy is challenging. Additionally, cancer protein markers such as prostate-specific antigen and carcinoma antigen-125 can either be expressed at low levels even in advanced cancer or be expressed in normal cells (Connal et al., 2023).

10.4.1 Artificial intelligence

Artificial intelligence (AI) is a computational and machine-based novel approach to recognizing patterns, processing data, and predicting outcomes. When combined with existing technologies for biomarker discovery, AI analyzes large complex datasets to identify multiple microbial taxa and specific combinations of microbiota that can accurately predict cancer (Novielli et al., 2024).

In a study by Novielli et al. (2024), machine learning, a subset of AI, was used to identify CRC biomarkers from fecal microbiome data. The study included three datasets involving 442 human stool samples from Canada, France, and the United States of America. These datasets had sequencing of the V4 region of the 16S rRNA. The obtained data were analyzed using the three algorithms: XGBoost, random forest, and support vector machine. The study found an association between gut microbiota and CRC, with the random forest algorithm showing the best results (Novielli et al., 2024).

10.4.2 Enzyme-linked immunosorbent assay

Enzyme-linked immunosorbent assay (ELISA) is an immunological assay used to detect and quantify antigens. Monoclonal or polyclonal antibodies detect specific or multiple epitopes of an antigen, respectively. Hence, it is used as a microbiome-based diagnostic tool by measuring host immune responses to microbial antigens. ELISA can help quantify circulating antibodies and microbial components in blood, thereby making microbial components serve as diagnostic biomarkers.

In CRC, an imbalance of the gut microbiome leads to disruption of the mucosal barrier and dissemination of microbes to other parts through circulation. Circulation of microbes initiates the production of antibodies against them and also the release of microbial components, such as LPS, in the bloodstream. ELISA-based detection of these antibodies and antigens helps determine the host–microbiome interaction.

In a study on *F. nucleatum* in CRC, Wang et al. (2016) employed ELISA to quantify anti-*F. nucleatum*-IgA and IgG levels in CRC patients compared to controls. The study found significantly higher levels of IgA and IgG in CRC patients. The sensitivity and specificity of ELISA for IgA were 36.43% and 92.71%, respectively. In contrast, the sensitivity and specificity for IgG were lower (Wang et al., 2016). Additionally, by combining CEA with anti-*F. nucleatum*-IgA, the CRC diagnosis was improved. Furthermore, combining anti-*F. nucleatum*-IgA and CEA with carbohydrate antigen 19-9 helped classify CRC stages I–II. Thus, the authors concluded that anti-*F. nucleatum*-IgA could be a potential diagnostic biomarker for CRC (Wang et al., 2016).

In another study, ELISA was used to detect serum S100 calcium-binding protein A12 (S100A12) and soluble receptor for advanced glycation end products (sRAGE), inflammatory markers, in elderly patients with CRC. The results indicated that S100A12 and sRAGE were significantly higher in CRC patients and correlated with gut microbiota dysbiosis. Additionally, postchemotherapy, their levels decreased significantly (Qiao et al., 2025).

10.4.3 Metabolomics

Metabolomics is the study of metabolites or small molecules (<2000 Da) of biological origin. Because each microbiota releases certain amounts and types of metabolites based on its surroundings, metabolomics can provide critical information about the functional state of the microbial community in response to stimuli or interactions (Bauermeister et al., 2022). In metabolomics, mass spectrometry (MS) is the most commonly used technique due to its high sensitivity and ability to detect and quantify diverse metabolites (Aksenov et al., 2017; Bauermeister et al., 2022). Utilizing gas/liquid chromatography with MS helps in studying polar and nonpolar metabolites, including volatile and nonvolatile compounds. The technique helps in the identification of individual substances being tested by separating a complex biological mixture. Nuclear Magnetic Resonance is another technique used to analyze metabolites, though with lower sensitivity than MS (Ganesan et al., 2023).

Sugimura et al. (2022) utilized liquid chromatography–MS/MS and targeted MS to identify antitumor molecules released by *L. gallinarum* in CRC tumor models. The results identified ILA in the *L. gallinarum* culture supernatant and the gut of mice infected with *L. gallinarum* as a key enriched metabolite with antitumor effects (Sugimura et al., 2022).

Zheng et al. (2023) found another method for biomarker profiling where a bowel evacuation approach was used to detect metabolite ions in urine. In this approach, the authors collected urine samples before and after the laxative use. They found 331 significantly affected metabolite ions, including 100 modified metabolites. This strategy can generate a microbiome-associated metabolite map (M3), which can be compared with disease-related metabolite profiles (Zheng et al., 2023).

10.4.4 Metagenomics

Metagenomics involves the study of microbial genetic material for its identification and classification. It differs from genomics in that it includes the genetic material of the whole microbial community, whereas in genomics, the genetic material of a specific organism is considered. Thus, metagenomics helps characterize complex microbiomes (Aguiar-Pulido et al., 2016).

Advancements in next-generation sequencing (NGS) have made it possible to study microbial communities by analyzing their genetic material. When combined with metabolomics (Fig. 10.2) and metatranscriptomics, the potential of metagenomics can be fully explored to provide information on gene expression and metabolic output (Aguiar-Pulido et al., 2016).

Despite the advancements in sequencing technologies, it is challenging to analyze huge metagenomic data because most of the software to analyze these data is available only on a 64-bit Linux system, which is difficult to understand or not available to researchers. Additionally, there are over 100 analysis tools and pipelines, thus indicating that there is no single standard protocol to analyze the metagenomic data. Examples of the tools include Galaxy, QIIME, Mothur, PathoScope, and MetaDEGalaxy (Aguiar-Pulido et al., 2016; Thang et al., 2019).

Galaxy provides access for users to the latest NGS protocols and bioinformatics tools in a graphical user interface to execute complex workflows. However, it needs substantial computational and storage resources (Aguiar-Pulido et al., 2016; Thang et al., 2019). QIIME consists of >150 Python scripts for taxonomic analysis of microbial DNA using marker genes such as 16S rRNA. It allows flexible construction of pipelines and is available in the Galaxy Toolshed (Aguiar-Pulido et al., 2016; Thang et al., 2019). Mothur targets microbial ecology as well as human microbiome communities. It provides domain-specific language to construct workflows, and

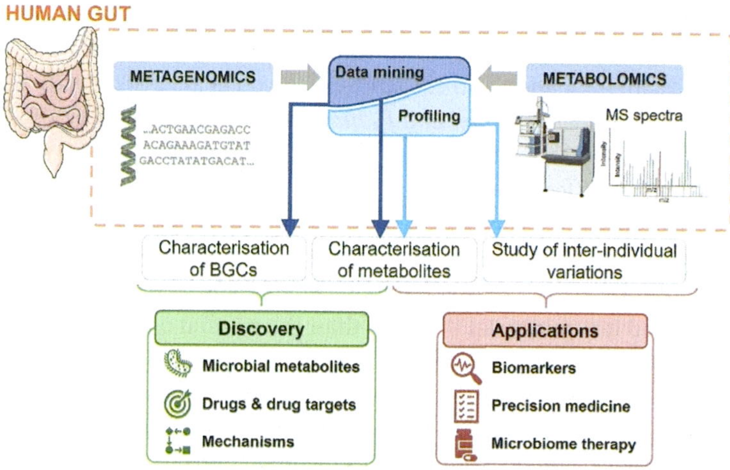

FIGURE 10.2 Metagenome – metabolome crosstalk for human gut microbiome study and its clinical applications. Both datasets can be mined to discover new metabolites, drugs, drug targets, and biological mechanisms. A profiling strategy can also be applied to seek microbial biomarkers of certain health conditions or treatment efficacy, identify how gut microbes modify disease prognosis, and use this knowledge to define personalized treatments based on precision medicine or microbiome therapies to counteract the effects of these microbes. *Source: From Puig-Castellví, F., Pacheco-Tapia, R., Deslande, M., Jia, M., Andrikopoulos, P., Chechi, K., Bonnefond, A., Froguel, P., & Dumas, M.-E., (2023). Advances in the integration of metabolomics and metagenomics for human gut microbiome and their clinical applications.* TrAC Trends in Analytical Chemistry. *167, 117248, https://doi.org/10.1016/j.trac.2023.117248. (This is an open-access article under the CC BY license). (http://creativecommons.org/licenses/by/4.0/).*

like QIIME, it focuses on marker genes such as 16S rRNA. PathoScope helps identify bacterial strains from raw sequences and generate statistical reports, including gene locations, abundance percentage, and protein products (Aguiar-Pulido et al., 2016). MetaDEGalaxy is a specialized pipeline within Galaxy that integrates the R packages phyloseq and DESeq2 (Thang et al., 2019), focusing on differential abundance analysis.

Different metagenomic techniques are used to study microbiomes depending on the research objective. Each technique differs in resolution, target, data complexity, and suitability for taxonomic and functional profiling. Below are the most commonly used methods described:

10.4.4.1 16S rDNA/rRNA sequencing

It is one of the cost-effective and computationally tractable technologies used to characterize microbiota. 16S rRNA is a ribosomal gene (~1.6 kb) in bacteria and archaea. It has nine variable regions (V1–V9), sharing 97%–99% identity in the bacterial genome of the same genus and species. Thus, it serves as a strong phylogenetic marker for molecular taxonomy by varying combinations of variable and conserved regions (Aitmanaitė et al., 2023; Chrisman et al., 2021; Guerrero-Preston et al., 2016; Ridlon et al., 2014). PCR and sequencing facilities make 16S rDNA/rRNA sequencing feasible and help determine new species, reclassify, rename, and determine phylogenetic relationships (Woo et al., 2008).

However, the success rate of species identification with 16S rDNA/rRNA sequencing is only between 62% and 92% due to blind spots within some major genera. Therefore, *groEL* is another gene used for species identification and classification (Woo et al., 2002, 2008). For example, the 16S rRNA of *Burkholderia pseudomallei* and *B. thailandensis* differ only by 1%. In comparison, the groEL gene differs by 2.4% between any strain of *B. pseudomallei* and any strain of *B. thailandensis.* Thus, these higher differences in groEL make it more suitable to distinguish species than 16S rRNA (Woo et al., 2002).

Guerrero-Preston et al. (2016) used a 16S rRNA V3–V5 marker gene approach to characterize saliva microbiota from head and neck squamous cell carcinoma patients. They found that the cancerous samples had less microbial diversity than the normal ones. Also, microbial diversity was reduced after surgery but increased in patients with recurrence, suggesting that the microbiota could be used as diagnostic and prognostic biomarkers in head and neck squamous cell carcinoma (Guerrero-Preston et al., 2016). Similarly, Yeo et al. (2024) found reduced microbial diversity in head and neck cancers compared to healthy controls. The authors used oral rinse and saliva samples for 16S rRNA sequencing because they serve as better diagnostic tools than swab samples, which are site-specific (Yeo et al., 2024). Another study, where a meta-analysis was performed using 16 studies on gastric cancer, found that a combination of genera can have good diagnostic efficacy and broad applicability (Chen et al., 2023).

Because most microbiota possess a higher amount of RNA than DNA, RNA sequencing provides better detection than DNA sequencing (Luo et al., 2024). However, it suffers from varying results based on sample types, study batches, primer sets, low throughput, and nonspecific taxonomic identification, thus limiting its reliability across studies (Jovel et al., 2016; Mannion et al., 2023; Yeo et al., 2024).

10.4.4.2 Internal transcribed spacer sequencing

In a eukaryotic cell, nuclear ribosomal DNA contains genes for 18S, 5.8S, and 28S rRNA. These coding genes are separated by noncoding genes (spacers) called internal transcribed spacers (ITS). ITS1 is located between genes for 18S and 5.8S rRNAs, and ITS2 is located between genes for 5.8S and 28S rRNAs. Being highly variable among different species, it makes an excellent biomarker to distinguish microbial species (Prahl et al., 2021). The ITS region is the official fungal barcode for fungal identification and classification (Bellemain et al., 2010).

Using ITS sequencing, Rittenour et al. (2014) found that phylum *Ascomycota, Basidiomycota,* and *Zygomycota* dominated the air and dust in the indoor environment of asthmatic children's homes in Kansas City, Missouri, USA. They also identified rarely documented fungal species of *Pleosporales,* an order of *Ascomycota.* Many *Basidiomycota* species were identified with ITS sequencing but not by viable or nonviable methods, thus indicating the higher sensitivity of ITS sequencing compared to viable and nonviable methods (Rittenour et al., 2014).

10.4.4.3 Pathogen-targeted sequencing

Pathogen-targeted sequencing (PTS) is a technique to identify disease-specific pathogens by sequencing specific microbial DNA. PTS provides advantages of detection sensitivity irrespective of the human genome, background bacteria, and pathogen genome size, as well as low cost, reduced sample transportation, and quantitative pathogen detection (Gao et al., 2021).

Metagenomic next-generation sequencing (mNGS) is one of the cost-effective methods to detect human pathogens in cerebrospinal fluid. However, in a study by Gao et al. (2021), PTS showed higher sensitivity than mNGS in detecting pathogens in cerebrospinal fluid. Together, both techniques detected nine positive samples out of 38 samples. In the remaining samples, 13 were detected as positive by PTS alone, and only four were detected as positive by mNGS alone. When comparing the positive and negative predictive values, PTS (70.8%) had a higher sensitivity rate than mNGS (41.7%) (Gao et al., 2021).

10.4.4.4 Shotgun metagenomics

Shotgun metagenomics, a whole-genome sequencing method, provides advantages over 16S rRNA sequencing in microbiome characterization by identifying bacterial and nonbacterial microbiomes, species- and strain-level resolution, and functional characterization (Mannion et al., 2023). Unlike 16S rRNA sequencing, where only 16S rRNA is sequenced, this method uses whole-genome sequencing to locate a genome in a phylogenetic tree. This also helps in the identification of novel species, which is not possible with 16S rRNA sequencing due to its limited segment (Aitmanaitė et al., 2023; Jovel et al., 2016).

For example, in the study by Jovel et al. (2016), 16S rRNA sequencing identified microbes well at the genus level, while at the species level, identification was limited due to the low resolution of the V4 region and the lack of a reference genome, thus misclassifying closely related species such as *C. sordelli* and *C. difficile.* Additionally, primers overrepresented genera like *Clostridium* and *Lactobacillus.* On the other hand, shotgun metagenomics showed species-level resolution with higher accuracy. It also resolved taxa in families like *Enterobacteriaceae* and *Peptostreptococcaceae,* which share >96% 16S rRNA similarity (Jovel et al., 2016).

Despite the benefit of shotgun metagenomics in identifying microbial species using whole-genome sequencing, its application is limited when an incomplete microbial genome is recovered. This is because, with an incomplete genome, microbial classification at the taxonomic level is hindered by the degree of conservation of the available sequences. Additionally, environmental contamination of the sample also limits the application of shotgun metagenomics and 16S rRNA sequencing (Jovel et al., 2016).

10.4.5 Metaproteomics

Metaproteomics is the large-scale study of protein expression, structure, and function in complex microbial communities within a given environment. Proteomics can provide information on their functional activity and interactions with the host, and in some cases, it can identify post-translational modifications of proteins. Thus, it can identify microbial proteins associated with cancer-related pathways and immune modulation.

A study on fresh and frozen-thawed stool samples from patients with inflammatory bowel diseases—Crohn's disease and ulcerative colitis—indicated that metaproteomics worked well on both types of samples. Using LC-tandem MS, the authors identified a total of 231,500 peptides and 43,521 protein subgroups across the 40 samples (20 fresh and 20 frozen-thawed). The correlation of metaproteomic profiles was strong (Pearson's $r > 0.9$) between the two types of samples (Henry et al., 2022). In another study, the authors used data-independent acquisition-based label-free quantitative proteomics to identify proteins in the fecal samples of CRC patients and healthy volunteers. Out of the total 30,062 protein groups identified and quantified, 341 protein groups were significantly higher in CRC patients than in healthy volunteers. These proteins were related to iron intake and transport, oxidative stress, and DNA replication, recombination, and repair. Thus, the authors concluded that metaproteomics can help in determining functional information on the intestinal microbiome, can support pathogenesis research, and shows promise for clinical diagnosis (Long et al., 2020).

Despite the increased application of metaproteomics in the gut microbiome, due to a lack of a comprehensive and standard metaproteomics workflow, limited studies are available on the oral microbiome. To overcome this drawback, Jiang et al. (2022) developed a free-flow isoelectric focusing–MS-based metaproteomics methodology for an in-depth analysis of the human oral microbiome in lung cancer. With this method, they found that, compared to conventional metaproteomics, this method reduced interfering peptide signals by 52.87%, and there was an increase in bacterial peptides and species by 94.97% and 44.90%, respectively. They also identified 3647 oral bacterial proteins and an imbalance and dysregulated functions of *F. nucleatum* and *Prevotella histicola* in immune response and cellular redox homeostasis (Jiang et al., 2022).

10.4.6 Metatranscriptomics

Metatranscriptomics is a culture-independent quantification of genes of a microbial community. It differs from metagenomics by identifying transcribed genes (mRNA) actively expressed at a given time in bacteria, archaea, eukaryotes, and viruses. Though less commonly used than metagenomics, it employs mapping transcriptomic tools to specialized databases with the help of alignment tools such as Bowtie2, Burrows–Wheeler Alignment, and Basic Local Alignment Search Tool. After that, the results are annotated using resources such as Gene Ontology, Kyoto Encyclopedia of Genes and Genomes, Clusters of Orthologous Groups, and Swiss-Prot. Following this, analyses are performed, such as enrichment or principal component analysis, based on phylogenetic analysis (Aguiar-Pulido et al., 2016; Zhang et al., 2021c).

Metatranscriptomics is highly subject-specific and body-site dependent, thus helping in determining local molecular activity. By combining human and microbial transcriptional profiles, it is possible to determine host–microbe interactions. However, for general mechanistic characterization, it is challenging to employ metatranscriptomics (Zhang et al., 2021c). Additionally, it remains underutilized due to the difficulty in isolating RNA molecules and preventing their degradation during processing. Furthermore, it also needs to be performed in depth to avoid under-detection of low-abundance transcripts. Consequently, metatranscriptomics-based biomarkers have not yet reached preclinical testing, highlighting the significant future potential of this approach (Zhang et al., 2021c).

10.5 Cancer therapy and microbiome

The microbiome influences the efficacy of cancer therapeutics, and understanding microbial signatures in the context of cancer therapy will provide opportunities to modulate the microbiome to enhance effectiveness, reduce drug resistance, and increase overall survival (Ting et al., 2022). Recent studies have suggested complex interactions between drugs and the microbiome, leading to a new field of study, "pharamcomicrobiomics" (Aziz et al., 2011), in which the gut microbiome influences clinical outcomes in patients, including cancer patients (Conti et al., 2023). Chemotherapy, immunotherapy, and radiation therapy in the context of the gut microbiome are discussed below.

10.5.1 Chemotherapeutics and microbiome modulation

Irinotecan, a standard chemotherapeutic drug used to treat metastatic CRC, is converted to a toxic compound by *Clostridium* clusters that secrete the enzyme β-glucuronidase, leading to severe side effects such as diarrhea (Stringer et al., 2014). β-glucuronidase inhibitors have been shown to reduce side effects without affecting irinotecan efficacy (Cheng et al., 2019). The role of microbiome modulation was further evidenced in a randomized, double-blind pilot study, in which probiotics prevented diarrhea associated with irinotecan treatment (Mego et al., 2015).

Cyclophosphamide, an alkylating chemotherapeutic agent, modulates the antitumor responses by altering the gut microbiome that aids in its action; cyclophosphamide increases the translocation of specific Gram-positive bacteria, such as *E. hirae* and *L. johnsonii,* into the secondary lymphoid organs, which in turn induces T-helper and memory cells (Viaud et al., 2013). In addition, Vlaud et al. (2013) showed that germ-free tumor-bearing mice or mice treated with antibiotics against Gram-positive bacteria were resistant to cyclophosphamide treatment, suggesting the critical role of these bacteria.

Gemcitabine, a nucleoside analog commonly used to treat pancreatic ductal adenocarcinoma, often becomes ineffective because patients develop resistance to the drug. Geller et al. (2017) showed that specific bacteria metabolize gemcitabine into an inactive form, thereby increasing resistance to the drug, and demonstrated that treatment with the antibiotic ciprofloxacin reverses this resistance.

Platinum-based chemotherapeutics, such as oxaliplatin and cisplatin, were shown to depend on the characteristics of commensal gut bacteria, such as *B. fragilis,* to modulate immune responses that promote their anticancer activity, and the activity of these drugs was lost in the absence of these immunogenic, nonenterotoxigenic bacteria (Roberti et al., 2020).

Doxorubicin, an anthracycline antibiotic, is commonly used as a chemotherapeutic to treat several solid tumors, but it leads to severe organ damage, including cardiotoxicity (Curigliano et al., 2016). Doxorubicin was shown to induce microbial dysbiosis by releasing toxic substances, such as LPSs, into the bloodstream, thereby promoting the production of inflammatory markers that result in systemic damage. Probiotics (Abu-Elsaad et al., 2015) and fecal microbiota transplant (An et al., 2021) treatments have shown improvement in doxorubicin-induced cardiotoxicity, highlighting the potential role of microbiome modulation in reducing toxic effects and improving drug efficacy.

These studies demonstrate cross-talk between chemotherapeutic drugs and the microbiome, which can affect overall survival in cancer patients. In addition, in recent years, several studies have shown the microbiome's role in modulating immune checkpoint inhibitors (ICIs), a key scientific breakthrough in successful cancer treatment (Lu et al., 2022).

10.5.2 Immune checkpoint inhibitors and microbiome modulation

Immunosurveillance evasion emerged as one of the hallmarks of cancer progression, and breakthrough developments in immunotherapy in the last decade have changed the landscape of cancer treatment (Waldman et al., 2020). ICIs that inactivate cytotoxic T lymphocyte antigen 4 (CTLA4) and PD-1 on T cells and release cancer cells from immune suppression have been highly successful in cancer therapy against various cancers, including melanoma, lung cancer, CRC, gastric cancer, and renal cell carcinoma (Hodi et al., 2010; Hwang et al., 2023). Despite the success of immunotherapy, only a small percentage of patients respond to ICIs, and this response has been shown to be associated with gut microbiota composition (Roy & Trinchieri, 2017; Sivan et al., 2015; Vétizou et al., 2015; Xie & Liu, 2024).

Anti-CTLA4 therapy that releases the brake on T-cell activation and has been demonstrated to modulate the microbiome to exert its effect. It was shown that ICI targeting CTLA4 promotes the growth of *Bacteroides* spp., which, in turn, further activates dendritic cells and Th1 cells to initiate tumor cell killing (Vétizou et al., 2015). When germ-free mice were recolonized with *Bacteroides* spp., it not only reversed immunoresistance but also protected them from immune-related adverse effects (Pitt et al., 2016; Vétizou et al., 2015), suggesting a correlation between microbial composition and its effects on the tumor microenvironment.

Anti-PD-1/programmed death-ligand 1 (PD-L1) therapy prevents PD-1 from binding PD-L1 and induces immune responses through cytokine release and T-cell activation (Hwang et al., 2023). When treated with anti-PD-1 therapy, patients with a unique, diverse gut microbiome responded to the ICI, facilitating stratification into responders versus nonresponders. The responders harbored diverse bacteria, such as *Ruminococcaceae, A. muciniphila*, and *Eubacterium*, which helped patients respond positively to anti-PD-1 treatment (Gopalakrishnan et al., 2018; Routy et al., 2018). When melanoma patients with anti-PD-1 therapy resistance undergo fecal microbiota transplant from responders, it results in a positive clinical response in a small percentage of the anti-PD-1-resistant patient population (Baruch et al., 2021). Probiotics are shown to be selectively effective in renal cell carcinoma, with improved progression-free survival when combined with anti-PD-1 (nivolumab) and anti-CTLA4 drugs(ipilimumab) (Dizman et al., 2022). All these studies indicate the influence of gut microbiome composition on immune modulation and the effect of ICIs.

10.5.3 Radiation and microbiome modulation

RT forms a key treatment modality for cancer patients, and it causes debilitating side effects on the gastrointestinal system. RT alters microbial composition, affecting sensitization and toxicity in patients. RT disrupts the microbiome, leading to decreased microbial diversity, reduced beneficial bacteria such as *Bifidobacteria* and *Faecalibacterium*, and increased harmful bacteria such as *Fusobacteria* and *Proteobacteria* (Fernandes et al., 2021; Wang et al., 2021). Metabolomics analysis has revealed that patients who respond to RT have increased levels of *Faecalibacterium*, which activate the cyclic guanosine monophosphate–adenosine monophosphate synthase (cGAS) and stimulator of interferon genes (STING) cGAS–STING pathway, which further modulates the immune response (Li et al., 2022). RT and the microbiome engage in bidirectional communication that can be modulated to increase RT sensitivity and reduce its toxic effects (Palkovsky et al., 2025). A combination of prebiotics and probiotics has helped patients treated with RT from RT-induced diarrhea (Scartoni et al., 2015). Fecal microbiota transplant in patients with chronic enteritis due to RT reduced intestinal damage and decreased symptoms of diarrhea, abdominal pain, rectal hemorrhage, and fecal incontinence, underscoring the impact of microbial modulation on RT-induced damage (Ding et al., 2020).

Microbiome signatures have the potential to serve as personalized or precision modulators and biomarkers for cancer therapy. Therefore, it is imperative to develop standardized techniques for identifying microbial biomarkers to enhance our understanding of the pharmacobiome.

10.6 Current challenges, prospects, and conclusion

The future of microbiome-based diagnostics and biomarkers is promising, with significant potential across various medical disciplines. As the field advances, microbiome profiling is expected to become a key component of precision medicine, complementing genomic and metabolomic data to help predict disease risk, guide personalized therapies, and monitor treatment responses. These diagnostics may allow for the noninvasive, early detection of diseases such as colorectal and pancreatic cancers, neurodegenerative conditions like Parkinson's, and autoimmune disorders, including inflammatory bowel disease. Integration with AI and multiomics approaches will enhance diagnostic accuracy by identifying subtle microbial patterns and building predictive algorithms. Technological innovations, such as portable sequencing tools, could enable real-time, point-of-care microbiome analysis in clinical settings.

Despite the promising future of microbiome-based diagnostics, several challenges currently hinder their clinical implementation. A major issue is the lack of standardization in sample collection, sequencing, and data analysis, which leads to inconsistent results across studies. Additionally, the microbiome's complexity and variability among individuals, influenced by factors such as diet, age, and environment, make it difficult to identify consistent biomarkers and require large, diverse, longitudinal studies. Another limitation is the predominance of correlational rather than causal findings, reducing clinical reliability. Experimental models and integration with host biology are being developed to uncover causal relationships. Furthermore, few microbiome-based diagnostics have been clinically validated or approved for medical use, highlighting the need for rigorous, multicenter clinical trials and collaboration with regulatory bodies. The interpretation of microbiome data also remains a barrier, requiring complex bioinformatics tools and expertise, though more accessible, clinician-friendly software platforms are in development. Ethical and privacy concerns related to the personal nature of microbiome data are being addressed through improved governance frameworks and data protection policies.

While the gut microbiome has received the most attention, future research is expanding into other microbial niches—such as the oral, skin, and vaginal microbiomes—which may yield additional diagnostic biomarkers. Additionally, the gut-brain axis presents new opportunities for microbiome-based diagnostics in mental health conditions like depression, anxiety, and post-traumatic stress disorder. Moving forward, efforts will be needed to establish regulatory standards, validate clinical tools, and ensure ethical use of patient microbiome data. Overall, microbiome-based diagnostics are expected to transform healthcare by offering earlier, more personalized, and less invasive approaches to disease detection and management.

References

Abu-Elsaad, N. M., Abd Elhameed, A. G., El-Karef, A., & Ibrahim, T. M. (2015). Yogurt containing the probacteria *Lactobacillus acidophilus* combined with natural antioxidants mitigates doxorubicin-induced cardiomyopathy in rats. *Journal of Medicinal Food, 18*(9), 950–959. https://doi.org/10.1089/jmf.2014.0104.

Aguiar-Pulido, V., Huang, W., Suarez-Ulloa, V., Cickovski, T., Mathee, K., & Narasimhan, G. (2016). Metagenomics, metatranscriptomics, and metabolomics approaches for microbiome analysis. *Evolutionary bioinformatics online, 12*(Suppl 1), 5–16. https://doi.org/10.4137/EBO.S36436.

Aitmanaitė, L., Širmonaitis, K., & Russo, G. (2023). Microbiomes, their function, and cancer: How metatranscriptomics can close the knowledge gap. *International Journal of Molecular Sciences, 24*(18), 13786. https://doi.org/10.3390/ijms241813786.

Ajouz, H., Mukherji, D., & Shamseddine, A. (2014). Secondary bile acids: An underrecognized cause of colon cancer. *World Journal of Surgical Oncology, 12*(1). https://doi.org/10.1186/1477-7819-12-164.

Akbar, N., Ahmed Khan, N., Sualeh Muhammad, J., & Siddiqui, R. (2022). The role of gut microbiome in cancer genesis and cancer prevention. *Health Sciences Review, 2*, 100010. https://doi.org/10.1016/j.hsr.2021.100010.

Aksenov, A. A., Silva, R. D., Knight, R., Lopes, N. P., & Dorrestein, P. C. (2017). Global chemical analysis of biology by mass spectrometry. *Nature Reviews Chemistry, 1*. https://doi.org/10.1038/s41570-017-0054.

Aktories, K., & Barbieri, J. T. (2005). Bacterial cytotoxins: Targeting eukaryotic switches. *Nature Reviews Microbiology, 3*(5), 397–410. https://doi.org/10.1038/nrmicro1150.

Alexander, E. M., Kreitler, D. F., Guidolin, V., Hurben, A. K., Drake, E., Villalta, P. W., Balbo, S., Gulick, A. M., & Aldrich, C. C. (2020). Biosynthesis, mechanism of action, and inhibition of the enterotoxin tilimycin produced by the opportunistic pathogen *Klebsiella oxytoca*. *ACS Infectious Diseases, 6*(7), 1976–1997. https://doi.org/10.1021/acsinfecdis.0c00326.

An, L., Wuri, J., Zheng, Z., Li, W., & Yan, T. (2021). Microbiota modulate doxorubicin induced cardiotoxicity. *European Journal of Pharmaceutical Sciences, 166*, 105977. https://doi.org/10.1016/j.ejps.2021.105977.

Anderson, N. M., & Simon, M. C. (2020). The tumor microenvironment. *Current Biology, 30*(16), R921. https://doi.org/10.1016/j.cub.2020.06.081.

Andersson, T., Bergdahl, G. E. ü, Saleh, K., Magnúsdóttir, H., Stødkilde, K., Brix Folsted Andersen, C., Lundqvist, K., Jensen, A., Brüggemann, H., & Lood, R. (2019). Common skin bacteria protect their host from oxidative stress through secreted antioxidant RoxP. *Scientific Reports., 9*(1). https://doi.org/10.1038/s41598-019-40471-3.

Ansari, S., & Yamaoka, Y. (2020). *Helicobacter pylori* virulence factor cytotoxin-associated gene A (CagA)-mediated gastric pathogenicity. *International Journal of Molecular Sciences, 21*(19), 7430. https://doi.org/10.3390/ijms21197430.

Arthur, J. C., Perez-Chanona, E., Mühlbauer, M., Tomkovich, S., Uronis, J. M., Fan, T. J., Campbell, B. J., Abujamel, T., Dogan, B., Rogers, A. B., Rhodes, J. M., Stintzi, A., Simpson, K. W., Hansen, J. J., Keku, T. O., Fodor, A. A., & Jobin, C. (2012). Intestinal inflammation targets cancer-inducing activity of the microbiota. *Science, 338*(6103), 120–123. https://doi.org/10.1126/science.1224820.

Aziz, R. K., Saad, R., & Rizkallah, M. R. (2011). PharmacoMicrobiomics or how bugs modulate drugs: An educational initiative to explore the effects of human microbiome on drugs. *BMC Bioinformatics, 12*(S7). https://doi.org/10.1186/1471-2105-12-s7-a10.

Azzimonti, B., Ballacchino, C., Zanetta, P., Cucci, M. A., Monge, C., Grattarola, M., Dianzani, C., Barrera, G., & Pizzimenti, S. (2023). Microbiota, oxidative stress, and skin cancer: An unexpected triangle. *Antioxidants., 12*(3), 546. https://doi.org/10.3390/antiox12030546.

Badawy, A. A. B. (2017). Kynurenine pathway of tryptophan metabolism: Regulatory and functional aspects. *International Journal of Tryptophan Research, 10*(1). https://doi.org/10.1177/1178646917691938.

Baghban, R., Roshangar, L., Jahanban-Esfahlan, R., Seidi, K., Ebrahimi-Kalan, A., Jaymand, M., Kolahian, S., Javaheri, T., & Zare, P. (2020). Tumor microenvironment complexity and therapeutic implications at a glance. *Cell Communication and Signaling, 18*(1). https://doi.org/10.1186/s12964-020-0530-4.

Baruch, E. N., Youngster, I., Ben-Betzalel, G., Ortenberg, R., Lahat, A., Katz, L., Adler, K., Dick-Necula, D., Raskin, S., Bloch, N., Rotin, D., Anafi, L., Avivi, C., Melnichenko, J., Steinberg-Silman, Y., Mamtani, R., Harati, H., Asher, N., Shapira-Frommer, R., … Boursi, B. (2021). Fecal microbiota transplant promotes response in immunotherapy-refractory melanoma patients. *Science, 371*(6529), 602–609. https://doi.org/10.1126/science.abb5920.

Bauermeister, A., Mannochio-Russo, H., Costa-Lotufo, L. V., Jarmusch, A. K., & Dorrestein, P. C. (2022). Mass spectrometry-based metabolomics in microbiome investigations. *Nature Reviews Microbiology, 20*(3), 143–160. https://doi.org/10.1038/s41579-021-00621-9.

Beaugerie, L., & Itzkowitz, S. H. (2015). Cancers complicating inflammatory bowel disease. *New England Journal of Medicine, 372*(15), 1441–1452. https://doi.org/10.1056/NEJMra1403718.

Bellemain, E., Carlsen, T., Brochmann, C., Coissac, E., Taberlet, P., & Kauserud, H. (2010). ITS as an environmental DNA barcode for fungi: An in silico approach reveals potential PCR biases. *BMC Microbiology, 10*(1), 189. https://doi.org/10.1186/1471-2180-10-189.

Bezine, E., Malaisé, Y., Loeuillet, A., Chevalier, M., Boutet-Robinet, E., Salles, B., Mirey, G., & Vignard, J. (2016). Cell resistance to the cytolethal distending toxin involves an association of DNA repair mechanisms. *Scientific Reports, 6*(1). https://doi.org/10.1038/srep36022.

Boffetta, P., & Nyberg, F. (2003). Contribution of environmental factors to cancer risk. *British Medical Bulletin, 68*(1), 71–94. https://doi.org/10.1093/bmp/ldg023.

Bong, A. H. L., & Monteith, G. R. (2018). Calcium signaling and the therapeutic targeting of cancer cells. *Biochimica et Biophysica Acta - Molecular Cell Research, 1865*(11), 1786–1794. https://doi.org/10.1016/j.bbamcr.2018.05.015.

Califf, R. M. (2018). Biomarker definitions and their applications. *Experimental Biology and Medicine (Maywood), 243*, 213–221. https://doi.org/10.1177/1535370217750088.

Capiod, S., & Skryma, P. (2007). Calcium signalling and cancer cell growth. *Subcellular Biochemistry, 45*, 405–427. https://doi.org/10.1007/978-1-4020-6191-2_15.

Chaisiriwong, L., Wanitphakdeedecha, R., Sitthinamsuwan, P., Sampattavanich, S., Chatsiricharoenkul, S., Manuskiatti, W., Panich, U., & Hrelia, S. (2016). A case-control study of involvement of oxidative DNA damage and alteration of antioxidant defense system in patients with basal cell carcinoma: Modulation by tumor removal. *Oxidative Medicine and Cellular Longevity, 2016*(1). https://doi.org/10.1155/2016/5934024.

Chen, F., Dai, X., Zhou, C. C., Li, K. X., Zhang, Y. J., Lou, X. Y., Zhu, Y. M., Sun, Y. L., Peng, B. X., & Cui, W. (2022). Integrated analysis of the faecal metagenome and serum metabolome reveals the role of gut microbiome-associated metabolites in the detection of colorectal cancer and adenoma. *Gut, 71*(7), 1315–1325. https://doi.org/10.1136/gutjnl-2020-323476.

Chen, J., Nie, S., Qiu, X., Zheng, S., Ni, C., Yuan, Y., Gong, Y., & Segata, N. (2023). Leveraging existing 16S rRNA microbial data to identify diagnostic biomarker in Chinese patients with gastric cancer: A systematic meta-analysis. *mSystems, 8*(5). https://doi.org/10.1128/msystems.00747-23.

Cheng, K. W., Tseng, C. H., Tzeng, C. C., Leu, Y. L., Cheng, T. C., Wang, J. Y., Chang, J. M., Lu, Y. C., Cheng, C. M., Chen, I. J., Cheng, Y. A., Chen, Y. L., & Cheng, T. L. (2019). Pharmacological inhibition of bacterial β-glucuronidase prevents irinotecan-induced diarrhea without impairing its antitumor efficacy *in vivo*. *Pharmacological Research, 139*, 41–49. https://doi.org/10.1016/j.phrs.2018.10.029.

Cheng, W. T., Kantilal, H. K., & Davamani, F. (2020a). The mechanism of *Bacteroides fragilis* toxin contributes to colon cancer formation. *Malaysian Journal of Medical Sciences, 27*(4), 9–21. https://doi.org/10.21315/mjms2020.27.4.2.

Cheng, Y., Ling, Z., & Li, L. (2020b). The intestinal microbiota and colorectal cancer. *Frontiers in Immunology, 11*. https://doi.org/10.3389/fimmu.2020.615056.

Chrisman, B. S., Paskov, K. M., Stockham, N., Jung, J. Y., Varma, M., Washington, P. Y., Tataru, C., Iwai, S., DeSantis, T. Z., David, M., & Wall, D. P. (2021). Improved detection of disease-associated gut microbes using 16S sequence-based biomarkers. *BMC Bioinformatics, 22*(1). https://doi.org/10.1186/s12859-021-04427-7.

Connal, S., Cameron, J. M., Sala, A., Brennan, P. M., Palmer, D. S., Palmer, J. D., Perlow, H., & Baker, M. J. (2023). Liquid biopsies: The future of cancer early detection. *Journal of Translational Medicine, 21*(1). https://doi.org/10.1186/s12967-023-03960-8.

Conti, G., D'Amico, F., Fabbrini, M., Brigidi, P., Barone, M., & Turroni, S. (2023). Pharmacomicrobiomics in anticancer therapies: Why the gut microbiota should be pointed out. *Genes, 14*(1), 55. https://doi.org/10.3390/genes14010055.

Curigliano, G., Cardinale, D., Dent, S., Criscitiello, C., Aseyev, O., Lenihan, D., & Cipolla, C. M. (2016). Cardiotoxicity of anticancer treatments: Epidemiology, detection, and management. *CA: A Cancer Journal for Clinicians, 66*(4), 309–325. https://doi.org/10.3322/caac.21341.

Dadgar-Zankbar, L., Shariati, A., Bostanghadiri, N., Elahi, Z., Mirkalantari, S., Razavi, S., Kamali, F., & Darban-Sarokhalil, D. (2023). Evaluation of enterotoxigenic *Bacteroides fragilis* correlation with the expression of cellular signaling pathway genes in Iranian patients with colorectal cancer. *Infectious Agents and Cancer, 18*(1). https://doi.org/10.1186/s13027-023-00523-w.

de la Vega, M. R., Chapman, E., & Zhang, D. D. (2018). NRF2 and the hallmarks of cancer. *Cancer Cell, 34*(1), 21–43. https://doi.org/10.1016/j.ccell.2018.03.022.

de Visser, K. E., & Joyce, J. A. (2023). The evolving tumor microenvironment: From cancer initiation to metastatic outgrowth. *Cancer Cell, 41*(3), 374–403. https://doi.org/10.1016/j.ccell.2023.02.016.

den Besten, G., Van Eunen, K., Groen, A. K., Venema, K., Reijngoud, D. J., & Bakker, B. M. (2013). The role of short-chain fatty acids in the interplay between diet, gut microbiota, and host energy metabolism. *Journal of Lipid Research, 54*(9), 2325–2340. https://doi.org/10.1194/jlr.R036012Netherlands.

Deng, Z., Mei, S. i, Ouyang, Z., Wang, R., Wang, L., Zou, B. o, Dai, J., Mao, K., Li, Q., Guo, Q., Yi, C., Meng, F., Xie, M., Zhang, X., Wang, R., Deng, T., Wang, Z., Li, X., Wang, Q., Liu, B., & Tian, X. (2025). Dysregulation of gut microbiota stimulates NETs-driven HCC intrahepatic metastasis: Therapeutic implications of healthy faecal microbiota transplantation. *Gut Microbes, 17*(1). https://doi.org/10.1080/19490976.2025.2476561.

DiMaio, D., Emu, B., Goodman, A. L., Mothes, W., & Justice, A. (2022). Cancer microbiology. *JNCI: Journal of the National Cancer Institute., 114*(5), 651–663. https://doi.org/10.1093/jnci/djab212.

Ding, S. Z., Goldberg, J. B., & Hatakeyama, M. (2010). *Helicobacter pylori* infection, oncogenic pathways and epigenetic mechanisms in gastric carcinogenesis. *Future Oncology, 6*(5), 851–862. https://doi.org/10.2217/fon.10.37.

Ding, X., Li, Q., Li, P., Chen, X., Xiang, L., Bi, L., Zhu, J., Huang, X., Cui, B., & Zhang, F. (2020). Fecal microbiota transplantation: A promising treatment for radiation enteritis? *Radiotherapy and Oncology, 143*, 12–18. https://doi.org/10.1016/j.radonc.2020.01.011.

Dizman, N., Meza, L., Bergerot, P., Alcantara, M., Dorff, T., Lyou, Y., Frankel, P., Cui, Y., Mira, V., Llamas, M., Hsu, J., Zengin, Z., Salgia, N., Salgia, S., Malhotra, J., Chawla, N., Chehrazi-Raffle, A., Muddasani, R., Gillece, J., … Pal, S. K. (2022). Nivolumab plus ipilimumab with or without live bacterial supplementation in metastatic renal cell carcinoma: A randomized phase 1 trial. *Nature Medicine, 28*(4), 704–712. https://doi.org/10.1038/s41591-022-01694-6.

Dougherty, M. W., & Jobin, C. (2021). Shining a light on colibactin biology. *Toxins., 13*(5), 346. https://doi.org/10.3390/toxins13050346.

Duan, Y., Xu, Y., Dou, Y., & Xu, D. (2025). *Helicobacter pylori* and gastric cancer: Mechanisms and new perspectives. *Journal of Hematology & Oncology, 18*(1). https://doi.org/10.1186/s13045-024-01654-2.

Dubinsky, V., Dotan, I., & Gophna, U. (2020). Carriage of colibactin-producing bacteria and colorectal cancer risk. *Trends in Microbiology, 28*(11), 874–876. https://doi.org/10.1016/j.tim.2020.05.015.

Duizer, C., & de Zoete, M. R. (2023). The role of microbiota-derived metabolites in colorectal cancer. *International Journal of Molecular Sciences, 24*(9), 8024. https://doi.org/10.3390/ijms24098024.

Ealla, K. K. R., Kumari, N., Chintalapani, S., Uppu, S., Sahu, V., Veeraraghavan, V. P., Ramani, P., & Govindool, S. R. (2024). Interplay between dental caries pathogens, periodontal pathogens, and sugar molecules: Approaches for prevention and treatment. *Archives of Microbiology, 206*(3). https://doi.org/10.1007/s00203-024-03856-1.

Elinav, E., Strowig, T., Kau, A. L., Henao-Mejia, J., Thaiss, C. A., Booth, C. J., Peaper, D. R., Bertin, J., Eisenbarth, S. C., Gordon, J. I., & Flavell, R. A. (2011). NLRP6 inflammasome regulates colonic microbial ecology and risk for colitis. *Cell, 145*(5), 745–757. https://doi.org/10.1016/j.cell.2011.04.022.

Fan, Y., Su, Q., Chen, J., Wang, Y., & He, S. (2022). Gut microbiome alterations affect glioma development and foxp3 expression in tumor microenvironment in mice. *Frontiers in Oncology, 12*. https://doi.org/10.3389/fonc.2022.836953.

Fernandes, A., Oliveira, A., Soares, R., & Barata, P. (2021). The effects of ionizing radiation on gut microbiota: A systematic review. *Nutrients, 13*(9), 3025. https://doi.org/10.3390/nu13093025.

Finn, O. J. (2012). Immuno-oncology: Understanding the function and dysfunction of the immune system in cancer. *Annals of Oncology, 23*(8), viii6–9. https://doi.org/10.1093/annonc/mds256.

Ganesan, R., Yoon, S. J., & Suk, K. T. (2023). Microbiome and metabolomics in liver cancer: Scientific technology. *International Journal of Molecular Sciences, 24*(1). https://doi.org/10.3390/ijms24010537.

Gao, D., Hu, Y., Jiang, X., Pu, H., Guo, Z., & Zhang, Y. (2021). Applying the pathogen-targeted next-generation sequencing method to pathogen identification in cerebrospinal fluid. *Annals of Translational Medicine, 9*(22), 1675. https://doi.org/10.21037/atm-21-5488.

García-Weber, D., Dangeard, A. S., Teixeira, V., Hauke, M., Carreaux, A., Josenhans, C., & Arrieumerlou, C. (2023). In vitro kinase assay reveals ADP-heptose-dependent ALPK1 autophosphorylation and altered kinase activity of disease-associated ALPK1 mutants. *Scientific Reports, 13*(1). https://doi.org/10.1038/s41598-023-33459-7.

Ge, Z., Rogers, A. B., Feng, Y., Lee, A., Xu, S., Taylor, N. S., & Fox, J. G. (2007). Bacterial cytolethal distending toxin promotes the development of dysplasia in a model of microbially induced hepatocarcinogenesis. *Cellular Microbiology, 9*(8), 2070–2080. https://doi.org/10.1111/j.1462-5822.2007.00939.x.

Geller, L. T., Barzily-Rokni, M., Danino, T., Jonas, O. H., Shental, N., Nejman, D., Gavert, N., Zwang, Y., Cooper, Z. A., Shee, K., Thaiss, C. A., Reuben, A., Livny, J., Avraham, R., Frederick, D. T., Ligorio, M., Chatman, K., Johnston, S. E., Mosher, C. M., … Straussman, R. (2017). Potential role of intratumor bacteria in mediating tumor resistance to the chemotherapeutic drug gemcitabine. *Science, 357*(6356), 1156–1160. https://doi.org/10.1126/science.aah5043.

Gok Yavuz, B., Datar, S., Chamseddine, S., Mohamed, Y. I., LaPelusa, M., Lee, S. S., Hu, Z. I., Koay, E. J., Cao, H. S. T., Jalal, P. K., Daniel-MacDougall, C., Hassan, M., Duda, D. G., Amin, H. M., & Kaseb, A. O. (2023). The gut microbiome as a biomarker and therapeutic target in hepatocellular carcinoma. *Cancers, 15*(19), 4875. https://doi.org/10.3390/cancers15194875.

Goldberg, A. A., Titorenko, V. I., Beach, A., & Sanderson, J. T. (2013). Bile acids induce apoptosis selectively in androgen-dependent and independent prostate cancer cells. *PeerJ, 1*(1), e122. https://doi.org/10.7717/peerj.122.

Gonzalez, H., Hagerling, C., & Werb, Z. (2018). Roles of the immune system in cancer: From tumor initiation to metastatic progression. *Genes & Development, 32*(19-20), 1267–1284. https://doi.org/10.1101/gad.314617.118.

Gopalakrishnan, V., Spencer, C. N., Nezi, L., Reuben, A., Andrews, M. C., Karpinets, T. V., Prieto, P. A., Vicente, D., Hoffman, K., Wei, S. C., Cogdill, A. P., Zhao, L., Hudgens, C. W., Hutchinson, D. S., Manzo, T., Petaccia De Macedo, M., Cotechini, T., Kumar, T., Chen, W. S., … Wargo, J. A. (2018). Gut microbiome modulates response to anti-PD-1 immunotherapy in melanoma patients. *Science, 359*(6371), 97–103. https://doi.org/10.1126/science.aan4236.

Gou, H., Zeng, R., Lau, H. C. H., & Yu, J. (2024). Gut microbial metabolites: Shaping future diagnosis and treatment against gastrointestinal cancer. *Pharmacological Research, 208*, 107373. https://doi.org/10.1016/j.phrs.2024.107373.

Guerrero-Preston, R., Godoy-Vitorino, F., Jedlicka, A., Rodríguez-Hilario, A., González, H., Bondy, J., Lawson, F., Folawiyo, O., Michailidi, C., Dziedzic, A., Thangavel, R., Hadar, T., Noordhuis, M. G., Westra, W., Koch, W., & Sidransky, D. (2016). 16S rRNA amplicon sequencing identifies microbiota associated with oral cancer, human papilloma virus infection and surgical treatment. *Oncotarget, 7*(32), 51320–51334. https://doi.org/10.18632/oncotarget.9710.

Gupta, A., Madani, R., & Mukhtar, H. (2010). *Streptococcus bovis* endocarditis, a silent sign for colonic tumour. *Colorectal Disease, 12*(3), 164–171. https://doi.org/10.1111/j.1463-1318.2009.01814.x.

Hanif, F., Muzaffar, K., Perveen, K., Malhi, S. M., & Simjee, S. U. (2017). Glioblastoma multiforme: A review of its epidemiology and pathogenesis through clinical presentation and treatment. *Asian Pacific Journal of Cancer Prevention, 18*(1), 3–9. https://doi.org/10.22034/APJCP.2017.18.1.3.

Hanus, M., Parada-Venegas, D., Landskron, G., Wielandt, A. M., Hurtado, C., Alvarez, K., Hermoso, M. A., López-Köstner, F., & De la Fuente, M. (2021). Immune system, microbiota, and microbial metabolites: The unresolved triad in colorectal cancer microenvironment. *Frontiers in Immunology, 12*. https://doi.org/10.3389/fimmu.2021.612826.

He, Z., Gharaibeh, R. Z., Newsome, R. C., Pope, J. L., Dougherty, M. W., Tomkovich, S., Pons, B., Mirey, G., Vignard, J., Hendrixson, D. R., & Jobin, C. (2019). *Campylobacter jejuni* promotes colorectal tumorigenesis through the action of cytolethal distending toxin. *Gut, 68*(2), 289–300. https://doi.org/10.1136/gutjnl-2018-317200.

Henry, C., Bassignani, A., Berland, M., Langella, O., Sokol, H., & Juste, C. (2022). Modern metaproteomics: A unique tool to characterize the active microbiome in health and diseases, and pave the road towards new biomarkers—Example of Crohn's disease and ulcerative colitis flare-ups. *Cells., 11*(8), 1340. https://doi.org/10.3390/cells11081340.

Herceg, Z., & Hainaut, P. (2007). Genetic and epigenetic alterations as biomarkers for cancer detection, diagnosis and prognosis. *Molecular Oncology, 1*(1), 26–41. https://doi.org/10.1016/j.molonc.2007.01.004.

Hodi, F. S., O'Day, S. J., McDermott, D. F., Weber, R. W., Sosman, J. A., Haanen, J. B., Gonzalez, R., Robert, C., Schadendorf, D., Hassel, J. C., Akerley, W., Van Den Eertwegh, A. J. M., Lutzky, J., Lorigan, P., Vaubel, J. M., Linette, G. P., Hogg, D., Ottensmeier, C. H., Lebbé, C., … Urba, W. J. (2010). Improved survival with ipilimumab in patients with metastatic melanoma. *New England Journal of Medicine, 363*(8), 711–723. https://doi.org/10.1056/NEJMoa1003466.

Holbert, C. E., Cullen, M. T., Casero, R. A., & Stewart, T. M. (2022). Polyamines in cancer: Integrating organismal metabolism and antitumour immunity. *Nature Reviews Cancer, 22*(8), 467–480. https://doi.org/10.1038/s41568-022-00473-2.

Hou, K., Wu, Z. X., Chen, X. Y., Wang, J. Q., Zhang, D., Xiao, C., Zhu, D., Koya, J. B., Wei, L., Li, J., & Chen, Z. S. (2022). Microbiota in health and diseases. *Signal Transduction and Targeted Therapy, 7*(1). https://doi.org/10.1038/s41392-022-00974-4.

Hou, X., Du, H., Deng, Y., Wang, H., Liu, J., Qiao, J., Liu, W., Shu, X., Sun, B., & Liu, Y. (2023). Gut microbiota mediated the individualized efficacy of temozolomide via immunomodulation in glioma. *Journal of Translational Medicine, 21*(1). https://doi.org/10.1186/s12967-023-04042-5.

Hwang, S. W., Kim, M. K., & Kweon, M. N. (2023). Gut microbiome on immune checkpoint inhibitor therapy and consequent immune-related colitis: A review. *Intestinal Research, 21*(4), 433–442. https://doi.org/10.5217/IR.2023.00019.

Jabłońska-Trypuć, A. (2023). The role of the microbiome in inflammation and carcinogenesis. *Frontiers in Bioscience - Elite, 15*(4). https://doi.org/10.31083/j.fbe1504028.

Jia, D., Kuang, Z., & Wang, L. (2024). The role of microbial indole metabolites in tumor. *Gut Microbes, 16*(1). https://doi.org/10.1080/19490976.2024.2409209.

Jiang, X., Zhang, Y., Wang, H., Wang, Z., Hu, S., Cao, C., & Xiao, H. (2022). In-depth metaproteomics analysis of oral microbiome for lung cancer. *Research, 2022.* https://doi.org/10.34133/2022/9781578.

Jovel, J., Patterson, J., Wang, W., Hotte, N., O'Keefe, S., Mitchel, T., Perry, T., Kao, D., Mason, A. L., Madsen, K. L., & Wong, G. K.-S. (2016). Characterization of the gut microbiome using 16S or shotgun metagenomics. *Frontiers in Microbiology, 7.* https://doi.org/10.3389/fmicb.2016.00459.

Kandalai, S., Li, H., Zhang, N., Peng, H., & Zheng, Q. (2023). The human microbiome and cancer: A diagnostic and therapeutic perspective. *Cancer Biology & Therapy, 24*(1). https://doi.org/10.1080/15384047.2023.2240084.

Keane, L., Cryan, J. F., & Gleeson, J. P. (2025). Exploiting the gut microbiome for brain tumour treatment. *Trends in Molecular Medicine, 31*(3), 213–223. https://doi.org/10.1016/j.molmed.2024.08.008.

Khamari, R., Trinh, A., Gabert, P. E., Corazao-Rozas, P., Riveros-Cruz, S., Balayssac, S., Malet-Martino, M., Dekiouk, S., Joncquel Chevalier Curt, M., Maboudou, P., Garçon, G., Ravasi, L., Guerreschi, P., Mortier, L., Quesnel, B., Marchetti, P., & Kluza, J. (2018). Glucose metabolism and NRF2 coordinate the antioxidant response in melanoma resistant to MAPK inhibitors. *Cell Death and Disease, 9*(3). https://doi.org/10.1038/s41419-018-0340-4.

Khan, A. A., Sirsat, A. T., Singh, H., & Cash, P. (2022). Microbiota and cancer: Current understanding and mechanistic implications. *Clinical and Translational Oncology, 24*(2), 193–202. https://doi.org/10.1007/s12094-021-02690-x.

Kim, E., Lisby, A., Ma, C., Lo, N., Ehmer, U., Hayer, K. E., Furth, E. E., & Viatour, P. (2019). Promotion of growth factor signaling as a critical function of β-catenin during HCC progression. *Nature Communications, 10*(1). https://doi.org/10.1038/s41467-019-09780-z.

Kim, Y. R., Oh, J. E., Kim, M. S., Kang, M. R., Park, S. W., Han, J. Y., Eom, H. S., Yoo, N. J., & Lee, S. H. (2010). Oncogenic NRF2 mutations in squamous cell carcinomas of oesophagus and skin. *Journal of Pathology, 220*(4), 446–451. https://doi.org/10.1002/path.2653.

Kong, C., Yan, X., Zhu, Y., Zhu, H., Luo, Y., Liu, P., Ferrandon, S., Kalady, M. F., Gao, R., He, J., Yin, F., Qu, X., Zheng, J., Gao, Y., Wei, Q., Ma, Y., Liu, J.-Y., & Qin, H. (2021). *Fusobacterium nucleatum* promotes the development of colorectal cancer by activating a cytochrome P450/epoxyoctadecenoic acid axis via TLR4/Keap1/NRF2 signaling. *Cancer Research, 81*(17), 4485–4498. https://doi.org/10.1158/0008-5472.can-21-0453.

Kovács, P., Csonka, T., Kovács, T., Sári, Z., Ujlaki, G., Sipos, A., Karányi, Z., Szeőcs, D., Hegedűs, C., Uray, K., Jankó, L., Kiss, M., Kiss, B., Laoui, D., Virág, L., Méhes, G., Bai, P., & Mikó, E. (2019). Lithocholic acid, a metabolite of the microbiome, increases oxidative stress in breast cancer. *Cancers, 11*(9), 1255. https://doi.org/10.3390/cancers11091255.

Kumari, N., Giri, P. S., & Rath, S. N. (2021). Adjuvant role of a T-type calcium channel blocker, TTA-A2, in lung cancer treatment with paclitaxel. *Cancer Drug Resistance, 4*(4), 996–1007. https://doi.org/10.20517/cdr.2021.54.

Kumari, N., Pullaguri, N., Rath, S. N., Bajaj, A., Sahu, V., & Ealla, K. K. R. (2024). Dysregulation of calcium homeostasis in cancer and its role in chemoresistance. *Cancer Drug Resistance, 7.* https://doi.org/10.20517/cdr.2023.145.

Kwong, T. N. Y., Wang, X., Nakatsu, G., Chow, T. C., Tipoe, T., Dai, R. Z. W., Tsoi, K. K. K., Wong, M. C. S., Tse, G., Chan, M. T. V., Chan, F. K. L., Ng, S. C., Wu, J. C. Y., Wu, W. K. K., Yu, J., Sung, J. J. Y., & Wong, S. H. (2018). Association between bacteremia from specific microbes and subsequent diagnosis of colorectal cancer. *Gastroenterology, 155*(2), 383. https://doi.org/10.1053/j.gastro.2018.04.028.

Lai, Y. R., Chang, Y. F., Ma, J., Chiu, C. H., Kuo, M. L., & Lai, C. H. (2021). From DNA damage to cancer progression: Potential effects of cytolethal distending toxin. *Frontiers in Immunology, 12.* https://doi.org/10.3389/fimmu.2021.760451.

Lamaudière, M. T. F., Arasaradnam, R., Weedall, G. D., & Morozov, I. Y. (2023). The colorectal cancer microbiota alter their transcriptome to adapt to the acidity, reactive oxygen species, and metabolite availability of gut microenvironments. *mSphere., 8*(2). https://doi.org/10.1128/msphere.00627-22.

Lee, Y. H., Tsai, K. W., Lu, K. C., Shih, L. J., & Hu, W. C. (2022). Cancer as a dysfunctional immune disorder: Pro-tumor TH1-like immune response and anti-tumor THαβ immune response based on the complete updated framework of host immunological pathways. *Biomedicines, 10*(10). https://doi.org/10.3390/biomedicines10102497.

Lenci, I., Milana, M., Signorello, A., Grassi, G., & Baiocchi, L. (2023). Secondary bile acids and the biliary epithelia: The good and the bad. *World Journal of Gastroenterology, 29*(2), 357–366. https://doi.org/10.3748/wjg.v29.i2.357.

Li, Z., Zhang, Y., Hong, W., Wang, B., Chen, Y., Yang, P., Zhou, J., Fan, J., Zeng, Z., & Du, S. (2022). Gut microbiota modulate radiotherapy-associated antitumor immune responses against hepatocellular carcinoma via STING signaling. *Gut Microbes, 14*(1). https://doi.org/10.1080/19490976.2022.2119055.

Liang, S., Mao, Y., Liao, M., Xu, Y., Chen, Y., Huang, X., Wei, C., Wu, C., Wang, Q., Pan, X., & Tang, W. (2020). Gut microbiome associated with APC gene mutation in patients with intestinal adenomatous polyps. *International Journal of Biological Sciences, 16*(1), 135–146. https://doi.org/10.7150/ijbs.37399.

Lin, H. J., Liu, H. H., Lin, C. D., Kao, M. C., Chen, Y. A., Chiang-Ni, C., Jiang, Z. P., Huang, M. Z., Lin, C. J., Lo, U. G., Lin, L. C., Lai, C. K., Lin, H., Hsieh, J. T., Chiu, C. H., & Lai, C. H. (2017). Cytolethal distending toxin enhances radiosensitivity in prostate cancer cells by regulating autophagy. *Frontiers in Cellular and Infection Microbiology, 7.* https://doi.org/10.3389/fcimb.2017.00223.

Ling, H., Sayer, J. M., Plosky, B. S., Yagi, H., Boudsocq, F., Woodgate, R., Jerina, D. M., & Yang, W. (2004). Crystal structure of a blenzo[a]pyrene diol epoxide adduct in a ternary complex with a DNA polymerase. *Proceedings of the National Academy of Sciences of the United States of America, 101*(8), 2265–2269. https://doi.org/10.1073/pnas.0308332100.

Liu, Y., Lau, H. C. H., & Yu, J. (2023). Microbial metabolites in colorectal tumorigenesis and cancer therapy. *Gut Microbes, 15*(1). https://doi.org/10.1080/19490976.2023.2203968.

Liu, Y., Zhang, S., Zhou, W., Hu, D., Xu, H., & Ji, G. (2022). Secondary bile acids and tumorigenesis in colorectal cancer. *Frontiers in Oncology, 12.* https://doi.org/10.3389/fonc.2022.813745.

Long, S., Yang, Y., Shen, C., Wang, Y., Deng, A., Qin, Q., & Qiao, L. (2020). Metaproteomics characterizes human gut microbiome function in colorectal cancer. *npj Biofilms and Microbiomes, 6*(1). https://doi.org/10.1038/s41522-020-0123-4.

Lu, R., Wu, S., Zhang, Y.-g, Xia, Y., Liu, X., Zheng, Y., Chen, H., Schaefer, K. L., Zhou, Z., Bissonnette, M., Li, L., & Sun, J. (2014). Enteric bacterial protein AvrA promotes colonic tumorigenesis and activates colonic beta-catenin signaling pathway. *Oncogenesis, 3*(6), e105. https://doi.org/10.1038/oncsis.2014.20.

Lu, R., Wu, S., Zhang, Y.-g, Xia, Y., Zhou, Z., Kato, I., Dong, H., Bissonnette, M., & Sun, J. (2016). *Salmonella* protein AvrA activates the STAT3 signaling pathway in colon cancer. *Neoplasia, 18*(5), 307–316. https://doi.org/10.1016/j.neo.2016.04.001.

Lu, Y., Yuan, X., Wang, M., He, Z., Li, H., Wang, J., & Li, Q. (2022). Gut microbiota influence immunotherapy responses: Mechanisms and therapeutic strategies. *Journal of Hematology & Oncology, 15*(1). https://doi.org/10.1186/s13045-022-01273-9.

Luo, F., Wang, X., Ye, C., & Sun, H. (2024). Microbial biomarkers in liquid biopsy for cancer: An overview and future directions. *Cancer Control, 31*. https://doi.org/10.1177/10732748241292019.

Luo, M., Hu, M., Xu, F., Wu, X., Dong, D., & Wang, W. (2020). Preventive effect of *Lactobacillus reuteri* on melanoma. *Biomedicine & Pharmacotherapy, 126*, 109929. https://doi.org/10.1016/j.biopha.2020.109929.

Magiatis, P., Pappas, P., Gaitanis, G., Mexia, N., Melliou, E., Galanou, M., Vlachos, C., Stathopoulou, K., Skaltsounis, A. L., Marselos, M., Velegraki, A., Denison, M. S., & Bassukas, I. D. (2013). *Malassezia* yeasts produce a collection of exceptionally potent activators of the Ah (Dioxin) receptor detected in diseased human skin. *Journal of Investigative Dermatology, 133*(8), 2023–2030. https://doi.org/10.1038/jid.2013.92.

Mannion, A., Sheh, A., Shen, Z., Dzink-Fox, J. A., Piazuelo, M. B., Wilson, K. T., Peek, R., & Fox, J. G. (2023). Shotgun metagenomics of gastric biopsies reveals compositional and functional microbiome shifts in high- and low-gastric-cancer-risk populations from Colombia, South America. *Gut Microbes., 15*(1). https://doi.org/10.1080/19490976.2023.2186677.

Matsuoka, Y., Yoshida, R., Kawahara, K., Sakata, J., Arita, H., Nkashima, H., Takahashi, N., Hirayama, M., Nagata, M., Hirosue, A., Kuwahara, Y., Fukumoto, M., Toya, R., Murakami, R., & Nakayama, H. (2022). The antioxidative stress regulator Nrf2 potentiates radioresistance of oral squamous cell carcinoma accompanied with metabolic modulation. *Laboratory Investigation, 102*(8), 896–907. https://doi.org/10.1038/s41374-022-00776-w.

Matsuzaki, T., Yokokura, T., & Azuma, I. (1987). Antimetastatic effect of *Lactobacillus casei* YIT9018 (LC 9018) on a highly metastatic variant of B16 melanoma in C57BL/6J mice. *Cancer Immunology Immunotherapy, 24*(2), 99–105. https://doi.org/10.1007/BF00205585.

Mego, M., Chovanec, J., Vochyanova-Andrezalova, I., Konkolovsky, P., Mikulova, M., Reckova, M., Miskovska, V., Bystricky, B., Beniak, J., Medvecova, L., Lagin, A., Svetlovska, D., Spanik, S., Zajac, V., Mardiak, J., & Drgona, L. (2015). Prevention of irinotecan induced diarrhea by probiotics: A randomized double blind, placebo controlled pilot study. *Complementary Therapies in Medicine, 23*(3), 356–362. https://doi.org/10.1016/j.ctim.2015.03.008.

Minghetti, L. (2004). Cyclooxygenase-2 (COX-2) in inflammatory and degenerative brain diseases. *Journal of Neuropathology & Experimental Neurology, 63*(9), 901–910. https://doi.org/10.1093/jnen/63.9.901.

Mirzaei, R., Afaghi, A., Babakhani, S., Sohrabi, M. R., Hosseini-Fard, S. R., Babolhavaeji, K., Akbari, S. K. A., Yousefimashouf, R., & Karampoor, S. (2021). Role of microbiota-derived short-chain fatty acids in cancer development and prevention. *Biomedicine & Pharmacotherapy, 139*, 111619. https://doi.org/10.1016/j.biopha.2021.111619.

Mohamed, Z. S., Wu, Q., Jacome, M. A., Chen, J., & Etame, A. B. (2025). The role of gut microbiome on glioblastoma oncogenesis and malignant evolution. *International Journal of Molecular Sciences, 26*(7). https://doi.org/10.3390/ijms26072935.

Neal, J. T., Peterson, T. S., Kent, M. L., & Guillemin, K. (2013). *H. pylori* virulence factor CagA increases intestinal cell proliferation by Wnt pathway activation in a transgenic zebrafish model. *Disease Models & Mechanisms, 6*(3). https://doi.org/10.1242/dmm.011163.

Neuper, T., Frauenlob, T., Dang, H. H., Krenn, P. W., Posselt, G., Regl, C., Fortelny, N., Schäpertöns, V., Unger, M. S., Üblagger, G., Neureiter, D., Mühlbacher, I., Weitzendorfer, M., Singhartinger, F., Emmanuel, K.,

Huber, C. G., Wessler, S., Aberger, F., & Horejs-Hoeck, J. (2024). ADP-heptose attenuates *Helicobacter pylori*-induced dendritic cell activation. *Gut Microbes, 16*(1). https://doi.org/10.1080/19490976.2024.2402543.

Novielli, P., Romano, D., Magarelli, M., Di Bitonto, P., Diacono, D., Chiatante, A., Lopalco, G., Sabella, D., Venerito, V., Filannino, P., Bellotti, R., De Angelis, M., Iannone, F., & Tangaro, S. (2024). Explainable artificial intelligence for microbiome data analysis in colorectal cancer biomarker identification. *Frontiers in Microbiology, 15*. https://doi.org/10.3389/fmicb.2024.1348974.

Nowotarski, S. L., Woster, P. M., & Casero, R. A. (2013). Polyamines and cancer: Implications for chemotherapy and chemoprevention. *Expert Reviews in Molecular Medicine, 15*, e3. https://doi.org/10.1017/erm.2013.3.

Ou, J., Carbonero, F., Zoetendal, E. G., DeLany, J. P., Wang, M., Newton, K., Gaskins, H. R., & O'Keefe, S. J. D. (2013). Diet, microbiota, and microbial metabolites in colon cancer risk in rural Africans and African Americans. *American Journal of Clinical Nutrition, 98*(1), 111–120. https://doi.org/10.3945/ajcn.112.056689.

Palframan, S. L., Kwok, T., & Gabriel, K. (2012). Vacuolating cytotoxin A (VacA), a key toxin for *Helicobacter pylori* pathogenesis. *Frontiers in Cellular and Infection Microbiology, 2*, 92. https://doi.org/10.3389/fcimb.2012.00092.

Palkovsky, M., Modrackova, N., Neuzil-Bunesova, V., Liberko, M., & Soumarova, R. (2025). The bidirectional impact of cancer radiotherapy and human microbiome: Microbiome as potential anti-tumor treatment efficacy and toxicity modulator. *In Vivo, 39*(1), 37–54. https://doi.org/10.21873/invivo.13803.

Patel, D., Murray, I. A., Dong, F., Annalora, A. J., Gowda, K., Coslo, D. M., Krzeminski, J., Koo, I., Hao, F., Amin, S. G., Marcus, C. B., Patterson, A. D., & Perdew, G. H. (2023). Induction of AHR signaling in response to the indolimine class of microbial stress metabolites. *Metabolites, 13*(9), 985. https://doi.org/10.3390/metabo13090985.

Pitt, J. M., Vétizou, M., Boneca, I. G., Lepage, P., Chamaillard, M., & Zitvogel, L. (2016). Enhancing the clinical coverage and anticancer efficacy of immune checkpoint blockade through manipulation of the gut microbiota. *Oncoimmunology, 6*(1), e1132137. https://doi.org/10.1080/2162402X.2015.1132137.

Pöltl, L., Kitsera, M., Raffl, S., Schild, S., Cosic, A., Kienesberger, S., Unterhauser, K., Raber, G., Lembacher-Fadum, C., Breinbauer, R., Gorkiewicz, G., Sebastian, C., Hoefler, G., & Zechner, E. L. (2023). Microbiota-derived genotoxin tilimycin generates colonic stem cell mutations. *Cell Reports, 42*(3), 112199. https://doi.org/10.1016/j.celrep.2023.112199.

Pomyen, Y., Budhu, A., Chaisaingmongkol, J., Forgues, M., Dang, H., Ruchirawat, M., Mahidol, C., Wang, X. W., Pupacdi, B., Rabibhadana, S., Phonphutkul, K., Lertprasertsuke, N., Chotirosniramit, A., Auewarakul, C. U., Ungtrakul, T., Budhisawasdi, V., Pairojkul, C., Sangrajang, S., Harris, C. C., … Wiltrout, R. (2021). Tumor metabolism and associated serum metabolites define prognostic subtypes of Asian hepatocellular carcinoma. *Scientific Reports, 11*(1). https://doi.org/10.1038/s41598-021-91560-1.

Prahl, R. E., Khan, S., Deo, R. C., & Ulaganathan, K. (2021). The role of internal transcribed spacer 2 secondary structures in classifying mycoparasitic *Ampelomyces*. *Plos One, 16*(6), e0253772. https://doi.org/10.1371/journal.pone.0253772.

Qasem, H. H., & El-Sayed, W. M. (2025). The bacterial microbiome and cancer: Development, diagnosis, treatment, and future directions. *Clinical and Experimental Medicine, 25*(1). https://doi.org/10.1007/s10238-024-01523-9.

Qiao, S. B., Niu, M. L., Liang, W. T., Zhang, L. J., Chen, X., & Zhu, Y. K. (2025). Analysis of serum S100A12, soluble advanced glycation end products receptor, and gut microbiome in elderly patients with colorectal cancer. *World Journal of Gastrointestinal Oncology, 17*(6). https://doi.org/10.4251/wjgo.v17.i6.106393.

Ramos, A., Sadeghi, S., & Tabatabaeian, H. (2021). Battling chemoresistance in cancer: Root causes and strategies to uproot them. *International Journal of Molecular Sciences, 22*(17), 9451. https://doi.org/10.3390/ijms22179451.

Ratsika, A., Pereira, J. S. C., Lynch, C. M. K., Clarke, G., & Cryan, J. F. (2023). Microbiota-immune-brain interactions: A lifespan perspective. *Current Opinion in Neurobiology, 78*, 102652. https://doi.org/10.1016/j.conb.2022.102652.

Raza, A., Khan, A. Q., Inchakalody, V. P., Mestiri, S., Yoosuf, Z. S. K. M., Bedhiafi, T., El-Ella, D. M. A., Taib, N., Hydrose, S., Akbar, S., Fernandes, Q., Al-Zaidan, L., Krishnankutty, R., Merhi, M., Uddin, S., & Dermime, S. (2022). Dynamic liquid biopsy components as predictive and prognostic biomarkers in colorectal cancer. *Journal of Experimental and Clinical Cancer Research, 41*(1). https://doi.org/10.1186/s13046-022-02318-0.

Reuter, S., Gupta, S. C., Chaturvedi, M. M., & Aggarwal, B. B. (2010). Oxidative stress, inflammation, and cancer: How are they linked? *Free Radical Biology and Medicine, 49*(11), 1603–1616. https://doi.org/10.1016/j.freeradbiomed.2010.09.006.

Ridlon, J. M., Kang, D. J., Hylemon, P. B., & Bajaj, J. S. (2014). Bile acids and the gut microbiome. *Current Opinion in Gastroenterology, 30*(3), 332–338. https://doi.org/10.1097/MOG.0000000000000057.

Rittenour, W. R., Ciaccio, C. E., Barnes, C. S., Kashon, M. L., Lemons, A. R., Beezhold, D. H., & Green, B. J. (2014). Internal transcribed spacer rRNA gene sequencing analysis of fungal diversity in Kansas City indoor environments. *Environmental Science. Processes & impacts., 16*(1), 33–43. https://doi.org/10.1039/c3em00441d.

Roberti, M. P., Yonekura, S., Duong, C. P. M., Picard, M., Ferrere, G., Tidjani Alou, M., Rauber, C., Iebba, V., Lehmann, C. H. K., Amon, L., Dudziak, D., Derosa, L., Routy, B., Flament, C., Richard, C., Daillère, R., Fluckiger, A., Van Seuningen, I., Chamaillard, M., … Zitvogel, L. (2020). Chemotherapy-induced ileal crypt apoptosis and the ileal microbiome shape immunosurveillance and prognosis of proximal colon cancer. *Nature Medicine, 26*(6), 919–931. https://doi.org/10.1038/s41591-020-0882-8.

Rosito, M., Maqbool, J., Reccagni, A., Giampaoli, O., Sciubba, F., Antonangeli, F., Scavizzi, F., Raspa, M., Cordella, F., Tondo, L., Di Angelantonio, S., Trettel, F., Miccheli, A., D'Alessandro, G., & Limatola, C. (2024). Antibiotics treatment promotes vasculogenesis in the brain of glioma-bearing mice. *Cell Death and Disease, 15*(3). https://doi.org/10.1038/s41419-024-06578-w.

Rous, P. (1911). A sarcoma of the fowl transmissible by an agent separable from the tumor cells. *Journal of Experimental Medicine, 13*(4), 397–411. https://doi.org/10.1084/jem.13.4.397.

Routy, B., Le Chatelier, E., Derosa, L., Duong, C. P. M., Alou, M. T., Daillère, R., Fluckiger, A., Messaoudene, M., Rauber, C., Roberti, M. P., Fidelle, M., Flament, C., Poirier-Colame, V., Opolon, P., Klein, C., Iribarren, K., Mondragón, L., Jacquelot, N., Qu, B., … Zitvogel, L. (2018). Gut microbiome influences efficacy of PD-1-based immunotherapy against epithelial tumors. *Science, 359*(6371), 91–97. https://doi.org/10.1126/science.aan3706.

Roy, S., & Trinchieri, G. (2017). Microbiota: A key orchestrator of cancer therapy. *Nature Reviews Cancer, 17*(5), 271–285. https://doi.org/10.1038/nrc.2017.13.

Sakatani, A., Hayashi, Y., Saiki, H., Kato, M., Uema, R., Inoue, T., Kimura, K., Yoshii, S., Tsujii, Y., Shinzaki, S., Iijima, H., & Takehara, T. (2023). A novel role for Helicobacter pylori cytotoxin-associated gene A in negative regulation of autophagy in human gastric cells. *BMC Gastroenterology, 23*(1). https://doi.org/10.1186/s12876-023-02944-8.

Scartoni, D., Desideri, I., Giacomelli, I., Di Cataldo, V., Di Brina, L., Mancuso, A., Furfaro, I., Bonomo, P., Simontacchi, G., & Livi, L. (2015). Nutritional supplement based on zinc, prebiotics, probiotics and vitamins to prevent radiation-related gastrointestinal disorders. *Anticancer Research, 35*(10), 5687–5692.

Sears, C. L., & Pardoll, D. M. (2011). Perspective: Alpha-bugs, their microbial partners, and the link to colon cancer. *Journal of Infectious Diseases, 203*(3), 306–311. https://doi.org/10.1093/jinfdis/jiq061.

Sivan, A., Corrales, L., Hubert, N., Williams, J. B., Aquino-Michaels, K., Earley, Z. M., Benyamin, F. W., Lei, Y. M., Jabri, B., Alegre, M.-L., Chang, E. B., & Gajewski, T. F. (2015). Commensal *Bifidobacterium* promotes antitumor immunity and facilitates anti-PD-L1 efficacy. *Science, 350*(6264), 1084–1089. https://doi.org/10.1126/science.aac4255.

Soda, K. (2011). The mechanisms by which polyamines accelerate tumor spread. *Journal of Experimental and Clinical Cancer Research, 30*(1). https://doi.org/10.1186/1756-9966-30-95.

Song, X., Xin, N., Wang, W., & Zhao, C. (2015). Wnt/β-catenin, an oncogenic pathway targeted by *H. pylori* in gastric carcinogenesis. *Oncotarget, 6*(34), 35579–35588. https://doi.org/10.18632/oncotarget.5758.

Stringer, A. M., Gibson, R. J., Logan, R. M., Bowen, J. M., Yeoh, A. S. J., & Keefe, D. M. K. (2014). Faecal microflora and β-glucuronidase expression are altered in an irinotecan-induced diarrhea model in rats. *Cancer Biology & Therapy, 7*(12), 1919–1925. https://doi.org/10.4161/cbt.7.12.6940.

Sugimura, N., Li, Q., Chu, E. S. H., Lau, H. C. H., Fong, W., Liu, W., Liang, C., Nakatsu, G., Su, A. C. Y., Coker, O. O., Wu, W. K. K., Chan, F. K. L., & Yu, J. (2022). *Lactobacillus gallinarum* modulates the gut microbiota and produces anti-cancer metabolites to protect against colorectal tumourigenesis. *Gut, 71*(10), 2011–2021. https://doi.org/10.1136/gutjnl-2020-323951.

Sun, C. Y., Young, G. H., Hsieh, Y. T., Chen, Y. H., Wu, M. S., Wu, V. C., Lee, J. H., & Lee, C. C. (2015). Protein-bound uremic toxins induce tissue remodeling by targeting the EGF receptor. *Journal of the American Society of Nephrology, 26*(2), 281–290. https://doi.org/10.1681/ASN.2014010021.

Sun, J., Chen, F., & Wu, G. (2023). Potential effects of gut microbiota on host cancers: Focus on immunity, DNA damage, cellular pathways, and anticancer therapy. *The ISME Journal, 17*(10), 1535–1551. https://doi.org/10.1038/s41396-023-01483-0.

Takeshima, H., & Ushijima, T. (2019). Accumulation of genetic and epigenetic alterations in normal cells and cancer risk. *npj Precision Oncology, 3*(1). https://doi.org/10.1038/s41698-019-0079-0.

Tannock, L. R., De Beer, M. C., Ji, A., Shridas, P., Noffsinger, V. P., Den Hartigh, L., Chait, A., De Beer, F. C., & Webb, N. R. (2018). Serum amyloid A3 is a high density lipoprotein-associated acute-phase protein. *Journal of Lipid Research, 59*(2), 339–347. https://doi.org/10.1194/jlr.M080887.

Glioblastoma Multiforme (2024). https://www.ncbi.nlm.nih.gov/books/NBK558954/. (Accessed: January 18, 2026)

Teh, B. T., Fearon, E. R., Genetic and epigenetic alterations in cancer Abeloff's clinical oncology. (2019), https://doi.org/10.1016/B978-0-323-47674-4.00014-1.

Tennoune, N., Andriamihaja, M., & Blachier, F. (2022). Production of indole and indole-related compounds by the intestinal microbiota and consequences for the host: The good, the bad, and the ugly. *Microorganisms, 10*(5), 930. https://doi.org/10.3390/microorganisms10050930.

Thang, M. W. C., Chua, X. Y., Price, G., Gorse, D., & Field, M. A. (2019). MetaDEGalaxy: Galaxy workflow for differential abundance analysis of 16s metagenomic data. *F1000Research, 8*. https://doi.org/10.12688/f1000research.18866.2.

Thomas*, T., & Thomas, T. J. (2001). Polyamines in cell growth and cell death: Molecular mechanisms and therapeutic applications. *Cellular and Molecular Life Sciences, 58*(2), 244–258. https://doi.org/10.1007/pl00000852.

Ting, N. L. N., Lau, H. C. H., & Yu, J. (2022). Cancer pharmacomicrobiomics: Targeting microbiota to optimise cancer therapy outcomes. *Gut, 71*(7), 1412–1425. https://doi.org/10.1136/gutjnl-2021-326264.

Tjalsma, H., Boleij, A., Marchesi, J. R., & Dutilh, B. E. (2012). A bacterial driver-passenger model for colorectal cancer: Beyond the usual suspects. *Nature Reviews Microbiology, 10*(8), 575–582. https://doi.org/10.1038/nrmicro2819.

Tofalo, R., Cocchi, S., & Suzzi, G. (2019). Polyamines and gut microbiota. *Frontiers in Nutrition, 6*. https://doi.org/10.3389/fnut.2019.00016.

Trivieri, N., Pracella, R., Cariglia, M. G., Panebianco, C., Parrella, P., Visioli, A., Giani, F., Soriano, A. A., Barile, C., Canistro, G., Latiano, T. P., Dimitri, L., Bazzocchi, F., Cassano, D., Vescovi, A. L., Pazienza, V., & Binda, E. (2020). BRAFV600E mutation impinges on gut microbial markers defining novel biomarkers for serrated colorectal cancer effective therapies. *Journal of Experimental and Clinical Cancer Research, 39*(1). https://doi.org/10.1186/s13046-020-01801-w.

Tsuji, A., Ikeda, Y., Yoshikawa, S., Taniguchi, K., Sawamura, H., Morikawa, S., Nakashima, M., Asai, T., & Matsuda, S. (2023). The tryptophan and kynurenine pathway involved in the development of immune-related diseases. *International Journal of Molecular Sciences, 24*(6), 5742. https://doi.org/10.3390/ijms24065742.

Uchino, Y., Goto, Y., Konishi, Y., Tanabe, K., Toda, H., Wada, M., Kita, Y., Beppu, M., Mori, S., Hijioka, H., Otsuka, T., Natsugoe, S., Hara, E., & Sugiura, T. (2021). Colorectal cancer patients have four specific bacterial species in oral and gut microbiota in common—A metagenomic comparison with healthy subjects. *Cancers, 13*(13), 3332. https://doi.org/10.3390/cancers13133332.

Unterhauser, K., Pöltl, L., Schneditz, G., Kienesberger, S., Glabonjat, R. A., Kitsera, M., Pletz, J., Josa-Prado, F., Dornisch, E., Lembacher-Fadum, C., Roier, S., Gorkiewicz, G., Lucena, D., Barasoain, I., Kroutil, W., Wiedner, M., Loizou, J. I., Breinbauer, R., Fernando Díaz, J., … Zechner, E. L. (2019). *Klebsiella oxytoca* enterotoxins tilimycin and tilivalline have distinct host DNA-damaging and microtubule-stabilizing activities. *Proceedings of the National Academy of Sciences, 116*(9), 3774–3783. https://doi.org/10.1073/pnas.1819154116.

Verma, M. (2017). Mechanistic and technical challenges in studying the human microbiome and cancer epidemiology. *Technology in Cancer Research & Treatment, 16*(2), 150–158. https://doi.org/10.1177/1533034616645219.

Vétizou, M., Pitt, J. M., Daillère, R., Lepage, P., Waldschmitt, N., Flament, C., Rusakiewicz, S., Routy, B., Roberti, M. P., Duong, C. P. M., Poirier-Colame, V., Roux, A., Becharef, S., Formenti, S., Golden, E., Cording, S., Eberl, G., Schlitzer, A., Ginhoux, F., … Zitvogel, L. (2015). Anticancer immunotherapy by CTLA-4 blockade relies on the gut microbiota. *Science., 350*(6264), 1079–1084. https://doi.org/10.1126/science.aad1329.

Viaud, S., Saccheri, F., Mignot, G., Yamazaki, T., Daillère, R., Hannani, D., Enot, D. P., Pfirschke, C., Engblom, C., Pittet, M. J., Schlitzer, A., Ginhoux, F., Apetoh, L., Chachaty, E., Woerther, P.-L., Eberl, G., Bérard, M., Ecobichon, C., Clermont, D., … Zitvogel, L. (2013). The intestinal microbiota modulates the anticancer immune effects of cyclophosphamide. *Science, 342*(6161), 971–976. https://doi.org/10.1126/science.1240537.

Voigt, A. Y., Emiola, A., Johnson, J. S., Fleming, E. S., Nguyen, H., Zhou, W., Tsai, K. Y., Fink, C., & Oh, J. (2022). Skin microbiome variation with cancer progression in human cutaneous squamous cell carcinoma. *Journal of Investigative Dermatology, 142*(10), 2773. https://doi.org/10.1016/j.jid.2022.03.017.

Wahlström, A., Sayin, S. I., Marschall, H. U., & Bäckhed, F. (2016). Intestinal crosstalk between bile acids and microbiota and its impact on host metabolism. *Cell Metabolism., 24*(1), 41–50. https://doi.org/10.1016/j.cmet.2016.05.005.

Waldman, A. D., Fritz, J. M., & Lenardo, M. J. (2020). A guide to cancer immunotherapy: From T cell basic science to clinical practice. *Nature Reviews Immunology, 20*(11), 651–668. https://doi.org/10.1038/s41577-020-0306-5.

Wang, H. F., Li, L. F., Guo, S. H., Zeng, Q. Y., Ning, F., Liu, W. L., & Zhang, G. (2016). Evaluation of antibody level against *Fusobacterium nucleatum* in the serological diagnosis of colorectal cancer. *Scientific Reports, 6*. https://doi.org/10.1038/srep33440.

Wang, L., Wang, X., Zhang, G., Ma, Y., Zhang, Q., Li, Z., Ran, J., Hou, X., Geng, Y., Yang, Z., Feng, S., Li, C., & Zhao, X. (2021). The impact of pelvic radiotherapy on the gut microbiome and its role in radiation-induced diarrhoea: A systematic review. *Radiation Oncology, 16*(1). https://doi.org/10.1186/s13014-021-01899-y.

Wang, X., Fang, Y., Liang, W., Cai, Y., Wong, C. C., Wang, J., Wang, N., Lau, H. C.-H., Jiao, Y., Zhou, X., Ye, L., Mo, M., Yang, T., Fan, M., Song, L., Zhou, H., Zhao, Q., Chu, E. S.-H., Liang, M., … Yu, J. (2025). Gut-liver translocation of pathogen *Klebsiella pneumoniae* promotes hepatocellular carcinoma in mice. *Nature Microbiology, 10*(1), 169–184. https://doi.org/10.1038/s41564-024-01890-9.

Wang, X., & Huycke, M. M. (2007). Extracellular superoxide production by *Enterococcus faecalis* promotes chromosomal instability in mammalian cells. *Gastroenterology, 132*(2), 551–561. https://doi.org/10.1053/j.gastro.2006.11.040.

Wibowo, B., Kalim, H., Khotimah, H., Sujuti, H., & Wibowo, R. (2023). The effect of *Salmonella* AvrA infection on colon cancer: An in-silico study. *Asian Pacific Journal of Cancer Prevention, 24*(1), 163–170. https://doi.org/10.31557/apjcp.2023.24.1.163.

Woo, P. C. Y., Lau, S. K. P., Teng, J. L. L., Tse, H., & Yuen, K.-Y. (2008). Then and now: Use of 16S rDNA gene sequencing for bacterial identification and discovery of novel bacteria in clinical microbiology laboratories. *Clinical Microbiology and Infection, 14*(10), 908–934. https://doi.org/10.1111/j.1469-0691.2008.02070.x.

Woo, P. C. Y., Woo, G. K. S., Lau, S. K. P., Wong, S. S. Y., & Yuen, K.- (2002). Single gene target bacterial identification. *Diagnostic Microbiology and Infectious Disease, 44*(2), 143–149. https://doi.org/10.1016/s0732-8893(02)00439-x.

World Health Organization Cancer. (2025). https://www.who.int/news-room/fact-sheets/detail/cancer. (Accessed 10 January, 2025).

Wilson, S., Jones, L., Couseens, C., & Hanna, K. (2002). The links between environmental factors, genetics, and the development of cancer. In Cancer and the environment: Gene-environment interaction. National Academies Press. https://www.ncbi.nlm.nih.gov/books/NBK220897/. (Accessed: February 6, 2025).

Wu, H., Zheng, X., Pan, T., Yang, X., Chen, X., Zhang, B., Peng, L., & Xie, C. (2022). Dynamic microbiome and metabolome analyses reveal the interaction between gut microbiota and anti-PD -1 based immunotherapy in hepatocellular carcinoma. *International Journal of Cancer, 151*(8), 1321–1334. https://doi.org/10.1002/ijc.34118.

Wu, X. Q., Ying, F., Chung, K. P. S., Leung, C. O. N., Leung, R. W. H., So, K. K. H., Lei, M. M. L., Chau, W. K., Tong, M., Yu, J., Wei, D., Tai, W. C. S., Ma, S., Lu, Y. Y., & Lee, T. K. W. (2025). Intestinal *Akkermansia muciniphila* complements the efficacy of PD1 therapy in MAFLD-related hepatocellular carcinoma. *Cell Reports Medicine, 6*(1), 101900. https://doi.org/10.1016/j.xcrm.2024.101900.

Wu, Y., Jiao, N., Zhu, R., Zhang, Y., Wu, D., Wang, A.-J., Fang, S., Tao, L., Li, Y., Cheng, S., He, X., Lan, P., Tian, C., Liu, N.-N., & Zhu, L. (2021). Identification of microbial markers across populations in early detection of colorectal cancer. *Nature Communications, 12*(1). https://doi.org/10.1038/s41467-021-23265-y.

Xavier, J. B., Young, V. B., Skufca, J., Ginty, F., Testerman, T., Pearson, A. T., Macklin, P., Mitchell, A., Shmulevich, I., Xie, L., Caporaso, J. G., Crandall, K. A., Simone, N. L., Godoy-Vitorino, F., Griffin, T. J., Whiteson, K. L., Gustafson, H. H., Slade, D. J., Schmidt, T. M., … Wargo, J. A. (2020). The cancer microbiome: Distinguishing direct and indirect effects requires a systemic view. *Trends in Cancer, 6*(3), 192–204. https://doi.org/10.1016/j.trecan.2020.01.004.

Xie, Y., & Liu, F. (2024). The role of the gut microbiota in tumor, immunity, and immunotherapy. *Frontiers in Immunology, 15*. https://doi.org/10.3389/fimmu.2024.1410928.

Xing, F., Hu, Q., Qin, Y., Xu, J., Zhang, B., Yu, X., & Wang, W. (2022). The relationship of Redox with hallmarks of cancer: The importance of homeostasis and context. *Frontiers in Oncology, 12*. https://doi.org/10.3389/fonc.2022.862743.

Yang, R., & Qian, L. (2022). Research on gut microbiota-derived secondary bile acids in cancer progression. *Integrative Cancer Therapies, 21*. https://doi.org/10.1177/15347354221114100.

Ye, Z., Petrof, E. O., Boone, D., Claud, E. C., & Sun, J. (2007). *Salmonella* effector AvrA regulation of colonic epithelial cell inflammation by deubiquitination. *American Journal of Pathology, 171*(3), 882–892. https://doi.org/10.2353/ajpath.2007.070220.

Yeo, K., Wu, F., Li, R., Smith, E., Wormald, P.-J., Valentine, R., James Psaltis, A., Vreugde, S., & Fenix, K. (2024). Is short-read 16S rRNA sequencing of oral microbiome sampling a suitable diagnostic tool for head and neck cancer? *Pathogens, 13*(10), 826. https://doi.org/10.3390/pathogens13100826.

Yu, L. X., & Schwabe, R. F. (2017). The gut microbiome and liver cancer: Mechanisms and clinical translation. *Nature Reviews Gastroenterology and Hepatology, 14*(9), 527–539. https://doi.org/10.1038/nrgastro.2017.72.

Yuan, L. Z., Shi, X., Tang, D., Zheng, S. P., Xiao, Z. M., & Wang, F. (2021). Construction and preservation of a stable and highly expressed recombinant *Helicobacter pylori* vacuolating cytotoxin A with apoptotic activity. *BMC Microbiology, 21*(1). https://doi.org/10.1186/s12866-021-02262-7.

Zaki, M. H., Boyd, K. L., Vogel, P., Kastan, M. B., Lamkanfi, M., & Kanneganti, T. D. (2010). The NLRP3 inflammasome protects against loss of epithelial integrity and mortality during experimental colitis. *Immunity, 32*(3), 379–391. https://doi.org/10.1016/j.immuni.2010.03.003.

Zechner, E. L., & Kienesberger, S. (2024). Microbiota-derived small molecule genotoxins: Host interactions and ecological impact in the gut ecosystem. *Gut Microbes, 16*(1). https://doi.org/10.1080/19490976.2024.2430423.

Zhang, G., & Sun, D. (2024). The synthesis of the novel *Escherichia coli* toxin—Colibactin and its mechanisms of tumorigenesis of colorectal cancer. *Frontiers in Microbiology, 15*. https://doi.org/10.3389/fmicb.2024.1501973.

Zhang, J., Zuo, K., Fang, C., Yin, X., Liu, X., Zhong, J., Li, K., Li, J., Xu, L., & Yang, X. (2021a). Altered synthesis of genes associated with short-chain fatty acids in the gut of patients with atrial fibrillation. *BMC Genomics, 22*(1). https://doi.org/10.1186/s12864-021-07944-0.

Zhang, Q., Zhao, Q., Li, T., Lu, L., Wang, F., Zhang, H., Liu, Z., Ma, H., Zhu, Q., Wang, J., Zhang, X., Pei, Y., Liu, Q., Xu, Y., Qie, J., Luan, X., Hu, Z., & Liu, X. (2023). *Lactobacillus plantarum*-derived indole-3-lactic acid ameliorates colorectal tumorigenesis via epigenetic regulation of CD8+ T cell immunity. *Cell Metabolism, 35*(6), 943. https://doi.org/10.1016/j.cmet.2023.04.015.

Zhang, X., Coker, O. O., Chu, E. S. H., Fu, K., Lau, H. C. H., Wang, Y. X., Chan, A. W. H., Wei, H., Yang, X., Sung, J. J. Y., & Yu, J. (2021b). Dietary cholesterol drives fatty liver-associated liver cancer by modulating gut microbiota and metabolites. *Gut, 70*(4), 761–774. https://doi.org/10.1136/gutjnl-2019-319664.

Zhang, Y., Tang, N., Zhou, H., & Zhu, Y. (2024). The role of microbial metabolites in endocrine tumorigenesis: From the mechanistic insights to potential therapeutic biomarkers. *Biomedicine & Pharmacotherapy, 172*, 116218. https://doi.org/10.1016/j.biopha.2024.116218.

Zhang, Y., Thompson, K. N., Branck, T., Yan, Y., Nguyen, L. H., Franzosa, E. A., & Huttenhower, C. (2021c). Metatranscriptomics for the human microbiome and microbial community functional profiling. *Annual Review of Biomedical Data Science, 4*, 279–311. https://doi.org/10.1146/annurev-biodatasci-031121-103035.

Zheng, H. C. (2017). The molecular mechanisms of chemoresistance in cancers. *Oncotarget, 8*(35), 59950–59964. https://doi.org/10.18632/oncotarget.19048.

Zheng, S., Zhou, L., Hoene, M., Peter, A., Birkenfeld, A. L., Weigert, C., Liu, X., Zhao, X., Xu, G., & Lehmann, R. (2023). A new biomarker profiling strategy for gut microbiome research: Valid association of metabolites to metabolism of microbiota detected by non-targeted metabolomics in human urine. *Metabolites., 13*(10), 1061. https://doi.org/10.3390/metabo13101061.

Zhong, X., Chen, O., Zhou, T. J., Lü, M., Wan, J., & Chen, T. (2021). Cytotoxin-associated gene A-positive *Helicobacter pylori* promotes autophagy in colon cancer cells by inhibiting miR-125b-5p. *Canadian Journal of Infectious Diseases and Medical Microbiology, 2021*, 1–9. https://doi.org/10.1155/2021/6622092.

Zhou, P., She, Y., Dong, N., Li, P., He, H., Borio, A., Wu, Q., Lu, S., Ding, X., Cao, Y., Xu, Y., Gao, W., Dong, M., Ding, J., Wang, D.-C., Zamyatina, A., & Shao, F. (2018). Alpha-kinase 1 is a cytosolic innate immune receptor for bacterial ADP-heptose. *Nature, 561*(7721), 122–126. https://doi.org/10.1038/s41586-018-0433-3.

Zhou, Y., Tao, L., Qiu, J., Xu, J., Yang, X., Zhang, Y., Tian, X., Guan, X., Cen, X., & Zhao, Y. (2024). Tumor biomarkers for diagnosis, prognosis and targeted therapy. *Signal Transduction and Targeted Therapy, 9*(1). https://doi.org/10.1038/s41392-024-01823-2.

Zwezerijnen-Jiwa, F. H., Sivov, H., Paizs, P., Zafeiropoulou, K., & Kinross, J. (2023). A systematic review of microbiome-derived biomarkers for early colorectal cancer detection. *Neoplasia, 36*, 100868. https://doi.org/10.1016/j.neo.2022.100868.

11

Modulatory effects of gut microbiome in cancer immunotherapy: A novel paradigm for blockade of immune checkpoint inhibitors

Pankaj Bhatt[a], Hardik Chaudhari[b], Paresh Prajapati[c], Harshal S. Anwane Dhote[d] and Shilpa Rani[e]

[a]COLLEGE OF PHARMACY, COER UNIVERSITY, ROORKEE, UTTARAKHAND, INDIA [b]DEPARTMENT OF PHARMACY, COLLIER PHARMACY, NAPLES, FL, UNITED STATES [c]DEPARTMENT OF PHARMACY, GUJARAT UNIVERSITY, AHMEDABAD, GUJARAT, INDIA [d]DEPARTMENT OF PHARMACEUTICAL CHEMISTRY, SGBAU, RAJASHRI COLLEGE OF PHARMACY, MEHKAR, MAHARASHTRA, INDIA [e]DEPARTMENT OF PHARMACY, RIMT UNIVERSITY MANDI GOBINDGARH, PUNJAB, INDIA

11.1 Introduction

Cancer immunotherapy has changed the face of oncology (Desai et al., 2016; Statovci et al., 2017). This is a way to use the body's own immune system to recognize and fight cancer cells, an alternative to chemo and radiation (Luca et al., 2020). The most exciting developments in this field are immune checkpoint inhibitors (ICIs), chimeric antigen receptor T-cell (CAR-T) therapy, and therapeutic vaccines (Niccolai et al., 2019). ICIs, which include programmed death 1 (PD-1) and programmed death ligand 1 (PD-L1) inhibitors, have shown great efficacy in solid tumors like melanoma and lung cancer (Corrêa-Oliveira et al., 2016). By blocking these checkpoints, ICIs reactivate exhausted T cells and allow them to mount an antitumor response (Luca et al., 2020). CAR-T therapy involves genetically modifying a patient's T cells to express receptors that target cancer antigens and has impressive results in hematological malignancies like acute lymphoblastic leukemia and certain types of lymphoma (Rosa et al., 2015; Round et al., 2011). Therapeutic vaccines aim to stimulate an immune response against tumor-specific antigens but have not yet reached the same level of success as ICIs and CAR-T therapies (Costantini et al., 2017). Even with progress in cancer immunotherapy, applying these treatments in real life is

The Microbiome and Cancer Treatment: Overcoming Resistance and Enhancing Efficacy.
DOI: https://doi.org/10.1016/B978-0-443-33206-7.00001-7

challenging (Luca et al., 2020). A major issue is that patients respond differently; some experience significant, lasting benefits, while others see little or no improvement (Hu et al., 2018). These differences can be due to factors such as the tumor itself, patient-specific traits, and environmental factors (Hu et al., 2018). Another concern is immune-related adverse events (irAEs), where the immune system attacks healthy tissues by mistake, causing problems like colitis, dermatitis, and pneumonitis (Kamada et al., 2013). Because these factors interact, cancer immunotherapy is complex and needs to be personalized to enhance effectiveness and reduce side effects (Bauer et al., 1963). Research shows the gut microbiome plays a key role in how the immune system reacts to cancer treatments (Benveniste et al., 1971; Ivanov & Littman, 2010). The gut microbiome consists of trillions of microorganisms in the digestive tract and can influence immune response through different mechanisms (Cummings et al., 1987). Studies have discovered that certain gut bacteria can boost the success of ICIs by activating T cells and affecting inflammatory pathways (Bauer et al., 1963; Nakajima et al., 2021). For example, bacteria like *Bifidobacterium* are associated with better results in PD-1 blockade therapy (Schafer et al., 2012). On the other hand, an imbalance in gut bacteria, known as dysbiosis, is linked to worse treatment outcomes and more irAEs (Brás et al., 2020). The connection between gut health and immunotherapy response suggests that modifying the gut microbiome might be an effective way to improve treatment outcomes (Heneka et al., 2015). Strategies like dietary changes, probiotics, fecal microbiota transplantation (FMT), and prebiotics are being studied to enhance the makeup of gut microorganisms in patients undergoing immunotherapy (Consalvi et al., 2021). Understanding how gut bacteria interact with the immune system and cancer may help researchers develop personalized treatment plans using these microbial markers to benefit patients (Román-Albasini et al., 2020; Szebeni et al., 2018). As exploration into the gut microbiome and cancer immunotherapy continues, incorporating microbiome modification into clinical trials could lead to improved and safer cancer treatments (Stadtmauer et al., 2020) (Fig. 11.1).

11.2 Immunomodulatory pathways

Immunomodulatory pathways are key to immune homeostasis so the physique can reply to one-of-a-kind ailments and illnesses (Macpherson et al., 2012). Immunomodulators, elements that pleasantly tune the immune system, are necessary in this process, supporting the body's battle against ailments and regaining balance (Lu et al., 2020; Younis et al., 2021). These complicated pathways contain many mechanisms, along with microbial metabolites, Toll-like receptor (TLR) signaling, dendritic cell activation, and T-cell differentiation (Gilotra et al., 2021). Microbial metabolites such as short-chain fatty acids (SCFAs), bile acids, and tryptophan derivatives modulate the immune system. SCFAs like acetate, propionate, and butyrate are produced via the intestine microbiota via the fermentation of dietary fibers and have various immunomodulatory effects (Arguello et al., 2015). These metabolites induce bigger lymphocyte proliferation, dispose of free radical species, and modulate immune cell differentiation and function (Castellano et al., 2013). For instance, butyrate inhibits nuclear factor kappa-light-chain-enhancer of activated B cells (NF-κB), a key transcription element involved in the expression of proinflammatory

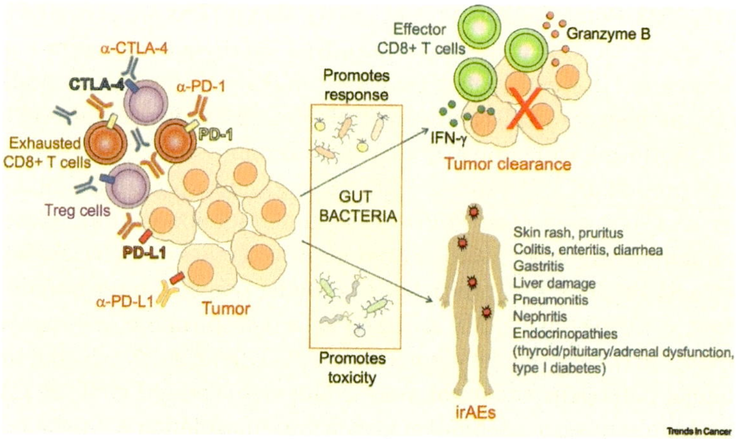

FIGURE 11.1 Gut microbiome modulation of immune checkpoint inhibitor responses in cancer. Immunotherapy: balancing efficacy and immune-related adverse events (irAEs). The dual role of gut bacteria in cancer immunotherapy is to enhance antitumor responses via effector $CD8^+$ T cells and IFN-γ production for tumor clearance. It also highlights the promotion of immune-related adverse events (irAEs) such as skin rash, colitis, and pneumonitis due to toxicity. The interplay between microbial influence, therapeutic efficacy, and irAEs underscores the need for personalized microbiome modulation strategies.

cytokines, decreasing the production of cytokines like interleukin-1 beta (IL-1β) and IL-18 and promoting the improvement of regulatory T cells (Tregs), which are necessary for immune tolerance and stopping autoimmune responses (Park et al., 2001). Bile acids, synthesized in the liver and modified via intestinal bacteria, additionally have immunomodulatory effects, activating particular receptors like Farnesoid X receptor (FXR) and TGR5 on immune cells and modulating immune responses (Gao et al., 2013; Shu et al., 2014). FXR activation can suppress proinflammatory cytokine production and promote Treg differentiation, whilst TGR5 activation can stimulate anti-inflammatory cytokine production, such as IL-10, by macrophages (Cho et al., 2003). Tryptophan, an imperative amino acid, is metabolized by intestinal microorganisms into compounds with immunomodulatory effects. Indoleamine 2,3-dioxygenase (IDO), for instance, catabolizes tryptophan into kynurenine, suppressing T-cell responses and promoting immune tolerance (Park et al., 2001). Kynurenine additionally prompts the aryl hydrocarbon receptor (AhR), modulating immune cells. Toll-like receptors (TLRs) and pattern recognition receptors (PRRs) of the innate immune system recognize pathogen-associated molecular patterns (PAMPs) and trigger signaling pathways to prompt immune responses (Rodríguez-Ramiro et al., 2012). TLR signaling is the place dendritic cell (DC) activation-and subsequent T-cell differentiation-really gets underway (Kraehenbuehl et al., 2022; Mukai et al., 2010). That's due to the fact that TLRs on immune cells like macrophages and DCs recognize PAMPs and set off the activation of transcription elements that force the expression of genes involved in immune responses (Salvadori et al., 2021). TLR2, in particular, prompts MAPK signaling pathways and NF-κB in macrophages, controlling the immune response. DCs are the bridge between innate and adaptive immunity. They specify a variety of TLRs and are tremendously responsive to TLR ligands (Liu et al., 2022; Pomatto-Watson et al., 2021). When TLRs are activated in DCs, you get maturation and activation, which results in improved expression of costimulatory molecules and cytokine secretion. Those activated DCs then migrate to the lymph nodes, where they present processed antigens to T cells and set off adaptive immune responses (Cho et al., 2003). Retinoic acid (RA) performs a function in both innate immunity and DC differentiation. It primes intestinal lamina propria DCs to express RALDH2 and end up CD103+ DCs, which in turn produce greater RA (Pietrocola et al., 2016). T-cell differentiation is quintessential in adaptive immunity. The immune response towards a unique antigen relies upon it (Lévesque et al., 2019). The stability between Th1, Th2, Th17, and Treg cells is what keeps immune homeostasis in check. Th1 cells produce cytokines like IFN-γ and TNF-α, which promote cell-mediated immunity (Ajona et al., 2020). Th17 cells secrete cytokines like IL-17 and IL-22, which assist in shielding against extracellular pathogens and autoimmune illnesses (Vernieri et al., 2022). Tregs are the ones that suppress immune responses and maintain immune tolerance. They specifically express Foxp3 and produce immunosuppressive cytokines like IL-10 and TGF-β (Wu et al., 2021). The stability between Th1/Th17 and Treg cells can be influenced by means of microbial metabolites, TLR signaling, and DC activation (Kroemer et al., 2015). SCFAs like butyrate sincerely promote Treg differentiation and suppress Th1 and Th17 differentiation. TLR signaling influences T-cell differentiation, with distinct TLR ligands advertising exceptional T-cell subsets (Groot et al., 2020). DCs play an indispensable role in the aid of presenting antigens and offering costimulatory signals. The cytokines they produce impact T-cell differentiation (Kroemer et al., 2018). Liver intestinal microbes and microbial-derived metabolites modify the development and modulation of the immune system (Kumar et al., 2021). Those pathways focusing on microbial metabolites, TLR signaling, DC activation and T-cell differentiation provide attainable aims to modulate the immune response. That influences protection towards pathogens, tissue restoration, and immune homeostasis (Ferrere et al., 2021) (Fig. 11.2).

11.3 Microbiome-immune checkpoint axis

The microbiome-immune checkpoint axis is a developing discipline of research that explores the complicated interaction between the intestinal microbiome, the immune system, and cancer therapies, mainly ICIs (Messaoudene et al., 2022; Zhang & Zhang, 2020). These inhibitors, focused on proteins like PD-1, PD-L1, and CTLA-4, have revolutionized most cancer treatment by the aid of reactivating immune cells to target tumors (Heinzerling et al., 2019). However, many sufferers no longer respond well, so we need to look into factors that affect their effectiveness (Shiravand et al., 2022). The intestinal microbiome has emerged as a key participant in ICI responses, with specific bacterial taxa and microbial metabolites playing essential roles in antitumor immunity. This complicated relationship entails modulating immune cell function, producing metabolites that have an effect on immune responses, and retaining the stability of the intestinal ecosystem, all of which affect ICI efficacy (Larroquette et al., 2021). Certain bacterial taxa like *Bifidobacterium, Akkermansia muciniphila*, and *Faecalibacterium* are key players in bettering PD-1/PD-L1 inhibitor efficacy (Yu et al., 2019). Specific *Bifidobacterium* species have been

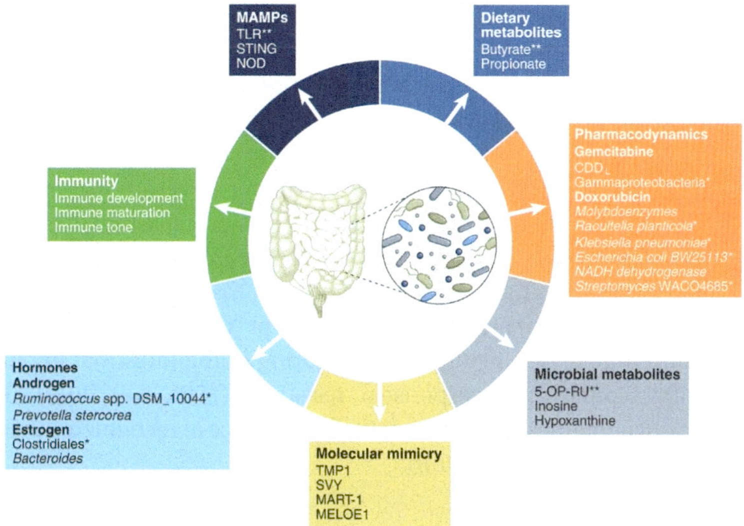

FIGURE 11.2 Hallmarks of the impact of the gut microbiome on immunity, health, and disease. The intricate effect of the gut microbiome on immunity, disease, and health, with respect to its role in hormone regulation, immune development, and pharmacodynamics. It shows the effect of individual bacteria and microbial metabolites such as butyrate on molecular mimicry and dietary metabolism. Important pathways that include Microbe-Associated Molecular Patterns (MAMPs), TLR signaling, and microbial pathogens' interaction with them are demonstrated to affect host response. *TLR*, toll-like receptor.

proven to raise ICI efficacy in preclinical research with the aid of activating DCs and facilitating CD8+ T cell infiltration into tumors, leading to elevated interferon-gamma (IFN-γ) production, which is integral for antitumor responses (Sivan et al., 2015). *A. muciniphila* has additionally been proven to improve responses to PD-1/PD-L1 inhibitors (Vétizou et al., 2015). Patients with greater tiers of *A. muciniphila* in their intestinal microbiome respond better to ICIs via the cGAS/STING pathway involved in innate immune sensing, resulting in antitumor immunity (Patel et al., 2021). *Faecalibacterium*, acknowledged for its anti-inflammatory properties and butyrate production, additionally influences ICI efficacy via modulating the intestinal environment and immune responses (Pio et al., 2019). Butyrate, produced by using *Faecalibacterium* and different fiber-fermenting gut microbes, produces Tregs, which are necessary for immune homeostasis and stopping immoderate inflammation (Younis et al., 2021). The intestinal microbiome also influences responses to CTLA-4 inhibitors, with research showing that its composition can affect responses to anti-CTLA-4 therapy (Mabbott et al., 2013; Macpherson et al., 2012). Disruption of the intestinal microbiome by way of antibiotics abrogates the antitumor outcomes of anti-CTLA-4 therapy in mouse models, highlighting the significance of a balanced intestinal microbiota for cure success (Stadtmauer et al., 2020). Specific bacterial species and microbial communities, like positive *Clostridiales* species and a combination of bacterial traces like *Parabacteroides, Alistipes,* and *Bacteroides*, have been proven to be related to higher responses to anti-CTLA-4 therapy, enhancing antitumor immunity through a range of mechanisms including modulating antigen-presenting cell characteristics and improving T-cell activation (Consalvi et al., 2021). The web page of microbial publicity additionally influences B cell repertoire development, with mucosal publicity inducing an IgA-dominant response and systemic publicity an IgM-IgG-dominant response, shaping adaptive immune responses with implications for CTLA-4 inhibitor efficacy (Brás et al., 2020). Longitudinal research of the intestinal microbiome in patients receiving ICB therapy has shown notable patterns of microbial species and pathways associated with progression-free survival (PFS) (Schafer et al., 2012). Higher stages of SCFA-producing species from the *Lachnospiraceae* family are considered in sufferers who have longer PFS after beginning ICB therapy and are associated with higher response rates and overall survival (Schafer et al., 2012). Patients with shorter PFS have greater degrees of *Clostridium spiroforme* and different *Lachnospiraceae* species and are resistant to ICB treatment (Cummings et al., 1987). These findings highlight the importance of longitudinal monitoring of the intestinal microbiome during ICB therapy to identify biomarkers of response or resistance (Hara et al., 2013). The specific microbial taxa and patient outcomes demonstrate the importance of recognizing these interactions to optimize immunotherapy (Hu et al., 2018).

11.4 Gut barrier integrity and systemic immunity

Immunomodulatory pathways are key to immune homeostasis, so the body can respond to ailments and illnesses (Jiang et al., 2021). Immunomodulators, elements that alter the immune system, are vital in this process (Castellano et al., 2013). These pathways contain many mechanisms, along with microbial metabolites, TLR signaling, DC activation, and T-cell differentiation (Liu et al., 2022). Microbial metabolites, such as SCFAs, bile acids, and tryptophan derivatives, play a massive position in modulating the immune system (Jiang et al., 2019). SCFAs produced via intestine microbiota through dietary fiber fermentation have an impact on immune cell differentiation and function by increasing lymphocyte proliferation and removing free radicals (Kroemer et al., 2015). Butyrate, for instance, inhibits NF-κB activation, reduces proinflammatory cytokine production, and promotes regulatory T cell (Treg) development, which is necessary for immune tolerance and stopping autoimmune responses (Heinzerling et al., 2019). Bile acids modified by means of intestinal microorganisms set off receptors like FXR and TGR5 on immune cells, modulating immune responses (Ferrere et al., 2021). FXR activation can decrease pro-inflammatory cytokine production and promote Treg development, whilst TGR5 activation stimulates anti-inflammatory cytokine production through macrophages (Groot et al., 2020). Tryptophan, a quintessential amino acid, is metabolized into compounds like kynurenine with the aid of indoleamine 2,3-dioxygenase (IDO), suppressing T-cell responses and promoting immune tolerance (Ajona et al., 2020). TLRs are pattern recognition receptors (PRRs) in the innate immune system that recognize PAMPs, triggering signaling cascades that set off immune responses (Salvadori et al., 2021). TLR signaling is vital for DC activation and subsequent T-cell differentiation. Upon PAMP recognition, TLRs spark off intracellular signaling pathways, leading to the activation of transcription elements like NF-κB and interferon regulatory elements (IRFs), which adjust the expression of genes involved in immune responses (Kroemer et al., 2015; Mukai et al., 2010). DCs bridge the innate and adaptive immune structures as expert antigen-presenting cells (Mabbott et al., 2013). TLR activation in DCs leads to their maturation and activation, growing the expression of co-stimulatory molecules and secreting cytokines (Román-Albasini et al., 2020). Activated DCs migrate to lymph nodes, offering processed antigens to T cells and initiating adaptive immune responses (Schafer et al., 2012). Retinoic acid (RA) modulates innate immunity and DC differentiation, priming DCs for better RA production. T-cell differentiation, vital for adaptive immunity, determines the immune response in opposition to unique antigens (Hu et al., 2018). The stability between T helper 1 (Th1), T helper two (Th2), T helper 17 (Th17), and Tregs is necessary for immune homeostasis (Statovci et al., 2017). Th1 cells promote cell-mediated immunity, Th17 cells protect against extracellular microorganisms and fungi, and are involved in autoimmune disease pathogenesis (Jiang et al., 2021). Tregs suppress immune responses and preserve immune tolerance, stopping autoimmune illnesses and controlling immoderate immune responses (Messaoudene et al., 2022). Microbial metabolites, TLR signaling, and DC activation modulate this balance (Yu et al., 2019). For example, SCFAs like butyrate promote Treg differentiation and suppress Th1 and Th17 cell differentiation (Pio et al., 2019). TLR signaling can additionally impact T-cell differentiation; unique TLR ligands promote unique T-cell subsets (Al-Khayri et al., 2022). DCs play a key function in T-cell differentiation by providing antigens and offering co-stimulatory signals. Cytokines produced by DCs also have an effect on T-cell differentiation (Younis et al., 2021). Natural killer (NK) cells contribute to mobile innate immunity by inducing mobile apoptosis in addition to specific antigen activation, which is inhibited by MHCI expression on nucleated cells (Gao et al., 2013). Properly stimulating these pathways and turning off immune responses after infections unravel are key to profitable decision and average health (Wu et al., 2021; Vernieri et al., 2022).

11.5 Probiotics and prebiotics

Probiotics and prebiotics are getting extra focus for intestinal health and overall wellness (Mukai et al., 2010). Probiotics are live microorganisms, normally bacteria, that are recommended when consumed in enough amounts, whilst prebiotics are non-digestible food factors that feed the beneficial microorganisms in the gut (Lim & Cha, 2011). Clinical use of probiotics is gaining momentum, specifically with precise strains like *Lactobacillus* spp., which have been studied substantially in many scientific trials (Ajona et al., 2020). These trials cover a range of conditions from gastrointestinal issues to immune system modulation (Kumar et al., 2021). A lot of research has been done, over 1000 scientific studies globally, for greater than 700 illnesses and conditions; probiotics are getting more and more popular (Patel et al., 2021). Notably, *Lactobacillus rhamnosus* GG and *Bifidobacterium animalis* ssp. Lactis BB12 is the most studied strain; they are the most used in probiotic research (Rodríguez-Ramiro et al., 2012). But probiotics can be stress-specific, so consequences differ throughout exclusive studies (Pomatto-Watson et al., 2021). This stress specificity is a main issue in probiotic research as it makes it hard to generalize findings throughout distinct populations and conditions (Kandere-Grzybowska et al., 2006). Also, many medical trials lack standardization of the precise strains used, dosages administered, and characteristics of the probiotic products themselves (Castellano et al., 2013). This can make it not possible to replicate outcomes and draw conclusions about the effectiveness of probiotics for unique fitness issues (Uematsu et al., 2008). The European Society for Paediatric Gastroenterology, Hepatology and Nutrition (ESPGHAN) has encouraged the restriction of probiotic use to positive prerequisites due to this variability in evidence (Nakajima et al., 2021). Moreover, meta-analyses of randomized controlled trials (RCTs) frequently yield conflicting outcomes due to variations in learning plan and populations (Luca et al., 2020). For instance, some research has proven big advantages of probiotics in decreasing signs of acute gastroenteritis and antibiotic-related diarrhea, while others have found no enormous distinction in contrast to placebo groups (Costantini et al., 2017). Such discrepancies spotlight the need for rigorous research designs that account for individual variability and, without a doubt, outline intervention parameters (Heneka et al., 2015). Also, many trials do not register their protocols earlier than participant recruitment, which raises issues about bias and methodological rigor (Csepregi et al., 2016). An assessment of medical trials confirmed that solely about 32% had been registered earlier than such as members, which is toward precise scientific exercise guidelines (Younis et al., 2021). This lack of preregistration can lead to selective reporting of effects primarily based on beneficial consequences brought up post hoc (Shu et al., 2014). Furthermore, excessive person variation amongst individuals can have an effect on trial outcomes; lifestyle choices and baseline health status can significantly affect how men and women respond to probiotic interventions (Kraehenbuehl et al., 2022). Addressing these boundaries requires higher-quality research designs that include stratification primarily based on person traits and standardized protocols for reporting results (Groot et al., 2020). Besides probiotics, synbiotics—combos of probiotics and prebiotics—are being investigated for their synergistic results on fitness outcomes (Heinzerling et al., 2019). Some research proposes that synbiotic supplementation can also enhance insulin sensitivity and metabolic profiles in persons with insulin resistance or metabolic syndrome (Jiang et al., 2019). But comparable challenges involving pressure specificity and standardization exist in synbiotic lookup as well (Vétizou et al., 2015). The more the extra physique of proof indicates advantages of probiotics and prebiotics; however, it additionally warns us to be cautious when deciphering consequences from medical trials due to stress-specific outcomes and lack of standardization in research design and product formulation (Pio et al., 2019). As we move ahead, it's necessary to comply with strict requirements for format and reporting to enable higher contrast between trials and to sooner or later understand how to use these biotic dealers in scientific practice (Heinzerling et al., 2019).

11.6 Fecal microbiota transplantation

FMT is a method in which fecal microorganisms and different microbes from a healthy donor are transferred to a recipient, typically to deal with *Clostridioides difficile* contamination (CDI) (Gao et al., 2013; Salvadori et al., 2021). It's been proven to be very effective, mainly in recurrent CDI, where it outperforms standard treatments like vancomycin (Ajona et al., 2020). The method requires cautious donor decision and stool pattern education to make sure security and efficacy (Messaoudene et al., 2022). While FMT is primarily recognized for treating CDI, its purposes extend to different gastrointestinal problems like colitis, constipation and irritable bowel syndrome, as well as neurological conditions like multiple sclerosis and Parkinson's disease (Jiang et al., 2019). The success rate of FMT for CDI is high: 85%–90% of patients improve after one treatment (Gopalakrishnan et al., 2018). FMT is a high-quality choice to extend antibiotic use, which can lead to antibiotic resistance (Mukai et al., 2010). Initially regarded as an ultimate motel due to its unconventional nature and risks, FMT is now increasingly more well-known as a fashionable therapy for relapsing CDI (Ferrere et al., 2021). The approach has gained traction in medical practice, with recent approvals for precise FMT products indicating growing recognition of its benefits (Gao et al., 2013). Optimal administration of FMT follows established guidelines that outline the steps for donor selection, sample guidance, and the proper transplantation process (Kroemer et al., 2015). The intestine microbiota is the key to FMT, a numerous array of organisms that make contributions to intestine health (Patel et al., 2021). Donor screening is rigorous, frequently involving shut spouses and children to make testing easier (Jiang et al., 2019). This screening procedure consists of clinical records comparison and laboratory checks for more than a few gastrointestinal pathogens (Cho et al., 2003). There's no standardized protocol for specimen prep; however, sparkling stool is desired to maximize bacterial viability (Kroemer et al., 2015). FMT works by displacing pathogenic organisms with recommended microorganisms through aggressive exclusion (Yu et al., 2019). In CDI, the pathogenic *C. difficile* can be countered by introducing healthy microbiota from the donor (Pio et al., 2019). Recent research advocates that bacteriophages and metabolites may additionally play a role in FMT beyond simply live bacteria (Hu et al., 2018). Restoring really useful SCFAs in the intestine after FMT is another location of interest, displaying the complexity of the intestinal microbiome (Statovci et al., 2017). Despite its promise, FMT has risks, including contamination and pathogen transmission via donor stool (Jiang et al., 2021). Thus, stringent screening measures are critical to ensuring donor protection and decreasing recipient risks (Luca et al., 2020). Regulatory troubles additionally encompass the use of FMT; feces have been designated an experimental drug in some areas since 2013, and standardization and long-term safety have become ongoing subjects of discussion (Csepregi et al., 2016). Aside from curing CDI, FMT is under investigation for advantages in treating gastrointestinal cancers and melanoma (Macpherson et al., 2012). The intestinal microbiome's manipulation of immunity shows that FMT has the promise to make most cancer treatments more effective by shaping the tumor microenvironment (Gilotra et al., 2021). Preclinical trials exhibit that FMT has the potential to make responses to immunotherapy in such cancers more effective with the aid of recognizing unique microbial signatures that are linked to treatment response (Mukai et al., 2010).

11.7 Dietary interventions

Dietary approaches, especially with an emphasis on high-fiber diets and polyphenols, have received promising results to enhance the effectiveness of immunotherapy, and ketogenic diets have been found to modulate microbial metabolite production (Kumar et al., 2021; Wu et al., 2021). The growing body of evidence suggests that dietary fiber profoundly regulates the intestinal Gut Microbiome (GMB) and consequently influences the response to immunotherapy (Yu et al., 2019). High-fiber diets have been linked with favorable PFS in melanoma sufferers under immune checkpoint blockade (ICB) (Patel et al., 2021). Clinical research exhibit that sufferers with an ordinary consumption of high-fiber diets are about 5 instances greater probably to reply favorably to anti-PD-1 therapy than these with a decrease consumption of dietary fibers (Pio et al., 2019). A mere elevation of solely 5 grams in dietary fiber consumption per day is related with a 30% reduction in disorder development risk (Wu et al., 2021). This favorable impact is due to dietary fiber facilitating recommended bacteria, like *Ruminococcaceae*, to generate SCFAs that have been observed to exert antitumor effects (Rodríguez-Ramiro et al., 2012). SCFAs such as butyrate are key to modulating immunity and boosting antitumor efficacy (Kroemer et al., 2015). High-fiber diets have been discovered to modulate the GMB to beautify an intratumoral IF-I/NK cell axis that enhances ICB efficacy and makes the tumor microenvironment more favorable to immunostimulatory phenotypes (Shiravand et al., 2022). It is not, however, an advantage uniformly recommended for all patients; prior composition of an individual's GMB before dietary intervention is crucial (Castellano et al., 2013). High-fiber diets will be more helpful for sufferers whose routine weight-loss program consists of little dietary fiber and has a dearth of microbial diversity with dominance by *Bacteroides* (Csepregi et al., 2016). Augmenting solely one ostensibly really useful taxon, like *Faecalibacterium prausnitzii*, will now not be adequate to result in higher than predicted outcomes (Schafer et al., 2012). Such findings expose the need for customized dietary techniques taking a person's unique composition of the GMB into consideration (Hara et al., 2013). Polyphenols play a tremendous role in intestinal microbiota and the modulation of the immune system (Hu et al., 2018). Polyphenols are found in an extensive range of plant-based vitamins and have anticancer outcomes via a multiplicity of mechanisms (Rosa et al., 2015). Polyphenols have the functionality to promote the boom of recommended intestinal microorganisms and beautify a symbiotic relationship that can enhance immunity (Round et al., 2011). Polyphenol-enriched diets, collectively with dietary fiber and monounsaturated fatty acids, are associated with higher response rates to immunotherapy (Bauer et al., 1963). Synergy between dietary fiber, polyphenols, and the intestinal microbiota is an area that is gaining a lot of interest in research (Schafer et al., 2012). A proresponse GMB and an eating regimen rich in dietary fiber together will likely yield beneficial effects on immunotherapy responses (Román-Albasini et al., 2020). Future research ought to intention at studying how to modulate efficiently the GMB through managed dietary interventions to optimize immunity (Mabbott et al., 2013). Unlike with high-fiber diets, ketogenic diets with low carbohydrate and excessive fats content material can have a big have an impact on on microbial metabolite production (Uematsu et al., 2008). Ketogenic diets have some promise in the area of cancer treatment, even though their affect on intestine microbiota and immunity is complicated and no longer nicely understood (Younis et al., 2021). Such diets have the achievable to exchange the intestine microbiota composition and end result in lowered manufacturing of SCFAs and different recommended metabolites (Castellano et al., 2013). Such a minimize can be quintessential for the efficacy of immunotherapy given that SCFAs are indispensable to modulate immunity (Gao et al., 2013). As such, extra lookup must be performed to decide the affect of ketogenic diets on intestine microbiota and standard impact on the efficacy of immunotherapy (Cho et al., 2003). A myriad of scientific trials is ongoing to decide the have an impact on of dietary interventions to anticancer immunity (Lévesque et al., 2019). Such trials are investigating the use of high-fiber diets as a approach aimed at optimizing the composition of the GMB to beautify the response to immunotherapy (Shu et al., 2014). As lookup goes on, future microbiome-focused dietary interventions will have to be optimized to be primarily based on patients' nonpublic GMB composition, tumor-intrinsic factors, and systemic fitness factors (Groot et al., 2020). The interface between weight loss plan and immunity suggests the viable to use dietary interventions to enhance the efficacy of most cancers treatment (Kumar et al., 2021). High-fiber diets now not solely inspire really useful microbial populations however additionally pork up metabolic pathways that want immunity in opposition to tumors (Heinzerling et al., 2019). Polyphenols supply extra degrees of complexity given that they have an impact on each microbial range and immunity via activating antioxidant movements and favoring modulation of inflammatory signaling pathways (Sivan et al., 2015). Furthermore, studying how a range of dietary patterns impact the composition of the GMB can end result in extra fine centered treatments in the subject of oncology (Gopalakrishnan et al., 2018). For example, taking a weight loss program that includes a lot of fruits, vegetables, complete grain, nuts, and healthful fat like that in the Mediterranean weight loss plan has been related with decrease irritation ranges than Western diets with a lot of processed foods (Patel et al., 2021). The discount is viewed to be a end result of the center of attention positioned inside plant-based diets that provide crucial vitamins alongside minimizing pro-inflammatory compounds (Jiang et al., 2019). The feature of prebiotics—compounds that promote the increase or activation of recommended microorganisms—must no longer be forgotten in dietary interventions for bettering the effectiveness of immunotherapy (Kumar et al., 2021). Through consumption of fibrous diets that act as prebiotics inside the gut, folks will be capable to have a effective affect upon mucosal immune activities (Kroemer et al., 2018). This have an effect on dampens enteric infection by means of elevating anti-inflammatory cytokines and reducing pro-inflammatory cytokines inside systemic circulation (Heinzerling et al., 2019). Additionally, undigested meals content material can be fermented to end up SCFAs such as butyrate inside the colon; these SCFAs are absorbed into circulation the place systemic motion upon one-of-a-kind mobile populations of the immune gadget occurs (Jiang et al., 2019). The ability of butyrate to promote T-regulatory cell (Treg) counts and suppress ranges of interferon-gamma (IFN-γ) highlights its promise of treating inflammatory conditions (Patel et al., 2021). Conversely, ketogenic diets carry about metabolic ameliorations that are probable to promote antitumor motion by means of wonderful mechanisms in contrast to these with high-fiber diets (Ajona et al., 2020). Ketogenic diets result in multiplied ranges of ketone our bodies like beta-hydroxybutyrate (BHB) that have been located to exert immunomodulatory features that may want to complement most cancers treatment options such as PD-1 blockade or CTLA-4 blockade (Mukai et al., 2010). In preclinical experiments with ketogenic diet-mice, scientists located higher T lymphocyte-dependent tumor manipulate over aggressive tumors like pores and skin melanomas and renal cancers (Shu et al., 2014). Results point out that ketogenic diets have the conceivable to beautify antitumor consequences when mixed with immunotherapies by means of boosting T-cell tumor-reactive characteristic in parallel with advisable adjustments in intestine microbiota (Gilotra et al., 2021). The metabolic transition induced by means of ketogenic diets—defined via much less glycemia with a parallel upward shove in ketone physique production—mirrors the stipulations created with the aid of fasting states that have promising promise in treating cancer

(Cho et al., 2003). Ketogenic diets can decrease tiers of circulating insulin-like boom component 1 (IGF-1) merchandising tumor growth, collectively with a surroundings conducive to superior T-cell activation in opposition to malignancies (Stadtmauer et al., 2020). Clinical trials to examine ketogenic food plan results to traditional healing procedures will higher exhibit dietary techniques that can be included into regimens towards most cancers effectively (Heneka et al., 2015). By reading shifts in fecal microbiota of sufferers with ketogenic interventions mixed with immunotherapy protocols like nivolumab or ipilimumab (anti-PD-1/anti-CTLA-4), scientists purpose to make better associations between ameliorations in intestine microbiota composition prompted with the aid of weight loss plan and therapeutic response (Luca et al., 2020).

11.8 Phage therapy and precision editing

Phage therapy, the place engineered bacteriophages are used to mainly goal and damage pathogenic bacteria, is a promising course in combating antibiotic-resistant infection (Đudarić et al., 2015). Bacteriophages, viruses that lyse and spoil bacteria, grant a selective technique of combating bacterial contamination barring unfavourable beneficial bacteria (Jiang et al., 2021). The emergence of antibiotic resistance has pushed pastime in phage remedy to new levels, main researchers to think about a number of techniques to beautify phage effectivity and host vary by way of genetic engineering (Hu et al., 2018). Bacteriophages are engineered through enhancing their genome to higher infect and lyse goal bacteria, evading bacterial protection strategies, and growing host range (Bauer et al., 1963). Gene-editing methods, such as homologous recombination and CRISPR-Cas systems, are used to edit phage genomes with preferred modifications precisely (Benveniste et al., 1971). A DNA template carrying preferred differences is delivered with the aid of homologous recombination to the host bacterium the place the template is integrated with the phage genome via recombination upon contamination with the bacterium (Cummings et al., 1987). The lambda crimson device made up of Exo, Beta, and Gam protein elements is an environment friendly device that can catalyze recombination of exogenous fragments with ease, main to improved effectivity in Escherichia coli phages (Schafer et al., 2012). However, recombination effectivity is restrained with the aid of inefficient transformation of host micro organism to take up DNA (Subramanian et al., 2015). BRED overcomes this hindrance by way of handing over phage DNA, template DNA, and exogenous recombination structures through electroporation to bacterial cells, substantially merchandising phage gene recombination, even in gram-positive micro organism with greater inflexible cell walls. CRISPR-Cas systems grant every other versatile tool to engineer phages, permitting centered and specific change of phage genomes (Uematsu et al., 2008). CRISPR-Cas structures are capable to distinguish between wild-type and engineered phages and to pick preferred phage variants (Macpherson et al., 2012). The engineered bacteriophages can also be made to counter bacterial phage resistance strategies, such as with the aid of altering phage tail fiber protein to understand choice bacterial receptors (Younis et al., 2021). Bacteriophage receptor-binding protein (RBP) amendment through altering the host vary figuring out areas (HRDRs) can alternate host vary and infectivity of the bacteriophages (Arguello et al., 2015). Evolutionary approaches, thru repeated culturing of wild-type phages with mutant lines or artificially inducing mutations in the place of the RBPs, can be utilized to alternate the bacteriophage RBPs (Park et al., 2001). Synthetic biology techniques have additionally been designed to decrease the specificity of phages and bacterial phage resistance emergence, such as structure-guided diagram and yeast-based systems to swap phage tail fiber protein (Shu et al., 2014). Concepts of customized phage remedy consist of phage determination or phage adaptation to extra efficiently infect micro organism that have been remoted at a affected person contamination site (Gao et al., 2013). One-size-fits-all methods are logistically and greater intricate than customized strategies however are extra straight away sustainable (Kandere-Grzybowska et al., 2006). Synbio and genetech advances have made phages with multiplied therapeutic practicable possible, and there is a promise of phage remedy techniques that are personalised to every affected person and infection (Pietrocola et al., 2016). As regulatory manners alter to comprise precision and customized phage therapy, engineered bacteriophages promise to assist overcome the growing hazard of antibiotic-resistant infection (Vernieri et al., 2022). Table 11.1 compiles current and concluded clinical trials in the exploration of the role of the gut microbiome in cancer immunotherapy. It outlines trial identifiers, study area, cancer targets, methodologies, and status, with a focus on observational and interventional strategies. References offer additional background to each trial result and implication.

11.9 Challenges and controversies

The world of contemporary medicine is full of complexities and controversy that influence the development and deployment of new therapies. Navigating such complexities, healthcare practitioners and scientists need to resolve the ethical, pragmatic, and scientific challenges that emerge in pursuing successful therapies (de Groot et al., 2020).

11.10 Interpatient variability

Individual variability in microbiome composition, the end result of a state-of-the-art play of genetic, geographical, and life-style factors, is a foremost venture in microbiome research and its attainable integration with customized medicine (Ferrere et al., 2021). The human microbiome, a complicated neighborhood of microorganisms occupying and masking the human body, performs a centralized feature in severa aspects of human health, ranging from immunity and metabolism to behaviors (Shiravand et al., 2022). But microbial neighborhood composition is vastly one-of-a-kind between individuals, and this contributes to variations in response to diet, drugs, and disease (Jiang et al., 2019). Genetic elements enter the equation with the aid of affecting the immune system of the host, intestine physiology, and nutrient absorption, all elements that have an oblique impact on the microbiome (Sivan et al., 2015). Some genes, for instance, can affect the production of antimicrobial peptides in the gut, exerting selective pressures that promote certain microbial species over others (Pio et al., 2019). The geographic area has a profound impact on microbiome composition due to variants in environmental exposure, dietary intake, and cultural practices (Kumar et al., 2021). People in one-of-a-kind areas are exposed to distinctive microorganisms in the soil, water, and air, and there are various

Table 11.1 Clinical trials evaluating microbial role/intervention as immunotherapy modulator in cancer.

Clinical trial Gov. identifier	Study time	Condition	Comment	Status	References
NCT02960282	Analysis of gut microbiome in fecal samples from metastatic cancer patients	Colorectal cancer (Stage IV)	Observational study focusing on biospecimen collection and laboratory biomarker analysis	Recruiting	Subramanian et al. (2015)
NCT03643289	Evaluating gut microbiome and metabolomics in melanoma Immunotherapy	Melanoma (Stage IV)	Observational study assessing gut microbiome diversity via metagenome sequencing pre- and posttreatment	Recruiting	Csepregi et al. (2016)
NCT03688347	Investigating the microbiome in lung cancer and other malignancies	Lung cancer and other cancers	Observational study analyzing nasal, oral, and fecal microbiomes, correlating with treatment responses and immunotherapy toxicities	Recruiting	Al-Khayri et al. (2022)

(*continued on next page*)

NCT03686202	Study on microbial ecosystem therapeutics (MET-4) in immunotherapy	Solid tumors	Interventional phase 1 study assessing safety, tolerability, and engraftment of MET-4 strains with immunotherapy	Recruiting	Mabbott et al. (2013)
NCT02592967	Safety and immunogenicity of JNJ-64041757 in NSCLC patients	Nonsmall cell lung cancer (Stages 3B and IV)	Interventional phase 1 study evaluating JNJ-64041757 as a standalone immunotherapy	Active	Uematsu et al. (2008)
NCT02625857	Safety and immunogenicity of JNJ-64041809 in metastatic prostate cancer	Castration-resistant prostate cancer	Interventional phase 1 study assessing JNJ-64041809 as a single immunotherapy	Completed	Macpherson et al. (2012)
NCT02843425	BE GONE Trial: Beans to enrich gut microbiome versus obesity	Colorectal cancer prevention	Interventional study evaluating the impact of fiber supplementation from beans on bacterial populations in cancer patients' diets	Recruiting	Szebeni et al. (2018)

patterns of colonization inside the gut (Castellano et al., 2013). In addition, dietary staples are special in unique areas and supply specific substrates to feed microbes and have an impact on the metabolic characteristics of the intestinal microbiome (Arguello et al., 2015). Lifestyle elements, diet, antimicrobial drug use, hygiene regimen, and degree of stress make a lot of contributions to interpatient variability (Lu et al., 2020). Diet, in general, influences microbiome composition profoundly, with special dietary patterns favoring the growth of distinct microbial species (Macpherson et al., 2012). High-fiber diets, for example, promote the growth of microorganisms that can ferment complex carbohydrates, whereas dietary consumption that is rich in saturated fats and highly processed foods can cause a change in the gingival microbiota and create dysbiosis (Al-Khayri et al., 2022). The use of antimicrobial tablets can have a dramatic effect on microbiome composition and decrease microbial richness and pick antibiotic resistance-promoting bacteria (Stadtmauer et al., 2020). Even practices such as handwashing and the use of sanitizers can affect the pores and skin microbiome and affect the transmission of microorganisms within a community (Román-Albasini et al., 2020). Temporal instability can impact the oral and stool microbial diversity (Benveniste et al., 1971). Higher intrapatient temporal variability of the oral SDI used to be related to extended contamination risk, and elevated stool SDI CVs had been related to expanded contamination risk ninety days post-IC (Bauer et al., 1963). Information about such elements is crucial to devise superb microbiome-based interventions that can be designed to meet the needs and circumstances of individuals (Jiang et al., 2021).

11.11 Technical limitations

The distinction between 16S rRNA sequencing and metagenomic sequencing highlights both technical obstacles and gaps in decision-making that scientists have to navigate when addressing microbial communities (Luca et al., 2020). 16S rRNA sequencing principally involves the amplification of a single area of the ribosomal RNA gene, as a consequence permitting bacterial taxa to be recognized at the family or genus level (Bauer et al., 1963). Though this is inexpensive and returns incredibly fast results, the technique tends to be missing in the depth that is critical to attain a holistic perception of difficult microbiomes (Cummings et al., 1987). Conversely, metagenomic sequencing aims at all the genomic content of a sample, permitting a more detailed evaluation that goes down to the species and even the stress level (Benveniste et al., 1971). Such functionality is very beneficial when surveying heterogeneous microbial populations or discovering new organisms that are currently represented in modern databases (Consalvi et al., 2021). Nonetheless, metagenomic sequencing has its shortcomings in that sequencing is more steeply priced and more computationally demanding due to the massive amount of data produced (Csepregi et al., 2016). Additionally, the presence of non-microbial DNA inside samples tends to make evaluation extra tedious because shotgun metagenomic sequencing fails to differentiate between microbial and host DNA and therefore can mask the real microbiome composition (Mabbott et al., 2013). This is in particular pertinent in human microbiome research where samples may also incorporate considerable quantities of human genetic material, such as pores and skin or oral swabs (Younis et al., 2021). In such cases, 16S rRNA sequencing may also grant clearer insights by way of focusing totally on microbial sequences. Another crucial factor to reflect on is the decision hole between these two techniques (Arguello et al., 2015). While 16S rRNA sequencing can efficiently pick out dominant bacterial populations, it frequently fails to detect less abundant taxa that may play imperative roles in fitness and sickness dynamics (Castellano et al., 2013). Metagenomic sequencing excels in this regard by presenting a more complete view of microbial diversity, which includes uncommon species that ought to be biologically significant (Shu et al., 2014). However, this accelerated decision comes at the price of complexity in information interpretation, as distinguishing between causative and correlative relationships inside microbiome research can be challenging (Gao et al., 2013). The concern in setting up causality versus correlation remains a contentious difficulty in microbiome research (Rodríguez-Ramiro et al., 2012). Many research records associations between precise microbial profiles and a number of fitness conditions; however, proving that these associations are causal rather than simply correlational requires rigorous experimental designs and longitudinal studies (Pomatto-Watson et al., 2021). The dynamic nature of microbial communities similarly complicates these analyses, as shifts in composition can take place due to environmental factors, dietary changes, or host interactions (Vernieri et al., 2022). Thus, whilst metagenomic sequencing gives improved decision-making and a broader grasp of microbial ecosystems, it additionally necessitates careful consideration of the study plan to draw significant conclusions about causality. Additionally, each method faces barriers associated with its respective databases and analytical tools (Kroemer et al., 2015). The precision of taxonomic classification relies upon the completeness of reference libraries; areas of lacking records inside reference libraries can result in misidentifications or underestimation of specific taxa (Ferrere et al., 2021). As scientists delve similarly and similarly afield to pattern the richness of microbial life, there is a need to proceed to construct upon and refine reference libraries and more effective bioinformatics equipment that can cope with state-of-the-art datasets produced through metagenomic strategies (Sivan et al., 2015). In conclusion, even though 16S rRNA sequencing is a beneficial tool utilized to make preliminary estimates of microbial diversity and community composition, its taxonomic shortcomings and failure to detect rare taxa display that alternative techniques like metagenomic sequencing are necessary (Vétizou et al., 2015). The latter now not only has greater depth but also offers information and interpretation complexity challenges to be conscious of in the layout of studies (Gopalakrishnan et al., 2018). As we understand more about the microbiome, overcoming these technical challenges will be vital to push research and translate findings to the hospital to make contributions to higher fitness advantages to humans (Mukai et al., 2010). Ultimately, the employment of each 16S rRNA and metagenomic sequencing strategies will provide a higher understanding of microbial communities and their characteristic in disease and health, and will lead to revolutionary therapy protocols to benefit from the strength of the microbiome (Rodríguez-Ramiro et al., 2012).

11.12 Regulatory and ethical hurdles

The hastily creating self-discipline of microbiome-based treatment plans is a challenge to outstanding regulatory and moral challenges that need to be met to supply assurance of patient protection and promote innovation (Castellano et al., 2013). The U.S. Food and Drug Administration (FDA) and the European Medicines Agency (EMA) are each proactively growing unique pointers for these new therapies, but broad chasms and uncertainties persist (Macpherson et al., 2012). The cutting-edge framework inside the FDA oversees products made of or affecting microbes, such as FMT, live biotherapeutic products, and live microbes in foods, to reflect the variety of purposes and workable consequences of microbiome research (Subramanian et al., 2015). The FDA approval of microbiome-based treatment options such as Rebyota and Vowst for recurrent *Clostridioides difficile* contamination (rCDI) is, in basic terms, the first step taken in overcoming the elaborate regulatory framework (Szebeni et al., 2018). One of the largest challenges is the full enlargement and harmonization of regulatory structures that are involved in the manufacturing improvement of stay biotherapeutic products (Heneka et al., 2015). These therapies, designed to address dysbiosis within the gut microbiome, require controlled manufacturing processes, defined analytical testing methods, and established clinical performance, necessitating clear regulatory guidance and expectations (Nakajima et al., 2021). The complexity of the gut microbiome, consisting of hundreds of bacterial species influencing gut activity, neural development, and drug response, makes it difficult to determine definitive links between the microbiome and human health (Hara et al., 2013). FMT, involving the transfer of fecal matter from a healthy donor to a recipient, presents unique safety concerns, particularly the risk of pathogen transmission (Luca et al., 2020). Although FMT has shown promise in treating rCDI and is recommended in both U.S. and European treatment guidelines for second or further CDI recurrence, the procedure carries inherent risks that require careful consideration (Hu et al., 2018). The FDA has issued statements on the risk of pathogen transmission associated with FMT, emphasizing the need for rigorous screening of stool donors for pathogens to mitigate potential risks (Rosa et al., 2015). Rebyota, administered by using enema, relies upon stool donors, and for that reason experiences scalability issues; however, it employs a novel *Microbiota Restoration Platform* to cut down contamination risk (Benveniste et al., 1971). The ethics associated with FMT are now not restricted to the transmission of pathogens to encompass problems of donor choice, informed consent, and the risk of long-term health consequences to recipients (Schafer et al., 2012). FMT remedy, no longer having been approved by regulatory agencies, provides many ethical, legal, and societal problems that will need to be overcome under an efficacious regulatory policy response (Hu et al., 2018). Maintaining accurate manufacturing exercise (GMP) and sufficient good measures to ensure consistency are key to overcoming issues of protection and public belief in microbiome modalities (Macpherson et al., 2012). Passing regulatory and analytical troubles with the improvement and manufacture of stay biotherapeutic products needs cooperation between regulatory and governmental agencies, industry, and academe (Arguello et al., 2015). Filling regulatory gaps, optimization of the analytics to better represent Live Biotherapeutic Products, and a definition of recommendations in medical trials will be imperative steps to propel the field (Lévesque et al., 2019). As microbiome modalities are developing, nonstop conversation and cooperation between stakeholders will be essential to make certain that such novel remedies are manufactured and utilized in a safe, ethical, and efficacious manner to benefit patients (Kumar et al., 2021).

11.13 Future directions

The future of microbiome personalization is very promising with the improvement of AI-based microbiome profiling to stratify patients (Sivan et al., 2015). As we acquire perception into the microbial populace that inhabits the human body, we become more conscious of the role the microbiome plays in health and disease and its effect on processes ranging from metabolism to immunity (Patel et al., 2021). AI applied sciences have the functionality to process copious quantities of microbiome information and become aware of wonderful microbial signatures that are linked to distinct conditions (Younis et al., 2021). This creates an extra correct mode of affected person stratification, where healthcare practitioners are capable of customizing interventions to suit patients based on their microbial profile (Uematsu et al., 2008). Utilizing a desktop to gain knowledge of algorithms, scientists are in a position to become aware of tricky patterns and relationships inside microbiome profiles that are now not detectable with traditional analysis (Mabbott et al., 2013). This now not only deepens our perception of the exclusive microbiomes and their effect upon patients but also enables the development of custom-made treatment techniques taking every patient's microbial profile into account (Luca et al., 2020). For example, people struggling with a precise intestinal disease should be helped with focused dietary plans or probiotherapy that aims to create an appropriate stability inside their microbiota (Costantini et al., 2017). AI-based profiling is additionally in a position to assist docs forecast responses to therapies, particularly in the discipline of treating tumors where the microbiome has been discovered to have a direct impact upon the efficacy of immunotherapy (Rosa et al., 2015). By reading the content material and practical competencies of a patient's microbiome, healthcare experts are capable of make knowledgeable picks pertaining to the plausible cures that will be most effective, with the possible to streamline redress and minimize side effects (Niccolai et al., 2019). In addition, personalized microbiome engineering would be extended to preventive medicine to pick out humans at risk of developing specific diseases based on their microbiome signature (Al-Khayri et al., 2022; Uematsu et al., 2008). This preventive method would result in early interventions that preserve a healthier microbiome and stop disorder development (Lu et al., 2020). As applied sciences proceed to improve, combining genomic sequencing with AI-based evaluation will proceed to enhance the capability to understand and manipulate the microbiome with a therapeutic aim (Arguello et al., 2015). Coupling state-of-the-art top-of-the-line sequencing applied sciences with superior bioinformatics will furnish scientists with the equipment to delve deeper into the purposeful roles of targeted microbial taxa, paving the way to progressive techniques that leverage the energy of the microbiome to customize medicine (Al-Khayri et al., 2022). Additionally, problems of ethics associated with customized microbiome engineering will have to be mentioned as we proceed forward (Castellano et al., 2013). Providing equal get entry to such modern-day applied sciences and making sure affected person privateness will be imperative to gaining public and constructing public have confidence and acceptance (Kandere-Grzybowska et al., 2006). Navigating these troubles will require cooperation between researchers, clinicians, and policymakers to strengthen rules that prioritize the affected person first and motivate innovation in microbiome science (Groot et al., 2020).

11.14 Conclusion

The gut microbiome has a profound effect on cancer immunotherapy by improving the effectiveness of ICIs, CAR-T cell therapy, and therapeutic vaccine treatment. Certain bacteria, e.g., *Bifidobacterium* and *A. muciniphila*, and metabolites like SCFAs promote antitumor immunity by stimulating T-cells and inflammatory modulation. Dysbiosis, by contrast, is associated with poor treatment response and increased irAEs and calls for microbial equilibrium. Interventions like a diet high in fiber, probiotics, prebiotics, FMT, and phage therapy hold promise to fine-tune the response to immunotherapy. Clinical trials demonstrate that dietary supplementation with high fiber improves PFS, and FMT can enhance the efficacy of ICI by remolding the tumor microenvironment. AI-assisted microbiome profiling further allows for personalized treatment by predicting microbial signatures of therapeutic efficacy. In spite of all this, interindividual variability, technical constraints in sequencing, and regulatory issues continue to be a hindrance. Standardized protocols and robust trial protocols are essential to overcome them, together with some ethical issues of equitable access and patient privacy. Modulation of the microbiome added to immunotherapy promises a new era in the field of oncology with better efficacy and fewer side effects. Multidisciplinary collaborative efforts by researchers, clinicians, and policymakers are essential to translate this knowledge into bedside practices and make microbiome-based interventions a pillar of personalized cancer treatment.

References

Ajona, D., Ortiz-Espinosa, S., Lozano, T., Exposito, F., Calvo, A., Valencia, K., Redrado, M., Remírez, A., Lecanda, F., Alignani, D., Lasarte, J. J., Macaya, I., Senent, Y., Bértolo, C., Sainz, C., Gil-Bazo, I., Eguren-Santamaría, I., Lopez-Picazo, J. M., Gonzalez, A., … Pio, R. (2020). Short-term starvation reduces IGF-1 levels to sensitize lung tumors to PD-1 immune checkpoint blockade. *Nature Cancer, 1*(1), 75–85. https://doi.org/10.1038/s43018-019-0007-9.

Al-Khayri, J. M., Sahana, G. R., Nagella, P., Joseph, B. V., Alessa, F. M., & Al-Mssallem, M. Q. (2022). Flavonoids as potential anti-inflammatory molecules: A review. *Molecules, 27*(9). https://doi.org/10.3390/molecules27092901.

Arguello, M. A., Schulze, K. J., Wu, L. S. F., Dreyfuss, M. L., Khatry, S. K., Christian, P., & West, K. P. (2015). Circulating IGF-1 may mediate improvements in haemoglobin associated with vitamin A status during pregnancy in rural Nepalese women. *Asia Pacific Journal of Clinical Nutrition, 24*(1), 128–137. https://doi.org/10.6133/apjcn.2015.24.1.12.

Bauer, H., Horowitz, R. E., Levenson, S. M., & Popper, H. (1963). The response of the lymphatic tissue to the microbial flora. Studies on germfree mice. *The American journal of pathology., 42*, 471–483.

Benveniste, J., Lespinats, G., Adam, C., & Salomon, J. C. (1971). Immunoglobulins in intact, immunized, and contaminated axenic mice: Study of serum IgA. *Journal of Immunology, 107*(6), 1647–1655.

Brás, J. P., Bravo, J., Freitas, J., Barbosa, M. A., Santos, S. G., Summavielle, T., & Almeida, M. I. (2020). TNF-alpha-induced microglia activation requires miR-342: Impact on NF-kB signaling and neurotoxicity. *Cell Death and Disease, 11*(6). https://doi.org/10.1038/s41419-020-2626-6.

Castellano, G., González-Santander, J. L., Lara, A., & Torrens, F. (2013). Classification of flavonoid compounds by using entropy of information theory. *Phytochemistry, 93*, 182–191. https://doi.org/10.1016/j.phytochem.2013.03.024.

Cho, S. Y., Park, S. J., Kwon, M. J., Jeong, T. S., Bok, S. H., Choi, W. Y., Jeong, W. I., Ryu, S. Y., Do, S. H., Lee, C. S., Song, J. C., & Jeong, K. S. (2003). Quercetin suppresses proinflammatory cytokines production through MAP kinases and NF-κB pathway in lipopolysaccharide-stimulated macrophage. *Molecular and Cellular Biochemistry, 243*(1-2), 153–160. https://doi.org/10.1023/A:1021624520740.

Consalvi, S., Poce, G., Ghelardini, C., Mannelli, L. D. iC., Patrignani, P., Bruno, A., Anzini, M., Calderone, V., Martelli, A., Testai, L., Giordani, A., & Biava, M. (2021). Therapeutic potential for coxibs-nitric oxide releasing hybrids in cystic fibrosis. *European Journal of Medicinal Chemistry, 210*, 112983. https://doi.org/10.1016/j.ejmech.2020.112983.

Corrêa-Oliveira, R., Fachi, J. L., Vieira, A., Sato, F. T., & Vinolo, M. A. R. (2016). Regulation of immune cell function by short-chain fatty acids. *Clinical and Translational Immunology, 5*(4). https://doi.org/10.1038/cti.2016.17.

Costantini, L., Molinari, R., Farinon, B., & Merendino, N. (2017). Impact of omega-3 fatty acids on the gut microbiota. *International Journal of Molecular Sciences, 18*(12), 2645. https://doi.org/10.3390/ijms18122645.

Csepregi, K., Neugart, S., Schreiner, M., & Hideg, É (2016). Comparative evaluation of total antioxidant capacities of plant polyphenols. *Molecules, 21*(2), 208. https://doi.org/10.3390/molecules21020208.

Cummings, J. H., Pomare, E. W., Branch, W. J., Naylor, C. P., & Macfarlane, G. T. (1987). Short chain fatty acids in human large intestine, portal, hepatic and venous blood. *Gut, 28*(10), 1221–1227. https://doi.org/10.1136/gut.28.10.1221.

de Groot, S., Lugtenberg, R. T., Cohen, D., Welters, M. J. P., Ehsan, I., Vreeswijk, M. P. G., Smit, V. T. H. B. M., Graaf, H., Heijns, J. B., Portielje, J. E. A., Wouw, A. J., Imholz, A. L. T., Kessels, L. W., Vrijaldenhoven, S., Baars, A., Kranenbarg, E. M.-K., Carpentier, M. D.-, Putter, H., Hoeven, J. J. M., … Kroep, J. R. (2020). Fasting mimicking diet as an adjunct to neoadjuvant chemotherapy for breast cancer in the multicentre randomized phase 2 DIRECT trial. *Nature Communications, 11*(1). https://doi.org/10.1038/s41467-020-16138-3.

Desai, M. S., Seekatz, A. M., Koropatkin, N. M., Kamada, N., Hickey, C. A., Wolter, M., Pudlo, N. A., Kitamoto, S., Terrapon, N., Muller, A., Young, V. B., Henrissat, B., Wilmes, P., Stappenbeck, T. S., Núñez, G., & Martens, E. C. (2016). A dietary fiber-deprived gut microbiota degrades the colonic mucus barrier and enhances pathogen susceptibility. *Cell, 167*(5), 1339. https://doi.org/10.1016/j.cell.2016.10.043.

Đudarić, L., Fužinac-Smojver, A., Muhvić, D., & Giacometti, J. (2015). The role of polyphenols on bone metabolism in osteoporosis. *Food Research International, 77*, 290–298. https://doi.org/10.1016/j.foodres.2015.10.017.

Ferrere, G., Alou, M. T., Liu, P., Goubet, A.-G., Fidelle, M., Kepp, O., Durand, S., Iebba, V., Fluckiger, A., Daillère, R., Thelemaque, C., Grajeda-Iglesias, C., Silva, C. A. C., Aprahamian, F., Lefevre, D., Zhao, L., Ryffel, B., Colomba, E., Arnedos, M., … Zitvogel, L. (2021). Ketogenic diet and ketone bodies enhance the anticancer effects of PD-1 blockade. *JCI Insight, 6*(2). https://doi.org/10.1172/jci.insight.145207.

Gao, Y., Li, W., Jia, L., Li, B., Chen, Y. C., & Tu, Y. (2013). Enhancement of (−)-epigallocatechin-3-gallate and theaflavin-3-3′-digallate induced apoptosis by ascorbic acid in human lung adenocarcinoma SPC-A-1 cells and esophageal carcinoma Eca-109 cells via MAPK pathways. *Biochemical and Biophysical Research Communications, 438*(2), 370–374. https://doi.org/10.1016/j.bbrc.2013.07.078.

Gilotra, N. A., Wand, A. L., Pillarisetty, A., Devraj, M., Pavlovic, N., Ahmed, S., Saad, E., Solnes, L., Garcia, C., Okada, D. R., Constantinescu, F., Mohammed, S. F., Griffin, J. M., Kasper, E. K., Chen, E. S., & Sheikh, F. H. (2021). Clinical and imaging response to tumor necrosis factor alpha inhibitors in treatment of cardiac sarcoidosis: A multicenter experience. *Journal of Cardiac Failure, 27*(1), 83–91. https://doi.org/10.1016/j.cardfail.2020.08.013.

Gopalakrishnan, V., Spencer, C. N., Nezi, L., Reuben, A., Andrews, M. C., Karpinets, T. V., Prieto, P. A., Vicente, D., Hoffman, K., Wei, S. C., Cogdill, A. P., Zhao, L., Hudgens, C. W., Hutchinson, D. S., Manzo, T., Petaccia de Macedo, M., Cotechini, T., Kumar, T., Chen, W. S., … Wargo, J. A. (2018). Gut microbiome modulates response to anti–PD-1 immunotherapy in melanoma patients. *Science, 359*(6371), 97–103. https://doi.org/10.1126/science.aan4236.

Hara, N., Alkanani, A. K., Ir, D., Robertson, C. E., Wagner, B. D., Frank, D. N., & Zipris, D. (2013). The role of the intestinal microbiota in type 1 diabetes. *Clinical Immunology, 146*(2), 112–119. https://doi.org/10.1016/j.clim.2012.12.001.

Heinzerling, L., Toni, G. S., Hundorfean, G., & Zimmer, L. (2019). *Checkpoint inhibitors: The diagnosis and treatment of side effects*: 116. Deutsches Ärzteblatt International https://doi.org/10.3238/ARZTEBL.2019.0119.

Heneka, M. T., Carson, M. J., Khoury, J. E., Landreth, G. E., Brosseron, F., Feinstein, D. L., Jacobs, A. H., Wyss-Coray, T., Vitorica, J., Ransohoff, R. M., Herrup, K., Frautschy, S. A., Finsen, B., Brown, G. C., Verkhratsky, A., Yamanaka, K., Koistinaho, J., Latz, E., Halle, A., … Kummer, M. P. (2015). Neuroinflammation in Alzheimer's disease. *The Lancet Neurology, 14*(4), 388–405. https://doi.org/10.1016/S1474-4422(15)70016-5.

Hu, L., Yin, C., Zhao, F., Ali, A., Ma, J., & Qian, A. (2018). Mesenchymal stem cells: Cell fate decision to osteoblast or adipocyte and application in osteoporosis treatment. *International Journal of Molecular Sciences, 19*(2), 360. https://doi.org/10.3390/ijms19020360.

Ivanov, I. I., & Littman, D. R. (2010). Segmented filamentous bacteria take the stage. *Mucosal Immunology, 3*(3), 209–212. https://doi.org/10.1038/mi.2010.3.

Kamada, N., Seo, S. U., Chen, G. Y., & Núñez, G. (2013). Role of the gut microbiota in immunity and inflammatory disease. *Nature Reviews Immunology, 13*(5), 321–335. https://doi.org/10.1038/nri3430.

Kraehenbuehl, L., Weng, C.-H., Eghbali, S., Wolchok, J. D., & Merghoub, T. (2022). Enhancing immunotherapy in cancer by targeting emerging immunomodulatory pathways. *Nature Reviews Clinical Oncology, 19*(1), 37–50. https://doi.org/10.1038/s41571-021-00552-7.

Kroemer, G., López-Otín, C., Madeo, F., & de Cabo, R. (2018). Carbotoxicity—Noxious effects of carbohydrates. *Cell, 175*(3), 605–614. https://doi.org/10.1016/j.cell.2018.07.044.

Kroemer, G., Senovilla, L., Galluzzi, L., André, F., & Zitvogel, L. (2015). Natural and therapy-induced immunosurveillance in breast cancer. *Nature Medicine, 21*(10), 1128–1138. https://doi.org/10.1038/nm.3944.

Kumar, S., Behl, T., Sachdeva, M., Sehgal, A., Kumari, S., Kumar, A., Kaur, G., Narayan Yadav, H., & Bungau, S. (2021). Implicating the effect of ketogenic diet as a preventive measure to obesity and diabetes mellitus. *Life Sciences, 264*, 118661. https://doi.org/10.1016/j.lfs.2020.118661.

Larroquette, M., Domblides, C., Lefort, F., Lasserre, M., Quivy, A., Sionneau, B., Bertolaso, P., Gross-Goupil, M., Ravaud, A., & Daste, A. (2021). Combining immune checkpoint inhibitors with chemotherapy in advanced solid tumours: A review. *European Journal of Cancer, 158*, 47–62. https://doi.org/10.1016/j.ejca.2021.09.013.

Lévesque, S., Le Naour, J., Pietrocola, F., Paillet, J., Kremer, M., Castoldi, F., Baracco, E. E., Wang, Y., Vacchelli, E., Stoll, G., Jolly, A., De La Grange, P., Zitvogel, L., Kroemer, G., & Pol, J. G. (2019). A synergistic triad of chemotherapy, immune checkpoint inhibitors, and caloric restriction mimetics eradicates tumors in mice. *OncoImmunology, 8*(11). https://doi.org/10.1080/2162402X.2019.1657375.

Lim, Y. C., & Cha, Y. Y. (2011). Epigallocatechin-3-gallate induces growth inhibition and apoptosis of human anaplastic thyroid carcinoma cells through suppression of EGFR/ERK pathway and cyclin B1/CDK1 complex. *Journal of Surgical Oncology, 104*(7), 776–780. https://doi.org/10.1002/jso.21999.

Liu, D., Huang, Y., Huang, C., Yang, S., Wei, X., Zhang, P., Guo, D., Lin, J., Xu, B., Li, C., He, H., He, J., Liu, S., Shi, L., Xue, Y., & Zhang, H. (2022). Calorie restriction with or without time-restricted eating in weight loss. *New England Journal of Medicine, 386*(16), 1495–1504. https://doi.org/10.1056/nejmoa2114833.

Lu, Y., Xue, J., Deng, T., Zhou, X., Yu, K., Deng, L., Huang, M., Yi, X., Liang, M., Wang, Y., Shen, H., Tong, R., Wang, W., Li, L., Song, J., Li, J., Su, X., Ding, Z., Gong, Y., … Mok, T. (2020). Safety and feasibility of CRISPR-edited T cells in patients with refractory non-small-cell lung cancer. *Nature Medicine, 26*(5), 732–740. https://doi.org/10.1038/s41591-020-0840-5.

Luca, S. V., Macovei, I., Bujor, A., Miron, A., Skalicka-Woźniak, K., Aprotosoaie, A. C., & Trifan, A. (2020). Bioactivity of dietary polyphenols: The role of metabolites. *Critical Reviews in Food Science and Nutrition, 60*(4), 626–659. https://doi.org/10.1080/10408398.2018.1546669.

Mabbott, N. A., Donaldson, D. S., Ohno, H., Williams, I. R., & Mahajan, A. (2013). Microfold (M) cells: Important immunosurveillance posts in the intestinal epithelium. *Mucosal Immunology, 6*(4), 666–677. https://doi.org/10.1038/mi.2013.30.

Macpherson, A. J., Geuking, M. B., Slack, E., Hapfelmeier, S., & McCoy, K. D. (2012). The habitat, double life, citizenship, and forgetfulness of IgA. *Immunological Reviews, 245*(1), 132–146. https://doi.org/10.1111/j.1600-065X.2011.01072.x.

Messaoudene, M., Pidgeon, R., Richard, C., Ponce, M., Diop, K., Benlaifaoui, M., Nolin-Lapalme, A., Cauchois, F., Malo, J., Belkaid, W., Isnard, S., Fradet, Y., Dridi, L., Velin, D., Oster, P., Raoult, D., Ghiringhelli, F., Boidot, R., Chevrier, S., ... Routy, B. (2022). A natural polyphenol exerts antitumor activity and circumvents anti–PD-1 resistance through effects on the gut microbiota. *Cancer Discovery, 12*(4), 1070–1087. https://doi.org/10.1158/2159-8290.cd-21-0808.

Mukai, R., Shirai, Y., Saito, N., Fukuda, I., Nishiumi, S., Yoshida, K.-, & Ashida, H. (2010). Suppression mechanisms of flavonoids on aryl hydrocarbon receptor-mediated signal transduction. *Archives of Biochemistry and Biophysics, 501*(1), 134–141. https://doi.org/10.1016/j.abb.2010.05.002.

Nakajima, Y., Chamoto, K., Oura, T., & Honjo, T. (2021). Critical role of the CD44lowCD62Llow CD8+ T cell subset in restoring antitumor immunity in aged mice. *Proceedings of the National Academy of Sciences of the United States of America, 118*(23). https://doi.org/10.1073/pnas.2103730118.

Niccolai, E., Baldi, S., Ricci, F., Russo, E., Nannini, G., Menicatti, M., Poli, G., Taddei, A., Bartolucci, G., Calabrò, A. S., Stingo, F. C., & Amedei, A. (2019). Evaluation and comparison of short chain fatty acids composition in gut diseases. *World Journal of Gastroenterology, 25*(36), 5543–5558. https://doi.org/10.3748/wjg.v25.i36.5543.

Park, J. W., Choi, Y. J., Suh, S. I., & Kwon, T. K. (2001). Involvement of ERK and protein tyrosine phosphatase signaling pathways in EGCG-induced cyclooxygenase-2 expression in Raw 264.7 cells. *Biochemical and Biophysical Research Communications, 286*(4), 721–725. ttps://doi.org/10.1006/bbrc.2001.5415.

Patel, P., Poudel, A., Kafle, S., Thapa Magar, M., & Cancarevic, I. (2021). Influence of microbiome and antibiotics on the efficacy of immune checkpoint inhibitors. *Cureus, 13*(8). https://doi.org/10.7759/cureus.16829.

Pietrocola, F., Pol, J., Vacchelli, E., Rao, S., Enot, D. P., Baracco, E. E., Levesque, S., Castoldi, F., Jacquelot, N., Yamazaki, T., Senovilla, L., Marino, G., Aranda, F., Durand, S., Sica, V., Chery, A., Lachkar, S., Sigl, V., Bloy, N., ... Kroemer, G. (2016). Caloric restriction mimetics enhance anticancer immunosurveillance. *Cancer Cell, 30*(1), 147–160. https://doi.org/10.1016/j.ccell.2016.05.016.

Pio, R., Ajona, D., Ortiz-Espinosa, S., Mantovani, A., & Lambris, J. D. (2019). Complementing the cancer-immunity cycle. *Frontiers in Immunology, 10*. https://doi.org/10.3389/fimmu.2019.00774.

Pomatto-Watson, L. C. D., Bodogai, M., Bosompra, O., Kato, J., Wong, S., Carpenter, M., Duregon, E., Chowdhury, D., Krishna, P., Ng, S., Ragonnaud, E., Salgado, R., Gonzalez Ericsson, P., Diaz-Ruiz, A., Bernier, M., Price, N. L., Biragyn, A., Longo, V. D., & de Cabo, R. (2021). Daily caloric restriction limits tumor growth more effectively than caloric cycling regardless of dietary composition. *Nature Communications, 12*(1). https://doi.org/10.1038/s41467-021-26431-4.

Rodríguez-Ramiro, I., Ramos, S., Bravo, L., Goya, L., & Ángeles Martín, M. (2012). Procyanidin B2 induces Nrf2 translocation and glutathione S-transferase P1 expression via ERKs and p38-MAPK pathways and protect human colonic cells against oxidative stress. *European Journal of Nutrition, 51*(7), 881–892. https://doi.org/10.1007/s00394-011-0269-1.

Román-Albasini, L., Díaz-Véliz, G., Olave, F. A., Aguayo, F. I., García-Rojo, G., Corrales, W. A., Silva, J. P., Ávalos, A. M., Rojas, P. S., Aliaga, E., & Fiedler, J. L. (2020). Antidepressant-relevant behavioral and synaptic molecular effects of long-term fasudil treatment in chronically stressed male rats. *Neurobiology of Stress, 13*. https://doi.org/10.1016/j.ynstr.2020.100234.

Rosa, V., Galgani, M., Santopaolo, M., Colamatteo, A., Laccetti, R., & Matarese, G. (2015). Nutritional control of immunity: Balancing the metabolic requirements with an appropriate immune function. *Seminars in Immunology, 27*(5), 300–309. https://doi.org/10.1016/j.smim.2015.10.001.

Round, J. L., Lee, S. M., Li, J., Tran, G., Jabri, B., Chatila, T. A., & Mazmanian, S. K. (2011). The toll-like receptor 2 pathway establishes colonization by a commensal of the human microbiota. *Science, 332*(6032), 974–977. https://doi.org/10.1126/science.1206095.

Salvadori, G., Mirisola, M. G., & Longo, V. D. (2021). Intermittent and periodic fasting, hormones, and cancer prevention. *Cancers, 13*(18), 4587. https://doi.org/10.3390/cancers13184587.

Schafer, D. P., Lehrman, E. K., Kautzman, A. G., Koyama, R., Mardinly, A. R., Yamasaki, R., Ransohoff, R. M., Greenberg, M. E., Barres, B. A., & Stevens, B. (2012). Microglia Sculpt postnatal neural circuits in an activity and complement-dependent manner. *Neuron, 74*(4), 691–705. https://doi.org/10.1016/j.neuron.2012.03.026.

Shiravand, Y., Khodadadi, F., Kashani, S. M. A., Hosseini-Fard, S. R., Hosseini, S., Sadeghirad, H., Ladwa, R., O'byrne, K., & Kulasinghe, A. (2022). Immune checkpoint inhibitors in cancer therapy. *Current Oncology, 29*(5), 3044–3060. https://doi.org/10.3390/curroncol29050247.

Shu, Z., Yu, M., Zeng, G., Zhang, X., Wu, L., & Tan, X. (2014). Epigallocatechin-3-gallate inhibits proliferation of human aortic smooth muscle cells via up-regulating expression of mitofusin 2. *European Journal of Cell Biology, 93*(4), 137–144. https://doi.org/10.1016/j.ejcb.2014.04.001.

Sivan, A., Corrales, L., Hubert, N., Williams, J. B., Aquino-Michaels, K., Earley, Z. M., Benyamin, F. W., Lei, Y. M., Jabri, B., Alegre, M. L., Chang, E. B., & Gajewski, T. F. (2015). Commensal *Bifidobacterium* promotes antitumor immunity and facilitates anti-PD-L1 efficacy. *Science, 350*(6264), 1084–1089. https://doi.org/10.1126/science.aac4255.

Stadtmauer, E. A., Fraietta, J. A., Davis, M. M., Cohen, A. D., Weber, K. L., Lancaster, E., Mangan, P. A., Kulikovskaya, I., Gupta, M., Chen, F., Tian, L., Gonzalez, V. E., Xu, J., Jung, I., Joseph Melenhorst, J., Plesa, G., Shea, J., Matlawski, T., Cervini, A., ... June, C. H. (2020). CRISPR-engineered T cells in patients with refractory cancer. *Science, 367*(6481). https://doi.org/10.1126/science.aba7365.

Statovci, D., Aguilera, M., MacSharry, J., & Melgar, S. (2017). The impact of Western diet and nutrients on the microbiota and immune response at mucosal interfaces. *Frontiers in Immunology, 8*. https://doi.org/10.3389/fimmu.2017.00838.

Subramanian, N., Torabi-Parizi, P., Gottschalk, R. A., Germain, R. N., & Dutta, B. (2015). Network representations of immune system complexity. *Wiley Interdisciplinary Reviews: Systems Biology and Medicine, 7*(1), 13–38. https://doi.org/10.1002/wsbm.1288.

Szebeni, J., Simberg, D., González-Fernández, Á., Barenholz, Y., & Dobrovolskaia, M. A. (2018). Roadmap and strategy for overcoming infusion reactions to nanomedicines. *Nature Nanotechnology, 13*(12), 1100–1108. https://doi.org/10.1038/s41565-018-0273-1.

Uematsu, S., Fujimoto, K., Jang, M. H., Yang, B. G., Jung, Y. J., Nishiyama, M., Sato, S., Tsujimura, T., Yamamoto, M., Yokota, Y., Kiyono, H., Miyasaka, M., Ishii, K. J., & Akira, S. (2008). Regulation of humoral and cellular gut immunity by lamina propria dendritic cells expressing Toll-like receptor 5. *Nature Immunology, 9*(7), 769–776. https://doi.org/10.1038/ni.1622.

Vernieri, C., Fucà, G., Ligorio, F., Huber, V., Vingiani, A., Iannelli, F., Raimondi, A., Rinchai, D., Frigè, G., Belfiore, A., Lalli, L., Chiodoni, C., Cancila, V., Zanardi, F., Ajazi, A., Cortellino, S., Vallacchi, V., Squarcina, P., Cova, A., ... de Braud, F. (2022). Fasting-mimicking diet is safe and reshapes metabolism and antitumor immunity in patients with cancer. *Cancer Discovery, 12*(1), 90–107. https://doi.org/10.1158/2159-8290.cd-21-0030.

Vétizou, M., Pitt, J. M., Daillère, R., Lepage, P., Waldschmitt, N., Flament, C., Rusakiewicz, S., Routy, B., Roberti, M. P., Duong, C. P. M., Poirier-Colame, V., Roux, A., Becharef, S., Formenti, S., Golden, E., Cording, S., Eberl, G., Schlitzer, A., Ginhoux, F., Mani, S., ... Zitvogel, L. (2015). Anticancer immunotherapy by CTLA-4 blockade relies on the gut microbiota. *Science, 350*(6264), 1079–1084. https://doi.org/10.1126/science.aad1329.

Wu, Q., Tian, A.-L., Li, B., Leduc, M., Forveille, S., Hamley, P., Galloway, W., Xie, W., Liu, P., Zhao, L., Zhang, S., Hui, P., Madeo, F., Tu, Y., Kepp, O., & Kroemer, G. (2021). IGF1 receptor inhibition amplifies the effects of cancer drugs by autophagy and immune-dependent mechanisms. *Journal for ImmunoTherapy of Cancer, 9*(6), e002722. https://doi.org/10.1136/jitc-2021-002722.

Younis, N. N., Mohamed, H. E., Shaheen, M. A., Abdelghafour, A. M., & Hammad, S. K. (2021). Inactivation of Wnt/β-catenin/renin angiotensin axis by tumor necrosis factor-alpha inhibitor, infliximab, ameliorates CKD induced in rats. *Biochemical Pharmacology, 185*. https://doi.org/10.1016/j.bcp.2021.114426.

Yu, C., Liu, X., Yang, J., Zhang, M., Jin, H., Ma, X., & Shi, H. (2019). Combination of immunotherapy with targeted therapy: Theory and practice in metastatic melanoma. *Frontiers in Immunology, 10*(MAY). https://doi.org/10.3389/fimmu.2019.00990.

Zhang, Y., & Zhang, Z. (2020). The history and advances in cancer immunotherapy: Understanding the characteristics of tumor-infiltrating immune cells and their therapeutic implications. *Cellular & Molecular Immunology, 17*(8), 807–821. https://doi.org/10.1038/s41423-020-0488-6.

12

Current challenges and future prospects for microbiome research in cancer treatment

Paras Jain and Prabhakar Kumar Verma

DEPARTMENT OF PHARMACEUTICAL SCIENCES, MAHARSHI DAYANAND UNIVERSITY, ROHTAK, HARYANA, INDIA

12.1 Introduction

Cancer, one of the major disease that spread globally and leads to mortality, currently extensive research is being conducted, and several strategies are being developed to limit tumor growth, which will result in the prevention of disease progression. There are several conventional methods like surgical intervention, radiotherapy, and cytotoxic chemotherapy. Also, there are several treatment options with good results, like immune checkpoint blockade, engineered T-cell therapy, and vaccines. Nevertheless, significant obstacles remain. Several patients experience drug resistance, disease relapse, metastatic spread, or debilitating adverse effects that compromise treatment success and quality of life. As a result, current research mainly focuses on designing safer, more individualized, and biologically targeted therapies to achieve more durable clinical outcomes (Liu & Zhang, 2022).

Recently, several scientists gained an interest in understanding how the microbiome contributes to cancer treatment responses. The human microbiome plays a vital role in regulating immune activity, metabolic processes, and overall physiological balance (Pandey & Khan, 2023). There are several studies that suggest that these microbes can significantly impact the effectiveness of anticancer interventions, including chemotherapy, immunotherapy, and molecularly targeted treatments. Consequently, several studies are still going on to identify the basic mechanism through which the microbiome shapes the specific therapeutic outcomes in oncology (Gupta et al., 2021).

Microbes and cancer have been linked historically for as long as 4000 years. Following the development of the germ hypothesis of infectious diseases, William Busch's 1868 report of spontaneous tumor regressions in S*treptococcus* pyogenes-infected patients marked the beginning of clinical studies on the role of microbes in cancer (Bor et al., 2019). Over the course of the ensuing century, many people rejected the role of bacteria in carcinogenesis and cancer treatment due to poor repeatability, erroneous microbiological claims, and high toxicity (Nallanchakravarthula et al., 2021).

The Microbiome and Cancer Treatment: Overcoming Resistance and Enhancing Efficacy.
DOI: https://doi.org/10.1016/B978-0-443-33206-7.00002-9

While few microorganisms directly cause cancer, many appear to be complicit in its development, frequently working through the host's immune system; on the other hand, several of them exhibit immune stimulatory qualities. Through modulation of primary and secondary lymphoid tissue activities, mechanistic investigations of interactions between the gut microbiota and immune system demonstrate potent impacts on anticancer immunity (Yadav & Chauhan, 2022). Toll-like receptor-initiated cytokine signaling is triggered by several of these routes, but antigenic mimicry with cancer cells and microbial metabolic effects are also significant. Microbial metabolites also control tumor somatic mutation patterns and alter the effectiveness of immune checkpoint inhibitors in preclinical settings.

Although there are still significant obstacles to overcome, a deeper understanding of the roles microorganisms play in cancer offers the opportunity to enhance every phase of the cancer care cycle. This development would be greatly aided by coordinated efforts to describe the microbiota associated with cancer in tumor, stool, and blood samples using gold-standard contamination controls. This would be comparable to the function of The Cancer Genome Atlas in describing the landscape of somatic mutations in cancer (Greathouse et al., 2022; Kiousi et al., 2023). The effectiveness of various microbiota modulation strategies, such as dietary changes or modified bacteria injected intratumorally, is presently being tested in extensive clinical trials. If these types of bacteria have the potential to treat cancer. Then the patients suffering from cancer mainly depend on the microbial perspective. So that the effective therapeutic result will be obtained, and the relationship between cancer, host, and microbes will be understandable.

There are several researchers who have investigated the relationship between the gut microbiota and cancer initiation, progression, metastasis, and therapeutic resistance. There is much evidence that supports the effectiveness of intestinal microbes and adverse reactions toward chemotherapy, as well as immunotherapy. In an experiment that involves a mouse model, designed to change the composition of gut microbiota so that the response obtained to immunotherapeutic agents is positive (Sepich-Poore et al., 2021). Due to its major involvement and contribution in maintaining physiological balance and disease processes, gut microbiota has become a major focus in biomedical research. Even several alterations in metabolic activity and microbial diversity increased the susceptibility to immune-related conditions like malignancies, inflammatory bowel disease, autoimmune disorders, and chronic inflammatory states. To support these investigations, several preclinical and clinical studies have already been reported. So that better outcomes result will be obtained in the form of treatment (Lou et al., 2021; Yadav & Verma, 2022).

For immune checkpoint inhibitor therapies, gut microbiota composition is combined with the therapeutic efficacy and toxicity profile. Sivan and colleagues provided data that supports the potential of PD-L1 blockade. Their investigations suggested that the presence of specific bacterial taxa, i.e., *Bifidobacterium* species, was associated with reduced tumor growth, enhanced T-cell infiltration, and amplified anticancer immune responses (Singh et al., 2023).

12.2 Microbiome and cancer

Unchecked cell division and the capacity of cancerous cells to infiltrate neighboring tissues and spread to other organs are characteristics of cancer. As the primary causes of tumor growth, genetic abnormalities and environmental exposures have historically been the focus of cancer research. Nonetheless, there is mounting evidence that dysbiosis, or microbial imbalance, is a major contributor to carcinogenesis. According to Mao et al. (2018), dysbiosis can interfere with immunological, inflammatory, and metabolic regulatory pathways. It can lead to the formation of genotoxic compounds that can harm the host DNA (Helmink et al., 2019).

There is a huge relationship between bacteria and cancer to be discovered and studied, most notably the microbiome and colorectal cancer (CRC). Some of the metabolites produced by the gut microbiota that trigger the host immune system to release genotoxic substances. In the development of CRC, these microbes and host-derived agents play a very crucial role. There are several studies that signify that overall reduction in bacterial load and microbial diversity in the fecal samples and intestinal mucosa along with CRC. For CRC spread and its development, bacterial species like *Escherichia coli* and *Fusobacterium nucleatum* have been linked together (Sánchez-Alcoholado et al., 2020).

12.2.1 Microbiome and breast cancer

As per the reports, breast cancer is one of the most diagnosed cancers in the world and occurs most prominently second in females and third in males. Bray et al. (2018) suggested that it is one of the main causes of fatalities that happen worldwide. Recent investigations have proven that there is a strong correlation between breast cancer and gut microbiota. Several studies indicated that patients with breast cancer had higher chances of having bacterial species like *Clostridium, Enterobacterium, Lactobacilli, Bacteroides,* and *Escherichia coli* (Ma et al., 2019). While on comparison with the normal tissues, breast cancer (malignant) has been found in higher amount of special microbes like *Methylobacterium radiotolerans.*

In advanced breast cancer patients, the bacterial burden is lowered overall, and there is a decline in gene expression that has been involved in antibacterial immune response. These results symbolize that an imbalance in the level of microbes makes the host's immune system weak and unable to fight against cancer cells. For the diagnosis of breast cancer, microbial composition assessment and bacterial burden are both the most important factors to provide significant information (Chen et al., 2019).

The huge risk of breast cancer is also affected by the gut microbiota, which is essential in regulating the estrogen levels of the patients. For tumor growth, increased estrogen levels and changes in microbial species are among the most important factors (Fernández et al., 2018). Members from the family *Bacteroidetes* phylum, i.e., produce an enzyme called β-glucuronidase that functions as enterohepatic recycling and subsequent reabsorption into the bloodstream (Ma et al., 2019). The term "estrobolome" means the overall collection of gut microbiota bacteria that function in estrogen metabolism.

12.2.2 Microbiome and prostate cancer

Prostate cancer globally ranks as fifth, especially in terms of mortality rate among males, and is the second most common type of cancer that is diagnosed. Major causes of this cancer are obesity, food choices, and poor physical activity that may affect its spread and progression

(Fujita et al., 2022). Recently, the role of microbiota in the treatment of prostate cancer has gained the interest of several researchers and scientists. Microbiome plays a vital role in its development and progression through direct and indirect pathways (Kustrimovic et al., 2023; Porter et al., 2018). Changes occur in the prostate and urinary tract microbiota due to indirect effects produced by the stomach microbiota.

Gut flora, one of the major factors that control androgens as well as hormone metabolism. Hormones like testosterone and dihydrotestosterone (DHT) are among the major factors in the growth and progression of prostate cancer. Through several ways, intestinal microbiota changes the androgen levels. They also take part in the biotransformation of substances like dietary and endogenous substrates into bioactive substances that may affect the hormonal balance of the body. Additionally, some bacteria produce enzymes that can transform steroids into active androgens (Pernigoni et al., 2023).

Gut microbiota also affects the immunological response and systemic inflammation, which in turn have an indirect impact on hormonal balance. Androgen homeostasis disruption connected with gut dysbiosis and chronic low-grade inflammation may affect the progression and development of cancer. Several chemicals that are produced by the bacteria may affect the host steroidogenesis (Pernigoni et al., 2023).

In the androgen production process, several steroidogenic enzymes are involved along with bacterial species. Development of prostate cancer and its progression may be affected by modulation, which also changes the androgen level circulation (Pernigoni et al., 2023). Reduction in the hormone, i.e., androgen, leads to inhibition of tumor formation as it is linked to the microbes (Fujita et al., 2023; Pernigoni et al., 2023). On the other hand, an imbalance in microbes leads to an increase in androgen levels, which also increases the chances of disease. Therefore, a balanced gut microbiota level is very necessary to control hormone levels as well as tumor growth.

For better treatment, the interaction between gut microbiota and androgen production is necessary. There are well-established treatment methods like hormone-based therapy and gut microbiota alteration, which would be very helpful in eradicating prostate cancer.

12.2.3 Microbiome and lung cancer

Lung cancer is one of the major causes of alteration of microbiome levels in the respiratory tract of patients (Zhao et al., 2021). *Proteobacteria, Firmicutes, Fusobacteria, Actinobacteria, and Bacteroidetes* cover all the bacterial species that are present in the healthy population. Species like *Pseudomonas,* Modestobacter, *Streptococcus, Prevotella, Veillonella, Haemophilus, and Neisseria* are predominantly found in very large quantities, especially in the respiratory tract of patients suffering from lung cancer (Wang et al., 2021).

Patients with squamous cell carcinoma and lung adenocarcinoma are commonly found with the *Selenomonas, Capnocytophaga, and Veillonella*-like species (Goto et al., 2020). ERK and PI3K signaling pathways have been combined with the *Streptococcus and Wechsler* (oral microbes) that promote lung cancer tumor growth (Tsay et al., 2018; Wang et al., 2021).

Lung cancer progression has also been linked to persistent infections brought on by *Helicobacter pylori* and *Mycobacterium tuberculosis.* Remarkably, only the lower airways of patients with lung cancer have been found to harbor *Bradyrhizobium japonicum*. Additional evidence suggests that some histological subtypes of lung cancers may be linked to differences in the composition of the microbiome. For instance, it has been found that some bacteria, such as *Acidovorax, Klebsiella, Rhodoferax, Comamonas,* and *Polarmonas,* are more abundant in small-cell carcinoma cases than in adenocarcinoma instances. Crucially, altering the pulmonary microbiota has been suggested as a possible tactic to inhibit or stop the growth of lung cancer (Wang et al., 2021).

12.3 Experience of cancer therapy by bacteria

According to experimental data, the widely used chemotherapeutic medication cyclophosphamide (CTX) can change the gut microbiota in mice, upsetting the microbial balance and permitting some Gram-positive bacteria to pass through the intestinal mucosa. This bacterial translocation encourages the production of Th17 cells with traits similar to Th1-type responses and boosts immunological activity within secondary lymphoid organs. Research based on genetic models involving species like *Caenorhabditis elegans* and *Escherichia coli* has shown the complex relationship between the microbes, host, and drugs like flouropyrimidine (anticancer drug). The overall results signify that there is a dynamic correlation between microbes and drug response in the treatment of cancer.

The findings indicate that bacterial pathways involved in the metabolism of vit. B6, B9, and ribonucleotides can significantly influence how *C. elegans* responds to fluoropyrimidine-based therapies. Because the human body is intricate and influenced by various internal and external factors, the impact of bacteria and dietary nutrients on treatment outcomes is not yet fully understood (Yang et al., 2024). Initial research involving mice treated with a combination of antibiotics suggests that changes in the microbiome may reduce the effectiveness of platinum chemotherapy and CpG oligonucleotide immunotherapy. When the microbiome is balanced and healthy, immunotherapy can suppress tumor growth by inducing myeloid cells to produce tumor necrosis factor (TNF) and activating CD8 T cells. This suggests that beneficial microbes improve patient outcomes by triggering tumor-associated myeloid cells to release inflammatory cytokines in response to immunotherapy, a process that involves activation of Toll-like receptor 4 (TLR4).

12.3.1 Microbial pathogens cause some types of cancer

Helicobacter pylori and several cancer-causing oncogenic viruses provide perhaps the strongest evidence that microbiota are neither passengers nor bystanders (Table 12.1). Gastric adenocarcinoma is closely associated with *H. pylori* infections. Gastrointestinal inflammation plays a role in this, with gastritis brought on by *H. pylori* being thought to be a sign of cancer (Din et al., 2023). To prove that *H. pylori* is an etiologic agent of gastritis and stomach ulcers, Dr Barry Marshall infected himself with the bacteria in his study that earned him the 2005 Nobel Prize in Physiology or Medicine. This is the reason why *H. pylori* is currently being eradicated from human populations worldwide. However, by altering stomach pH and reducing acid reflux, *H. pylori* protects against Barrett's esophagus and esophageal cancer (Bhatt et al., 2017; Wang et al., 2025). This illustrates

Table 12.1 Microbes, cancer type, their site, and MOA.

Microbe/genus	Associated cancer type	Tumor site/tissue	Notes/mechanism
Fusobacterium nucleatum	Colorectal cancer (CRC)	Colon, rectum	Promotes inflammation, immune evasion, and tumor progression
Peptostreptococcus anaerobius	Colorectal cancer	Colon	Activates oncogenic signaling pathways and modulates tumor microenvironment
Bacteroides fragilis (enterotoxigenic)	Colorectal cancer	Colon	Produces BFT toxin that induces DNA damage and inflammation
Helicobacter pylori	Gastric cancer	Stomach	Chronic infection causes gastritis, atrophy, and gastric carcinoma
Salmonella enterica	Gallbladder, colon	Gallbladder, colon	Chronic infection may induce DNA damage and tumor-promoting inflammation
Escherichia coli (pks+ strains)	Colorectal cancer	Colon	Produces colibactin, a genotoxin that induces DNA double-strand breaks
Enterococcus hirae	Various solid tumors (murine models)	Systemic/tumor microenvironment	Modulates $CD8^+$ T cell responses; improves chemotherapy efficacy
Barnesiella intestinihominis	Various solid tumors (murine models)	Tumor microenvironment	Enhances T cell infiltration and chemotherapy response
Lactobacillus johnsonii	Sarcoma (murine models)	Tumor microenvironment	Supports immunostimulatory effects of cyclophosphamide
Lactobacillus murinus	Sarcoma (murine models)	Tumor microenvironment	Promotes antitumor immune responses during chemotherapy
Clostridium spp.	Colorectal cancer, liver metastases	Colon, liver	Butyrate production with anti-inflammatory and anticancer effects
Faecalibacterium prausnitzii	Colorectal cancer	Colon	Butyrate-producing, anti-inflammatory, supports gut barrier
Streptococcus bovis	Colorectal cancer	Colon	Chronic colonization linked to tumor-promoting inflammation

(*continued on next page*)

Table 12.1 Microbes, cancer type, their site, and MOA—cont'd

Microbe/genus	Associated cancer type	Tumor site/tissue	Notes/mechanism
Mycobacterium tuberculosis	Lung cancer (association)	Lungs	Chronic infection and inflammation may contribute to carcinogenesis
Human papillomavirus (HPV)	Cervical, oropharyngeal cancer	Cervix, oropharynx	Viral oncoproteins E6/E7 inhibit tumor suppressors p53/pRb
Epstein–Barr virus (EBV)	Nasopharyngeal carcinoma, gastric cancer, lymphoma	Nasopharynx, stomach, lymphoid tissue	Latent infection drives oncogenic pathways
Hepatitis B virus (HBV)	Hepatocellular carcinoma	Liver	Chronic infection causes cirrhosis and hepatocarcinogenesis
Hepatitis C virus (HCV)	Hepatocellular carcinoma	Liver	Chronic viral infection induces inflammation, fibrosis, and cancer

how the interaction between supposedly harmful microorganisms and their human host can be far more nuanced than first thought. This is especially true for bacterial drivers of carcinogenesis. The development and spread of tumors linked to microbial dysbiosis are multifactorial processes that occur after "multiple hits," in contrast to viruses, which express constitutively active viral mimics of cellular proto-oncogenes (Dave et al., 2012). Not every person Table 12.1 infected with oncogenic microorganisms goes on to acquire cancer. Along with environmental conditions, genetic variation in the host and microorganism impacts the occurrence and severity of cancer. For instance, only strains of *H. pylori* that possess the cytotoxin-associated gene A (cagA) virulence factor effectively cause gastritis and stomach cancer. The immune response is influenced by host genetics, which is another significant factor in determining whether an infected person gets cancer. Aside from diet and lifestyle factors, including obesity, alcoholism, and tobacco use, chronic inflammation is thought to be a particularly significant risk factor (Elinav et al., 2019; Ting et al., 2022). Microbes and their cancer sites are shown in Table 12.1.

12.3.2 Potentially promoting the growth and progression of cancer

Using models of pancreatic, colon, and melanoma with tumors implanted under the skin and in the liver, showed that the suppression of tumor growth by antibiotics depended on the presence of adaptive immune cells. This antitumor effect was reduced in Rag1-deficient mice, which lack mature T and B lymphocytes. Mechanistically, altering the microbiota led to an increase in T cells producing interferon-gamma (IFN-γ) and a reduction in T cells that produce interleukin 17a (IL-17a) and IL-10. Targeting harmful bacteria could help restore immune system functions and improve the success of cancer treatments. Various cancers, such as colorectal, esophageal, gastric, head and neck squamous cell carcinoma, and pancreatic cancer, have been associated with *Fusobacterium nucleatum* (Irfan et al., 2020). Studies involving mouse models and cell cultures have demonstrated that the FadA adhesin protein on *F. nucleatum* binds to E-cadherin, a type of epithelial cadherin, activating -catenin signaling pathways. Tumor growth is encouraged by this interaction, which also influences inflammatory reactions and aids in the development of cancer. A synthetic peptide that inhibits *F. nucleatum's* adhesion to E-cadherin inhibits the proliferation of CRC cells. In CRC patients, there is a huge increase in the amount of fadA found in their colon tissues as compared to the healthy population (McQuade et al., 2019). Apart from this, fadA is an important factor for the inflammatory and cancer-related disease processes because of the elevated levels of Wnt7b and NFkB2 in the RNA analysis of patients.

As per the studies, it is the *F. nucleatum* that promotes the growth and progression of colorectal tumors. Also, there is one of the most important components, i.e., Fap2 adhesion, that allows the organisms to concentrate within tumor tissues. It is the Fap2 that destroys immune surveillance and undermines anticancer action. By decreasing the cytotoxic action of natural killer (NK) cells and inducing apoptosis in human lymphocytes by interacting with the TIGIT receptor. (Chattaraj et al., 2023; Eslami et al., 2025). *F. nucleatum* is responsible for the decline in chemotherapy sensitivity in CRC, which leads to tumor growth. Its amount is increased in patients who have received chemotherapy.

According to the mechanistic study, it disrupted the TLR4–MYD88 signaling cascade, thereby decreasing the expression levels of miR-18a* and miR-4800. These changes at the molecular level increase the chemoresistance by inducing autophagy. The result analysis of the treatment given may be increased by some interventions that target these signaling pathways. Species like *Peptostreptococcus anaerobius* have been linked with the CRC. This bacterium utilizes a surface protein, putative cell wall binding repeat 2 (PCWBR2), to selectively bind to cancerous colorectal cells, while showing little to no affinity for normal colonic epithelial cells, suggesting a preferential interaction with tumor tissue. It interacts with the 2/1 integrin receptor on colonic cells, leading to activation of the PI3K-Akt signaling pathway. This activation subsequently promotes inflammation and cell growth through the natural factor kappa B (NF-κB) signaling cascade (Yang et al., 2021). *Peptostreptococcus anaerobius* has been found to promote tumor growth by encouraging cell proliferation and fostering a proinflammatory environment within tumors through the recruitment of tumor-infiltrating myeloid-derived suppressor cells (MDSCs) and tumor-associated macrophages (TAMs). Therefore, future studies should investigate the impact of this bacterial species on the effectiveness of chemotherapy and cancer immunotherapy treatments. In addition, radiation therapy exerts a potent immune-modulating effect by enhancing tumor-associated antigen cross-presentation, which activates IFN-γ and cytotoxic CD8+ T cells. Treatment with vancomycin, an antibiotic targeting Gram-positive bacteria, has been shown to increase CD8+ T cell infiltration and IFN-γ expression in mice, thereby improving the antitumor effects of radiotherapy . The study involving melanoma and lung cancer models found that adding sodium butyrate, an important metabolite from Gram-positive bacteria, negated the observed effect. This indicates that the presence and levels of Gram-positive bacteria could affect how patients respond to radiation therapy. Fig. 12.1 depicts how gut microbiota show their effects on tumorogenesis.

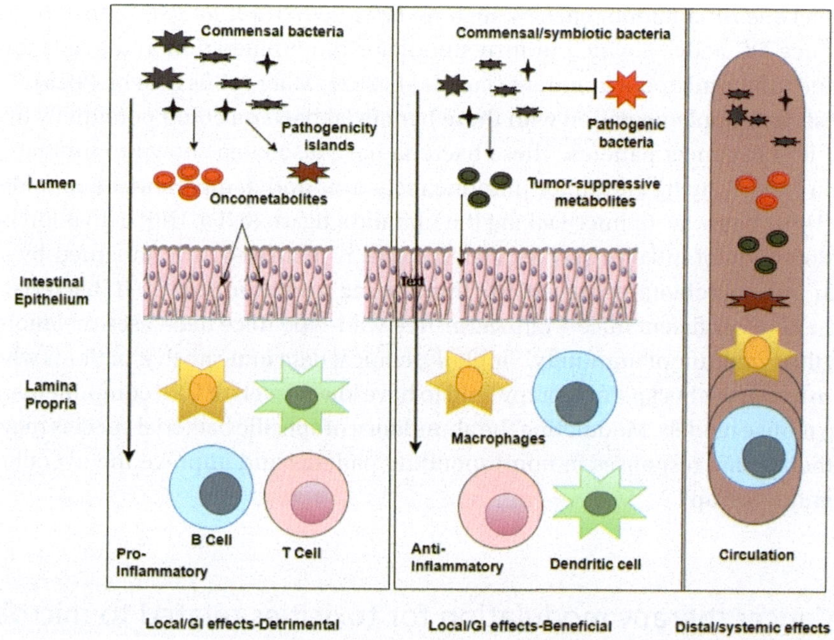

FIGURE 12.1 Gut microbiota effects on cancer in GIT. *GIT*, gastrointestinal tract. Impact of gut microbiota on gastrointestinal cancer development, progression, and therapeutic response through immune modulation, inflammation, and microbial metabolite interactions.

12.4 Microbial biomarkers for efficacy in treatment

Several bacterial species, such as *Lactobacillus johnsonii, Enterococcus hirae, and Barnesiella intestinihominis,* have been shown in animal studies to enhance the antitumor immune response elicited by cyclophosphamide (CTX) (Roy et al., 2025). Mechanistically,*B. intestinihominis* accumulates in the colon and promotes the infiltration of γδ T cells that secrete IFN-γ within tumors. In contrast, *E. hirae* translocates from the small intestine to secondary lymphoid organs, where it increases the ratio of cytotoxic $CD8^+$ T cells to regulatory T cells (Tregs) in tumor tissues. The effectiveness of CTX in controlling tumor growth depends on an intact gut microbiota; antibiotic treatment that disrupts these microbial communities reduces CTX efficacy, whereas oral administration of *E. hirae* can restore its antitumor activity. Additionally, a protein containing a nucleotide-binding oligomerization domain was identified as an inhibitor of *E. hirae* and *B. intestinihominis* in a separate mouse model. Various *Bacteroides* species also influence the antitumor efficacy of anticytotoxic T-lymphocyte associated protein 4 (CTLA-4) therapy. In germ-free or antibiotic-treated mice, anti-CTLA-4 treatment is ineffective; however, colonization with *Bacteroides fragilis* restores responsiveness by promoting Th1-type immune responses in lymph nodes and supporting the development of dendritic cells (DCs) within tumors. Similar observations in cancer patients indicate that T cell responses triggered by *Bacteroides thetaiotaomicron* or *B. fragilis* correlate with improved outcomes following

CTLA-4 blockade. In addition, species such as *Bifidobacterium longum* and *Bifidobacterium breve* enhance DC activity, which in turn stimulates the proliferation and activation of $CD8^+$ T cells in the tumor microenvironment (Jain et al., 2021; Mafe & Büsselberg, 2025). These findings suggest that supplementation with these beneficial bacteria could potentially improve the efficacy of ICIs in cancer patients. These bacteria have also been shown to inhibit melanoma progression by enhancing antitumor immune responses and dampening the unfolded protein response (UPR) pathway. In mice lacking the ubiquitin ligase RNF5, UPR activation is reduced, and the expression of inflammasome-related genes is increased, accompanied by significant changes in gut microbiota composition. Introducing a consortium of 11 bacterial strains—enriched in RNF5-deficient mice—into germ-free wild-type mice decreases melanoma growth and strengthens antitumor immunity. Similarly, clinical data indicate that patients who respond favorably to immune checkpoint therapy tend to have lower levels of UPR components, mirroring findings in mouse models. Modulating the abundance of specific bacterial species may therefore enhance therapeutic responses in nonresponding patients and improve the overall efficacy of cancer immunotherapy

12.4.1 Cancer therapy modulation for toxicities related to microbiota

The microbiota is changed by gastrointestinal (GI) surgery, which includes preoperative washing with oral and intravenous antibiotics. This might result in issues such as anastomotic leakage and infection (Chen et al., 2019; Ma et al., 2024). Microbiota modification is very helpful to solve these kinds of issues, as some investigations suggest that bacterial species like *Lactobacillus* and *Akkermansia muciniphila* regulate the intestinal wound healing process through a mechanism that depends upon the O_2 species and receptors (formyl peptide). The effect of *Bacteroides thetaiotaomicron* in controlling the expression of genes related to angiogenesis, mucosal barrier fortification, and nutrient absorption was also demonstrated by a study employing germ-free mice colonized with the bacteria. Pathogenic bacteria like *Serratia marcescens* and *Pseudomonas aeruginosa* encourage the development of anastomotic leaks, in contrast to these helpful bacteria that preserve intestinal function and epithelial integrity (Jalil et al., 2023; Tsigalou et al., 2023). Thus, the likelihood of problems may be reduced by selectively inhibiting pathogens while concurrently preserving "good" bacteria before or after surgery.

Like surgery, taking ICIs can have negative side effects, such as colitis. According to metagenomic sequencing, patients with cancer who have colitis brought on by checkpoint inhibition exhibit different profiles of certain bacteria (Cammarota et al., 2020). Research has shown that cancer patients treated with ipilimumab who have increased levels of Bacteroidetes and microbial genes involved in polyamine transport and B vitamin synthesis tend to be more resistant to developing colitis (Zhao et al., 2023). The risk of ipilimumab-induced colitis in patients may be predicted by the found microbial biomarkers. Studies indicate that fecal microbiota transplantation (FMT) and the use of a bacterial cocktail comprising *Bacteroidales* and *Burkholderiales* can both mitigate colitis induced by ICI in cancer patients and in mice subjected to antibiotic treatment, respectively (Li et al., 2022). Although FMT shows fewer adverse effects compared to corticosteroids, anti-TNF, and anti-integrin therapies, and effectively reduces inflammation and ulcer formation, the small sample size and limited mechanistic understanding call for more extensive validation.

As per the fecal samples results of patients undergoing radiation therapy, individuals with radiation enteropathy exhibited an enrichment of particular microbial taxa, such as *Clostridium IV* and *Roseburia*, but a decreased diversity of bacteria. FMT has been found to improve GI tract function and strengthen the epithelial barrier, thereby reducing gastrointestinal damage caused by radiation and enhancing the survival rates in mice exposed to radiation (Zhang et al., 2023). Importantly, FMT promotes increased levels of intestinal trefoil factor (TFF3/ITF1), Pgk1, Glut1 (Slc2a1), Muc2, and multidrug resistance protein 1 (MDR1), which together help to thicken the mucus layer in these irradiated animals.

Additionally, FMT reduces the toxicity of radiation to the bone marrow. When combined, the treatment notably improves the survival outcomes of irradiated mice more effectively than FMT or bone marrow transplantation by themselves. This suggests that FMT could serve as a radioprotective agent, potentially enhancing the treatment success for cancer patients receiving radiation therapy (Herrera-Quintana et al., 2024a).

FMT carries dangers despite its protective impact against toxicities brought on by cancer therapy. Through FMT, pathogens could be spread to the recipients. Therefore, thorough microbiological screening is necessary to exclude the possibility of spreading recognized diseases, particularly those that are resistant to antibiotics (Do et al., 2013). Finding the situations for which FMT has genuine clinical potential is still difficult, though. Predicting a patient's reaction to FMT is impossible due to a lack of information and understanding of the function of FMT in cancer. For patients to benefit fully from FMT, it is crucial to conduct more studies investigating the microbial compositions of donors and recipients, as well as the mechanisms involved.

12.4.2 Antibiotics or other methods for bacterial depletion

Due to their role in carcinogenesis, carcinogenic bacteria have been eliminated in a number of ways to stop cancer or slow the formation of tumors. The part that *H. pylori* plays in gastric carcinogenesis is well known among these pathogens (Oyovwi et al., 2025). The risk of early-stage gastric cancer is decreased when *H. pylori* is eradicated in the population with a combination of antibiotics like amoxicillin and clarithromycin.

During an examination of 490,510 control cases and 125,441 cancer cases, a positive correlation was found between antibiotic use and cancer risk (Guan et al., 2024). Therapies involving monoclonal antibodies, antibiotics, and monotherapy decreased the rate of survival of patients suffering from renal carcinoma, indicating that commensal removal compromises the effectiveness of ICIs. Patients often experience unintended harm due to the conventional use of antibiotics, which disrupts the balance of the beneficial microbiome. To reduce this disturbance and ensure effective cancer therapies, innovative approaches are needed. One promising strategy involves using the CRISPR- Cas9 system, delivered via bacteriophages, to selectively target specific bacteria at the intersection of the microbiome and cancer. The use of dextran nanoparticles carrying irinotecan and chemically linked to azide-modified phages that specifically target *F. nucleatum* within tumors has been shown to improve the chemotherapy outcomes against CRC Herrera-Quintana et al.,2024a, 2024b, 2024c). Since this phage therapy is confined to gastrointestinal tumors, it likely results in fewer side effects compared to broader treatments. With the approval of an increasing number of nanomedicines for various medical uses, current clinical trials continue to confirm the effectiveness of nanoparticles in delivering drugs. Nanotechnologies can be utilized to distribute anticancer medications in a regulated way or to target germs linked to tumors, which will reduce patient adverse effects. Due to the significant role of nanotechnology in cancer prevention and therapy, it is essential to concentrate research on assessing the toxic effects, adverse reactions, and subsequent biological pathways triggered by nanoparticles (Chen & Tsao, 2013).

12.4.3 Probiotics bacteria compositional modulation in cancer

Probiotics and prebiotics are among the most prominent subjects for clinical trials, especially in the case of cancer. While some studies found that patients taking probiotics had better clinical outcomes, others could not find any evidence of a meaningful effect of probiotics (Ratiner et al., 2024). As per the reports (Prakash & Xia, 2023), microbial profile data of bacterial species like *B. lactis* and *L. acidophilus* are changed in the case of patients with CRC. Probiotics have demonstrated significant potential in modulating gut microbiota composition and inhibiting cancer progression. Specifically, probiotic supplementation has been shown to reduce the abundance of bacterial genera associated with CRC, such as *Fusobacterium* and *Peptostreptococcus*, while increasing beneficial butyrate-producing bacteria, including *Faecalibacterium* and members of the order *Clostridiales*. It is well known that bacteria that produce butyrate have anti-inflammatory and antitumorigenic properties in the gut environment. In addition to microbial regulation, probiotics have been shown to inhibit the growth of tumors in animal models. For example, Yamamoto et al. (2022) demonstrated that probiotics not only altered microbial profiles but also slowed cancer spread in vivo. Similarly, recent studies showed that the probiotic mixture VSL#3 reduced intestinal inflammation during diethylnitrosamine (DEN) treatment, preserved intestinal mucosal integrity, and inhibited tumor formation in a DEN-induced rat model of hepatocarcinogenesis. Reduction of Th17 cells in the tumor microenvironment, the formulation of probiotic prohep decreased the formation of hepatocellular carcinoma (HCC), as per a different study that involves the use of a subcutaneous transplantation mouse model. It is the probiotics that lead to the conditions related to HCC development. As per the 108 clinical trial study that evaluated the therapeutic potential of VSL#3 in patients with cirrhosis109 or nonalcoholic fatty liver disease (Ma et al., 2024).

A recent study suggested that protection against radiation provided by *Lactobacillus rhamnosus,* how? In their study, tumor-bearing mice were treated with either phosphate-buffered saline (PBS) alone, radiation alone, LGG alone, or LGG administered before radiation exposure. The outcome showed that lipoteichoic acid (LTA), which is released by LGG, attaches to pericryptal macrophages' TLR2 and stimulates the chemokine CXCL12. CXCL12 then attaches itself to CXCR4 on mesenchymal stem cells that express cyclo-oxygenase-2, causing them to migrate It acts on the pericryptal region to produce prostaglandin E2, which helps protect epithelial stem cells from damage caused by radiation. However, this method has yet to be confirmed in human studies.

Probiotics may alter the host's inflammatory state in addition to providing radioprotection, which could affect how well cancer treatment works. Several scientific studies have questioned the effectiveness of probiotics in cancer treatment. For instance, in patients undergoing surgery for head and neck cancer, those who received a combination of *Lactobacillus* and *Bifidobacterium* strains did not experience improved clinical outcomes compared to those given a placebo (Fang et al., 2025). Both groups exhibited similar levels of inflammatory markers and diamine oxidase—which indicates gut barrier function—as well as comparable rates of postoperative infections. Variations in the host genome and microbiota between individuals may account for the contradictory findings of clinical trials.

Probiotic colonization and function affect the host's native microbiota, gene expression profile and other factors (Herrera-Quintana et al., 2024a, 2024b, 2024c; Li et al., 2022). Due to several differences, the identification of the clinical benefits is very difficult in cancer patients. Probiotics clinical trials in a large number have several limitations, like small sample sizes, short treatment periods, and insufficient patient follow-up to identify the long-term effects of probiotics (Sharma et al., 2021). Therefore, a thorough study is required to determine the effectiveness of probiotic therapy, especially in cancer patients. A recent study showed the effects of 11-strain probiotics and an FMT on the postantibiotic restoration of the human and mouse microbiota. The outcomes showed that a rapid and complete recovery is given by an FMT, while probiotics pause the microbiome restoration processes. Based on this discovery, patients who have been treated with antibiotics may benefit from using an FMT rather than probiotics to restore their microbiota (Bwanga et al., 2023; Park et al., 2022).

12.5 Organoids offer more detailed mechanistic understanding of how the gut microbiota contributes to cancer development

Pluripotent stem cells or tissue-derived organoids preserve many of the traits of their parent tissues, such as histology and marker expression. Organoids are used for drug screening and disease modeling because of these characteristics. The limitations of current research employing mouse models or cell lines are addressed by organoids, including Fig. 12.1, Table 12.1, and Table 12.2, the incompatibility of human samples, and the inherent discrepancies between rodent models and human physiology. Compared to two-dimensional culture, the incorporation of bacteria into organoid culture provides a richer mechanistic understanding and enables the investigation of host-bacteria interactions (Lee et al., 2023). Research has demonstrated that *H. pylori* can promote tumor development by directly injecting the bacteria into human gastric organoids. The bacterial protein CagA was found to interact with the c-Met receptor on epithelial cells, triggering its phosphorylation and encouraging the growth of these cells (Mohseni & Ghorbani, 2024). In a related experiment, DCs derived from human monocytes were cultured alongside gastric organoids and then exposed to *H. pylori*. Findings suggested that the DCs' movement toward the organoids makes possible interaction with the gastric epithelial cells. Bacterial infection is more prone to replicate in vivo with the aid of the coculture method. When

Table 12.2 Bacterial strains, cancer type. Mechanism and clinical trial stages.

S. no.	Bacterial strain/construct	Targeted cancer type	Therapeutic payload/mechanism	Clinical trial phase	References/source
1.	*Listeria monocytogenes* (LADD)	Castration-resistant prostate cancer	Tumor-associated antigens; stimulates T-cell immune response	Phase II	ClinicalTrials.gov
2.	*Listeria monocytogenes* (LADD)	Nonsmall cell lung cancer	Tumor antigens; immune activation	Phase I	ClinicalTrials.gov
3.	*Salmonella typhimurium* VNP20009	Metastatic melanoma, metastatic renal cell carcinoma	Tumor colonization; immune stimulation	Phase I	Toso et al. (2002)
4.	*Salmonella typhimurium* VNP20009	Melanoma	Tumor-targeted colonization and immune modulation	Phase I	Heimann and Rosenberg (2003)
5.	*Salmonella typhimurium* VNP20009 expressing TAPET-CD (cytosine deaminase)	Head and neck carcinoma; esophageal adenocarcinoma	Prodrug activation (5-fluorocytosine → 5-fluorouracil)	Phase I	Nemunaitis et al. (2003)
6.	*Salmonella typhimurium* VNP20009 expressing IL-2	Liver cancer	Cytokine delivery to tumor microenvironment to enhance T-cell activity	Phase I	ClinicalTrials.gov
7.	*Salmonella typhimurium* Ty21a VXM01	Pancreatic cancer	VEGFR2-targeting DNA vaccine; antiangiogenic immune response	Phase I	Schmitz-Winnenthal et al. (2018)
8.	Mixed bacterial vaccine	Various malignant tumors	Combination of tumor-associated antigens; immune stimulation	Phase I	ClinicalTrials.gov
9.	*Salmonella typhimurium* VNP20009	Advanced metastatic solid tumors	Tumor colonization; immunomodulatory activity	Phase I	ClinicalTrials.gov
10.	*Salmonella typhimurium* VNP20009	Solid tumors	Tumor-targeted bacterial therapy	Phase I	ClinicalTrials.gov
11.	*Salmonella typhimurium* VNP20009	Metastatic tumors	Tumor homing; immune activation	Phase I	ClinicalTrials.gov

H. pylori is present, DCs are drawn to the stomach mucosa to aid in *H. pylori* phagocytosis. To improve functional development, mixing of organoids is done through coculturing method that leads to greater structural complexity (Kunjalwar et al., 2024; Yang & Guo, 2024). Organoids produced from the tissues of patients will be used as models for forecasting tumors that may help with a variety of treatments.

12.5.1 Treatment

Immunomodulation is one of the primary mechanisms driving these varied responses. Studies from the recently published data suggested that the preclinical experiments performed with animal and cell culture models, human clinical trials, and meta-analysis studies showed that the gut microbiota influences how the host reacts to a variety of cancer treatments (Schorr et al., 2023). In addition to this, dysbiosis causes disparate therapeutic responses. For example, Patents with diseases like hematological malignancies, along with allogeneic hematopoietic stem cell transplantation, showed predictive intestinal diversity with low mortality (Alsahafi et al., 2019).

12.5.2 Immunotherapy

T-lymphocytes, the main regulators of the adaptive immune system, play a vital role in detecting and destroying cancer cells. A secondary signal is required to make it fully active. This signal is located on the cells of antigens, which function in conjunction with the antigen to enable the sequential activation of T cells. It is delivered through additional surface molecules present on the antigen. There are several immune checkpoints that make T-lymphocytes associated with CTLA-4, PD-1, and its ligand. These all play a very crucial role in preventing autoimmune diseases by suppressing immune responses (Singh et al., 2025; Yamamoto et al., 2022).

Cancer cells and components of the tumor stroma often take advantage of immune checkpoint pathways by upregulating inhibitory molecules that suppress antitumor immune responses. Through this mechanism, malignant cells can escape immune detection and destruction. ICIs, a kind of monoclonal antibody that is approved by the USFDA, prevent the suppression of the immune system. Inhibitory signaling pathways that typically limit T-cell activation are blocked by drugs that target CTLA-4 (like ipilimumab) and PD-1 or its receptor PD-L1 (like nivolumab and pembrolizumab). ICIs make the immune system destroy cancer cells by breaking up these regulatory connections and restoring T-cell actions. Several studies signify that these medications are very beneficial in the treatment of cancers like bladder cancer, renal cell carcinoma (RCC), nonsmall cell lung cancer, Hodgkin lymphoma, and melanoma (Addissouky et al., 2023; Bejarano et al., 2021).

A variation occurs in patient responses, especially when ICIs are used for the treatment. A recent research study suggested that the gut microbiota connected to the host immune system is a very crucial part in determining the outcome. Several interactions between the immunotherapy and gut microbiota lead to variation in therapeutic response to ICIs (Elmore et al., 2021). This idea has received strong support from preclinical research. Two separate studies showed that variations in gut microbiota composition affected the effectiveness of immune checkpoint inhibition in mouse melanoma models. Genetically identical C57BL/6 mice from two separate suppliers—Taconic and The Jackson Laboratory (JAX)—showed varied tumor growth patterns in a study. Interestingly, JAX mice responded better to anti-PD-L1 medication and showed slower melanoma progression than Taconic mice. Rather than hereditary causes, these disparities were ascribed to changes in their gut microbial compositions. Furthermore, fecal microbiota transplantation from JAX mice into Taconic mice enhanced the latter's responsiveness to anti-PD-L1 treatment. The investigators identified *Bifidobacterium* as a key contributor, demonstrating that supplementation with this genus alone improved therapeutic efficacy. Mechanistically, *Bifidobacterium* appeared to enhance DC function, thereby promoting $CD8^+$ T-cell-mediated antitumor immunity (Khakimova et al., 2019; Wu et al., 2024).

Study suggested that alterations in gut microbiome due to the intake of anti-CTLA-4 result in a reduction in *Bacteroidales* and *Burkholderiales* and an increase in *Clostridiales*. To counteract the lack of anti-CTLA-4 effectiveness in reducing tumor size under germ-free conditions, *B. fragilis* and/or *B. thetaiotaomicron* were introduced. These bacteria enhanced tumor-targeted immune responses by promoting DC maturation and modulating IL-12-driven TH1 responses. Although the two studies involved different immune checkpoint inhibitors and identified distinct microbial populations, they shared similar mechanisms—namely, the activation of DCs and the improved function of tumor-infiltrating effector T cells (Fosgerau & Hoffmann, 2015).

Immune checkpoint inhibitors are effective treatments but are often associated with gastrointestinal and liver-related side effects. The complex interplay between a patient's genetic makeup, immune system activity, environmental factors, and the gut microbiome contributes to the common immune-related adverse effects of hepatitis, diarrhea, and inflammation of the intestines seen with these therapies. Compared to people without colitis who are also receiving ipilimumab, patients who acquire new-onset, immune-mediated colitis as a result of treatment with anti-CTLA-4 monoclonal antibodies exhibit a reduced presence of Bacteroidetes in their gut microbiome. The protection against colitis appears to be associated with microbial pathways involved in polyamine transport and the biosynthesis of vitamins B1, B2, and B5. These microbial features were found in higher abundance in individuals who did not develop colitis during the treatment (Sheikh et al., 2023; Xu et al., 2019).

TLR9 on immune cells is liganded by synthetic CpG oligonucleotides (CpG-ON), which boost immunological responses. CpG-ON combined with blocking IL-10 receptor antibodies offers a therapeutic benefit when paired with peptide vaccinations, resulting in decreased tumor volume and longer human survival. Through the production of proinflammatory cytokines, CpG-ON and IL-10R antibodies reduce the tumor burden in mice tumors. When mice are treated with antibiotics or raised in germ-free conditions, their effectiveness is reduced (Ma et al., 2019; Zhou et al., 2021).

12.5.3 Chemotherapy

Alterations in the gut microbiome are a common consequence of cytotoxic chemotherapy, although the precise clinical implications of these microbial shifts for long-term prognosis remain incompletely defined. Increasingly, however, preclinical evidence indicates that the baseline composition and functional capacity of the microbiota can substantially influence the therapeutic efficacy of several conventional chemotherapeutic agents. In murine models, the antitumor activity of oxaliplatin—a platinum-based compound widely used in gastrointestinal malignancies—has been shown to depend, at least in part, on the presence of an intact and immunologically active microbiota. Broad-spectrum antibiotic disruption of gut bacteria resulted in significant transcriptional changes in the host, including upregulation of genes linked to tumor metabolism and progression and suppression of phagocytic function, antigen presentation pathways, and inflammatory signaling (Hadrich, 2018).

Proinflammatory activity in the tumor microenvironment was similarly inhibited by antibiotic-mediated microbial depletion, which decreased the recruitment of immune cells necessary for efficient tumor regression. Reactive oxygen species (ROS) production within tumors is a key mechanism behind oxaliplatin's effectiveness. ROS production was considerably reduced in germ-free or antibiotic-treated mice, which was associated with less DNA damage in cancerous cells and a less effective treatment response. These results imply that microbiota-driven immunomodulatory mechanisms play a role in chemotherapy-induced tumor control in addition to its direct cytotoxic effects on cancer cells. Because immune activation mediated by commensal bacteria appears to contribute significantly to chemotherapeutic results, the traditional difference between immunotherapy and chemotherapy may not be as strict as previously thought (Guan et al., 2023; You et al., 2022).

Another striking illustration of the interaction between microbiota and chemotherapy is cyclophosphamide (CP), an alkylating drug with a wide range of oncologic applications. By shrinking tiny intestinal villi and impairing barrier function, CP damages intestinal epithelial integrity. This harm makes it easier for certain commensal bacteria to go into secondary lymphoid organs, where they promote the growth of immunological and inflammatory effector cells (Ma et al., 2024). Both germ-free mice and animals treated with antibiotics to eradicate gut microbiota demonstrated a significant decrease in the anticancer activity of CP in experimental models. The significance of certain bacterial taxa was highlighted by the fact that the decrease in treatment efficacy was more noticeable when antibiotics that predominantly affected Gram-negative organisms were given than when those that targeted Gram-positive organisms.

Several Gram-positive species, such as segmented filamentous bacteria, *L. hirae, L. murinus,* and *L. johnsonii,* were found to be important mediators of CP-induced antitumor immunity in a nonmetastatic sarcoma mouse model. Further research showed that *Enterococcus hirae* translocation was linked to a higher intratumoral $CD8^+$ T cell to regulatory T cell (Treg) ratio, indicating a change toward a tumor microenvironment that is more immunostimulatory. Furthermore, it has been demonstrated that the Gram-negative bacterium *Barnesiella intestinihominis* increases the anticancer effects of CP by encouraging the infiltration of T cells that produce interferon-γ into tumor tissues (Zaatry et al., 2024).

Crucially, encouraging clinical correlations have been found through translational observations in individuals with advanced lung and ovarian malignancies. Longer progression-free survival was typically observed in those who developed TH1 memory immune responses that were selectively targeted against *E. hirae* and *Barnesiella intestinihominis,* but not against unrelated microbial species. These results suggest that specific microbial consortia may be purposefully included in supplemental treatment approaches. To strengthen anticancer immunity, cyclophosphamide or other alkylating drugs may be given with a carefully crafted microbiota "cocktail," which is enriched for advantageous *Enterococcus* and *Barnesiella* strains. In the future, using just live bacteria might not be required; purified immunomodulatory metabolites or molecular components made from these organisms might be safer and easier to manage adjuvants. All of these research demonstrate the increasing understanding that the gut microbiota plays an active role in the response to chemotherapy rather than being a passive observer. Integrating microbial modulation into standard oncologic protocols may therefore represent a promising strategy to enhance therapeutic efficacy while moving toward a more personalized model of cancer treatment (Addissouky et al., 2023; Lu et al., 2024).

12.6 Oncological drug targets derived from microbial sources

In order to create chemotherapies and targeted medicines, the biotechnology and pharmaceutical sectors currently concentrate on cellular targets. However, microbiota may also be a target for drugs in the not-too-distant future. Additionally, microbial drug targets may help reduce the harmful GI tract side effects of several chemotherapeutics. Certain adverse effects, such those caused by irinotecan (camptothecin), are severe enough to restrict the dosage or length of treatment. Irinotecan is a chemotherapy drug commonly used to treat pancreatic and CRCs. It works by inhibiting topoisomerase I, an enzyme crucial for DNA replication, and mainly targets rapidly dividing cancer cells. When administered, irinotecan acts as a prodrug and is converted inside the body to its active form, SN38. The liver then modifies SN38 by attaching glucuronic acid, producing an inactive compound called SN38-G. This inactive form is excreted into the GI tract, where certain bacteria produce enzymes known as glucuronidases. By eliminating the glucuronic acid, these enzymes cause the gut's SN38 to become active again. It's interesting to note that bacteria use the liberated glucuronic acid as fuel. Regular dose adjustments and dose de-escalation are necessary since increased SN38 levels in the intestines cause severe and even fatal diarrhea (Barh et al., 2020; Bejarano et al., 2021; Verma et al., 2022).

When compared to typical mice with complete microbiota, germ-free animals show less GI damage and can withstand greater dosages of irinotecan. Neomycin administered concurrently with irinotecan was found to have a little therapeutic benefit in reducing side effects in a clinical investigation (Wang et al., 2018). Broad-spectrum antibiotics can unintentionally eliminate many beneficial gut bacteria, creating an environment where harmful pathogens such as *C. difficile* can thrive. A potential solution involves developing small-molecule inhibitors that specifically block bacterial glucuronidases without harming the bacteria or mammalian cells. Importantly, these inhibitors do not affect human glucuronidases. In preclinical studies, mice treated with these inhibitors alongside irinotecan were protected from experiencing diarrhea caused by the drug (Gambirasi et al., 2024; Yang et al., 2023). The GI tract is also negatively impacted by various chemotherapy drugs. For instance, doxorubicin and irinotecan are comparable in that microbiota is necessary for GI injury. According to these results, focusing on the microbiota may reduce the toxicity of some chemotherapeutics (Liu et al., 2021; Tiwari et al., 2025).

12.6.1 Using bacteria as vehicles for drug delivery in clinical trials

For targeted drug delivery in cancer treatment, bacteria become the novel platforms as they have the potential to make colonies of tumor cells. It is very difficult for immune cells to reach areas of hypoxia and necrosis of the tumor. Bacterial species like *Salmonella, Listeria,* and *Clostridium* selectively accumulate and reduce toxic action along with local pharmacological action. These species are present in the tumor. For drug delivery of cancer, bacteria are useful as they have the potential to target tumor cells. As per the preclinical research data, bacterial species that are genetically modified can be designed in such a way that they can secrete therapeutic compounds in a regulated way.

For example, to design tumor antigens, improve immune detection, cytokines like IL-2, to promote T-cell-mediated antitumor immunity, or enzymes like cytosine deaminase to locally activate prodrugs, genetically modified microbes are used. Scientists can use the applications of synthetic biology to provide safety and accuracy in the treatment given to the patient and design regulatory circuits that decrease the number of bacterial species in the tumor. A number of bacterial platforms have advanced to clinical trials in the early stages. Tests on individuals with nonsmall cell lung cancer and castration-resistant prostate cancer have shown that *Listeria monocytogenes* (live-attenuated double-deleted, or LADD) is safe and activates the immune system specifically in tumors. Similarly, several strains of *Salmonella typhimurium,* such as VNP20009 and Ty21a VXM01, have been assessed in clinical trials aimed at liver cancer, pancreatic cancer, RCC, metastatic melanoma, and other solid tumors. To improve local antitumor activity and lessen systemic side effects, some of these strains have been further modified to express therapeutic proteins such as cytosine deaminase or IL-2. In an effort to stimulate more comprehensive antitumor immune responses, mixed bacterial vaccinations combining multiple species have also been studied. Despite several development techniques, still there are so many hurdles in the oncological treatment procedures especially when we talk about bacterial drug delivery.

Drawbacks like systemic infection prevention, bacterial virulence management, and host immune response management, as they can destroy bacteria before they reach the tumor location area. Still, obstacles like patient safety, regulatory issues, and weak immune response persist. However, the employment of microbes to deliver drugs is a new and potentially revolutionary method of treating cancer. There are some special types of bacteria that have the power to comply with the traditional techniques like chemotherapy, immunotherapy, etc. These techniques are then combined with the tumor-targeting capabilities, immunostimulatory potential, and their potential to transport therapeutic payloads. There is still research going on in search of effective and safe treatment for cancer. In this direction, a therapy called bacteria-mediated therapeutics may be used for cancer treatment patients individually.

William B. Coley, in 1891, introduced different forms of immunotherapy for cancer along with the incorporation of infections with species like *Serratia marcescens* and *Streptococcus pyogenes* (Alum et al., 2025; Karumuru et al., 2025). Since then, a variety of bacterial species have been explored for their therapeutic potency and are being tested in clinical trials involving human patients (Table 12.2).

12.7 Current challenges

Due to the rising significance of the microbiome in treating a variety of human ailments, bacteria are receiving more and more attention in a variety of medical sectors (Guo et al., 2023). Bacteria are great prospects for treating various tumor types because of their unique genetic traits, capacity to flourish in low-oxygen tumor conditions, and capacity to specifically target cancer cells. Even though genetically modified bacteria have increased the accuracy of tumor targeting, a single anticancer medication might not be sufficient to completely eradicate cancer, suggesting the necessity for a combination of therapeutic approaches. This is due to the wide range of genetic and histologic variations among malignancies (Lu et al., 2021). To develop a medication for cancer treatment, a combinatorial approach can be used. Bacterial toxicity continues to be a major barrier to the clinical development of bacteria-based cancer therapy (BBCT). Numerous bacterial species naturally create endotoxins, exotoxins, and other virulence-associated chemicals that can result in organ failure, septic shock, severe systemic inflammation, or even death. These safety considerations severely limit the therapeutic window of live bacterial platforms. To tackle this issue, there is increasing research on the creation of genetically engineered and attenuated bacterial strains that reduce pathogenicity while retaining the capacity to target tumors (Elmore et al., 2021; Mendes & Vale, 2023).

Genetic attenuation strategies often involve the deletion or silencing of genes that produce virulence, the production of toxins, or unregulated growth. These modifications offer a difficult therapeutic trade-off even though they can significantly improve safety profiles. When virulence is decreased, the bacterium's capacity to effectively colonize tumors, initiate immunological activation, or deliver direct cytotoxic effects is often compromised. This highlights how crucial it is to carefully balance maintaining sufficient antitumor activity with lowering the possibility of damage. Therapeutic bacterial strains have been shown to be very responsive to modifications in their virulence determinants, and even little adjustments may have a big impact on how they work biologically in the tumor microenvironment. An additional layer of complexity is offered by microbe-associated molecular patterns (MAMPs), which are crucial for immunological recognition. Peptidoglycan, flagellin, and lipopolysaccharide (LPS) are examples of structural components that interact with host pattern recognition receptors, such as Toll-like receptors (TLRs), to initiate immune responses. The host's immune response may be significantly impacted by changes made to these structural motifs during bacterial modification. LPS's interaction with TLR4, for example, may be impacted by modifications to its lipid A component. Hexa-acylated lipid A variants may have better TLR4 binding due to their structural composition, which could bolster immune responses against malignancies. However, these modifications may also alter the physiology of bacteria, affecting membrane stability, growth kinetics, and metabolic fitness. Therefore, to avoid severe inflammatory damage while preserving therapeutic efficacy, careful management is required when creating LPS or other surface molecules.

For the treatment of cancer, BBCT shows new potential methods, but their regular optimization is necessary for their safe clinical applications. Toxicology, genetic stability, immunological compatibility, and antimicrobial resistance must all be addressed if modified bacteria are to serve as predictable and controllable medicinal agents. Modification in bacteria can serve as expected and restrained medicinal agents and address the toxicology, genetic stability, immunological compatibility, and antimicrobial resistance. To overcome these obstacles and move bacterial treatments closer to wider clinical adoption, it will be essential to continue developing synthetic biology in conjunction with thorough preclinical validation and well-planned clinical trials.

12.8 Future prospects

Microbe-based cancer therapies and their advancement mainly depend upon the approaches of genetic engineering that increase cancer specificity, biosafety, and therapeutic profile precision. Today, there are several modern tools available in the synthetic biology area, like CRISPR-Cas systems, programmable gene circuits, and inducible promoters that permit specific design of microbial strains that are capable of responding to oncological environment cues, i.e., hypoxia, acidic pH, elevated lactate levels, and aberrant metabolic signaling. At this molecular level, engineered microbes can be customized and changed in such a way that they can align with the immunological, genomic, and patient's tumor metabolic characteristics. So that they can support the long-term goals of oncology.

The inherent ability of some bacterial species to locate tumors is a particularly attractive trait. There are many anaerobes, like facultative or obligate, that accumulate in the tumors, especially in the region of hypoxia and necrosis areas that are very often poorly penetrated by conventional techniques like chemotherapy and radiotherapy. A significant advantage given by this natural tropism is that it allows several microbes to serve as vehicles for antitumor agents, involving cytotoxic proteins, immune-modulating cytokines, prodrug-converting enzymes, and tumor-targeting peptides. In a therapeutic optimized model, only those bacterial strains would be selected that are nonpathogenic and well characterized. They served as foundational platforms, along with minimizing systemic toxicity and preserving efficacy. To reduce off-target effects and enhance safety profiles, these strains might subsequently be further modified to express therapeutic payloads in a spatially and temporally regulated way.

Microorganism-based therapies are unlikely to be used as stand-alone treatments for maximum therapeutic benefit; instead, they may be used as supplementary elements in multimodal regimens. BBBCT may work in concert with immune checkpoint inhibitors, chemotherapy, radiation, or adoptive cell therapies. Microbial colonization, for instance, may improve antigen presentation, trigger local immune activation, and change the tumor microenvironment from immunosuppressive to immunostimulatory, all of which could improve the effectiveness of immunotherapies. Furthermore, although many modified bacteria preferentially concentrate in hypoxic tumor cores, to achieve complete tumor eradication, tumor regions with higher oxygen concentrations may require combination techniques that combine microbial therapy with additional systemic or targeted treatments.

Genetic flexibility and plasticity are among the advantages of microbial systems. Several microbes that are very different from many synthetic drug delivery systems in that they can amplify therapeutic signals, self-replicate within tumors, and dynamically adapt to changes in their environment. Due to the huge development in synthetic biology, safety measures that restrict bacterial survival outside of the tumor microenvironment, such as auxotrophic requirements or kill-switch mechanisms, can now be included. Safety measures are required for biosafety concerns and enhancing clinical acceptance. Programmable lysis mechanisms and quorum-sensing circuits can be made to release therapeutic medications only once sufficient tumor colonization has occurred, which would increase precision and reduce systemic exposure.

There are several hurdles that need to be overcome in techniques like BBCT's, especially before they were used for cancer treatment. Major concerns involve inflammation, toxicity, risk of sepsis, and unintentional immunological activation. Well-planned clinical studies are required to establish an ideal dosage regimen, long-term safety, and clinical benefits. Additionally, regulatory frameworks need to change to account for the special qualities of living, replicating treatments, which are very different from those of traditional small-molecule medications or biologics. GMOs are intentionally used on patients, but they raise several questions regarding ethical and societal perceptions that need to be handled very carefully through good communication and risk assessment.

In higher phases of clinical trials, a small number of microbial populations have been studied despite the fact that several animal studies have shown good anticancer results. The potential of BBCT will be very crucial due to less coordination amongst microbiologists, oncologists, immunologists, bioengineers, and regulatory agencies. It is the translational study, clinical studies, and standardized manufacturing methods that will close the gap between the results and outcomes of experiments and practical therapeutic use.

12.9 Conclusion

In conclusion, new research has demonstrated that bacteria can attach to tumors, stop their growth, and, in certain situations, completely destroy them. Nevertheless, it is challenging to cure cancers with a single bacterium therapy due to their variety. Due to their ability to activate the host immune response, bacteria are now being explored as promising tools in cancer therapy. Researchers are utilizing them both as potent adjuvants in immunotherapy and as targeted delivery systems for anticancer agents such as paclitaxel, 5-fluorouracil, small interfering RNA (siRNA), and doxorubicin-loaded hybrid micelles. Additionally, bacteria are being employed to transport photosensitizers like indocyanine green (ICG) and palladium-based nanoparticles directly to tumor sites. Another strategy to allay safety worries is to use bacterial outer membrane vesicles, which can transport a variety of chemotherapy medications into tumors, in place of the bacterial vector. Although this idea has not received much attention up to this point, its enormous potential is noteworthy. Furthermore, oral bacterial formulations have recently been used to treat cancer. However, the gastrointestinal tract's abundance of metabolic enzymes and acidic gastric environment severely impair therapeutic efficacy, necessitating more research to alter bacterial formulations.

There are certain bacteria that possess a unique capacity to preferentially localize and proliferate within tumor microenvironments, where they can also activate antitumor immune mechanisms. To increase their demand in oncology, bacteria can be engineered in such a way that they function as a targeted delivery system for pharmacotherapeutic agents. As per William Coley's concepts, to design bacteria-based oncology therapies, significant progress has been made, with ongoing research continuing to refine their safety and efficacy profiles. Significant advances in genetic engineering and synthetic biology enable more specific tumor designs, while several bacterial therapeutics are available for future oncology treatment.

References

Addissouky, T. A., El Tantawy El Sayed, I., Ali, M. M. A., Alubiady, M. H. S., & Wang, Y. (2023). Harnessing innovation for the future of breast cancer management. *Clinical Research in Oncology, 1*(1), 10–17. https://doi.org/10.46439/oncology.1.004.

Alsahafi, E., Begg, K., Amelio, I., Raulf, N., Lucarelli, P., Sauter, T., & Tavassoli, M. (2019). Clinical update on head and neck cancer: Molecular biology and ongoing challenges. *Cell Death & Disease, 10*(8). https://doi.org/10.1038/s41419-019-1769-9.

Alum, E. U., Uti, D. E., Ugwu, O. P.-C., Alum, B. N., Edeh, F. O., & Ainebyoona, C. (2025). Unveiling the microbial orchestra: Exploring the role of microbiota in cancer development and treatment. *Discover Oncology, 16*(1). https://doi.org/10.1007/s12672-025-02352-2.

Barh, D., Soares, S., Tiwari, S., & Azevedo, V. (2020). *Pan-genomics: Applications, challenges, and future prospects.* (pp. 1–450). Elsevier. https://doi.org/10.1016/B978-0-12-817076-2.09992-3.

Bejarano, L., Jordão, M. J. C., & Joyce, J. A. (2021). Therapeutic targeting of the tumor microenvironment. *Cancer Discovery, 11*(4), 933–959. https://doi.org/10.1158/2159-8290.cd-20-1808.

Bhatt, A. P., Redinbo, M. R., & Bultman, S. J. (2017). The role of the microbiome in cancer development and therapy. *CA: A Cancer Journal for Clinicians, 67*(4), 326–344. https://doi.org/10.3322/caac.21398.

Bor, G., Azmi, I. D. M., & Yaghmur, A. (2019). Nanomedicines for cancer therapy: Current status, challenges and future prospects. *Therapeutic Delivery, 10*(2), 113–132. https://doi.org/10.4155/tde-2018-0062.

Bray, F., Ferlay, J., Soerjomataram, I., Siegel, R. L., Torre, L. A., & Jemal, A. (2018). Global cancer statistics 2018: GLOBOCAN estimates of incidence and mortality worldwide for 36 cancers in 185 countries. *CA Cancer Journal for Clinicians, 68*(6), 394–424. https://doi.org/10.3322/caac.21492.

Cammarota, G., Ianiro, G., Ahern, A., Carbone, C., Temko, A., Claesson, M. J., Gasbarrini, A., & Tortora, G. (2020). Gut microbiome, big data and machine learning to promote precision medicine for cancer. *Nature Reviews Gastroenterology & Hepatology, 17*(10), 635–648. https://doi.org/10.1038/s41575-020-0327-3.

Chattaraj, S., Mitra, D., Chattaraj, A., Chattaraj, M., Kundu, M., Ganguly, A., & Mohapatra, P. K. D. (2023). Antioncogenic potential of probiotics: Challenges and future prospective. *Indian Journal of Microbiology Research, 10*(1), 1–10. https://doi.org/10.18231/j.ijmr.2023.001.

Chen, J., Douglass, J., Prasath, V., Neace, M., Atrchian, S., Manjili, M. H., Shokouhi, S., & Habibi, M. (2019). The microbiome and breast cancer: A review. *Breast Cancer Research and Treatment, 178*(3), 493–496. https://doi.org/10.1007/s10549-019-05407-5.

Chen, Y. E., & Tsao, H. (2013). The skin microbiome: Current perspectives and future challenges. *Journal of the American Academy of Dermatology, 69*(1), 143. https://doi.org/10.1016/j.jaad.2013.01.016.

Dave, M., Higgins, P. D., Middha, S., & Rioux, K. P. (2012). The human gut microbiome: Current knowledge, challenges, and future directions. *Translational Research, 160*(4), 246–257. https://doi.org/10.1016/j.trsl.2012.05.003.

Din, S. R. U, Saeed, S., Khan, S. U., Arbi, F. M., Xuefang, G., & Zhong, M. (2023). Bacteria-driven cancer therapy: Exploring advancements and challenges. *Critical Reviews in Oncology/Hematology, 191*, 104141. https://doi.org/10.1016/j.critrevonc.2023.104141.

Do, T., Devine, D., & Marsh, P. D. (2013). Oral biofilms: Molecular analysis, challenges, and future prospects in dental diagnostics. *Clinical, Cosmetic and Investigational Dentistry, 5*, 11–19. https://doi.org/10.2147/CCIDE.S31005.

Elinav, E., Garrett, W. S., Trinchieri, G., & Wargo, J. (2019). The cancer microbiome. *Nature Reviews Cancer, 19*(7), 371–376. https://doi.org/10.1038/s41568-019-0155-3.

Elmore, L. W., Greer, S. F., Daniels, E. C., Saxe, C. C., Melner, M. H., Krawiec, G. M., Cance, W. G., & Phelps, W. C. (2021). Blueprint for cancer research: Critical gaps and opportunities. *CA: A Cancer Journal for Clinicians, 71*(2), 107–139. https://doi.org/10.3322/caac.21652.

Eslami, M., Naderian, R., Bahar, A., Babaeizad, A., Gheshlagh, S. R., Oksenych, V., & Tahmesbi, H. (2025). Microbiota as diagnostic biomarkers: Advancing early cancer detection and personalized therapeutic approaches through microbiome profiling. *Frontiers in Immunology, 16*. https://doi.org/10.3389/fimmu.2025.1559480.

Fang, P., Yang, J., Zhang, H., Shuai, D., Li, M., Chen, L., & Liu, L. (2025). Emerging roles of intratumoral microbiota: A key to novel cancer therapies. *Frontiers in Oncology, 15*. https://doi.org/10.3389/fonc.2025.1506577.

Fernández, M. F., Reina-Pérez, I., Manuel Astorga, J., Rodríguez-Carrillo, A., Plaza-Díaz, J., & Fontana, L. (2018). Breast cancer and its relationship with the microbiota. *International Journal of Environmental Research and Public Health, 15*(8), 1747. https://doi.org/10.3390/ijerph15081747.

Fosgerau, K., & Hoffmann, T. (2015). Peptide therapeutics: Current status and future directions. *Drug Discovery Today, 20*(1), 122–128. https://doi.org/10.1016/j.drudis.2014.10.003.

Fujita, K., Matsushita, M., Banno, E., De Velasco, M. A., Hatano, K., Nonomura, N., & Uemura, H. (2022). Gut microbiome and prostate cancer. *International Journal of Urology, 29*(8), 793–798. https://doi.org/10.1111/iju.14894.

Gambirasi, M., Safa, A., Vruzhaj, I., Giacomin, A., Sartor, F., & Toffoli, G. (2024). Oral administration of cancer vaccines: Challenges and future perspectives. *Vaccines, 12*(1), 26. https://doi.org/10.3390/vaccines12010026.

Greathouse, K. L., Wyatt, M., Johnson, A. J., Toy, E. P., Khan, J. M., Dunn, K., Clegg, D. J., & Reddy, S. (2022). Diet-microbiome interactions in cancer treatment: Opportunities and challenges for precision nutrition in cancer. *Neoplasia, 29*, 100800. https://doi.org/10.1016/j.neo.2022.100800.

Guan, W.-L., He, Y., & Xu, R.-H. (2023). Gastric cancer treatment: Recent progress and future perspectives. *Journal of Hematology & Oncology, 16*(1). https://doi.org/10.1186/s13045-023-01451-3.

Guan, Y., Wu, D., Wang, H., & Liu, N. N. (2024). Microbiome-driven anticancer therapy: A step forward from natural products. *mLife, 3*(2), 219–230. https://doi.org/10.1002/mlf2.12118.

Guo, C., Kong, L., Xiao, L., Liu, K., Cui, H., Xin, Q., Gu, X., Jiang, C., & Wu, J. (2023). The impact of the gut microbiome on tumor immunotherapy: From mechanism to application strategies. *Cell & Bioscience, 13*(1). https://doi.org/10.1186/s13578-023-01135-y.

Gupta, K. H., Nowicki, C., Giurini, E. F., Marzo, A. L., & Zloza, A. (2021). Bacterial-based cancer therapy (BBCT): Recent advances, current challenges, and future prospects for cancer immunotherapy. *Vaccines, 9*(12), 1497. https://doi.org/10.3390/vaccines9121497.

Hadrich, D. (2018). Microbiome research is becoming the key to better understanding health and nutrition. *Frontiers in Genetics, 9*. https://doi.org/10.3389/fgene.2018.00212.

Heimann, D.M., Rosenberg, S.A. (2003). Continuous intravenous administration of live genetically modified salmonella typhimurium in patients with metastatic melanoma. *Journal of Immunotherapy* (Hagerstown, Md.: 1997). *26*(2):179. doi:10.1097/00002371-200303000-00011.

Helmink, B. A., Khan, M. A. W., Hermann, A., Gopalakrishnan, V., & Wargo, J. A. (2019). The microbiome, cancer, and cancer therapy. *Nature Medicine, 25*(3), 377–388. https://doi.org/10.1038/s41591-019-0377-7.

Herrera-Quintana, L., Vázquez-Lorente, H., Lopez-Garzon, M., Cortés-Martín, A., & Plaza-Diaz, J. (2024a). Cancer and the microbiome of the human body. *Nutrients, 16*(16), 2790. https://doi.org/10.3390/nu16162790.

Herrera-Quintana, L., Vázquez-Lorente, H., Silva, R. C. M. C., Olivares-Arancibia, J., Reyes-Amigo, T., Pires, B. R. B., & Plaza-Diaz, J. (2024b). The role of the microbiome and of radiotherapy-derived metabolites in breast cancer. *Cancers, 16*(21), 3671. https://doi.org/10.3390/cancers16213671.

Herrera-Quintana, L., Vázquez-Lorente, H., & Plaza-Diaz, J. (2024c). Breast cancer: Extracellular matrix and microbiome interactions. *International Journal of Molecular Sciences, 25*(13), 7226. https://doi.org/10.3390/ijms25137226.

Irfan, M., Delgado, R. Z. R., & Frias-Lopez, J. (2020). The oral microbiome and cancer. *Frontiers in Immunology, 11*. https://doi.org/10.3389/fimmu.2020.591088.

Jain, T., Sharma, P., Are, A. C., Vickers, S. M., & Dudeja, V. (2021). New insights into the cancer–microbiome–immune axis: Decrypting a decade of discoveries. *Frontiers in Immunology, 12*. https://doi.org/10.3389/fimmu.2021.622064.

Jalil, A. T., Thabit, S. N., Hanan, Z. K., Alasheqi, M. Q., Al-Azzawi, A. K. J., Zabibah, R. S., & Fadhil, A. A. (2023). Modulating gut microbiota using nanotechnology to increase anticancer efficacy of the treatments. *Macromolecular Research, 31*(8), 739–752. https://doi.org/10.1007/s13233-023-00168-z.

Karumuru, V., Dhasmana, A., Mamidi, N., Chauhan, S. C., & Yallapu, M. M. (2025). Unveiling the potential of urolithin A in cancer therapy: Mechanistic insights to future perspectives of nanomedicine. *Nanotheranostics, 9*(2), 121–143. https://doi.org/10.7150/ntno.110966.

Khakimova, G. G., Tryakin, A. A., Zabotina, T. N., Tsukanov, A. S., Aliev, V. A., & Gutorov, S. L. (2019). The role of the intestinal microbiome in the immunotherapy of colon cancer. *Malignant Tumours, 9*(2), 5–11. https://doi.org/10.18027/2224-5057-2019-9-2-5-11.

Kiousi, D. E., Kouroutzidou, A. Z., Neanidis, K., Karavanis, E., Matthaios, D., Pappa, A., & Galanis, A. (2023). The role of the gut microbiome in cancer immunotherapy: Current knowledge and future directions. *Cancers, 15*(7), 2101. https://doi.org/10.3390/cancers15072101.

Kunjalwar, R., Keerti, A., Chaudhari, A., Sahoo, K., & Meshram, S. (2024). Microbial therapeutics in oncology: A comprehensive review of bacterial role in cancer treatment. *Cureus, 16*(10). https://doi.org/10.7759/cureus.70920.

Kustrimovic, N., Bombelli, R., Baci, D., & Mortara, L. (2023). Microbiome and prostate cancer: A novel target for prevention and treatment. *International Journal of Molecular Sciences, 24*(2), 1511. https://doi.org/10.3390/ijms24021511.

Lee, P. Y., Azhan, F. S. M., & Low, T. Y. (2023). Biomarkers for colorectal cancer chemotherapy: Recent updates and future perspective. *Malaysian Journal of Pathology, 45*(3), 317–331. http://www.mjpath.org.my/2023/v45n3/colorectal-cancer-chemotherapy.pdf.

Li, J., Zhang, A., Wu, F. F., & Wang, X.-j. (2022). Alterations in the gut microbiota and their metabolites in colorectal cancer: Recent progress and future prospects. *Frontiers in Oncology, 12*. https://doi.org/10.3389/fonc.2022.841552.

Liu, J., Liu, C., & Yue, J. (2021). Radiotherapy and the gut microbiome: Facts and fiction. *Radiation Oncology, 16*(1). https://doi.org/10.1186/s13014-020-01735-9.

Liu, J., & Zhang, Y. (2022). Intratumor microbiome in cancer progression: Current developments, challenges and future trends. *Biomarker Research, 10*(1). https://doi.org/10.1186/s40364-022-00381-5.

Lou, X., Chen, Z., He, Z., Sun, M., & Sun, J. (2021). Bacteria-mediated synergistic cancer therapy: Small microbiome has a big hope. *Nano-Micro Letters, 13*(1). https://doi.org/10.1007/s40820-020-00560-9.

Lu, H., Wang, Q., Liu, W., Wen, Z., & Li, Y. (2021). Precision strategies for cancer treatment by modifying the tumor-related bacteria. *Applied Microbiology and Biotechnology, 105*(16-17), 6183–6197. https://doi.org/10.1007/s00253-021-11491-9.

Lu, W., Aihaiti, A., Abudukeranmu, P., Liu, Y., & Gao, H. (2024). Unravelling the role of intratumoral bacteria in digestive system cancers: Current insights and future perspectives. *Journal of Translational Medicine, 22*(1). https://doi.org/10.1186/s12967-024-05320-6.

Ma, L., Guo, H., Zhao, Y., Liu, Z., Wang, C., Bu, J., Sun, T., & Wei, J. (2024). Liquid biopsy in cancer: Current status, challenges and future prospects. *Signal Transduction and Targeted Therapy, 9*(1). https://doi.org/10.1038/s41392-024-02021-w.

Ma, W., Mao, Q., Xia, W., Dong, G., Yu, C., & Jiang, F. (2019). Gut microbiota shapes the efficiency of cancer therapy. *Frontiers in Microbiology, 10*. https://doi.org/10.3389/fmicb.2019.01050.

Mafe, A. N., & Büsselberg, D. (2025). The effect of microbiome-derived metabolites in inflammation-related cancer prevention and treatment. *Biomolecules, 15*(5), 688. https://doi.org/10.3390/biom15050688.

Mao, Q., Jiang, F., Yin, R., Wang, J., Xia, W., Dong, G., Ma, W., Yang, Y., Xu, L., & Hu, J. (2018). Interplay between the lung microbiome and lung cancer. *Cancer Letters, 415*, 40–48. https://doi.org/10.1016/j.canlet.2017.11.036.

McQuade, J. L., Daniel, C. R., Helmink, B. A., & Wargo, J. A. (2019). Modulating the microbiome to improve therapeutic response in cancer. *The Lancet Oncology, 20*(2), e77. https://doi.org/10.1016/s1470-2045(18)30952-5.

Mendes, I., & Vale, N. (2023). How can the microbiome induce carcinogenesis and modulate drug resistance in cancer therapy? *International Journal of Molecular Sciences, 24*(14), 11855. https://doi.org/10.3390/ijms241411855.

Mohseni, P., & Ghorbani, A. (2024). Exploring the synergy of artificial intelligence in microbiology: Advancements, challenges, and future prospects. *Computational and Structural Biotechnology Reports, 1*, 100005. https://doi.org/10.1016/j.csbr.2024.100005.

Nallanchakravarthula, S., Amruta, N., & Ramamurthy, C. (2021). Cancer microbiome: Opportunities and challenges. *Endocrine, Metabolic & Immune Disorders - Drug Targets, 21*(2), 215–229. https://doi.org/10.2174/1871530320999200818134942.

Nemunaitis, J. (2003). GVAX (GMCSF gene modified tumor vaccine) in advanced stage non small cell lung cancer. *Journal of controlled release, 91*(1–2), 225–231.

Oyovwi, M. O., Ben-Azu, B., & Babawale, K. H. (2025). Therapeutic potential of microbiome modulation in reproductive cancers. *Medical Oncology, 42*(5). https://doi.org/10.1007/s12032-025-02708-2.

Pandey, P., & Khan, F. (2023). Gut microbiome in cancer immunotherapy: Current trends, translational challenges and future possibilities. *Biochimica et Biophysica Acta (BBA) - General Subjects, 1867*(9), 130401. https://doi.org/10.1016/j.bbagen.2023.130401.

Park, E. M., Chelvanambi, M., Bhutiani, N., Kroemer, G., Zitvogel, L., & Wargo, J. A. (2022). Targeting the gut and tumor microbiota in cancer. *Nature Medicine, 28*(4), 690–703. https://doi.org/10.1038/s41591-022-01779-2.

Pernigoni, N., Guo, C., Gallagher, L., Yuan, W., Colucci, M., Troiani, M., Liu, L., Maraccani, L., Guccini, I., Migliorini, D., de Bono, J., & Alimonti, A. (2023). The potential role of the microbiota in prostate cancer pathogenesis and treatment. *Nature Reviews Urology, 20*(12), 706–718. https://doi.org/10.1038/s41585-023-00795-2.

Porter, C. M., Shrestha, E., Peiffer, L. B., & Sfanos, K. S. (2018). The microbiome in prostate inflammation and prostate cancer. *Prostate Cancer and Prostatic Diseases, 21*(3), 345–354. https://doi.org/10.1038/s41391-018-0041-1.

Prakash, Y. S., & Xai, Y. (2023). Microbiome in colonic carcinogenesis. *Wiley, Comprehensive Physiology, 13*, 4685–4708. https://doi.org/10.1002/cphy.c210052.

Ratiner, K., Ciocan, D., Abdeen, S. K., & Elinav, E. (2024). Utilization of the microbiome in personalized medicine. *Nature Reviews Microbiology, 22*(5), 291–308. https://doi.org/10.1038/s41579-023-00998-9.

Roy, B., Cao, K., Singh, C. O., Fang, X., Yang, H., & Wei, D. (2025). Advances in gut microbiota-related treatment strategies for managing colorectal cancer in humans. *Cancer Biology & Medicine, 22*(2), 93–112. https://doi.org/10.20892/j.issn.2095-3941.2024.0263.

Sánchez-Alcoholado, L., Ramos-Molina, B., Otero, A., Laborda-Illanes, A., Ordóñez, R., Medina, J. A., Gómez-Millán, J., & Queipo-Ortuño, M. I. (2020). The role of the gut microbiome in colorectal cancer development and therapy response. *Cancers, 12*(6), 1406. https://doi.org/10.3390/cancers12061406.

Schmitz-Winnenthal, F. H., Hohmann, N., Schmidt, T., Podola, L., Friedrich, T., Lubenau, H., … Beckhove, P. (2018). A phase 1 trial extension to assess immunologic efficacy and safety of prime-boost vaccination with VXM01, an oral T cell vaccine against VEGFR2, in patients with advanced pancreatic cancer. *Oncoimmunology, 7*(4), e1303584.

Schorr, L., Mathies, M., Elinav, E., & Puschhof, J. (2023). Intracellular bacteria in cancer—Prospects and debates. *npj Biofilms and Microbiomes, 9*(1). https://doi.org/10.1038/s41522-023-00446-9.

Sepich-Poore, G. D., Zitvogel, L., Straussman, R., Hasty, J., Wargo, J. A., & Knight, R. (2021). The microbiome and human cancer. *Science, 371*(6536). https://doi.org/10.1126/science.abc4552.

Sharma, V., Sharma, N., Sheikh, I., Kumar, V., Sehrawat, N., Yadav, M., Ram, G., Sankhyan, A., & Sharma, A. K. (2021). Probiotics and prebiotics having broad spectrum anticancer therapeutic potential: Recent trends and future perspectives. *Current Pharmacology Reports, 7*(2), 67–79. https://doi.org/10.1007/s40495-021-00252-x.

Sheikh, M., Roshandel, G., McCormack, V., & Malekzadeh, R. (2023). Current status and future prospects for esophageal cancer. *Cancers, 15*(3), 765. https://doi.org/10.3390/cancers15030765.

Singh, A., Alexander, S. G., & Martin, S. (2023). Gut microbiome homeostasis and the future of probiotics in cancer immunotherapy. *Frontiers in Immunology, 14*. https://doi.org/10.3389/fimmu.2023.1114499.

Singh, V., Shirbhate, E., Kore, R., Vishwakarma, S., Parveen, S., Veerasamy, R., Tiwari, A. K., & Rajak, H. (2025). Microbial metabolites-induced epigenetic modifications for inhibition of colorectal cancer: Current status and future perspectives. *Mini-Reviews in Medicinal Chemistry, 25*(1), 76–93. https://doi.org/10.2174/0113895575320344240625080555.

Ting, N. L.-N., Lau, H. C.-H., & Yu, J. (2022). Cancer pharmacomicrobiomics: Targeting microbiota to optimise cancer therapy outcomes. *Gut, 71*(7), 1412–1425. https://doi.org/10.1136/gutjnl-2021-326264.

Tiwari, A., Anshu, Kumar, C., & Zaid, M. (2025). Unravelling the herbal formulation of floating microspheres for gut microbiome modulation: Current challenges and future prospects. *Current Pharmaceutical Research*, 144–162. https://doi.org/10.63785/cpr.2025.1.1.144162.

Toso, J. F., Gill, V. J., Hwu, P., Marincola, F. M., Restifo, N. P., Schwartzentruber, D. J., … Rosenberg, S. A. (2002). Phase I study of the intravenous administration of attenuated Salmonella typhimurium to patients with metastatic melanoma. *Journal of clinical oncology, 20*(1), 142–152.

Tsay, J. C. J., Wu, B. G., Badri, M. H., Clemente, J. C., Shen, N., Meyn, P., Li, Y., Yie, T. A., Lhakhang, T., Olsen, E., Murthy, V., Michaud, G., Sulaiman, I., Tsirigos, A., Heguy, A., Pass, H., Weiden, M. D., Rom, W. N., Sterman, D. H., … Segal, L. N. (2018). Airway microbiota is associated with upregulation of the PI3K pathway in lung cancer. *American Journal of Respiratory and Critical Care Medicine, 198*(9), 1188–1198. https://doi.org/10.1164/rccm.201710-2118OC.

Tsigalou, C., Konstantinidis, T., Aloizou, A. M., Bezirtzoglou, E., & Tsakris, A. (2023). Future therapeutic prospects in dealing with autoimmune diseases: Treatment based on the microbiome model. In *Role of microorganisms in pathogenesis and management of autoimmune diseases: Volume II: Kidney, central nervous system, eye, blood, blood vessels and bowel: 2* (pp. 489–520). Springer. https://doi.org/10.1007/978-981-19-4800-8_25.

Verma, N., Thapa, K., & Dua, K. (2022). Microbiome in inflammatory lung diseases: Challenges and future prospects. In *Microbiome in inflammatory lung diseases* (pp. 339–358). Springer Nature. https://doi.org/10.1007/978-981-16-8957-4_19.

Wang, D., Cheng, J., Zhang, J., Zhou, F., He, X., Shi, Y., & Tao, Y. (2021). The role of respiratory microbiota in lung cancer. *International Journal of Biological Sciences, 17*(13), 3646–3658. https://doi.org/10.7150/ijbs.51376.

Wang, N., Wu, S., Huang, L., Hu, Y., He, X., He, J., Hu, B., Xu, Y., Rong, Y., Yuan, C., Zeng, X., & Wang, F. (2025). Intratumoral microbiome: Implications for immune modulation and innovative therapeutic strategies in cancer. *Journal of Biomedical Science, 32*(1). https://doi.org/10.1186/s12929-025-01117-x.

Wang, Y., Deng, W., Li, N., Neri, S., Sharma, A., Jiang, W., & Lin, S. H. (2018). Combining immunotherapy and radiotherapy for cancer treatment: Current challenges and future directions. *Frontiers in Pharmacology, 9*. https://doi.org/10.3389/fphar.2018.00185.

Wu, Y., Wang, P., Zhao, X., Liu, T., Situ, B., & Zheng, L. (2024). Dynamic interplay of intratumoral microbiota within the colorectal cancer microenvironment. *VIEW, 5*(1). https://doi.org/10.1002/viw.20230100.

Xu, J., Yang, P., Xue, S., Sharma, B., Sanchez-Martin, M., Wang, F., Beaty, K. A., Dehan, E., & Parikh, B. (2019). Translating cancer genomics into precision medicine with artificial intelligence: Applications, challenges and future perspectives. *Human Genetics, 138*(2), 109–124. https://doi.org/10.1007/s00439-019-01970-5.

Yadav, M., & Verma, A. K. (2022). Microbiota targeted via nanotechnology for lung cancer therapy: Challenges and Future perspectives. In *Microbiome in inflammatory lung diseases* (pp. 359–377). Springer Nature. https://doi.org/10.1007/978-981-16-8957-4_20.

Yadav, M., & Singh Chauhan, N. (2022). Microbiome therapeutics: Exploring the present scenario and challenges. *Gastroenterology Report, 10*. https://doi.org/10.1093/gastro/goab046.

Yamamoto, Y., Kanayama, N., Nakayama, Y., & Matsushima, N. (2022). Current status, issues and future prospects of personalized medicine for each disease. *Journal of Personalized Medicine, 12*(3), 444. https://doi.org/10.3390/jpm12030444.

Yang, L., Wang, Q. i, He, L., & Sun, X. (2024). The critical role of tumor microbiome in cancer immunotherapy. *Cancer Biology & Therapy, 25*(1). https://doi.org/10.1080/15384047.2024.2301801.

Yang, M., Yang, F., Chen, W., Liu, S., Qiu, L., & Chen, J. (2021). Bacteria-mediated cancer therapies: Opportunities and challenges. *Biomaterials Science, 9*(17), 5732–5744. https://doi.org/10.1039/d1bm00634g.

Yang, Q., Wang, B., Zheng, Q., Li, H., Meng, X., Zhou, F., & Zhang, L. (2023). A review of gut microbiota-derived metabolites in tumor progression and cancer therapy. *Advanced Science, 10*(15). https://doi.org/10.1002/advs.202207366.

Yang, T., & Guo, L. (2024). Advancing gastric cancer treatment: Nanotechnology innovations and future prospects. *Cell Biology and Toxicology, 40*(1). https://doi.org/10.1007/s10565-024-09943-9.

You, L., Zhou, J., Xin, Z., Spencer Hauck, J., Na, F., Tang, J., Zhou, X., Lei, Z., & Ying, B. (2022). Novel directions of precision oncology: Circulating microbial DNA emerging in cancer-microbiome areas. *Precision Clinical Medicine, 5*(1). https://doi.org/10.1093/pcmedi/pbac005.

Zaatry, R., Herren, R., Gefen, T., & Geva-Zatorsky, N. (2024). Microbiome and infectious disease: Diagnostics to therapeutics. *Microbes and Infection, 26*(7), 105345. https://doi.org/10.1016/j.micinf.2024.105345.

Zhang, W., Yang, F., Mao, S., Wang, R., Chen, H., Ran, Y., Liu, S., Wu, P., Yan, Y., Li, W., Zhang, J., & Yao, X. (2023). Bladder cancer-associated microbiota: Recent advances and future perspectives. *Heliyon, 9*(1), e13012. https://doi.org/10.1016/j.heliyon.2023.e13012.

Zhao, M., Jiang, G., Zhou, H. u, Li, J., Xiang, W., Li, S., Wang, H., & Zhou, J. (2023). Gut microbiota: A potential target for improved cancer therapy. *Journal of Cancer Research and Clinical Oncology, 149*(1), 541–552. https://doi.org/10.1007/s00432-022-04546-5.

Zhao, Y., Liu, Y., Li, S., Peng, Z., Liu, X., Chen, J., & Zheng, X. (2021). Role of lung and gut microbiota on lung cancer pathogenesis. *Journal of Cancer Research and Clinical Oncology, 147*(8), 2177–2186. https://doi.org/10.1007/s00432-021-03644-0.

Zhou, C.-B., Zhou, Y.-L., & Fang, J.-Y. (2021). Gut microbiota in cancer immune response and immunotherapy. *Trends in Cancer., 7*(7), 647–660. https://doi.org/10.1016/j.trecan.2021.01.010.

Index

Page numbers followed by "*f*" and "*t*" indicate, figures and tables respectively.

Printed and bound by CPI Group (UK) Ltd, Croydon, CR0 4YY
25/09/2026
02223047-0013